PROGRESS IN BRAIN RESEARCH

VOLUME 84

CHOLINERGIC NEUROTRANSMISSION:
FUNCTIONAL AND CLINICAL ASPECTS

Recent volumes in PROGRESS IN BRAIN RESEARCH

PROGRESS IN BRAIN RESEARCH

VOLUME 84

CHOLINERGIC NEUROTRANSMISSION: FUNCTIONAL AND CLINICAL ASPECTS

Proceedings of Nobel Symposium 76

EDITED BY

STEN-MAGNUS AQUILONIUS

and

PER-GÖRAN GILLBERG

Department of Neurology, University Hospital, Uppsala, Sweden

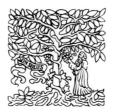

ELSEVIER
AMSTERDAM – NEW YORK – OXFORD
1990

ISBN 0-444-81148-6 (volume)
ISBN 0-444-80104-9 (series)

Published by
Elsevier Science Publishers B.V. (Biomedical Division)
P.O. Box 211
1000 AE Amsterdam
The Netherlands

Sole distributors for the USA and Canada:
Elsevier Science Publishing Company, Inc.
655 Avenue of the Americas
New York, NY 10010
USA

Library of Congress Cataloging in Publication Data

Cholinergic neurotransmission: functional and clinical aspects/
    edited by Sten-Magnus Aquilonius and Per-Göran Gillberg.
        p.   cm. -- (Progress in brain research; v. 84)
    Includes bibliographical references.
    Includes index.
    ISBN 0-444-81148-6 (alk. paper)
        1. Cholinergic mechanisms. 2. Muscarinic receptors.
3. Acetylcholine--Physiological effect. 4. Nicotinic receptors.
5. Myasthenia gravis--Pathophysiology. I. Aquilonius, Sten-Magnus.
II. Gillberg, Per-Göran. III. Series.
        [DNLM: 1. Nervous System Diseases--drug therapy. 2. Neural
Transmission. 3. Neuromuscular Junction--physiology.
4. Parasympathomimetics--therapeutic use. 5. Receptors,
Cholinergic--physiology. W1 PR667J v. 84 / WL 102.8 C547]
QP376.P7 vol. 84
612.8'2 s--dc20
[612.8'042]
DNLM/DLC
for Library of Congress   90-3988
                                                                              CIP

This book is printed on acid-free paper
Printed in The Netherlands

List of Contributors

P. Aas, Norwegian Defence Research Establishment, Division for Environmental Toxicology, P.O. Box 25, N-2007 Kjeller, Norway.

A. Adem, Department of Pharmacology, Uppsala University, Box 591, 751 24 Uppsala, Sweden

B. Ahrén, Departments of Pharmacology and Surgery, Lund University, Sölvegatan 10, S-223 62 Lund, Sweden

I. Alafuzoff, Department of Pathology, Karolinska Institute, S-10401 Stockholm, Sweden

F.J. Alvarez, Preclinical Research, Sandoz Ltd., CH-4002 Basle, Switzerland

K.-E. Andersson, Departments of Clinical Pharmacology, University Hospital, S-221 85 Lund, Sweden

S.H. Appel, Department of Neurology, Baylor College of Medicine, Houston, TX 77030, U.S.A.

S.-M. Aquilonius, Hospital Pharmacy, Departments of Anesthesiology and Neurology, University Hospital, S-751 85 Uppsala, Sweden

H. Askmark, Department of Neurology, University Hospital, S-751 85 Uppsala, Sweden

T. Bartfai, Department of Biochemistry, Arrhenius Laboratory, S-10691 Stockholm, Sweden

S. Berrard, Laboratoire de Neurobiologie Cellulaire et Moléculaire, CNRS, 1, Avenue de la Terrasse, 91198 Gif sur Yvette, France

R. Bertorelli, Laboratory of Cholinergic Neuropharmacology, Istituto di Ricerche Farmacologiche "Mario Negri", Via Eritrea 62, 20157 Milan, Italy

H. Boddeke, Preclinical Research, Sandoz Ltd., CH-4002 Basle, Switzerland

A. Brice, Laboratoire de Neurobiologie Cellulaire et Moléculaire, CNRS, 1, Avenue de la Terrasse, 91198 Gif sur Yvette, France

J.H. Brown, Department of Pharmacology M-36, University of California, San Diego, La Jolla, CA 92093, U.S.A.

G. Bucht, Department of Geriatric Medicine, Umeå University, Umeå, Sweden

R. Burke, Department of Neurology, Columbia University, New York, NY 10032-3784, U.S.A.

A.B. Cachelin, MRC Receptor Mechanisms Group, Department of Pharmacology, University College London, Gower Street, London WC1E 6BT, U.K.

F. Casamenti, Department of Preclinical and Clinical Pharmacology, University of Florence, Viale Morgagni 65, 50134 Florence, Italy

G. Chinaglia, Institute of Pathology, Department of Neuropathology, University of Basle, CH-4003 Basle, Switzerland

D. Colquhoun, MRC Receptor Mechanisms Group, Department of Pharmacology, University College London, Gower Street, London WC1E 6BT, U.K.

S. Consolo, Laboratory of Cholinergic Neuropharmacology, Istituto di Ricerche Farmacologiche "Mario Negri", Via Eritrea 62, 20157 Milan, Italy

J. Crawley, Unit of Behavioral Neuropharmacology, National Institute of Mental Health, Bethesda, MD 20892, U.S.A.

A.C. Cuello, Department of Pharmacology and Therapeutics, McGill University, 3655 Drummond Street, Montreal, Quebec, H3G 1Y6 Canada

K.L. Davis, Department of Psychiatry, The Mount Sinai School of Medicine, 100 St. & Fifth Avenue, New York, NY 10029, U.S.A.

J. Delforge, Service Hospitalier Frédéric Joliot, URA CEA-CNRS 1285, Département de Biologie, Commissariat à l'Energie Atomique, 91406 Orsay, France

A.G. Engel, Neuromuscular Research Laboratory, Mayo Clinic and Mayo Foundation, Rochester, MN 55905, U.S.A.

J.I. Engelhardt, Department of Neurology, Baylor College of Medicine, Houston, TX 77030, U.S.A.

H. Eriksson, Unit of Neurochemistry and Neurotoxicology, University of Stockholm, S-106 91 Stockholm, Sweden

S. Fahn, Neurological Institute, 710 West 168th Street, New York, NY 10032, U.S.A.

G. Fisone, Department of Biochemistry, Arrhenius Laboratory, S-106 91, Sweden, and Laboratory of Cholinergic Neuropharmacology, Istituto di Recherche Farmacologiche "Mario Negri", 20157 Milan, Italy

L. Garofalo, Department of Pharmacology and Therapeutics, McGill University, 3655 Drummond Street, Montreal, Quebec, H3G 1Y6 Canada

E. Giacobini, Department of Pharmacology, Southern Illinois University, School of Medicine, P.O. Box 19230, Springfield, IL 62794–9230, U.S.A.

P.-G. Gillberg, Department of Neurology, University Hospital, S-751 85 Uppsala, Sweden

J.C. Gillin, Department of Psychiatry, University of California, San Diego School of Medicine, 3350 La Jolla Village Drive, San Diego, CA 92161, U.S.A.

M.G. Giovannini, Department of Preclinical and Clinical Pharmacology, University of Florence, Viale Morgagni 65, 50134 Florence, Italy

E. Giraldo, Department of Biochemistry, Istituto De Angeli, Boehringer-Ingelheim Italia, Milan, Italy

C.G. Gottfries, Department of Psychiatry and Neurochemistry, St. Jörgen's Hospital, S-422 03 Hisings Backa, Sweden

E. Habert, Laboratoire de Neurobiologie Cellulaire et Moléculaire, CNRS, 1, Avenue de la Terrasse, 91198 Gif sur Yvette, France

J. Häggblad, Unit of Neurochemistry and Neurotoxicology, University of Stockholm, 106 91 Stockholm, Sweden

J.V. Halliwell, Department of Physiology, Royal Free Hospital School of Medicine, University of London, Rowland Hill Street, London NW3 2PF, U.K.

I. Hanin, Department of Pharmacology and Experimental Therapeutics, Loyola University of Chicago School of Medicine, 2160 South First Avenue, Maywood, IL 60153, U.S.A.

V. Haroutunian, Psychiatry Service, The Bronx Veterans Administration Medical Center, 2130 W. Kinsbridge Road, Bronx, NY 10468, U.S.A.

P. Hartvig, Hospital Pharmacy, Department of Anesthesiology, University Hospital of Uppsala, S-751 85 Uppsala, Sweden

H. Hedlund, Department of Urology, University Hospital, S-221 85 Lund, Sweden

E. Heilbronn, Unit of Neurochemistry and Neurotoxicology, University of Stockholm, S-106 91 Stockholm, Sweden

T. Hökfelt, Department of Histology and Neurobiology, Karolinska Institut, Box 60400, S-10401 Stockholm, Sweden

M. Israel, Département de Neurochimie, Laboratoire de Neurobiologie, Cellulaire et Moléculaire, Centre National de la Recherche Scientifique, 91190 Gif sur Yvette, France

K. Jakob, Department of Neurology, Baylor College of Medicine, Houston, TX 77030, U.S.A.

M. Janier, Service Hospitalier Frédéric Joliot, URA CEA-CNRS 1285, Département de Biologie, Commissariat à l'Energie Atomique, 91406 Orsay, France

D.J. Jenden, Department of Pharmacology and Brain Research Institute, UCLA School of Medicine, Los Angeles, CA 90024-1735, U.S.A.

A. Karczmar, Department of Pharmacology, Loyola University Medical Center, 2160 South First Avenue, Maywood, IL 60153, U.S.A.

S. Karlsson, Department of Surgery, Lund University, Sölvegatan 10, S-223 62 Lund, Sweden

M. Khalili-Varasteh, Service Hospitalier Frédéric Joliot, URA CEA-CNRS 1285, Département de Biologie, Commissariat à l'Energie Atomique, 91406 Orsay, France

H. Ladinsky, Department of Biochemistry, Istituto de Angeli, Boehringer Ingelheim Milano, Via Serio 15, I-20139 Milan, Italy

D.G. Lambert, Department of Pharmacology and Therapeutics (MSB), University of Leicester, University Road, Leicester LE1 9HN, U.K.

B. Långstrom, Department of Organic Chemistry, Uppsala University, Box 591, 751 24 Uppsala, Sweden

D. Leguludec, Service Hospitalier Frédéric Joliot, URA CEA-CNRS 1285, Département de Biologie, Commissariat à l'Energie Atomique, 91406 Orsay, France

B. Lindh, Department of Anatomy, Karolinska Institut, Box 60400, S-10401 Stockholm, Sweden

S. Lindskog, Department of Pharmacology, Lund University, Sölvegatan 10, S-223 62 Lund, Sweden

B. Lindström, Department of Drugs, National Board of Health and Welfare, Uppsala, Sweden

H. Lundh, Department of Neurology, Halmstadt Hospital, S-30185 Halmstad, Sweden

J. Mallet, Laboratoire de Neurobiologie Cellulaire et Moléculaire, Centre National de la Recherche Scientifique, F-991 90 Gif-sur-Yvette, France

C.G. Marshall, MRC Receptor Mechanisms Group, Department of Pharmacology, University College London, Gower Street, London WC1E 6BT, U.K.

E. Martinson, Department of Pharmacology M-036, University of California, San Diego, La Jolla, CA 92093, U.S.A.

A. Mathie, MRC Receptor Mechanisms Group, Department of Pharmacology, University College London, Gower Street, London WC1E 6BT, U.K.

D. Maysinger, Department of Pharmacology and Therapeutics, McGill University, 3655 Drummond Street, Montreal, Quebec, H3G 1Y6 Canada

M. Mazière, Service Hospitalier Frédéric Joliot, URA CEA-CNRS 1285, Département de Biologie, Commissariat à l'Energie Atomique, 91406 Orsay, France

J. Meldolesi, Department of Medical Pharmacology, "B. Ceccarelli" Center for the Study of Peripheral Neuropathies and Neuromuscular Diseases, CNR Center of Cytopharmacology, University of Milan, Via Vanvitelli 32, 20129 Milan, Italy

G. Mengod, Preclinical Research, Sandoz Ltd., CH-4002 Basle, Switzerland

M.-M. Mesulam, Department of Neurology, Beth Israel Hospital, 330 Brookline Avenue, Boston, MA 02215, U.S.A.

P.C. Molenaar, Department of Pharmacology, Sylvius Laboratory, University of Leiden, P.O. Box 9503, 2300 RA Leiden, The Netherlands

E. Monferini, Department of Biochemistry, Istituto De Angeli, Boehringer-Ingelheim Italia, Milan, Italy

N. Morel, Département de Neurochimie, Laboratoire de Neurobiologie, Cellulaire et Moléculaire, Centre National de la Recherche Scientifique, 91190 Gif sur Yvette, France

A. Nagel, Neuromuscular Research Laboratory, Mayo Clinic and Mayo Foundation, Rochester, MN 55905, U.S.A.

S.R. Nahorski, Department of Pharmacology and Therapeutics, University of Leicester, University Road, Leicester LE1 9HN, U.K.

O. Nilsson, Department of Neurology, University Hospital, S-221 85 Lund, Sweden

L. Nilsson-Håkansson, Department of Pharmacology, Uppsala University, S-751 24 Uppsala, Sweden

A. Nordberg, Department of Pharmacology, Uppsala University, Box 591, S-751 24 Uppsala, Sweden

D.C. Ogden, MRC Receptor Mechanisms Group, Department of Pharmacology, University College London, Gower Street, London WC1E 6BT, U.K.

P.O. Osterman, Department of Neurology, Uppsala University, Akademiska Sjukhuset, S-751 85 Uppsala, Sweden

J.M. Palacios, Preclinical Research, Sandoz Ltd., CH-4002 Basle, Switzerland

E. Palazzi, Laboratory of Cholinergic Neuropharmacology, Istituto di Ricerche Farmacologiche "Mario Negri", Via Eritrea 62, 20157 Milan, Italy

F. Pedata, Department of Preclinical and Clinical Pharmacology, University of Florence, Viale Morgagni 65, 50134 Florence, Italy

C. Pepeu, Department of Preclinical and Clinical Pharmacology, University of Florence, Viale Morgagni 65, 50134 Florence, Italy

E.P. Pioro, Department of Pharmacology and Therapeutics, McGill University, 3655 Drummond Street, Montreal, Quebec, H3G 1Y6 Canada

M. Poo, Department of Biological Sciences, Columbia University, New York, NY 10027, U.S.A.

C. Prenant, Service Hospitalier Frédéric Joliot, URA CEA-CNRS 1285, Département de Biologie, Commissariat à l'Energie Atomique, 91406 Orsay, France

A. Probst, Institute of Pathology, Department of Neuropathology, University of Basle, CH-4003 Basle, Switzerland

B. Raynaud, Laboratoire de Pharmacologie et de Toxicologie Fondamentales, CNRS, Toulouse, France

A. Ribeiro Da Silva, Department of Pharmacology and Therapeutics, McGill University, 3655 Drummond Street, Montreal, Quebec, H3G 1Y6 Canada

I. Rosén, Department of Clinical Neurophysiology, University Hospital, S-22185 Lund, Sweden

A.C. Santucci, Psychiatry Service, The Bronx Veterans Administration Medical Center, 2130 W. Kinsbridge Road, Bronx, NY 10468, U.S.A.

G.B. Schiavi, Department of Biochemistry, Istituto De Angeli, Boehringer-Ingelheim, Italia, Milan, Italy

M.I. Schimerlik, Department of Biochemistry and Biophysics, Oregon State University, Corvallis, OR 97331-6503, U.S.A.

P.J. Shiromani, Department of Psychiatry, University of California, San Diego School of Medicine, 3350 La Jolla Village Drive, San Diego, CA 92161, U.S.A.

C.R. Slater, Division of Neurobiology, University of Newcastle upon Tyne, Westgate Road, Newcastle upon Tyne NE4 6BE, U.K.

H. Soreq, Department of Biological Chemistry, The Life Sciences Institute, The Hebrew University, Jerusalem (91904), Israel

L. Steinman, Departments of Neurology, Pediatrics and Genetics, Stanford University, Stanford, CA 94305, U.S.A.

Y. Stern, The Neurological Institute of New York, Columbia-Presbyterian Medical Center, New York, NY 10032-3784, U.S.A.

A. Syrota, Service Hospitalier Frédéric Joliot, URA CEA-CNRS 1285, Département de Biologie, Commissariat à l'Energie Atomique, 91406 Orsay, France

N. Tabti, Department of Biological Sciences, Columbia University, New York, NY 10027, U.S.A.

S. Thesleff, Department of Pharmacology, University of Lund, Sölvegatan 10, S-223 62 Lund, Sweden

F. Torri Tarelli, Department of Medical Pharmacology, "B. Ceccarelli" Center for the Study of Peripheral Neuropathies and Neuromuscular Diseases, CNR Center of Cytopharmacology, University of Milan, Via Vanvitelli 32, 20129 Milan, Italy

J. Trejo, Department of Pharmacology M-036, University of California, San Diego, La Jolla, CA 92093, U.S.A.

I. Trilivas, Department of Pharmacology M-036, University of California, San Diego, La Jolla, CA 92093, U.S.A.

S. Tuček, Institute of Physiology, Czechoslovak Academy of Sciences, Vldeňská 1083, 14220 Prague, Czechoslovakia

O. Uchitel, Faculty of Medicine, University of Buenos Aires, Buenos Aires, Argentina

F. Valtorta, Department of Medical Pharmacology, "B. Ceccarelli" Center for the Study of Peripheral Neuropathies and Neuromuscular Diseases, CNR Center of Cytopharmacology, University of Milan, Via Vanvitelli 32, 20129 Milan, Italy

M.G. Vannucchi, Department of Preclinical and Clinical Pharmacology, University of Florence, Viale Morgagni 65, 50134 Florence, Italy

J. Velazquez-Moctezuma, Department of Reproduction Biology, Universidad Autonoma Metropolitana-Iztapalapa, Avenue Michoacan Y Purisima, Dele Iztapalapa Mexico, DF-9340 Mexico

P. Vernier, Laboratoire de Neurobiologie Cellulaire et Moléculaire, CNRS 1, Avenue de la Terrasse, 91198 Gif sur Yvette, France

M. Viitanen, Department of Geriatric Medicine, Karolinska Institute, S-10401 Stockholm, Sweden

M.T. Vilaró, Preclinical Research, Sandoz Ltd., CH-4002 Basle, Switzerland

A. Villa, Department of Medical Pharmacology, "B. Ceccarelli" Center for the Study of Peripheral Neuropathies and Neuromuscular Diseases, CNR Center of Cytopharmacology, University of Milan, Via Vanvitelli, 32, 20129 Milan, Italy

T.J. Walls, Newcastle General Hospital, Newcastle upon Tyne NE4 6BE, U.K.

M. Weber, Laboratoire de Pharmacologie et de Toxicologie Fondamentales, CNRS, Toulouse, France

V.P. Whittaker, Arbeitsgruppe Neurochemie, Max-Planck-Institut für biophysikalische Chemie, P.O. Box 2841, D-3400 Göttingen, F.R.G.

K.H. Wiederhold, Preclinical Research, Sandoz Ltd., CH-4002 Basle, Switzerland

L. Wiklund, Hospital Pharmacy, Departments of Anesthesiology and Neurology, University Hospital, S-751 85 Uppsala, Sweden

B. Winblad, Department of Geriatric Medicine, Karolinska Institute, S-10401 Stockholm, Sweden

H. Zakut, Department of Obstetrics and Gynecology, The Edith Wolfson Medical Center, The Sackler Faculty of Medicine of the Tel Aviv University, Holon (58100), Israel

Preface

When organizing the Nobel symposium "Cholinergic Neurotransmission: Functional and Clinical Aspects", which took place on Lidingö Island, Stockholm, August 1989, we had in our minds the very first international meeting devoted to cholinergic mechanisms which was excellently organized in Sweden by Professor Edith Heilbronn and collaborators 20 years ago. With this background four well-known figures in cholinergic neuroscience were asked to contribute by giving their views on important achievements in cholinergic research in the period 1969–1989.

The aim of the main part of the proceedings from the symposium is to describe the cholinergic research-front of today with emphasis on the basic principles which guide us in clinical applications. In the spectrum of disorders met with daily in clinical neurology, altered cholinergic function is pathophysiologically important in a number of diseases, e.g., myasthenia gravis and myasthenic syndromes, disorders of movement and dementia. Furthermore, cholinergic mechanisms are involved in the regulation of pain, mood and sleep.

The chapters are organized to guide the reader from molecular biology through basic cholinergic pharmacology into clinically oriented contributions. Also, at the end of each chapter a group of scientists formulate their ideas on future prospects of research on cholinergic mechanisms in their different areas of interest.

We wish to express our sincere thanks to the advisory board with Professors T. Bartfai, Stockholm, C.-G. Gottfries, Gothenburg, E. Heillbron, Stockholm, and S. Thesleff, Lund.

The symposium was sponsored by the Nobel Foundation through its Nobel Symposium Fund. IBM graciously put its conference center, IBM Nordic Education Center, and its facilities at the disposal of the symposium.

Sten-Magnus Aquilonius
Per-Göran Gillberg
Uppsala,
Spring 1990

Contents

B. Autonomic Nervous System

Section III – Cholinergic Mechanisms in the Central Nervous Sytem

Section IV – Achievements in Cholinergic Research 1969–1989

SECTION I

Molecules and Principles in Cholinergic Synaptology

S.-M. Aquilonius and P.-G. Gillberg (Eds.)
Progress in Brain Research, Vol. 84
© 1990 Elsevier Science Publishers B.V. (Biomedical Division)

CHAPTER 1

Choline acetyltransferase: a molecular genetic approach

Jacques Mallet [1], Sylvie Berrard [1], Alexis Brice [1], Estelle Habert [1], Brigitte Raynaud [2],
Philippe Vernier [1] and Michel Weber [2]

[1] *Laboratoire de Neurobiologie Cellulaire et Moléculaire, CNRS, 1, Avenue de la Terrasse, 91198 Gif sur Yvette Cedex,
and* [2] *Laboratoire de Pharmacologie et de Toxicologie Fondamentales, CNRS, Toulouse, France*

Introduction

Choline acetyltransferase (ChAT) constitutes the only specific marker available to date for cholinergic neurons (Tucek, 1988). The paucity of the enzyme, whose purification from rat brain required about a 10^6-fold enrichment, has limited its biochemical and structural analysis. Such studies have now been facilitated by molecular genetic approaches which, in addition, make it possible to analyse in molecular terms the regulation of the expression of the enzyme during development and as a result of nerve activity. Furthermore, cholinergic neurons are implicated in degenerative diseases and the role played by ChAT in the process is not clear (Borroni et al., 1989). Here, we summarize recent findings in the study of ChAT following cloning of mammalian ChAT and discuss potential directions of research.

Molecular cloning and sequence of porcine and rat ChAT enzyme: comparison with the *Drosophila* enzyme

The choice of the starting material to isolate a particular cDNA is crucial when dealing with proteins such as ChAT which are expressed at a very low abundance. In an initial series of experiments, several tissues were tested for ChAT activity and striatum was found to exhibit the highest level (Table 1), which was 1.6-fold that of the ventral spinal cord (VSC). However, when *Xenopus* oocytes, which provide a convenient system to express proteins from exogenous mRNAs, were injected with the mRNAs prepared from various tissues, a 10-fold higher activity was obtained with VSC mRNAs than with striatum mRNAs (Berrard et al., 1989). These experiments suggested that ChAT mRNA was 10-fold more prominent in

TABLE I

ChAT acitivity in several rat tissues and in oocytes injected with 50 ng of the corresponding poly(A)$^+$ RNA

	ChAT activity of tissues (pmol/min/mg protein)	ChAT activity of microinjected oocytes (fmol/min/oocyte)
Striatum	1805 ± 95 ($n = 9$)	24
Ventral spinal cord	1111 ± 42 ($n = 6$)	234
Brainstem	1159 ± 38 ($n = 2$)	–
Brain	644 ± 57 ($n = 2$)	91
Hippocampus	362 ± 60 ($n = 2$)	0
Cerebellum	57 ± 4 ($n = 4$)	0
Liver	0 ($n = 2$)	–

ChAT activity was measured in tissues by the method of Fonnum (1976). Mean values of *n* experiments are shown. In injected oocytes, ChAT activity was measured according to Smith et al. (1979). Mean values of duplicates of a single experiment are shown (Berrard et al. 1986).

4

VSC than in striatum and that the former was the material of choice to generate a cDNA library from which to isolate a ChAT cDNA clone.

This finding, which was at first sight surprising, can be explained by the neuroanatomical differences between the two structures, taking into account the fact that ribosomes are largely confined to cell bodies. The long axons of cholinergic motor neurons from the VSC provide a dense innervation of the skeletal muscles. Therefore, although ChAT activity in VSC is only about half that found in the striatum, a large pool of ChAT mRNA in the VSC cell bodies is required to maintain a high level of synthesis of the enzyme, which has to be transported over long distances. In contrast, the cholinergic neurons of the striatum are interneurons and ChAT activity is more closely related to the corresponding mRNA level in this structure. This discordance between the

relative levels of mRNA and enzyme activity in different structures has also been found for tyrosine hydroxylase (TH) when comparing the adrenal medulla and locus coeruleus or substantia nigra (Faucon Biguet et al., 1986).

A ChAT cDNA clone was first isolated from VSC λgt 10 cDNA library, taking advantage of ten amino acids of the N-terminal sequence of porcine brain enzyme obtained by Braun et al. (1987). A 2120 basepair (bp) ChAT clone which contains the full 1923 bp coding sequence was obtained. The corresponding mRNA directed the synthesis of an active ChAT enzyme in *Xenopus* oocyte, as well as in a rabbit reticulocyte lysate (Berrard et al., 1987). The amino acid sequence deduced from the nucleotide sequence is shown in Fig. 1.

The porcine clone was then used to screen a λgt 11 library generated from rat brain. A 2.300

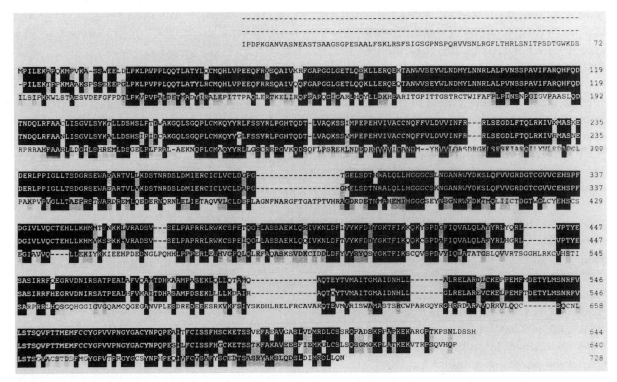

Fig. 1. Comparison of amino acid sequences for rat (upper line), porcine (middle line) and *Drosophila* (lower line) ChAT, predicted from their respective nucleotide sequences. Black and shaded boxes represent identical and homologous residues, respectively.

bp insert was isolated with the complete ChAT coding sequence of 1932 bp, 9 bp longer than that of porcine. The open reading frame encodes a protein of 644 amino acids with a calculated molecular weight of 72 319 and an isoelectric value of 7.93.

The comparison of amino acid sequences deduced from rat, porcine (Berrard et al., 1987), and *Drosophila* (Itoh et al., 1986) cDNAs is shown in Fig. 1. Only a single gap is required to align rat and porcine protein sequences, which exhibit 85% identity and 90% homology when homologous amino acid replacement is considered (Dayhoff et al., 1978). These values are similar to that of 83% found when the nucleotide coding sequences are compared. In contrast, twelve gaps have to be introduced for maximum alignment when comparison includes the *Drosophila* sequence. Under these conditions, the rat and porcine ChAT display 31 and 32% identity with the *Drosophila* sequence, whereas homology, as defined above, is 50 and 51%, respectively. No other significant homology with known proteins was found using the GenBank and National Biomedical Research Foundation protein sequence data bases.

Biochemical studies have shown that one histidine is involved in the catalytic reaction (Malthe-Sorenssen, 1976). We shall note that the three histidine residues at positions 195, 301 and 334 are conserved in the three sequences. This prediction can now be tested experimentally by in vitro mutagenesis.

High level expression of ChAT enzyme in eucaryotic host cells

High levels of expression of exogenous proteins can be obtained in both procaryotic and eucaryotic cells, using a variety of expression vectors. We have first chosen to express the rat enzyme in insect cells, taking advantage of the baculovirus transfer vector pAcYM1, derived from the nuclear polyhedrosis virus *Autographa californica* (AcNPV). This invertebrate expression system has been shown to generate a high level of recombi-

nant proteins and the post-translational modifications appear to be adequately performed in contrast to bacteria. The baculovirus system has been described in several reviews (Luckow and Summers, 1988; Yong Kang, 1988) and the details will not be presented here. The complete rat ChAT cDNA, whose sequence is shown in Fig. 1, was placed under the control of the strong AcNPV polyhedrin promoter, which directs the expression of the ChAT protein. The enzyme activity was analysed 40 h after infection of the *Sodoptera frugiperda* cell line, when cells enter into the lytic cycle. A high level of ChAT activity, 100-fold that of striatum, was observed in the cytosol of infected cells, whereas no activity could be detected in the membrane fraction. Biochemical experiments suggest that the enzyme also exists in a membrane-bound form, with different isoelectric point and molecular weight (Benishin and Carrol, 1983). Our results suggest that if a membrane-bound protein does exist, it derives from a different form of mRNA which could arise by an alternative splicing. Indeed, all modes of attachment characterized to date have been found to occur in the baculovirus system.

Comparison of the cytosolic protein pattern of the infected cells with control cells reveals the presence of a major band at 65 kDa which corresponds to ChAT (Fig. 2). Although the calculated molecular masses of rat and porcine are 71 kDa and 72 kDa respectively, previous studies have shown that the protein migrates at 65 kDa on SDS polyacrylamide gel. Its enzymatic characteristics are identical to that of the native enzyme analysed from rat brain homogenate (Tucek, 1988). The enzyme has recently been purified to homogeneity by a two-step procedure (results not shown). Experiments are now in progress to test, both in vivo and in vitro, whether the enzyme can be phosphorylated. Indeed, putative serine and threonine phosphorylation sites (Cohen, 1985) are located at positions 217, 327, 365 and 466 in the rat sequence, and are conserved in that of porcine.

The availability of ChAT in large amounts should facilitate crystallization of the enzyme for

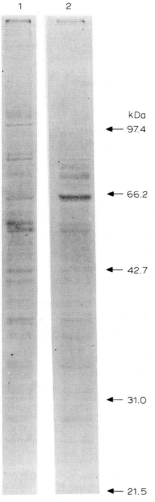

Fig. 2. Sodium dodecyl sulfate–polyacrylamide gel of cytosolic proteins synthesized by baculovirus-infected *Sodoptera frugiperda* cells. Total cell extracts were separated by gel electrophoresis and stained according to the Laemmli procedure. Lane 1, control cells: Lane 2, infected cells.

X-ray studies. This analysis, together with mutagenesis experiments, will elucidate the structure of the active site in molecular terms and the precise mechanism of the enzymatic reaction.

Phenotypic plasticity of ChAT expression in superior cervical ganglia

ChAT, as well as TH, the rate-limiting enzyme in catecholamine synthesis, have received much attention in the context of the phenotypic expression of neurotransmitters. Studies on the ontogeny of the autonomic nervous system have revealed that neurons can change their phenotype from, for example, adrenergic to cholinergic, depending on the nature of their environment (Patterson, 1978). This mechanism may now be analysed in molecular terms with primary cultures of neurons from superior cervical ganglia (SCG) of newborn rat (Potter et al., 1986). In this system the expression of neurotransmitters can be modified by several external signals. In the presence of muscle conditioned medium (CM) the expression of TH in these cells is depressed while that of ChAT is stimulated (Patterson, 1978; Swerts et al., 1983). In contrast, chronic depolarization of cultured sympathetic neurons by K^+, veratridine or electrical stimulation blocks the increase in ChAT activity and fosters noradrenergic differentiation (Swerts and Weber, 1984).

Sympathetic neurons dissociated from newborn rat SCG were first grown in the presence of cytosine arabinoside to eliminate ganglionic non-neuronal cells. We then exposed these neurons to three different conditions: (1) normal medium, (2) normal medium supplemented with 50% CM; and (3) high K^+ (40 mM) medium. After 18 days of culture, the levels of ChAT and TH mRNAs were compared by Northern blot assays (Fig. 3). The level of the latter was strikingly decreased in the presence of CM, while it was increased by high K^+. In contrast, ChAT mRNA was detectable only in the cultures grown in the presence of CM. In the two other media, no signal was discernible (Fig. 3) (Brice et al., 1989).

These results demonstrate that the changes in enzymatic activity are accompanied by measurable changes in mRNA levels. Therefore, neurotransmitter plasticity is not controlled, at least in this situation, exclusively by translational or post-translational events. Further experiments will, however, be necessary to establish whether de novo transcription occurs, since the observed results could also reflect enhanced stability of the mRNA. It should be noted that a clear signal was

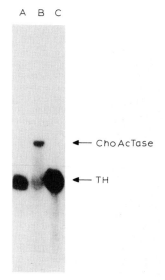

A B C

← ChoAcTase

← TH

Fig. 3. Effect of culture medium on ChAT and TH mRNA expression in rat SCG. Northern blot analysis was performed on 4 μg of total RNA extracted from SCG cultured for 18 days. Hybridization was carried out with radiolabelled rat ChAT and TH cDNA probes. Lane A, normal medium; Lane B, muscle-conditioned medium; Lane C, 40 mM K⁺ medium.

Modulation of ChAT gene expression by neuronal lesions in the rat striatum

The adaptative changes promoted in the striatum by a 6-hydroxydopamine lesion of the nigrostriatal dopaminergic pathway in the rat (Ungerstedt, 1971) provide a convenient model to study the modulation of gene expression of striatal neurons, and in particular cholinergic neurons. We have compared the ChAT mRNA levels, 25 days after a nigral lesion, with the levels of glutamic acid decarboxylase (GAD) and proenkephalin (PPE) mRNAs on the same blot of striatal poly(A)⁺ RNA. ChAT mRNA was found to be elevated 4-fold in the deafferented striatum as compared to control, an increase which is more prominent than that of GAD and PPE mRNA (Fig. 4). However, in the same animals, the ChAT enzymatic activity was not modified by the deafferentation. Although it is attractive to propose that an increase

observed for ChAT mRNA only in the presence of CM. Although ChAT activity is detectable in normal medium, no corresponding mRNA was revealed by Northern blot analysis (Fig. 3). A more sensitive assay, such as the recently developed amplification method (Saiki et al., 1985), may prove useful in this investigation. In normal medium ChAT activity could be restricted to a few cells which may not express catecholamines. However, this possibility is unlikely, since ample studies with CM have shown that most cells have the potential to express at least a dual adrenergic-cholinergic function, a property characteristic of the transitional state, which appears to extend over a period of several days (Potter et al., 1986). In this context, it would be informative to compare by in situ hybridization the expression of ChAT and TH mRNA in individual neurons.

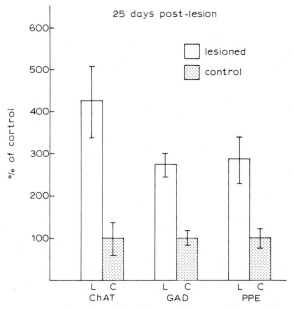

Fig. 4. Modulation of mRNA encoding GAD, PPE, ChAT, 25 days after a 6-OHDA nigral lesion. Poly(A)⁺ RNA, extracted from two pools of five lesioned and control striata, was analysed on the same blot. Amounts of specific mRNA in deafferented striata are expressed as a percent of mRNA levels measured in control striata. Means of two independent experiments are presented.

8

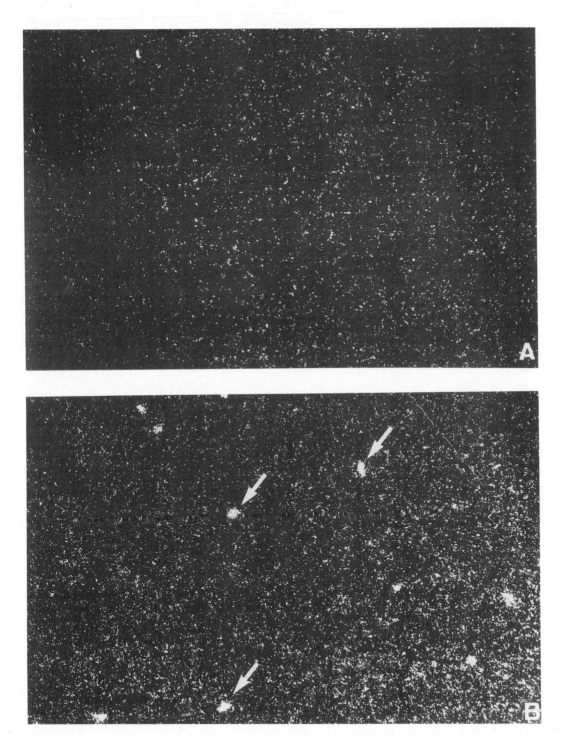

Fig. 5. In situ hybridization on rat striatum sections. Dark-field view of adjacent frontal sections hybridized with (A) a control pBR 322 probe and (B) a ChAT cDNA probe, labelled with cytidine 5′-(thio)triphosphates. Hybridization conditions were as described by Berod et al. (1987).

in the protein turnover could account for this observation, a more careful analysis is needed before firm conclusions can be drawn. In particular, the modulation of the expression of the ChAT mRNA at the cellular level would be most informative. With this in mind we have recently succeeded in visualizing cholinergic neurons on striatal slices of rat with the ChAT probe (Fig. 5). The above results, taken together, suggest that dopamine exerts an overall tonic inhibition on the activity of GABA-, enkephalin- and acetylcholine-containing neurons. The neurons react to the suppression of this influence, and develop a long-term adaptation with a modulation of gene expression. The signals which control this regulation and their precise role in the adaptive processes remain to be elucidated.

Perspectives

The identification of a cDNA clone encoding a complete mammalian ChAT enzyme opens new avenues in the study of the cholinergic system. Regardless of the possible existence of both a membrane-bound and a soluble form of ChAT, it will be of practical interest to examine whether the enzyme exists in multiple forms generated from the alternative splicing of a single pre-messenger RNA. Such a situation has recently been found to occur in the case of human TH. The ability to differentially express various forms of the enzyme that exhibit distinct specific activities represents an attractive means of regulating neurotransmitter availability at particular synapses. Such a possible diversity could also be developmentally regulated or be tissue-specific.

The porcine and rat ChAT cDNA hybridize with human ChAT mRNA, which will facilitate the isolation of the human gene. These probes will be more appropriate for analysing the regulation of the expression of the ChAT gene under various physiological conditions as well as in pathological situations such as Alzheimer's disease and amyotrophic lateral sclerosis, for which there is no animal model.

Biochemical studies in baculovirus can be complemented by the establishment of stable mammalian cell lines expressing ChAT. This approach will allow the identification of the elements necessary to produce cells which express and release acetylcholine. Ultimately, these cells may be grafted into the CNS, and may prove efficient in compensating for cholinergic deficits.

References

Benishin, C.G. and Caroll, P.T. (1983) Multiple forms of choline-o-acetyltransferase in mouse and rat brain: solubilization and characterization. *J. Neurochem.*, 41: 1030–1039.

Berod, A., Faucon Biguet, N., Dumas, S., Bloch, B. and Mallet, J. (1987) Modulation of tyrosine hydroxylase gene expression in the central nervous system visualized by in situ hybridization. *Proc. Natl. Acad. Sci. USA*, 84: 1699–1703.

Berrard, S., Faucon Biguet, N., Gregoire, D., Blanot, F., Smith, J. and Mallet, J. (1986) Synthesis of catalytically active choline acetyltransferase in *Xenopus* oocytes injected with messenger RNA from rat central nervous system. *Neurosci. Lett.*, 72: 93–98.

Berrard, S., Brice, A., Lottspeich, F., Braun, A., Barde, Y.-A. and Mallet, J. (1987) cDNA cloning and complete sequence of porcine choline acetyltransferase: In vitro translation of the corresponding RNA yields an active protein. *Proc. Natl. Acad. Sci. USA*, 84: 9280–9284.

Berrard, S., Brice, A. and Mallet, J. (1989) Molecular genetic approach to the study of mammalian choline acetyltransferase. *Brain Res. Bull.*, 22: 147–153.

Borroni, E., Derrington, E. and Whittaker, V.P. (1989) Chol-1: A cholinergic-specific ganglioside of possible significance in central nervous system neurochemistry and neuropathology. (Abstr.) *J. Neurochem.*, 52 (Suppl.), S34.

Braun, A., Barde, Y.-A., Lottspeich, F., Mewes, W. and Thoenen, H. (1987) N-terminal sequence of pig brain choline acetyltransferase purified by a rapid procedure. *J. Neurochem.*, 48: 16–21.

Brice, A., Berrard, S., Raynaud, B., Ansieau, S., Coppola, T., Weber, M.-J. and Mallet, J. (1989) Complete sequence of a cDNA encoding an active rat choline acetyltransferase: a tool to investigate the plasticity of cholinergic phenotype expression. *J. Neurosci. Res.*, 23: 266–273.

Cohen, P. (1985) The role of protein phosphorylation in the hormonal control of enzyme activity. *Eur. J. Biochem.*, 151: 439–448.

Dayhoff, M.O., Schwartz, R.M. and Orcutt, B.C. (1978) In M.O. Dayhoff (Ed.), *Atlas of protein sequence and structure, Vol. 5*, suppl. 3. National Biomedical Research Foundation, Washington, DC, pp. 345–352.

Faucon Biguet, N., Buda, M., Lamouroux, A., Samolyk, D. and Mallet, J. (1986) Time course of the changes of TH mRNA in rat brain and adrenal medulla after a single injection of reserpine. *EMBO J.*, 5: 287–291.

10

Fonnum, F. (1975) A rapid radiochemical method for the determination of choline acetyltransferase. *J. Neurochem.*, 24: 404–409.

Grima, B., Lamouroux, A., Blanot, F., Faucon Biguet, N. and Mallet, J. (1985) Complete coding sequence of rat tyrosin hydroxylase mRNA. *Proc. Natl. Acad. Sci. USA*, 82: 617–621.

Itoh, N., Slemmon, J.R., Hawke, D.H., Williamson, R., Morita, E., Itakura, K., Roberts, E., Shively, J.E., Crawford, G.D. and Salvaterra, P.M. (1986) Cloning of *Drosophila* choline acetyltransferase cDNA. *Proc. Natl. Acad. Sci. USA*, 83: 4081–4085.

Kang, C.Y. (1989) Baculovirus vectors for expression of foreign genes. *Adv. Virus Res.*, 35: 177–192.

Lamouroux, A., Faucon Biguet, N., Samolyk, D., Privat, A., Salomon, J.C., Pujol, J.-F. and Mallet, J. (1982) Identification of cDNA clones coding for rat tyrosine hydroxylase. *Proc. Natl. Acad. Sci. USA*, 79: 3881–3885.

Luckow, V.A. and Summers, M.D. (1988) Trends in the development of baculovirus expression vectors. *Biotechnology, 6:* 47–55.

Malthe-Sorenssen, D. (1976) Choline acetyltransferase—evidence for acetyl transfer by a histidine residue. *J. Neurochem.*, 27: 873–881.

Patterson, P.H. (1978) Environmental determination of autonomic neurotransmitter functions. *Annu. Rev. Neurosci.*, 1: 1–17.

Potter, D.D., Landis, S.C., Matsumoto, S.G. and Furshpan, E.J. (1986) Synaptic functions in rat sympathtic neurons in microcultures. II. Adrenergic/cholinergic dual status and plasticity. *J. Neurosci.*, 6: 1080–1098.

Saiki, R.K., Sharf, S., Faloona, F., Mullis, K.B., Horn, G.T., Erlich, H.A. and Arnheim N. (1985) Enzymatic amplification of α-globin genomic sequences and restriction site analysis for diagnosis of sickle cell anemia. *Science*, 230: 1350–1352.

Smith, J., Fauquet, M., Ziller, C. and Le Douarin, N.M. (1979) Acetyl choline synthesis by mesencephalic neural crest in the process of migration in vivo. *Nature (Lond.)*, 282, 853–855.

Swerts, J.P., Le Van Thaï, A., Vigny, A. and Weber, M.J. (1983) Regulation of enzymes responsible for neurotransmitter synthesis and degradation in cultured rat sympathetic neurons. I. Effects of muscle conditioned medium. *Dev. Biol.*, 100: 1–11.

Swerts, J.P. and Weber, M.J. (1984) Regulation of enzymes responsible for neurotransmitter synthesis and degradation in cultured rat sympathetic neurons. III. Effects of sodium butyrate. *Dev. Biol.*, 106: 282–288.

Tucek, S. (1988) Choline acetyltransferase and the synthesis of acetylcholine. In V.P. Whittaker (Ed.), *Handbook of Experimental Pharmacology, Vol. 86: The Cholinergic Synapse*. Berlin, Springer Verlag, pp. 125–165.

Ungerstedt, U. (1971) Postsynaptic supersensitivity after 6-hydroxydopamine induced degeneration of nigrostriaral dopaminnergic system. *Acta Physiol. Scand., Suppl.*, 367: 95–122.

S.-M. Aquilonius and P.-G. Gillberg (Eds.)
Progress in Brain Research, Vol. 84
© 1990 Elsevier Science Publishers B.V. (Biomedical Division)

CHAPTER 2

Structure and function of muscarinic receptors

Michael I. Schimerlik

Department of Biochemistry and Biophysics, Oregon State University, Corvallis, OR 97331-6503, U.S.A.

Introduction

Early pharmacological studies by Sir Henry Dale (1914) resulted in the characterization of cholinergic responses as either nicotinic or muscarinic in nature. This was followed by Otto Loewi's discovery of Vagusstoff (Loewi, 1921), demonstrating that acetylcholine (ACh) was the neurotransmitter which mediated the negative chronotropic and negative inotropic effects of vagal stimulation on the heartbeat. More recently, muscarinic receptors (mAChRs) have been shown to couple to physiological responses in the central and peripheral nervous system, smooth muscle, secretory glands and several clonal cell lines in addition to those in the heart (Schimerlik, 1989). At this time there appear to be at least five distinct subtypes of mAChR. Although this article will attempt to summarize results from several laboratories regarding the structure and function of the five mAChR subtypes, specific examples, particularly concerning physical characterization of the receptor protein, will be taken from work done in the author's laboratory utilizing the M_2 subtype from porcine atria.

Physiological responses

Depending on the particular system under consideration, muscarinic receptors can couple to physiological responses which are either excitatory or inhibitory in nature. In heart preparations, addition of ACh caused a reduction in the level of adenosine $3',5'$-cyclic monophosphate (cAMP) (Murad et al., 1962). Muscarinic inhibition of adenylyl cyclase was shown to require guanosine triphosphate (GTP) (Jacobs et al., 1979) and is now known to be mediated by one or more of a class of signal-transducing proteins called guanine nucleotide binding proteins (G-proteins) (Gilman, 1987). G-proteins that regulate adenylyl cyclase are heterotrimers consisting of differing G_α subunits and similar $G_{\beta\gamma}$ subunits. The role of the hormone-receptor complex is to promote the release of a tightly bound molecule of guanosine diphosphate (GDP) from the G_α subunit of the heterotrimer (Gilman, 1987). The binding of GTP to the vacant guanine nucleotide binding site results in the dissociation of the heterotrimer into $G_\alpha \cdot$ GTP plus $G_{\beta\gamma}$ subunits which then regulate various cellular effector systems or ion channels. Activity is terminated by the hydrolysis of GTP to GDP and phosphate by the GTPase activity of the G_α subunit followed by subunit reassociation to give the G-protein $\cdot$ GDP complex. The stimulatory G-protein, G_s, activates adenylyl cyclase, while the inhibitory G-protein, G_i, or the 'other' G-protein, G_o, inhibits the enzyme. Hormonal inhibition of adenylyl cyclase may occur by the liberation of excess $G_{\beta\gamma}$ subunits from G_i or G_o which promote $G_{s\alpha}$ reassociation to form the inactive heterotrimer (Katada et al., 1984), by competition of $G_{i\alpha}$ with $G_{s\alpha}$ for a binding site on the enzyme or by direct binding of $G_{i\beta\gamma}$ to a site on the enzyme (Katada et al., 1986). Pertussis toxin-catalysed ADP-ribosylation of G_i functionally uncouples mAChR-mediated inhibition of adenylyl cyclase in the heart (Kurose and Ui, 1983). In 1321 N1 human astrocytes, however, mAChRs attenuate cAMP levels by a different mechanism: activation of a calcium-sensitive phosphodiesterase (Tanner et al., 1986). Since astrocytes contain the M_4 mAChR subtypes while the M_2 subtype is found in heart, it can be seen that different mAChR subtypes may couple to different physiological effector systems (cloning and expression of mAChR genes, below).

A second biochemical response initiated by muscarinic agonists is the stimulation of inositol phospholipid (IP) metabolism. The activation of phospholipase C by mAChRs is guanine nucleotide-dependent (Haslam and Davidson, 1984) and is mediated by an as yet unisolated G-protein(s). That the identity of this G protein may depend on the system under consideration has been demonstrated by differing susceptibilities to uncoupling by treatment with pertussis or cholera toxins. Chick heart (Masters et al., 1985) and 1321 N1 astrocytes (Hepler and Harden, 1986) PI responses were not sensitive to pertussis toxin while the PI response of mast cells (Nakamura and Ui, 1985) was pertussis toxin-sensitive. The PI response of Flow 9000 pituitary tumor cells was sensitive to cholera toxin treatment but not treatment with pertussis toxin (Lo and Hughes, 1987).

Phospholipase C acts on phosphatidylinositol 4,5-bisphosphate to give inositol 1,4,5-triphosphate (IP_3) and diacylglycerol (DG). IP_3 can act to release Ca^{2+} from the endoplasmic reticulum (Streb et al., 1983), while DG activates protein kinase C (Nishizuka, 1988). DG may then be metabolized by the action of diacylglycerol lipase to release arachidonic acid, an eicosanoid precursor. Arachidonate can also arise from phospholipase A_2 action in a process mediated by a pertussis toxin-sensitive G-protein (Nakashima et al., 1988). Although muscarinic agonists have been shown to cause arachidonate release in cerebellar cortex slices (Reichman et al., 1987), it is not yet known whether this occurred by one or both of the above-mentioned pathways.

In addition to activating G-protein-dependent second-messenger systems, G-protein subunits may act directly on ion channels. The system most extensively studied in this respect has been the mAChR-activated inward rectifying potassium channel in the heart. Initial results from patch clamping experiments were contradictory, with one group suggesting that the α subunit of G_i activated the inward rectifying potassium channel (Yatani et al., 1987) and a second proposing a role for the $\beta\gamma$ subunits (Logothetis et al., 1987). As of this time, the controversy is not yet completely resolved; however, the α subunit is active at lower concentrations (Codina et al., 1987) than $\beta\gamma$, antibodies against $G_{i\alpha}$ block channel activation in inside-out patches (Yatani et al., 1988a), and recombinant $G_{i\alpha}$ subunits open the channel (Yatani et al., 1988b). These results strongly suggest that the $G_{i\alpha}$ subunit can directly interact with and activate the inward rectifying potassium channel in atria. More recently, it has been proposed that the $\beta\gamma$ subunit may activate the inward rectifying potassium channel in heart by activation of a phospholipase A_2. This results in increased levels of an arachidonic acid metabolite(s) which may act as a second messenger (Kim et al., 1989; Kurachi et al., 1989) to open the channel.

Ligand binding properties of muscarinic receptors

Interactions of ligands with mAChRs have been characterized utilizing radiolabeled antagonists such as L-quinuclidinyl benzilate (Yamamura and Synder, 1974) or labeled agonists such as *cis*-methyldioxolane (Galper et al., 1987). Antagonist binding appears to be consistent with a two-step kinetic mechanism (Jarv et al., 1979; Schimerlik and Searles, 1980), while agonists and GTP appeared to add in a random manner to form the agonist · mAChR · G protein · GTP complex (Galper et al., 1987). Agonist binding properties have been interpreted in terms of a ternary complex model (Ehlert, 1985) where the free mAChR binds agonist with low affinity while the mAChR · G-protein complex has high affinity for agonists.

Guanine nucleotide binding to the G-protein results in uncoupling of the mAChR from the G-protein with a return to the low-affinity agonist state. The interconversion of the mAChR from low- to high-affinity form for agonists has not been observed (Schreiber et al., 1985; Galper et al., 1987), suggesting that the mAChR and G-protein are either pre-coupled in the membrane or that the interaction between them was too fast to be observed.

Muscarinic receptor subtypes were first identified by the binding properties of the antagonist pirenzepine (Hammer et al., 1980), which permitted classification into high-affinity (M_1) and low-affinity (M_2) subtypes. The M_2 subtype was further subclassified into cardiac and glandular mAChRs based on the binding of AF-DX116 (Hammer et al., 1986), which binds more tightly to the cardiac subtype, and p-F-HHSiD (Lambrecht et al., 1988), which has a higher affinity for the smooth muscle and glandular M_2 mAChRs. Studies with cell lines expressing the five recombinant subtypes have shown, however, that it is not possible to differentiate between all five subtypes based on ligand binding properties alone (Peralta et al., 1987b; Buckley et al., 1989).

Purification and characterization of muscarinic receptors

Muscarinic receptors have been purified from porcine atria (Peterson et al., 1984), porcine cerebellum (Haga and Haga, 1985), rat forebrain (Berrie et al., 1985) and chick heart (Kwatra and Hosey, 1986). The procedures were somewhat different for each group; however, all laboratories utilized affinity chromatography on 3-(2'-amino-benzhydryloxy) tropane agarose, a method invented by Haga and Haga (1983). The results of hydrodynamic and compositional analysis of the purified porcine atrial mAChR are summarized in Table I. In either Triton X-405 or dodecyl β-maltoside the protein appeared roughly spherical with a frictional ratio of 1.2 and bound large quantities of detergent (1–2.5 g of detergent per

TABLE I

Properties of purified porcine atrial muscarinic receptor

Parameter	Triton X-405	Dodecyl β-D-maltoside
Stokes radius (Å)	43	53
Frictional ratio	1.21	1.22
Bound detergent (g/g)	1.01	2.54
Molecular mass (daltons)	68 000	72 000
Carbohydrate by weight (%)	26%	
Molecular weight of polypeptide chain	55 000	

Data are summarized from Peterson et al. (1986, 1988).

gram of protein), confirming the hydrophobic nature of the molecule. The molecular mass of protein plus carbohydrate was about 70 kDa and compositional analysis showed that the molecule was about 26% carbohydrate by weight, resulting in an estimation of the molecular mass of the protein portion of the molecule to be about 55 kDa. The mAChR is an acidic molecule with a pI of about 4.6 (Repke and Matthes, 1980).

Cloning and expression of muscarinic receptor genes

At this time, the amino acid sequences of five distinct mAChR subtypes have been deduced from clones isolated from human, rat and porcine cDNA and genomic libraries (Kubo et al., 1986a,b; Peralta et al., 1987a,b; Bonner et al., 1987, 1988). Southern analysis of rat and human genomic DNA has suggested that there may be up to four additional muscarinic subtypes in the rat and one additional human subtype (Bonner et al., 1987). The expression of mAChR subtypes appears to be relatively tissue and/or cell line specific (Bonner et al., 1987; Peralta et al., 1987b).

Hydropathy analysis of the amino acid sequence data from the five mAChR subtypes, shown in Fig. 1 for the porcine atrial mAChR, suggested a common structural motif in which the proteins have seven transmembrane regions. By

14

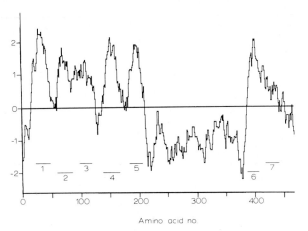

Fig. 1. Hydropathy analysis of porcine M_2 muscarinic acetylcholine receptor. Relative hydropathy of the amino acid sequence was analysed by the method of Kyte and Doolittle (1982) using a nineteen amino acid window. The bars indicate the putative transmembrane sequences and are numbered one to seven from the amino to the carboxyl terminus of the molecule.

analogy with rhodopsin (Ovchinnikov, 1982), the amino terminus is located outside the cell and the carboxyl terminus intracellularly. Fig. 2 shows the deduced amino acid sequence and proposed topology of the porcine atrial mAChR. Potential sites of N-linked glycosylation, given by the sequence N-X-S or T, are located at the amino terminal and potential phosphorylation sites can be found in the large intracellular loop between transmembrane regions five and six. Cytosolic loops one-two and three-four and the seven transmembrane regions have a high degree of amino acid identity amongst the mAChR subtypes; however, there is little sequence identity in the cytosolic loop connecting transmembrane regions five and six. Therefore this region may play a unique role in coupling mAChR subtypes to specific effector systems and/or in the regulation of the various subtypes. All subtypes contain three aspartic acid

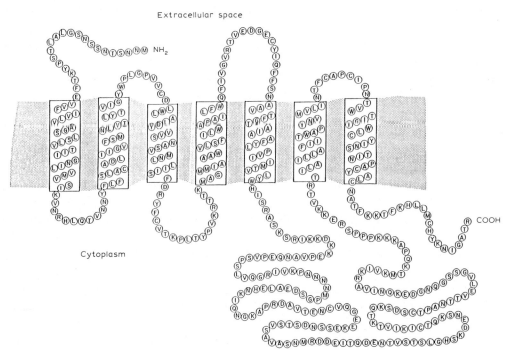

Fig. 2. Amino acid sequence and topography of the porcine M_2 muscarinic receptor. Amino acids are identified using standard one-letter abbreviations.

residues located just outside or within transmembrane regions two and three (aspartates 69, 97 and 103 for the porcine mAChR; Fig. 2). Peptide mapping studies after affinity alkylation with propylbenzilylcholine mustard have led Curtis et al. (1989) to propose that either or both of the two aspartates at the top of transmembrane helix two (aspartate 97 and 103 for the porcine mAChR) may act as the negative counter ion for the positively charged amino group of muscarinic ligands.

Expression of the genes coding for the five mAChR subtypes has permitted analysis of the ligand binding properties for the proteins as well as a determination of their specificity for effector systems. Expression of the M_1 and M_2 subtypes in *Xenopus* oocytes resulted in the expected ligand specificity for pirenzepine (M_1, high affinity; M_2, low affinity) and both mAChR subtypes coupled to a calcium-dependent increase in chloride conductance. In addition, the M_2 subtype activated a second channel in which current was carried by sodium and potassium ions (Kubo et al., 1986a; Fukuda et al., 1987). Expression of the M_2 subtype in Chinese hamster ovary cells (Ashkenazi et al., 1987) showed that the protein could couple to both inhibition of adenylyl cyclase and stimulation of IP metabolism. The M_2 mAChR was more tightly coupled to inhibition of adenylyl cyclase and the responses appeared to be mediated by different G proteins. Analysis of M_1–M_4 mAChRs expressed in embryonic kidney cells (Peralta et al., 1988), NG108-15 cells (Fukuda et al., 1988) and A9 L cells (Conklin et al., 1988) showed that the M_1 and M_4 subtypes coupled preferentially to the stimulation of IP metabolism, while M_2 and M_3 were selective for inhibition of adenylyl cyclase. The M_5 subtype, expressed in Chinese hamster ovary cells, coupled preferentially to the stimulation of IP metabolism (Bonner et al., 1988). The properties of the various subtypes are summarized in Table II.

Reconstitution of muscarinic receptors with G-proteins

Reconstitution of purified porcine brain mAChRs (Haga et al., 1985) or bovine brain mAChRs resolved from G-proteins by ion-exchange chromatography (Florio and Sternweis, 1985) with G_i and G_o resulted in preparations that showed agonist-stimulated GTPase activity and high-affinity guanine nucleotide-sensitive muscarinic agonist binding, respectively. Purified brain mAChRs reconstituted effectively with G_i and G_o (Haga et al., 1986) as well as G_n (Haga et al., 1989), a G protein most likely corresponding to G_{i2}. Studies with resolved subunits of G_o (Florio and Sternweis, 1989) showed that both G protein subunits were required for agonist-stimulated guanine nucleotide exchange. Agonists increased the association rate constant for GTP but decreased the rate of GDP association with G_o, suggesting a differential effect on the two guanine nucleotides.

Reconstitution of purified porcine atrial mAChRs with purified atrial G_i also demonstrated guanine nucleotide-sensitive high-affinity agonist binding (Tota et al., 1987). The data from

TABLE II

Properties of muscarinic receptor subtypes

Subtype	A.A. number	Molecular weight	Physiological response
M_1	460	51387	Stimulation of PI metabolism
M_2	466	51681	Inhibition of adenylyl cyclase
M_3	479	53014	Inhibition of adenylyl cyclase
M_4	590	66085	Stimulation of PI metabolism
M_5	532	60120	Stimulation of PI metabolism

Data are for the human subtypes.

TABLE III

Kinetic and thermodynamic analysis of the properties of reconstituted porcine atrial G_i and porcine atrial muscarinic receptors

Parameter/ligand	Carbachol	L-Hyoscyamine	Ratio
k_{cat} (min^{-1})	2.2	0.2	11
K_{EFF}^{GTP} (nM)	33	–	–
K_m^{GTP} (nM)	31	10	3.1
K_{off}^{GDP} (min^{-1})	4.5	0.1	45
K_D^{GDP} (nM)	500	10	50
K_D^{GTP} (nM)	10	10	1
$K_D^{GTP_\gamma S}$ (pM)	332	454	0.7

a series of kinetic and thermodynamic measurements on this reconstituted system are summarized in Table III. In the presence of the antagonist L-hyoscyamine, the dissociation of GDP appeared to be the sole rate-limiting step in the steady-state mechanism for GTP hydrolysis ($k_{cat} \approx K_{off}^{GDP}$); however in the presence of the agonist carbachol, k_{cat} was increased by about 11-fold, while K_{off}^{GDP} was increased 45-fold. These results suggest that GDP release is no longer solely rate-limiting in the presence of carbachol. The IC$_{50}$ for GTP in inducing the conversion of high-affinity mAChR for carbachol to low affinity (K_{EFF}^{GTP}) was approximately equal to the K_m for GTP (31 nM) for the agonist-stimulated GTPase activity. Finally, the affinity of GDP for G_i in the presence of the mAChR · carbachol complex was decreased by about 50-fold, consistant with the 45-fold increase in the rate of GDP dissociation; however, the affinity of GTP and GTP$_\gamma$S was unaffected by muscarinic ligands. These results suggest that the agonist · mAChR complex selectively weakens the binding of GDP to G_i mainly by increasing the dissociation rate constant for that ligand. This would then promote a feed-forward mechanism whereby bound GDP is exchanged for GTP.

Additional studies of the reconstituted system showed that the mAChR could be phosphorylated by cAMP-dependent protein kinase A (Rosenbaum et al., 1987). The phosphorylation stoichiometry was altered by muscarinic ligands only when the agonist-occupied mAChR was phosphorylated in the presence of G_i. These results suggested that the mAChR receptor has a unique conformation in the presence of both an agonist and G_i such that the extent of phosphorylation by cAMP-dependent protein kinase is increased.

The reconstituted system has also been used to define the mechanism of action of partial versus full muscarinic agonists. The GTPase activity of G_i was measured at varying levels of mAChR in the presence of saturating concentrations of the full agonist carbachol or the partial agonist pilocarpine. Analysis of the data showed that at saturating receptor concentrations, both ligands gave about the same value for the turnover number of the GTPase activity of G_i (5.0 min^{-1} for carbachol, 6.4 min^{-1} for pilocarpine); however, the receptor-agonist complex bound about 4-fold more weakly to G_i in the presence of the partial agonist ($K_d = 3.1$ nM) than in the presence of the full agonist ($K_d = 0.8$ nM). These results indicated that the difference between full and partial agonists in this system was due to weaker binding of the agonist · mAChR to G_i, resulting in a lower steady-state level of activated G-protein.

Conclusions

Over the past decade, our knowledge of the structure and mechanism of action of mAChRs has increased enormously. The detailed mechanism of receptor interactions with G-proteins has yet to be elucidated, as has the manner in which the various G-proteins interact with effector systems in the cell. These goals are complicated by the multiplicity of receptor subtypes, G-proteins and effector systems with which they interact and the apparent tissue specificity exhibited by the various components of the muscarinic signaling system.

Acknowledgements

The author would like to acknowledge the expert typing skills of Barbara Hanson and the support of his research by USPHS grants HL23632 and ES00210.

References

Ashkenazi, A., Winslow, J.W., Peralta, E.G., Peterson, G.L., Schimerlik, M.I., Capon, D.J. and Ramachandrin, J. (1987) An M2 muscarinic receptor subtype coupled to both adenylyl cyclase and phosphoinositide turnover. *Science,* 238: 672–674.

Berrie, C.P., Birdsall, N.J.M., Dadi, H.K., Hulme, E.C., Morris, R.J., Stockton, J.M. and Wheatley, M. (1985) Purification of the muscarinic acetylcholine receptor from rat forebrain. *Biochem. Soc. Trans.,* 13: 1101–1103.

Bonner, T.I., Buckley, N.J., Young, A.C. and Brann, M.R. (1987) Identification of a family of muscarinic acetylcholine receptor genes. *Science,* 237: 527–532.

Bonner, T.I., Young, A.C., Brann, M.R. and Buckley, N.J. (1988) Cloning and expression of the human and rat m5 muscarinic acetylcholine receptor genes. *Neuron,* 1: 403–410.

Buckley, N.J., Bonner, T.I., Buckley, C.M. and Brann, M.R. (1989) Antagonist binding properties of five cloned muscarinic receptors expressed in CHO-K1 cells. *Mol. Pharmacol.,* 35: 469–476.

Codina, J., Yatani, A., Grenet, D., Brown, A.M. and Birnbaumer, L. (1987) The α subunit of the GTP binding protein G_K opens atrial potassium channels. *Science,* 236: 442–445.

Conklin, B.R., Brann, M.R., Buckley, N.J., Ma, A.L., Bonner, T.I. and Axelrod, J. (1988) Stimulation of arachidonic acid release and inhibition of mitogenesis by cloned genes for muscarinic receptor subtypes stably expressed in A9 L cells. *Proc. Natl. Acad. Sci. USA,* 85: 8698–8702.

Curtis, C.A.M., Wheatley, M., Bansal, S., Birdsall, N.J.M., Eveleigh, P., Pedder, E.K., Poyner, D. and Hulme, E.C. (1989) Propylbenzilylcholine labels an acidic residue in transmembrane helix 3 of the muscarinic receptor. *J. Biol. Chem.,* 264: 489–495.

Dale, H.H. (1914) The action of certain esters and esters of choline, and their relation to muscarine. *J. Pharmacol. Exp. Ther.,* 6: 147–190.

Ehlert, F.J. (1985) The relationship between muscarinic receptor occupancy and adenylate cyclase inhibition in the rabbit myocardium. *Mol. Pharmacol.,* 28: 410–421.

Florio, V.A. and Sternweis, P.C. (1985) Reconstitution of resolved muscarinic cholinergic receptors with purified GTP-binding proteins. *J. Biol. Chem.,* 260: 3477–3483.

Florio, V. and Sternweis, P.C. (1989) Mechanisms of muscarinic receptor action on G_o in reconstituted phospholipid vesicles. *J. Biol. Chem.,* 264: 3909–3915.

Fukuda, K., Kubo, T., Akiba, I., Maeda, A., Mishina, M. and Numa, S. (1987) Molecular distinction between muscarinic acetylcholine receptor subtypes. *Nature (Lond.),* 327: 623–625.

Fukuda, K., Higashida, H., Kubo, T., Maeda, A., Akiba, I., Bujo, H., Mishina, M. and Numa, S. (1988) Selective coupling with K^+ currents of muscarinic acetylcholine receptor subtypes in NG108-15 cells. *Nature (Lond.),* 335: 355–358.

Galper, J.B., Haigh, L.S., Hart, A.C., O'Hara, D.S. and Livingstone, D.S. (1987) Muscarinic cholinergic receptors in the embryonic chick heart: interaction of agonist, receptor, and guanine nucleotides studied by an improved assay for direct binding of the muscarinic agonist [^{3}H]*cis*-methyldioxolane. *Mol. Pharmacol.,* 32: 230–240.

Gilman, A.G. (1987) G proteins: transducers of receptor-generated signals. *Annu. Rev. Biochem.,* 56: 615–649.

Haga, K. and Haga, T. (1983) Affinity chromatography of the muscarinic receptor. *J. Biol. Chem.,* 258: 13575–13579.

Haga, K. and Haga, T. (1985) Purification of the muscarinic acetylcholine receptor from porcine brain. *J. Biol. Chem.,* 260: 7927–7935.

Haga, K., Haga, T., Ichiyama, A., Katada, T., Kurose, H. and Ui, M. (1985) Functional reconstitution of purified muscarinic receptors and inhibitory guanine nucleotide regulatory protein. *Nature (Lond.),* 316: 731–733.

Haga, K., Haga, T. and Ichiyama, A. (1986) Reconstitution of the muscarinic acetylcholine receptor. Guanine nucleotide-sensitive high affinity binding of agonists to purified muscarinic receptors reconstituted with GTP-binding proteins (G_i and G_o). *J. Biol. Chem.,* 261: 10133–10140.

Haga, K., Uchiyama, H., Haga, T., Ichiyama, A., Kangawa, K. and Matsuo, H. (1989) Cerebral muscarinic acetylcholine receptors interact with three kinds of GTP-binding proteins in a reconstituted system of purified components. *Mol. Pharmacol.,* 35: 286–294.

Hammer, R., Berrie, C.P., Birdsall, N.J.M., Burgen, A.S.V. and Hulme, E.C. (1980) Pirenzepine distinguishes between different subclasses of muscarinic receptors. *Nature (Lond.),* 283: 90–92.

Hammer, R., Giraldo, E., Schiavi, G.B., Monferini, L. and Ladinsky, H. (1986) Binding profile of a novel cardioselective muscarine receptor antagonist, AF-DX116, to membranes of peripheral tissues and brain in the rat. *Life Sci.,* 38: 1653–1662.

Haslam, R.J. and Davidson, M.M.L. (1984) Receptor-induced diacylglycerol formation in permeabilized platelets; possible role for a GTP-binding protein. *J. Rec. Res.,* 4: 605–629.

Hepler, J.R. and Harden, T.K. (1986) Guanine nucleotide-dependent-pertussis toxin-insensitive stimulation of inositol phosphate formation by carbachol in a membrane preparation from human astrocytoma cells. *Biochem. J.,* 239: 141–146.

Jakobs, K.H., Aktories, K. and Schultz, G. (1979) GTP-dependent inhibition of cardiac adenylate cyclase by muscarinic cholinergic agonists. *Naunyn-Schmiedeberg's Arch. Pharmacol.,* 310: 113–119.

Järv, J., Hedlund, B. and Bartfai, T. (1979) Isomerization of the muscarinic receptor-antagonist complex. *J. Biol. Chem.,* 254: 5595–5598.

Katada, T., Bokoch, G.M., Smigel, M.D., Ui, M. and Gilman, A.G. (1984) The inhibitory guanine nucleotide-binding regulatory component of adenylate cyclase. *J. Biol. Chem.,* 259: 3586–3595.

Katada, T., Oinuma, M. and Ui, M. (1986) Mechanisms for inhibition of the catalytic activity of adenylate cyclase by the guanine nucleotide-binding protein serving as the substrate of islet-activating protein, pertussis toxin. *J. Biol. Chem.,* 261: 5215–5221.

Kim, D., Lewis, D.L., Graziadei, L., Neer, E.J., Bar-Sagi, D. and Clapham, D.E. (1989) G-protein βγ-subunits activate the cardiac muscarinic K$^+$ channel via phospholipase A$_2$. *Nature (Lond.)*, 337: 557–560.

Kubo, T., Fukuda, K., Mikami, A., Maeda, A., Takahashi, H., Mishina, M., Haga, T., Haga, K., Ichiyama, A., Kangawa, K., Kojima, M., Matsuo, H., Hirose, T. and Numa, S. (1986a) Cloning sequencing and expression of complementary DNA encoding the muscarinic acetylcholine receptor. *Nature (Lond.)*, 323: 411–416.

Kubo, T., Maeda, A., Sugimoto, K., Akiba, T., Mikami, A., Takahashi, H., Haga, T., Haga, K., Ichiyama, A., Kangawa, K., Matsui, H., Hirose, T. and Numa, S. (1986b) Primary structure of porcine cardiac muscarinic acetylcholine receptor deduced from the cDNA sequence. *FEBS. Lett.*, 209: 367–372.

Kurachi, Y., Ito, H., Sugimoto, T., Shimizu, T., Miki, I. and Ui, M. (1989) Arachidonate metabolites as intracellular modulators of the G-protein-gated cardiac K$^+$ channel. *Nature (Lond.)*, 337: 555–557.

Kurose, H. and Ui, M. (1983) Functional uncoupling of muscarinic receptors from adneylate cyclase in rat cardiac membranes by the active component of islet-activating protein, pertussis toxin. *J. Cyclic Nucl. Protein Phosphorylation Res.*, 9: 305–310.

Kwatra, M.M. and Hosey, M.M. (1986) Phosphorylation of the cardiac muscarinic receptor in intact chick heart and its regulation by a muscarinic agonist. *J. Biol. Chem.*, 261: 12429–12432.

Kyte, J. and Doolittle, R.F. (1982) A simple method for displaying the hydrophobic character of a protein. *J. Mol. Biol.*, 157: 105–132.

Lambrecht, G., Feifel, R., Forth, B., Strohmann, C., Tacko, R. and Mutschler, E. (1988) p-Fluoro-hexahydrosila-difenidol: the first M2β-selective muscarinic antagonist. *Eur. J. Pharmacol.*, 152: 193–194.

Lo, W.W.Y. and Hughes, J. (1988) A novel cholera toxin-sensitive G-protein (G$_c$) regulating receptor-mediated phosphoinositide signalling in human pituitary cloned cells. *FEBS Lett.*, 220; 327–331.

Loewi, O. (1921) Uber humorale Übertragbarkeit der Herznervenwirkung. *Pfluegers Arch. Physiol.*, 189: 239–242.

Logothetis, D.E., Kurachi, Y., Galper, J., Neer, E.J. and Clapham, D.E. (1987) The βγ subunits of GTP-binding proteins activate the muscarinic K$^+$ channel in heart. *Nature (Lond.)*, 325: 321–326.

Masters, S.B., Martin, M.W., Harden, T.K. and Brown, J.H. (1985) Pertussis toxin does not inhibit muscarinic-receptor-mediated phosphoinositide hydrolysis or calcium mobilization. *Biochem. J.*, 227: 933–937.

Murad, F., Chi, Y.-M., Rall, T.W. and Sutherland, E.W. (1962) The effect of catecholamines and choline esters on the formation of adenosine 3′,5′-phosphate by preparations from cardiac muscle and liver. *J. Biol. Chem.*, 237: 1233–1238.

Nakamura, T. and Ui, M. (1985) Simultaneous inhibitions of inositol phospholipid breakdown, arachidonic acid release,
and histamine secretion in mast cells by islet-activating protein, pertussis toxin. *J. Biol. Chem.*, 260: 3584–3595.

Nakashima, S., Nagata, K.-I., Ueeda, K. and Nozawa, Y. (1988) Stimulation of arachidonic acid release by guanine nucleotides in saponin-permeabilized neutrophils: evidence for involvement of GTP-binding proteins in phospholipase A$_2$ activation. *Arch. Biochem. Biophys.*, 261: 375–383.

Nishizuka, Y. (1988) The molecular heterogeneity of protein kinase C and its implications for cellular regulation. *Nature (Lond.)*, 334: 661–665.

Ovchinnikov, Y.A. (1982) Rhodopsin and bacteriorhodopsin: structure-function relationships. *FEBS Lett.*, 148: 179–191.

Peralta, E.G., Winslow, J.W., Peterson, G.L., Smith, D.H., Ashkenazi, A., Ramachandran, J., Schimerlik, M.I. and Capon, D.J. (1987a) Primary structure and biochemical properties of an M$_2$ muscarinic receptor. *Science*, 236: 600–605.

Peralta, E.G., Ashkenazi, A., Winslow, J.W., Ramachandran, J. and Capon, D.J. (1987b) Distinct primary structures, ligand binding properties and tissue-specific expression of four human muscarinic acetylcholine receptors. *EMBO J.*, 6: 3923–3929.

Peralta, E.G., Ashkenazi, A., Winslow, J.W., Ramachandran, J. and Capon, D.J. (1988) Differential regulation of PI hydrolysis and adenylyl cyclase by muscarinic receptor subtype. *Nature (Lond.)*, 334: 434–437.

Peterson, G.L., Herron, G.S., Yamaki, M., Fullerton, D.S. and Schimerlik, M.I. (1984) Purification of the muscarinic acetylcholine receptor from porcine atria. *Proc. Natl. Acad. Sci. USA*, 81: 4993–4997.

Peterson, G.L., Rosenbaum, L.C., Broderick, D.J. and Schimerlik, M.I. (1986) Physical properties of the purified cardiac muscarinic receptor. *Biochemistry*, 25: 3189–3202.

Peterson, G.L., Rosenbaum, L.C. and Schimerlik, M.I. (1988) Solubilization and hydrodynamic properties of pig atrial muscarinic acetylcholine receptor in dodecyl β-D-maltoside. *Biochem. J.*, 255: 553–560.

Repke, H. and Matthies, H. (1980) Biochemical characterization of solubilized muscarinic acetylcholine receptors. *Brain Res. Bull.*, 5: 703–709.

Rosenbaum, L.C., Malencik, D.A., Anderson, S.R., Tota, M.R. and Schimerlik, M.I. (1987) Phosphorylation of the porcine atrial muscarinic acetylcholine receptor by cyclic AMP dependent protein kinase. *Biochemistry*, 26: 8183–8188.

Schimerlik, M.I. (1989) Structure and regulation of muscarinic receptors. *Annu. Rev. Physiol.*, 51: 217–227.

Schimerlik, M.I. and Searles, R.P. (1980) Ligand interactions with the membrane-bound porcine atrial muscarinic receptor. *Biochemistry*, 19: 3407–3413.

Schreiber, G., Henis, Y.I. and Sokolovsky, M. (1985) Rate constants of agonist binding to muscarinic receptor in rat brain medulla. *J. Biol. Chem.*, 260: 8795–8802.

Streb, H., Irvine, R.F., Berridge, M.J. and Schultz, I. (1983) Release of Ca^{2+} from a nonmitochondrial intracellular store in pancreatic acinar cells by inositol-1,4,5-triphosphate. *Nature (Lond.)*, 306: 67–68.

Tanner, L.I., Harden, T.K., Wells, J.N. and Martin, M.W.

(1986) Identification of the phosphodiesterase regulated by muscarinic cholinergic receptors of 1321 N1 human astrocytoma cells. *Mol. Pharmacol.,* 29: 455–460.

Tota, M.R., Kahler, K. and Schimerlik, M.I. (1987) Reconstitution of the purified porcine atrial muscarinic receptor with purified porcine atrial inhibitory guanine nucleotide binding protein. *Biochemistry,* 26: 8175–8182.

Yamamura, H.I. and Snyder, S.H. (1974) Muscarinic cholinergic binding in rat brain. *Proc. Natl. Acad. Sci. USA,* 71: 1725–1729.

Yatani, A., Codina, J., Brown, A.M. and Birnbaumer, L. (1987) Direct activation of mammalian atrial muscarinic potassium channels by GTP regulatory protein G_K. *Science,* 235: 207–211.

Yatani, A., Hamm, H., Codina, J., Mazzoni, M.R., Birnbaumer, L. and Brown, A.M. (1988a) A monoclonal antibody to the α subunit of G_K blocks muscarinic activation of atrial K^+ channels. *Science,* 241: 828–831.

Yatani, A., Mattera, R., Codina, J., Graf, R., Okabe, K., Padrell, E., Iyengar, R., Brown, A.M. and Birnbaumer, L. (1988b) The G protein-gated atrial K^+ channel is stimulated by three distinct $G_{i\alpha}$-subunits. *Nature (Lond.),* 336: 680–682.

S.-M. Aquilonius and P.-G. Gillberg (Eds.)
Progress in Brain Research, Vol. 84
© 1990 Elsevier Science Publishers B.V. (Biomedical Division)

CHAPTER 3

Multiple pathways for signal transduction through the muscarinic cholinergic receptor

Joan Heller Brown, Ioanna Trilivas, JoAnn Trejo and Elizabeth Martinson

Department of Pharmacology M-036, University of California San Diego, La Jolla, CA 92093, U.S.A.

Introduction

There are a number of different molecular mechanisms by which signals from the muscarinic cholinergic receptor (mAChR) are transduced into cellular responses. There are also at least three pharmacologically distinct mAChR subtypes (Table I), which appear to correspond to the receptors encoded by the M_1, M_2 and M_3 genes * recently cloned in several laboratories (Kubo et al., 1986; Bonner et al., 1987; Peralta et al., 1987a,b). In the peripheral nervous system, M_1 receptors are primarily found in ganglia, where they decrease K^+ conductance and thereby generate a slow excitatory postsynaptic potential (North, 1986). The M_2 receptor is the predominant mAChR subtype found in mammalian cardiac muscle. This recep-

tor subtype appears to operate by coupling through a pertussis toxin-sensitive G-protein to the inhibition of adenylate cyclase or to the activation of K^+ channels, thereby decreasing cardiac rate and contractility (Nathanson, 1987). The receptors in gland and smooth muscle do not have the pharmacological characteristics of either M_1 or M_2 mAChR and can be tentatively classified together as M_3 mAChR receptors (Doods et al., 1987; Giraldo et al., 1988). Glandular secretion and smooth muscle contractile responses to acetylcholine appear to be mediated through M_3 receptors coupled to a signal transduction pathway involving the hydrolysis of inositol phospholipids, the mobilization of Ca^{2+}, the formation of diacylglycerol (DAG), and the activation of protein kinase C (PKC).

We have been interested in understanding the regulation and functions of the inositol phospholipid pathway because of its central role in

---

* The terminology used here is that of Bonner et al. (1987).

TABLE I

Localization and probable relationships of pharmacologically-defined muscarinic receptor subtypes to functional responses

Receptor subtype	Tissue	Signal transduction pathway	Response
M_1	Ganglia	Decrease K^+ conductance	Slow depolarization
M_2	Heart	Increase K^+ conductance; inhibit adenylate cyclase	Decrease rate; decrease contractility
M_3	Smooth muscle [a]	Increase phosphoinositide turnover and mobilize Ca^{2+}	Contraction
	Gland		Secretion

[a] Some smooth muscle receptors are of the pharmacologically defined M_2 subtype.

mediating parasympathetic responses. To this end we have studied a cultured cell line in which the mAChR appear to be of the M_3 subtype and to regulate phosphoinositide (PI) hydrolysis and calcium mobilization (Masters et al., 1984 1985; McDonough et al., 1988) without affecting adenylate cyclase activity (Meeker and Harden, 1982; Hepler et al., 1987). The studies described below demonstrate that phosphatidylcholine (PC) is also hydrolysed in response to mAChR stimulation and that this metabolic pathway contributes significantly to DAG formation. We also present data suggesting that protein kinase C activation by mAChR stimulation leads to induction of the proto-oncogene c-*fos*.

Experimental procedures

1321N1 astrocytoma cells were grown in 35-mm plates in Dulbecco's modified Eagle's medium supplemented with 5% fetal calf serum and 0.5% penicillin/streptomycin. Cultures were used at confluency (7 days of subculture, yielding roughly 10^6 cells/plate), except for studies of c-*fos* induction in which we used subconfluent (5-day) cells which were serum-starved for 24 h.

Phosphoinositide hydrolysis was studied by labeling cells with [^{3}H]inositol and separating inositol phosphates as described (Masters et al., 1985). Cytosolic [Ca^{2+}] was determined with fura-2 (McDonough et al., 1988). To study the release of PC metabolites from [^{3}H]choline-labeled 1321N1 cells, monolayers were labeled overnight with 1–10 μCi [^{3}H]choline. The medium was analysed for tritiated choline, phosphocholine, glycerophosphocholine and other water-soluble PC metabolites by extraction with tetraphenylboron/heptanone (Wetzel and Brown, 1983) or by TLC (Yavin, 1976), as described in Martinson et al. (1989). DAG mass was measured using diglyceride kinase following the procedure of Preiss et al. (1986). Phosphatidylethanol (PEth) formation from fatty acid-labeled lipids was measured by stimulating cells in the presence of 0.5% ethanol

and separating phospholipids as described (Liscovitch, 1989).

Protein kinase C redistribution was assessed by measuring [^{3}H]phorbol dibutyrate ([^{3}H]PDB) binding to intact cells as described by Trilivas and Brown (1989). For Western analysis, cell lysates were added to SDS-PAGE sample buffer containing 200 mM dithiothreitol as a reducing agent. After boiling for 5 min, samples were resolved by SDS-PAGE (Laemmli, 1970) and electrophoretically transferred to nitrocellulose membrane. Blots were incubated at room temperature with mouse monoclonal anti-PKC antibody (Amersham, 1:100 dilution in PBS), washed in PBS containing 0.1% Tween 20, and incubated with anti-mouse Ig-alkaline phosphatase conjugate (BioRad, 1:3000 dilution) for 1 h at room temperature.

For measurement of RNA by Northern blotting, cells were harvested in 4 M guanidine isothiocyanate and total RNA was isolated by centrifugation through cesium chloride (Chirgwin et al., 1979). RNA was separated by electrophoresis in 1% agarose gels containing 2.2 M formaldehyde and transferred to Hybond-N nylon membrane. The c-*fos*-specific RNA sequences were detected by hybridization with commercially available probes (Oncor Probes, Inc.) labeled by random priming (Pharmacia) with [α-^{32}P]dCTP. The RNA blots were hybridized by addition of $1-3 \times 10^6$ cpm/ml of labeled probe and incubated at 42°C overnight. Blots were washed with $0.1 \times SSC/0.1\%$ SDS over a temperature range of 42°C to 65°C.

Results and Discussion

Relationship between inositol phospholipid hydrolysis and Ca^{2+} mobilization

When 1321N1 cells are stimulated with the stable acetylcholine analogue carbachol there is a very rapid increase in inositol 1,4,5-trisphosphate (Ambler et al., 1987) and an immediate increase in cytosolic calcium (McDonough et al., 1988). The calcium is mobilized from an intracellular store which is easily depleted by treatment with agonist or with a low concentration (100 nM) of ionomycin (Martinson et al., 1989). Two types of experiment provide evidence that the mobilization of calcium results from the formation of InsP$_3$. First, a series of cholinergic agonists vary in their efficacies for stimulating phosphoinositide hydrolysis: acetylcholine and carbachol are full agonists, bethanechol and methacholine are partial agonists, and oxotremorine and pilocarpine do not stimulate PI hydrolysis. These agonists exhibit the same differences in relative efficacy for mobilizing calcium (Masters et al., 1984; Evans et al., 1985). The correlation between the magnitude of the PI response and the extent of calcium mobilization suggests that these are related responses. More direct evidence for a causal relationship between InsP$_3$ formation and Ca^{2+} mobilization comes from our experiments with phorbol esters. Acute treatment of 1321N1 cells with the phorbol ester PMA completely inhibits mAChR-mediated InsP$_3$ formation and concomitantly abolishes the rise in intracellular Ca^{2+} (Orellana et al., 1985; Orellana et al., 1987).

Protein kinase C redistribution and its regulation by intracellular Ca^{2+}

The other limb of the inositol phospholipid signal transduction pathway involves the activation of protein kinase C, presumed to be mediated by DAG. To determine whether protein kinase C was regulated in response to mAChR stimulation in 1321N1 cells, we examined changes in membrane-associated [^{3}H]phorbol dibutyrate ([^{3}H]-PDB) binding. These studies were carried out by measuring binding to intact cells rather than by preparing particulate and soluble fractions. Carbachol leads to a marked and rapid increase in the number of [^{3}H]PDB binding sites, reflecting an increase in the amount of PKC associated with the cell membrane (Trilivas and Brown, 1989). The increase in membrane-associated PKC is also transient, returning to near basal values within several minutes. When the effect of carbachol on cytosolic Ca^{2+} is prevented (by depleting the calcium pool or by buffering the calcium rise with quin-2) carbachol no longer increases membrane-

associated [^{3}H]PDB binding. These data demonstrate that the increase in calcium caused by mAChR activation in the intact cell is essential for PKC redistribution. In addition, the increase in [^{3}H]PDB binding precedes any measurable increase in the mass of DAG, normally considered to be the activator of PKC.

Diacylglycerol is formed slowly in response to carbachol

The increase in diacylglycerol that follows stimulation with carbachol has a time course different from that seen for InsP$_3$ formation, Ca^{2+} mobilization or PKC redistribution. Not only is there a lag of several minutes before DAG mass increases above the basal level, but DAG is elevated for at least 30 min in the continued presence of carbachol (Fig. 1). When [^{3}H]myristic acid is used to label the precursor phospholipids there is also a lag before one sees increases in radiolabeled DAG (Martinson et al., 1989). Thus, it appears that most of the DAG is generated through a process that is slower than phosphoinositide hydrolysis. Recent work from several laboratories suggests that phosphatidylcholine is also a substrate for hormonally regulated phospholipases (Besterman et al., 1986; Bocckino et

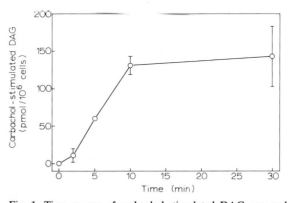

Fig. 1. Time course of carbachol-stimulated DAG accumulation in 1321N1 cells. The diacylglycerol concentration was determined using the mass assay as described in Experimental procedures. Data shown are for the carbachol-stimulated increase in DAG. A basal value of about 260 pmol/10^6 cells has been subtracted.

al., 1987; Pai et al., 1988; Löffelholz, 1989; Martin and Michaelis, 1989). Several growth factors and hormones as well as phorbol esters have been shown to stimulate PC hydrolysis and there is considerable interest in the role of this metabolic pathway in the generation of DAG.

Phosphatidylcholine hydrolysis occurs via phospholipases C and D

We examined the effect of mAChR stimulation on phosphatidylcholine metabolism in 1321N1 cells (Martinson et al., 1989). In these studies we labeled cell lipids overnight with [³H]choline, which was rapidly phosphorylated to phosphocholine and subsequently incorporated into phosphatidylcholine (and, to a small extent, sphingomyelin). There was no detectable formation of acetylcholine in these cells. We then mea-

sured the release of [³H]choline-containing metabolites into the cell medium. Carbachol increases both [³H]choline and [³H]phosphocholine release from labeled lipids (Fig. 2; see also Martinson et al., 1989). There is no increase in the release of these compounds from the cytoplasmic pool.

Phosphocholine is not converted to choline in either intact or permeabilized cells, indicating that the choline is formed independently of phosphocholine. Other evidence that [³H]choline and [³H]phosphocholine release occur through separate metabolic pathways is that they are differently affected by PKC down-regulation (see below) and they have different kinetics of release. Phosphocholine release is most marked during the first 2 min of stimulation with carbachol and increases little thereafter. In contrast, choline release increases more slowly and continues for at least 15 min of stimulation. We have focused our attention on the regulation of choline formation, since it occurs with a time course most like that for formation of DAG.

The concentration-response relationship for carbachol-stimulated [³H]choline formation is nearly identical to that for PKC redistribution (Fig. 3). The EC_{50} values for both of these responses are approximately 15 μM. Interestingly, we find an identical concentration-response relationship for DAG formation. The EC_{50} for inositol trisphosphate formation is approximately 6-times higher. These data do not prove casual relationships but do indicate a close correspondence between PKC redistribution, choline formation and DAG production. The relative efficacy of several agonists for stimulating choline release and DAG formation was also compared. Carbachol is a full agonist (comparable to oxotremorine-M) for stimulating PC hydrolysis and DAG formation, while oxotremorine and pilocarpine do not evoke either response.

Phosphocholine is the metabolite expected to result from the action of a PC-specific phospholipase C, while the release of choline suggests that there is hydrolysis of PC by a phospholipase D.

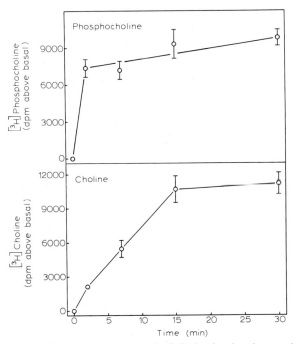

Fig. 2. Time course of carbachol-stimulated release of [³H]choline and [³H]phosphocholine in 1321N1 cells. Cells were labeled overnight with [³H]choline and the [³H]phosphocholine and [³H]choline in the cell medium were separated by extraction with tetraphenylboron/heptanone. The basal values for [³H]phosphocholine and [³H]choline have been subtracted.

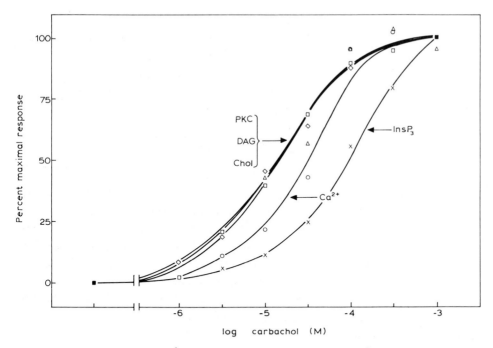

Fig. 3. Dose-response curves for [³H]choline release, PKC redistribution ([³H]PDB binding), DAG mass, cytosolic Ca^{2+} elevation (fura-2) and InsP₃ accumulation. The EC_{50} values were $\approx 15\ \mu M$ for choline, PKC and DAG, $\approx 30\ \mu M$ for Ca^{2+} and $\approx 90\ \mu M$ for InsP₃.

We used two approaches to determine whether carbachol activates a phospholipase D in 1321N1 cells. First we examined the formation of phosphatidic acid (PA), which is the other product of hydrolysis of PC by phospholipase D. When cells are labeled overnight with [³H]arachidonate and then challenged with carbachol there is rapid formation of radiolabeled PA. Radiolabeled DAG also increases, but more slowly than PA, suggesting that it is a product rather than the precursor of

TABLE II

Carbachol and PMA stimulate formation of [³H]phosphatidylethanol (PEth)

	[³H]PEth (cpm)
Control	$200\pm\ \ 180$
Carbachol	$1\,800\pm\ \ 550$
PMA	$5\,400\pm1\,500$

Cell lipids were labeled with [³H]myristate. Cells were then stimulated with 1 mM carbachol or 1 μM PMA for 30 min in the presence of 0.5% ethanol. The labeled PEth and PA were separated by TLC.

PA (Martinson et al., 1989). A second approach utilizes the ability of phospholipase D to catalyse a transphosphatidylation reaction involving PC. When phospholipase D is activated in the presence of ethanol, a novel phospholipid (phosphatidylethanol) is formed from PC. In 1321N1 cells carbachol causes a marked increase in the formation of this metabolite from [³H]myristate-labeled PC (Table II).

Protein kinase C involvement in phospholipase D activation

The phorbol ester PMA also has effects on PC metabolism. Unlike carbachol, it increases only [³H]choline (and not [³H]phosphocholine) release and therefore appears to stimulate PC hydrolysis exclusively via activation of phospholipase D. Like carbachol, PMA rapidly increases PA formation and this precedes the formation of DAG from labeled PC (Martinson et al., 1989). PMA also stimulates [³H]PEth formation, providing further evidence that a phospholipase D is activated (Ta-

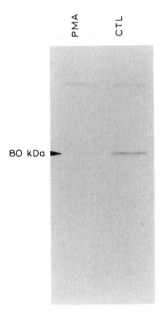

Fig. 4. Western blot analysis of PKC in control and PMA-down-regulated 1321N1 cells. Cells were cultured overnight in the presence of 1 μM PMA. Protein kinase C was detected using a commercially available monoclonal antibody and visualized by using an anti-mouse Ig-alkaline phosphatase conjugate.

ble II). The effects of PMA are presumably mediated through the activation of protein kinase C, and they suggest that activation of PKC may also mediate mAChR-stimulated hydrolysis of PC.

To test the involvement of protein kinase C in the action of carbachol we used long-term PMA treatment to down-regulate PKC. Following a 16-h treatment with 1 μM PMA, there is no detectable protein kinase C in the whole cell lysate (Fig. 4).

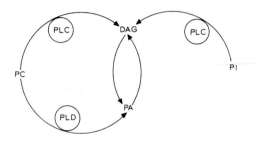

Fig. 5. Pathways for hormonally stimulated formation of diacylglycerol from phospholipids.

TABLE III

Effect of PKC down-regulation on carbachol-stimulated responses in 1321N1 cells

	Control	PKC-down-regulated
[³H]Choline	1.91	0.85
[³H]PEth	1.35	0.90
DAG	1.42	1.08

Data are expressed as fold stimulation.

Under these conditions, carbachol still stimulates the release of [³H]phosphocholine, but its effect on [³H]choline release is abolished (Table III; see also Martinson et al., 1989). The down-regulation of protein kinase C also blocks the increases in [³H]PEth formation in response to carbachol (Table III). These observations suggest that carbachol regulates phospholipase D through a mechanism requiring protein kinase C.

Contributions of PI and PC to DAG formation

Stimulation of the mAChR in 1321N1 cells could elevate DAG through at least three possible routes (Fig. 5). One is through the breakdown of PI and the polyphosphoinositides by a PI-specific phospholipase C. A second is through the hydrolysis of PC by a PC-specific phospholipase C. Both of these responses occur rapidly, however, while the time course of DAG accumulation shows a marked lag. Thus, phospholipase C activation may lead to a local increase in DAG that is adequate to initially activate protein kinase C but insufficient to be detected as an increase in mass at the whole-cell level.

A third route for DAG formation is through the action of phospholipase D followed by dephosphorylation of PA to DAG. There is growing evidence that a phospholipase D can hydrolyse PC (see Löffelholz et al., 1989), but PI is not generally considered a substrate for phospholipase D. If the PC-selective phospholipase D pathway shown in Fig. 5 contributes to carbachol-stimulated DAG formation, the loss of this pathway subsequent to PKC down-regulation should decrease DAG formation. Indeed, we find that the increase in DAG

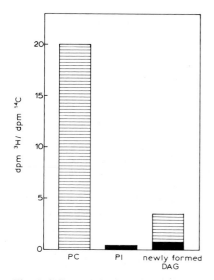

Fig. 6. Cells were double-labeled overnight with [³H]myristate and [¹⁴C]arachidonate. The ratios of ³H/¹⁴C in PC and PI were 20 and 0.4. The ratio in the *newly formed* DAG column was calculated by subtracting the ³H and ¹⁴C in DAG from unstimulated cells from that found after stimulation with carbachol.

seen 5 min after the addition of carbachol is markedly attenuated in PKC-down-regulated cells (Table III).

Another approach to examining the contributions of PI and PC to DAG formation utilizes differential fatty acid labeling of the precursor phospholipids. Cells are grown overnight in the presence of [³H]myristic acid and [¹⁴C]arachidonic acid, which incorporate selectively into PI and PC (Fig. 6). DAG that is formed in response to carbachol would be expected to have a fatty acid ratio resembling that of its lipid precursor. The ratio of [³H]myristate/[¹⁴C]arachidonate in DAG formed during 7 min of carbachol treatment is 3.5. This is not what one would expect if PC (ratio = 20) was the sole source of DAG, nor is it what one would see if PI (ratio = 0.4) was the exclusive source of DAG. A more quantitative assessment of the contributions of PC and PI to the newly formed DAG requires knowledge of the relative specific activities of the two phospholipids. Using this information, and assuming that PC and PI are the sole sources of the DAG formed in response to

carbachol, we calculate that approximately 80% of the DAG formed at 7 min is from PC and 20% arises from PI (Martinson et al., 1989). Thus, this approach confirms that most of the mass of DAG formed following mAChR stimulation is derived from PC rather than from PI.

Involvement of protein kinase C in mAChR-stimulated growth responses

A wide variety of agents, including mitogens and several neurotransmitters, induce the expression of the proto-oncogene c-*fos* in mammalian cells. The expression of c-*fos* has been hypothesized to be important for the transition of cells from quiescence to renewed cell growth. Blackshear and his colleagues reported that carbachol, like phorbol esters and EGF, induces c-*fos* in 1321N1 cells (Blackshear et al., 1987). Surprisingly, their data suggested that this was not a consequence of the increased Ca²⁺ and protein kinase C activation elicited by mAChR stimulation.

We re-examined the ability of mAChR stimulation to induce c-*fos* in 1321N1 cells. Carbachol causes more than a 15-fold increase in c-*fos* mRNA in these cells (Table IV). Serum and ionomycin have effects comparable to those of carbachol, whereas PMA appears to be less effective at inducing c-*fos*. When PKC is down-regulated by overnight treatment of the cells with 1 μM PMA,

TABLE IV

Effects of carbachol, PMA, serum and ionomycin on c-*fos* mRNA levels

	Normal	PKC down-regulated
Control	1	1
Carbachol (1 mM)	17	1
PMA (1 μM)	6	1
Serum (5%)	16	ND
Ionomycin (1 μM)	22	ND

Levels of c-*fos* mRNA were determined by Northern analysis and quantitated by radio-analytic scanning. Values are expressed as fold increase relative to control. To down-regulate PKC cells were treated with 1 μM PMA for 16 h.
ND = not determined.

the subsequent induction of c-*fos* by carbachol is blocked. This suggests that carbachol induces c-*fos* via activation of protein kinase C.

Conclusions

The 1321N1 astrocytoma cell has muscarinic receptors which stimulate the cascade of responses typically associated with the actions of Ca^{2+}-mobilizing hormones. The active isomer of $InsP_3$ is formed, Ca^{2+} is released from intracellular stores, diacylglycerol is elevated, and protein kinase C is redistributed to the membrane. In the studies described here we present evidence that two additional cellular responses are activated, apparently as a consequence of the activation of protein kinase C. First, mAChR stimulation increases the hydrolysis of phosphatidylcholine by a phospholipase D, resulting in the formation of choline and phosphatidic acid. The choline formed from PC could be important in ACh synthesis under certain conditions, as discussed by Löffelholz (1989). There is also considerable evidence for a second messenger role for phosphatidic acid, possibly acting as a mitogen (Moolenaar et al., 1986), and as a Ca^{2+} ionophore (Putney et al., 1980). In addition, the PA formed by this route is converted to DAG; indeed our studies suggest that this is the main source of DAG in mAChR-stimulated 1321N1 cells. The second consequence of PKC activation that we have described is an increase in c-*fos* mRNA. How c-*fos* is induced has not been fully elucidated, but it is clear that there is a PKC-responsive promoter region in the c-*fos* gene (Fisch et al., 1987). The interaction of c-*fos* with jun/AP-1 leads to transcription of several specific genes (Chiu et al., 1988; Schonthal et al., 1988). We are currently examining the possibility that the increase in c-*fos* serves as a "third messenger" for the induction of other gene products, particularly growth factors which may be secreted from astrocytes when they are stimulated. It will also be of interest to determine whether the activation of mAChR induces c-*fos* in neuronal cells, whether this is a signal for transcription of specific proteins, and whether this response occurs only in cells containing mAChR subtypes that couple to phospholipid metabolism.

References

Ambler, S.K., Solski, P.A., Brown, J.H. and Taylor, P. (1987) Receptor-mediated inositol phosphate formation in relation to calcium mobilization: A comparison of two cell lines. *Mol. Pharmacol.*, 32: 376–383.

Besterman, J.M., Duronio, V. and Cuatrecasas, P. (1986) Rapid formation of diacylglycerol from phosphatidylcholine: a pathway for generation of a second messenger. *Proc. Natl. Acad. Sci. USA*, 83: 6785–6789.

Blackshear, P.J., Stumpo, D.J., Huang, J.-K., Nemenoff, R.A. and Spach, D.H. (1987) Protein kinase C-dependent and -independent pathways of proto-oncogene induction in human astrocytoma cells. *J. Biol. Chem.*, 262: 7774–7781.

Bocckino, S.B., Blackmore, P.F., Wilson, P.B. and Exton, J.H. (1987) Phosphatidate accumulation in hormone-treated hepatocytes via a phospholipase D mechanism. *J. Biol. Chem.*, 262: 15309–15315.

Bonner, T.I., Buckley, N.J., Young, A.C. and Brann, M.R. (1987) Identification of a family of muscarinic acetylcholine receptor genes. *Science*, 237: 527–532.

Chirgwin, J.M., Przybyla, A.E., MacDonald, R.J. and Rutter, W.J. (1979) Isolation of biologically active ribonucleic acid from sources enriched in ribonuclease. *Biochemistry*, 18: 5294–5299.

Chiu, R., Boyle, W.J., Meek, J., Smeal, T., Hunter, T. and Karin, M. (1988) The c-fos protein interacts with c-Jun/AP-1 to stimulate transcription of AP-1 responsive genes. *Cell*, 54: 541–552.

Doods, H.N., Mathy, M.-J., Davidesko, D., van Charldorp, K.J., de Jonge, A. and van Zweiten, P.A. (1987) Selectivity of muscarinic antagonists in radioligand and in vivo experiments for the putative M1, M2 and M3 receptors. *J. Pharmacol. Exp. Ther.*, 242: 257–262.

Evans, T., Hepler, J.R., Masters, S.B., Brown, J.H. and Harden, T.K. (1985) Guanine nucleotide regulation of agonist binding to muscarinic cholinergic receptors: Regulation to efficacy of agonists for stimulation of phosphoinositide breakdown and Ca^{2+} mobilization. *Biochem. J.*, 232: 751–757.

Fisch, T.M., Prywes, R. and Roeder, R.G. (1987) c-fos sequences necessary for basal expression and induction by epidermal growth factor, 12-O-tetradecanoyl phorbol-13-acetate, and the calcium ionophore. *Mol. Cell. Biol.*, 7: 3490–3502.

Giraldo, E., Vigano, M.A., Hammer, R. and Ladinsky, H. (1988) Characterization of muscarinic receptors in guinea pig ileum longitudinal smooth muscle. *Mol. Pharmacol.*, 33: 617–625.

Hepler, J.R., Hughes, A.R. and Harden, T.K. (1987) Evidence that muscarinic cholinergic receptors selectively interact with either cyclic AMP or the inositol phosphate second messenger response systems. *Biochem. J.,* 247: 793–796.

Kubo, T., Fukuda, K., Mikami, A., Maeda, A., Takahashi, H., Mishina, M., Haga, T., Haga, K., Ichiyama, A., Kangawa, K., Kojima, M., Matsuo, H., Hirose, T. and Numa, S. (1986) Cloning, sequence and expression of complementary DNA encoding the muscarinic acetylcholine receptor. *Nature,* 323: 411–416.

Laemmli, U.K. (1970) Cleavage of structural proteins during the assembly of the head of bacteriophage T4. *Nature,* 227: 680–685.

Liscovitch, M. (1989) Phosphatidylethanol biosynthesis in ethanol-exposed NG108-15 neuroblastoma X glioma hybrid cells. Evidence for activation of a phospholipase D phosphatidyltransferase activity by protein kinase C. *J. Biol. Chem.,* 264: 1450–1456.

Löffelholz, K. (1989) Receptor regulation of choline phospholipid hydrolysis. A novel source of diacylglycerol and phosphatidic acid. *Biochem. Pharmacol.,* 38: 1543–1549.

Martin, T.W. and Michaelis, K. (1989) P2-purinergic agonists stimulate phosphodiesteratic cleavage of phosphatidylcholine in endothelial cells. Evidence for activation of phospholipase D. *J. Biol. Chem.,* 264: 8847–8856.

Martinson, E.A., Goldstein, D. and Brown, J.H. (1989) Muscarinic receptor activation of phosphatidylcholine hydrolysis. Relationship to phosphoinositide hydrolysis and diacylglycerol metabolism. *J. Biol. Chem.,* 264: 14748–14754.

Masters, S.B., Harden, T.K. and Brown, J.H. (1984) Relationships between phosphoinositide and calcium responses to muscarinic agonists in astrocytoma cells. *Mol. Pharmacol.,* 26: 149–155.

Masters, S.B., Quinn, M.T. and Brown, J.H. (1985) Agonist-induced desensitization of muscarinic receptor-mediated calcium efflux without concomitant desensitization of phosphoinositide hydrolysis. *Mol. Pharmacol.,* 27: 325–332.

McDonough, P.M., Eubanks, J.H. and Brown, J.H. (1988) Desensitization and recovery of muscarinic and histaminergic calcium mobilization: Evidence for a common hormone sensitive calcium store in 1321N1 astrocytoma cells. *Biochem. J.,* 249: 135–141.

Meeker, R.B. and Harden, T.K. (1982) Muscarinic cholinergic receptor-mediated control of cyclic AMP metabolism: Agonist-induced changes in nucleotide synthesis and degradation. *Mol. Pharmacol.,* 23: 384–392.

Moolenaar, W.H., Kruijer, W., Tilly, B.C., Verlaan, I., Bierman, A.J. and de Laat, S.W. (1986) Growth factor-like action of phosphatidic acid. *Nature,* 323: 171–173.

Nathanson, N.M. (1987) Molecular properties of the muscarinic acetylcholine receptor. *Annu. Rev. Neurosci.,* 10: 195–236.

North, R.A. (1986) Muscarinic receptors and membrane ion conductances. *Trends Pharmacol. Sci.,* Suppl: 19–22.

Orellana, S., Solski, P.A. and Brown, J.H. (1987) Guanosine 5′-O-(thiotriphosphate)-dependent inositol trisphosphate formation in membranes is inhibited by phorbol ester and protein kinase C. *J. Biol. Chem.,* 262: 1638–1643.

Orellana, S.A., Solski, P.A. and Brown, J.H. (1985) Phorbol ester inhibits phosphoinositide hydrolysis and calcium mobilization in cultured astrocytoma cells. *J. Biol. Chem.,* 260: 5236–5239.

Pai, J.-K., Siegel, M.I., Egan, R.W. and Billah, M.M. (1988) Phospholipase D catalyzes phospholipid metabolism in chemotactic peptide-stimulated HL-60 granulocytes. *J. Biol. Chem.,* 263: 12472–12477.

Peralta, E.G., Ashkenazi, A., Winslow, J.W., Smith, D.H., Ramachandran, J. and Capon, D.J. (1987a) Distinct primary structures, ligand-binding properties and tissue-specific expression of four human muscarinic acetylcholine receptors. *EMBO J.,* 6: 3923–3929.

Peralta, E.G., Winslow, J.W., Peterson, G.L., Smith, D.H., Ashkenazi, A., Ramachandran, J., Schimerlik, M.I. and Capon, D.J. (1987b) Primary structure and biochemical properties of an M2 muscarinic receptor. *Science,* 236: 600–605.

Preiss, J., Loomis, C.R., Bishop, W.R., Stein, R., Niedel, J.E. and Bell, R.M. (1986) Quantitative measurement of sn-1, 2-diacylglycerols present in platelets, hepatocytes, and ras- and sis- transformed normal rat kidney cells. *J. Biol. Chem.,* 261: 8597–8600.

Putney, J.W., Weiss, S.J., Van De Walle, C.M. and Haddas, R.A. (1980) Is phosphatidic acid a calcium ionophore under neurohumoral control?. *Nature,* 284: 345–347.

Schonthal, A., Herrlich, P., Rahmsdorf, H.J. and Ponta, H. (1988) Requirement for fos gene expression in the transcriptional activation of collagenase by other oncogenes and phorbol esters. *Cell,* 54: 325–334.

Trilivas, I. and Brown, J.H. (1989) Increases in intracellular Ca^{2+} regulate the binding of [^{3}H]phorbol 12,13-dibutyrate to intact 1321N1 astrocytoma cells. *J. Biol. Chem.,* 264: 3102–3107.

Wetzel, G.T. and Brown, J.H. (1983) Relationships between choline uptake, acetylcholine synthesis and acetylcholine release in isolated rat atria. *J. Pharmacol. Exp. Ther.,* 226: 343–348.

Yavin, E. (1976) Regulation of phospholipid metabolism in differentiating cells from rat brain cerebral hemispheres in culture: Patterns of acetylcholine, phosphocholine and choline phosphoglycerides labelling from [*methyl*-^{14}C]choline. *J. Biol. Chem.,* 251: 1392–1397.

S.-M. Aquilonius and P.-G. Gillberg (Eds.)
Progress in Brain Research, Vol. 84
© 1990 Elsevier Science Publishers B.V. (Biomedical Division)

CHAPTER 4

Second-messenger responses associated with stimulation of neuronal muscarinic receptors expressed by a human neuroblastoma SH-SY5Y

David G. Lambert and Stefan. R. Nahorski

Department of Pharmacology and Therapeutics (MSB), University of Leicester, University Road, Leicester, LE1 9HN, U.K.

Introduction

Stimulation of neuronal muscarinic receptors leads to a multiplicity of intracellular events, including stimulation of phosphoinositide hydrolysis (Fisher, 1985; Nahorski et al., 1986), release of intracellular stored Ca^{2+} (Nahorski, 1988), modulation of Ca^{2+} channel activity (Meldolesi and Pozzan, 1987), inhibition of cAMP production (Harden et al., 1985) and modulation of K^+ channel activity (Christie and North, 1987). In the main these cellular events should not be considered as isolated responses but as a complex interacting network of signals modulating neuronal function. This chapter will be largely concerned with muscarinic receptor stimulation of phosphoinositide hydroly-

sis, release of intracellular stored Ca^{2+} and modulation of Ca^{2+} channel activity.

Differential linkage of muscarinic receptor subtypes to phosphoinositide hydrolysis and cAMP turnover

It has been known for many years that muscarinic receptors are not homogeneous and, with the development of antagonists which display various degrees of selectivity between subtypes, muscarinic receptors have been classified as m1, m2 cardiac, m2 gland (which is also termed m3). These classifications have been made largely with three selective antagonists, pirenzepine, AF-DX 116 and 4-DAMP. Pirenzepine binds with high affinity to

TABLE I

Pharmacological and functional classification of muscarinic m1–m5 receptor subtypes

Subtype [a]	Common name	Central location	PZP	Affinity for		Linkage to	
				AFDX-116	4-DAMP	PI	Cyclase
m1	M_1	CX/HP	H	L	L	S	O/S
m2	M_2 (heart)	CER/TH	L	H	L	O	I
m3	M_3 (gland)	CX/HP	L	L	H	S	O/S
m4	–	CX/HP	L [b]	H [b]	–	O	I
m5	–	–	L [b]	L	–	S	O/S

[a] Nomenclature used by Bonner et al. (1987, 1988).
[b] Low slope.
CX = cortex, HP = hippocampus, CER = cerebellum, TH = thalamus, H = high affinity, L = low affinity, S = stimulates, I = inhibits, O = no effect (for references see text).

the m1 subtype, whilst AF-DX 116 and 4-DAMP display high affinity for the m2 and m3 subtypes respectively. Recently molecular biology has added a further two subtypes. Although these cannot currently be distinguished pharmacologically using the available selective antagonists, their affinity for pirenzepine and AF-DX 116 are shown along with that for the m1–m3 subtypes in Table I. Early work with cultured 1321N1 astrocytoma and NG108-15 neuroblastoma × glioma hybrids showed differential linkage to phosphoinositide hydrolysis and adenylate cyclase inhibition (Harden et al., 1985). It is now clear from the work of many groups (Peralta et al., 1988; Fukuda et al., 1988; Bonner et al., 1987, 1988) that the preferred linkage of m1, m3 and m5 subtypes is to stimulate phosphoinositide turnover, whilst that of the m2 and m4 subtypes is to inhibit adenylate cyclase (Table I). It should be noted that the word "preferred" is used here and that certainly in the case of the m3 subtype a modest stimulation of cAMP production can be observed, although it is not known whether this is a primary or secondary response (Baumgold and Fishman, 1988). To date there are no reports of preferential linkage of muscarinic receptor subtypes to increased $[Ca^{2+}]_i$.

Muscarinic receptor-mediated phosphoinositide hydrolysis and increased $[Ca^{2+}]_i$

When a muscarinic agonist occupies either m1, m3 or m5 receptor subtypes, there is an increased turnover of inositol lipids in the plasma membrane and the consequent liberation of water-soluble inositol phosphates into the cytosol (Brown et al., 1984; Lazareno et al., 1985; Barnard, 1988). The initial reaction in this series of events is the muscarinic receptor–G-protein-linked stimulation of phospholipase C. The substrate for phospholipase C is a specific membrane lipid, phosphatidylinositol 4,5-bisphosphate, which is hydrolysed to yield two biologically active messengers, diacylglycerol and $Ins(1,4,5)P_3$ (Berridge, 1987). Diacylglycerol activates protein kinase C, which then goes on to phosphorylate a variety of cellular

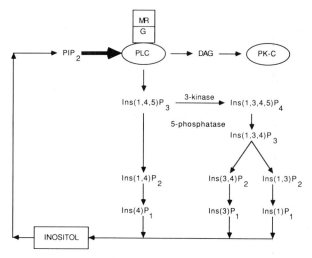

Fig. 1. Synthesis and metabolism of $Ins(1,4,5)P_3$. Abbreviations: PIP_2, phosphatidlyinositol 4,5-bisphosphate; MR, muscarinic receptor; G, G-protein; PLC, phospholipase C; PKC, protein kinase C; DAG, diacylglycerol. Phosphate positions on the inositol ring are indicated in brackets (modified from Nahorski, 1988).

regulatory proteins. There is now little doubt that $Ins(1,4,5)P_3$ releases Ca^{2+} from nonmitochondrial intracellular stores identified as the endoplasmic reticulum or more specialized calciosome (Streb et al., 1983; Volpe et al., 1988). $Ins(1,4,5)P_3$ is metabolized in the cell by two different routes (Fig. 1), involving either phosphorylation through 3-kinase activity to $Ins(1,3,4,5)P_4$ or dephosphorylation via 5-phosphatase to $Ins(1,4)P_2$. $Ins(1,3,4,5)P_4$ is produced rapidly and has been shown to have some biological activity, namely the possible opening of Ca^{2+} channels (see Nahorski, 1988). $Ins(1,3,4,5)P_4$ is dephosphorylated to $Ins(1,3,4)P_3$ via 5-phosphatase and then to $Ins(1,3)P_2$ and $Ins(3,4)P_2$. The bisphosphates generated by either route are then further dephosphorylated to monophosphates and inositol, which is then reincorporated into membrane phospholipids.

Agonists could increase $[Ca^{2+}]_i$ by a number of mechanisms. These include release of Ca^{2+} from an internal store, opening of membrane Ca^{2+} channels, inhibition of Ca^{2+}-ATP-ase activity and inhibition of Na/Ca^{2+} antiporter (Fig. 2) (Blaustein, 1988) and our understanding of these mechanisms has been greatly assisted by the use of fluorescent indicator dyes such as fura 2 (Cobbold and Rink, 1987). The most extensively characterized of these routes with muscarinic receptors is the release of internal stored Ca^{2+} and Ca^{2+} channel opening. Increased generation of Ins $(1,4,5)P_3$ (which is associated with muscarinic m1, m3 and m5 receptor occupation) causes a rapid transient release of intracellular bound Ca^{2+} into the cytoplasm. This method of increasing $[Ca^{2+}]_i$ has been reported in 1321N1 astrocytoma cells (McDonough et al., 1988), pancreatic acinar cells (Pandol et al., 1987; Muallem et al., 1988), parietal cells (Negulescu and Machin, 1988), PC12 cells (Gatti et al., 1988) and parotid acinar cells (Merritt and Rink, 1987; Merritt and Hallam, 1988; Takemura and Putney, 1989). The involvement of extracellular Ca^{2+} is clearly observed in 1321N1 astrocytoma cells (McDonough et al., 1988), parotid (Merritt and Rink, 1987; Merritt and Hallam, 1988) and parietal (Negulescu and Machin, 1988) cells, which show a biphasic $[Ca^{2+}]_i$ profile in approx. 1 mM external Ca^{2+} which is converted to a simple monophasic response in Ca^{2+}-free conditions. As shown by Hallam and Rink (1985), entry of Ca^{2+} across the plasma membrane can be monitored using the divalent cation

Mn^{2+}, which quenches fura 2 fluorescence at all excitation wavelengths. Since there are no internal stores of Mn^{2+}, muscarinic agonist-stimulated quenching is indicative of agonist-stimulated Ca^{2+} entry or Ca^{2+} channel opening. In at least two cell types, namely the parotid (Gray, 1988) and insulinoma cells (Prentki et al., 1988), muscarinic stimulation leads to oscillations in $[Ca^{2+}]_i$ with periods of 5 min for the former and 12–25 min for the latter. Various mechanisms for this oscillatory behaviour have been proposed (Berridge and Gallione, 1988). It is worth noting at this point a curious report (Schlegel et al., 1985) in which carbachol reduced $[Ca^{2+}]_i$. In this study pituitary GH_3 cells reduced their resting $[Ca^{2+}]_i$ from 110 nM to 63 nM in the presence of 10 μM carbachol: this reduction was blocked by atropine. The authors suggest that the underlying mechanism involved may be related to cAMP generation in these cells and indicates the possibility of crosstalk between cAMP generation and Ca^{2+} homeostasis.

Muscarinic receptors and second messengers in cultured neuronal cells

In view of the extraordinary complexity of interpreting neurochemical data in conventional brain slice preparations and the tedious preparation of primary cultured neurons (Gallo et al., 1982; McCarthy and deVellis 1980) many groups have moved to the use of clonal neuroblastoma cell lines. These cell lines serve as model homogeneous populations of cells expressing many of the properties of neuronal cells. N1E-115 mouse neuroblastoma cells express a relatively low density of muscarinic (probably m1) receptors linked to phosphoinositide metabolism (Fisher and Snider, 1987), whilst the other commonly used cell line, NG108-15 neuroblastoma × glioma hybrids, expresses muscarinic receptors that inhibit adenylate cyclase but do not stimulate phosphoinositide metabolism (Harden et al., 1985). Recently three human neuroblastoma cells expressing muscarinic binding sites have been described. IMR32 cells possess a high density of (probably m2) muscarinic

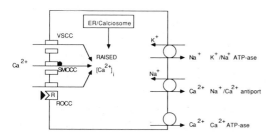

Fig. 2. Mechanisms by which a stimulus can increase $[Ca^{2+}]_i$. $[Ca^{2+}]_i$ can be raised by release of Ca^{2+} from the endoplasmic reticulum (ER) or calciosome or via Ca^{2+} entry through voltage-sensitive (VSCC), second-messenger-operated (SMOCC), or receptor-operated (ROCC) Ca^{2+} channels. Inhibition of the Ca^{2+}-ATPase will tend to increase $[Ca^{2+}]_i$, as will inhibition of the Na^+/Ca^{2+} antiporter. The Na^+/Ca^{2+} antiporter may be inhibited directly or indirectly via inhibition of the Na^+/K^{K+}-ATPase (this increases the $[Na^+]_i$ and inactivates the Na^+/Ca^{2+} antiporter).

receptors (Clementi et al., 1986) and NB-OK1 neuroblastoma cells express a high proportion of m1 receptors (Waelbroeck et al., 1988). It is not known at present whether either of these cell populations possess receptor linkage to phosphoinositide/cAMP/Ca^{2+} metabolism.

The SK-N-SH human neuroblastoma was derived from the bone marrow metastases of a 4-year-old girl (Biedler et al., 1973). These cells have been shown to have muscarinic receptors linked to phosphoinositide hydrolysis, increased $[Ca^{2+}]_i$ and increased cAMP (see below). The receptor subtype expressed by this neuroblastoma has been extensively characterized by Fisher and colleagues (Fisher and Snider, 1987; Fisher and Heacock, 1988; Fisher, 1988) as m3, displaying low affinity for pirenzepine and AF-DX 116 and high affinity for 4-DAMP. Fisher and Heacock (1988) and Fisher and Snider (1987) have also shown that the carbachol-stimulated [^{3}H]InsP$_1$ production is inhibited by these selective antagonists with the same affinities, indicating a functional correlation with the direct binding studies. We have recently reported low-affinity pirenzepine binding to whole cell and membrane preparations of SK-N-SH cells (Lambert et al., 1989) and a time-dependent increase in the production of [^{3}H]InsP$_1$, -InsP$_2$ and -InsP$_3$ (Baird et al., 1989). This increase in the individual inositol phosphates has also recently been reported by Baumgold and White (1989) and Fisher et al. (1989).

Muscarinic receptor occupation in these cells with oxotremorine-M increases $[Ca^{2+}]_i$ some 4-fold from a resting value of 59 nM to 293 nM at 1 mM oxotremorine-M. Half-maximum stimulation occurred at some 8 μM. The $[Ca^{2+}]_i$ response was biphasic and could be converted to a simple monophasic profile by the addition of EGTA. The time course of the initial spike phase was mirrored by an increase in [^{3}H]InsP$_3$ (Fisher et al., 1989). We have also shown that carbachol induces a biphasic increase in $[Ca^{2+}]_i$, rising from 109 nM to 640 nM in response to 1 mM carbachol. Half-maximum stimulation occurred at 11 μM carbachol (Baird et al., 1989).

As noted earlier, muscarinic m3 receptors have a preferred functional linkage to the stimulation of phosphoinositide hydrolysis. However, this receptor subtype (based on the classification by Fisher and Heacock, 1988) has been shown to be linked to a weak stimulation of cAMP production (Baumgold and Fishman, 1988). Oxotremorine and carbachol produced a 1.5–4-fold increase in cAMP production. This increase was pertussis toxin-insensitive and did not involve a G_i-like G-protein: the mechanism for this stimulation (direct or indirect) is unknown.

Although many important studies have been undertaken with these cells they have one major drawback. The SK-N-SH cell line contains at least two morphologically distinct cell types, only one of which is neuroblast-like. Ross and Biedler (1985) have selected cloned neuronal and non-neuronal cell lines from SK-N-SH cells that are phenotypically relatively stable. The subclones include the non-neuronal SH-EP1 and SH-SY5Y neuroblast-like cell (Fig. 3). Although the latter may resemble sympathetic ganglion cells their membranes possess GTP-binding protein alpha subunits in proportions similar to those found in human frontal cortex and suggest that they provide a more suitable model of central neurons than the other more commonly used cell lines (Klinz et al., 1987). In the differentiated state these cells release

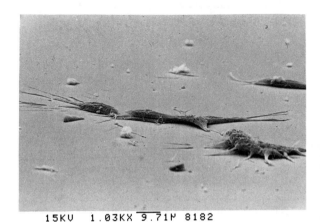

15KU   1.03KX 9.71P 8182

Fig. 3. Scanning electron micrograph of 2-day-old culture of undifferentiated SH-SY5Y human neuroblastoma cells.

noradrenaline in response to acetylcholine (Scott et al., 1986). The remainder of this chapter will be devoted to a description of the second messenger responses associated with muscarinic stimulation of SH-SY5Y cells and where there is discussion of the SH-SY5Y cells used in our laboratory, this will be limited to undifferentiated cells.

Receptor classification of SH-SY5Y cells

There is much controversy at present as to the nature of the muscarinic receptor subtype expressed by SH-SY5Y cells. Adem et al. (1987) reported a mixed m1 (34%) and m2 (66%) receptor expression by SH-SY5Y cells (although the m2 subtype was classified pharmacologically based only upon pirenzepine displacing with low affinity and could equally well be the m3 subtype). On the other hand, Serra et al. (1988) reported homogeneous m1 receptor expression by this neuroblastoma. We have recently learnt of two other variations, firstly where the SH-SY5Y cell expresses 70% m1 and 30% m2 receptors (A. Michel, Syntex, Palo Alto, CA, USA, personal communication) and the second in which the neuroblastoma expresses homogeneous m3 receptors (S.K Fisher, University of Michigan, Ann Arbor, MI, USA, personal communication). This homogeneous m3 receptor expression agrees with previous work for the parent SK-N-SH (Fisher and Heacock 1988) and is in agreement with our own findings for the SH-SY5Y clone where pirenzepine, AF-DX 116 and 4-DAMP displayed K_i values of 2.45×10^{-7}, 1.51×10^{-6} and 2.08×10^{-9} M, respectively, all with slope factors of unity (Lambert et al., 1989). Why there should be such variation in receptor expression is open to conjecture. It could be related to different sources of cells (our stock was from Dr. J. Biedler, Sloane Kettering Institute, NY, USA) or to different culture conditions. This latter postulate suggests that the environment may induce differential gene expression and clearly this idea needs further study. One point is clear: when using SH-SY5Y cells, receptor expression should be determined empirically.

Muscarinic stimulation of phosphoinositide metabolism in SH-SY5Y cells

Muscarinic receptors associated with the SH-SY5Y cell are coupled to phosphoinositide hydrolysis. Serra et al. (1988) show that carbachol causes a 50-fold increase in inositol phosphate formation in the presence of 10 mM Li^+ (Li^+ is used to inhibit the dephosphorylation of inositol monophosphates and hence acts as a means of amplification). In this study carbachol-stimulated inositol phosphate formation was inhibited dose-dependently by pirenzepine with a K_i of 11 nM. This value is consistent with the pharmacological classification of the m1 receptor and agrees with the direct binding studies also reported in this paper (Serra et al., 1988). The stimulation of phosphoinositide metabolism shown by Serra et al. (1988) is also reported to be pertussis toxin-sensitive (involving a pertissus toxin-sensitive G_i-like protein); however, in this study a significant effect was only observed with high concentrations (1 and 10 μg/ml) of pertussis toxin (Mei et al., 1988). We have also reported that carbachol increases the production of total [^{3}H] inositol phosphates (in the presence of 5 mM Li^+) dose-dependently with an EC_{50} of 7.5 μM. Maximum stimulation occurred in response to 1 mM carbachol (Fig. 4). Carbachol also increases the production of individual [^{3}H]inositol phosphates (absence of Li^+), $InsP_3$ peaking first, followed by $InsP_2$ and $InsP_4$ and then $InsP_1$, consistent with the schema shown in Fig. 1. The increase in $InsP_3$ is clearly biphasic, (Fig. 5) when measured either by the production of [^{3}H]$InsP_3$ or by mass D-Ins(1,4,5)P_3 measurements using a radioreceptor assay (Challiss et al., 1988). $InsP_3$ peaks at 5–10 s then declines to a new steady state above basal within approx. 1 min. HPLC analysis of [^{3}H]$InsP_3$ produced at 5 s confirms a substantial increase in Ins (1,4,5)P_3 production (Fig. 6). The basal mass level of Ins(1,4,5)P_3 in SH-SY5Y cells is relatively high (15 pmol/mg protein, rising to 154 pmol/mg protein at 10 s in response to 1 mM carbachol) but resembles that recently reported in brain slices

(Challiss et al., 1988), bovine tracheal smooth muscle (Chilvers et al. 1989) and NG108 and NIH3T3 cells (Fu et al., 1988). These data indicate that if homogeneously distributed in the cell, resting concentrations in excess of 1 μM could occur. These data taken together with the observation that Ins(1,4,5)P_3 releases stored Ca^{2+} (assayed as $^{45}Ca^{2+}$ release) in permeabilized SH-SY5Y cells (Safrany and Nahorski, unpublished data) at submicromolar concentrations suggest that Ins(1,4,5)P_3 must be compartmentalized in resting cells.

The involvement of a G-protein (G_p) in the coupling of the muscarinic receptor to phospholi-

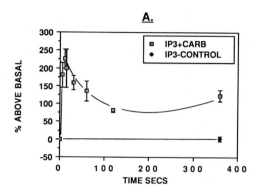

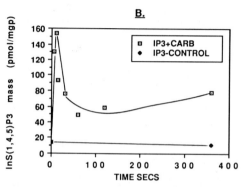

Fig. 5. Time course for the production of [^{3}H]InsP$_3$ (A) and Ins(1,4,5)P$_3$ mass (B) in response to 1 mM carbachol. For [^{3}H]InsP$_3$ cells were preincubated for 48 h with 4 μCi/ml [^{3}H]inositol. Reaction was terminated with trichloroacetic acid (1 M) and the inositol phosphates were extracted with freon/octylamine. [^{3}H]InsP$_3$ was separated by conventional anion-exchange chromatography (for method see Baird et al., 1989). For Ins(1,4,5)P$_3$ mass determinations the reaction was terminated and inositol phosphates were extracted as above. Ins(1,4,5)P$_3$ mass was quantitated using a radioreceptor assay (for method see Challiss et al., 1988).

pase C in these cells has been shown recently (Wojcikiewicz and Nahorski, 1989a,b, and unpublished data) where GTPγS, a stable analogue of GTP, was shown to increase the production of [^{3}H]inositol phosphates in electroporated SH-SY5Y cells. GTPγS also enhances the response to both full and partial agonists (carbachol and arecoline).

Muscarinic receptors linked to increased [Ca^{2+}]$_i$ in SH-SY5Y cells

Heikkila et al. (1987) have shown that SH-SY5Y cells loaded with quin2 exhibit a biphasic increase

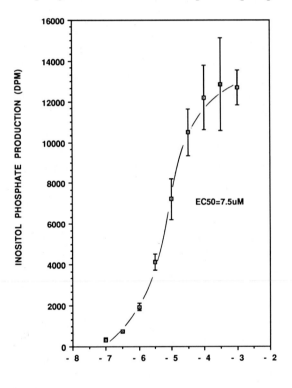

Fig. 4. Carbachol dose-related increase in inositol phosphate production in SH-SY5Y cells. Freshly harvested SH-SY5Y cells were preincubated in Krebs bicarbonate (pH 7.4) buffer supplemented with 5μCi/ml [^{3}H]inositol for 60 min. The cells were subsequently carbachol-stimulated for 30 min in the continued presence of [^{3}H]inositol and 5 mM Li$^+$. Reaction was terminated and the water-soluble inositol phosphates were extracted with chloroform/methanol/acid. Inositol phosphates were separated by conventional anion-exchange chromatography (for method, see Baird et al., 1989)

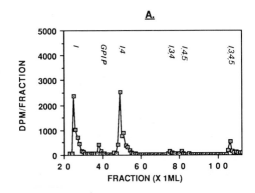

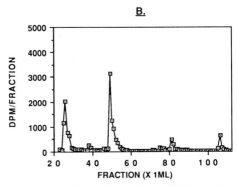

Fig. 6. Typical HPLC profile for [^{3}H]inositol phosphates produced in control (A) and carbachol-treated (1 mM, 5s) (B) SH-SY5Y cells. Reactions were terminated and inositol phosphates were extracted as described in Fig. 1. Neutral extracts were subjected to HPLC (Partisil SAX) and eluted with ammonium phosphate. The elution profiles were compared with known standards (for method see Batty et al., 1989).

in [Ca^{2+}]$_i$, rising from 100 to 170 nM in response to 0.1 mM acetylcholine, persisting for at least 5 min. Removal of the extracellular Ca^{2+} reduced the response considerably, [Ca^{2+}]$_i$ rising from only 30 to 50 nM. The EC_{50} for the increase in [Ca^{2+}]$_i$ seen in the presence of Ca^{2+} was 1 μM, whilst in parallel studies methacholine had an EC_{50} of 0.3 μM and nicotine was without effect. In a more recent study Akerman (1989) has shown that carbachol (0.1 mM) caused a transient increase in [Ca^{2+}]$_i$ in SH-SY5Y cells loaded with fura 2, rising from 120 to 440 nM. The EC_{50} for this monophasic response was about 4 μM. Depletion of the intracellular stores with EGTA and ionomycin or BAPTA caused a dramatic reduction in carbachol stimulated increases in [Ca^{2+}]$_i$,

suggesting that carbachol was mobilizing Ca^{2+} from an intracellular store, and that the difference between this and the Ca^{2+} transient seen in the presence of external Ca^{2+} must be due to Ca^{2+} entry.

We have extensively characterized the [Ca^{2+}]$_i$ response to muscarinic agonists in fura 2-loaded SH-SY5Y cells (Lambert and Nahorski, 1989a,b, 1990 and unpublished data), in which the Ca^{2+} signal is biphasic: our data are described below. Addition of the full agonists carbachol and muscarine (1 mM) causes a rapid initial spike in [Ca^{2+}]$_i$, maximal after some 8–10 s. This peak then declined slowly to reach a new plateau phase above basal values. The partial agonist arecoline produced a greatly reduced spike [Ca^{2+}]$_i$ compared to carbachol and muscarine; the plateau phase remained largely unaltered (at 1 mM) (Fig. 7). The EC_{50} for carbachol- and muscarine-stimulated plateau phase [Ca^{2+}]$_i$ lies approximately one log to the left of the EC_{50} for the corresponding spike [Ca^{2+}]$_i$, suggesting that two separate control mechanisms are operative (see below). Preincubation of SH-SY5Y cells with atropine abolishes the carbachol-stimulated rise in [Ca^{2+}]$_i$. When examining atropine inhibition of the carbachol-stimulated [Ca^{2+}]$_i$ spike, a K_i for atropine of 0.26 nM is observed. These data confirm the involvement of muscarinic receptors; however, the inhibition curve is of low slope (slope factor 0.62), suggesting that atropine might be discriminating two responses at the spike phase [Ca^{2+}]$_i$.

Removal of extracellular Ca^{2+} has a number of consequences: the basal [Ca^{2+}]$_i$ is reduced, the level of the carbachol-stimulated [Ca^{2+}]$_i$ spike is reduced and most strikingly the plateau-phase [Ca^{2+}]$_i$ is completely abolished (Fig. 8). We propose that the spike-phase [Ca^{2+}]$_i$ is due to the release of intracellular stored Ca^{2+}, since the time course is mirrored by that of Ins(1,4,5)P$_3$ production and these cells possess an Ins(1,4,5)P$_3$-sensitive Ca^{2+} release site (Nahorski and Potter, 1989; Safrany and Nahorski, unpublished data). The plateau-phase [Ca^{2+}]$_i$ is due to Ca^{2+} entry across the palsma membrane: this is shown by its depen-

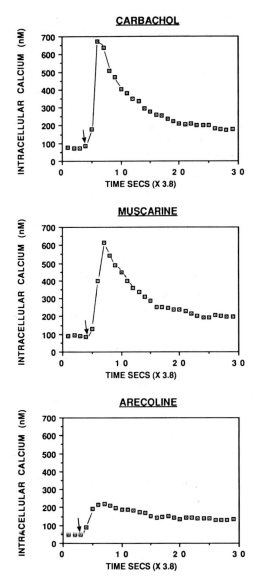

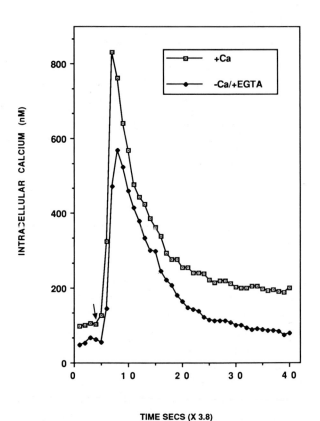

Fig. 7. Effect of muscarinic agonists (1 mM) carbachol, muscarine (full agonists) and arecoline (partial agonist) on $[Ca^{2+}]_i$ in fura 2-loaded SH-SY5Y cells. $[Ca^{2+}]_i$ was measured at 37°C in fura 2-loaded SH-SY5Y cells. Fura 2 fluorescence was monitored in a Perkin Elmer LS5B spectrofluorimeter. The ratio of fluorescence at 340/380 nm excitation (measured at 509 nm emission) was used to calculate $[Ca^{2+}]_i$ (Grynkiewicz et al., 1985). The time taken to drive between the 340 and 380 nm excitation intensities was 3.8 s. Agonist addition is indicated by the arrow.

lam and Rink, 1985). Ca^{2+} does not enter through a verapamil-, +PN-200-110- or conotoxin-blockable Ca^{2+} channel. This latter point implies that the direct involvement of L- or N-type Ca^{2+} channels in carbachol-stimulated Ca^{2+} entry can be ruled out. It should be noted, however, that Akerman (1989) has observed increased bis-oxonol fluorescence in SH-SY5Y cells stimulated with carbachol (this is indicative of depolarization); however, it should also be noted that in these cells a plateau-phase $[Ca^{2+}]_i$ was not observed. Mn^{2+} quenching experiments (in which we use 340 and 360 nm excitation intensities; the latter, the isosbestic point for fura 2, is insensitive to changes in Ca^{2+} but is Mn^{2+}-quenchable) reveal that quenching (Ca^{2+} entry) occurs early on during the dis-

Fig. 8. Removal of extracellular Ca^{2+} abolishes the 1 mM carbachol-stimulated plateau phase $[Ca^{2+}]_i$. $[Ca^{2+}]_i$ was calculated as in Fig 7. Agonist addition is indicated by the arrow. Modified from Lambert and Nahorski, 1990.

dence on extracellular Ca^{2+}, its inhibition by Ni^{2+} and the presence of agonist-stimulated quenching (of fura 2 fluorescence) in Mn^{2+}-treated cells (Hal-

charge of the internal stores. This could explain the low slope of the atropine inhibition curve described above if Ca^{2+} release and Ca^{2+} entry are occurring in concert. It thus seems clear that the spike phase is due to the release of Ca^{2+} from the internal store and that the plateau phase is due to Ca^{2+} entry. The mechanism for Ca^{2+} entry and the channel used is unclear. It is unlikely that the channel is voltage-sensitive but is blocked by Ni^{2+} and it is possible that a non-selective cation channel may be opening (Fasolato et al., 1988; Benham and Tsien, 1987). The channel could be second-messenger-operated (Meldolesi and Pozzan, 1987), involving $Ins(1,4,5)P_3$ or $Ins(1,3,4,5)P_4$ (since a plateau is observed in the production of $InsP_3$) but again this seems unlikely, since low concentrations of carbachol which may not produce an inositol phosphate response still induce a plateau-phase-like $[Ca^{2+}]_i$ response. Experiments

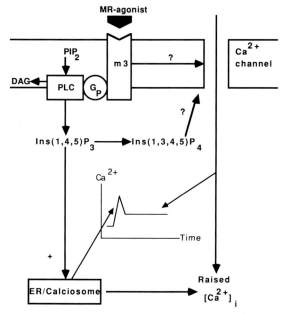

Fig. 9. Proposed relationship between phosphoinositide metabolism and elevated $[Ca^{2+}]_i$ in SH-SY5Y human neuroblastoma cells. A muscarinic (MR) agonist binds to m3 muscarinic receptor; this leads to a G-protein (Gp)-linked stimulation of phospholipase C (PLC). $Ins(1,4,5)P_3$ is generated, liberating Ca^{2+} from an intracellular store (ER/calciosome). This is the spike phase seen in the $[Ca^{2+}]_i$ profile. Extracellular Ca^{2+} enters (giving the plateau phase $[Ca^{2+}]_i$) through an as yet undefined route (see text)

currently under way also rule out a linkage of the muscarinic receptor to the Ca^{2+} channel through a pertussis toxin-sensitive G-protein, since this toxin does not interfere with the plateau (or spike) phase $[Ca^{2+}]_i$ (Lambert and Nahorski, unpublished data).

A careful analysis of the relationship between muscarinic receptor occupation and response in these cells indicates the possible presence of a receptor reserve for both inositol phosphate production and increased $[Ca^{2+}]_i$. This is shown by the lower K_i for carbachol binding of 30 μM, compared to the EC_{50} values for carbachol-stimulated inositol phosphate production of 7.5 μM and increased $[Ca^{2+}]_i$ of 7.6 μM (spike). These data also indicate that amplification between inositol phosphate production and mobilization of $[Ca^{2+}]_i$ is unlikely in these cells. The results of our studies with SH-SY5Y cells to date on phosphoinositide metabolism and elevated $[Ca^{2+}]_i$ are shown in Fig. 9.

Conclusions

The SH-SY5Y cell is a useful model neuronal system in which to study second messenger responses associated with muscarinic receptors, since the cell line expresses a homogeneous m3 receptor complement that subserves phosphoinositide hydrolysis, Ca^{2+} release from internal stores and Ca^{2+} channel opening. These studies as well as those in a variety of other preparations clearly illustrate the diversity of second messenger responses associated with muscarinic receptor subtypes. The recent availability of cells with transfected muscarinic receptors (Buckley et al., 1989) coupled with single cell imaging will, one hopes, allow further characterization of the linkage of m1–m5 subtypes to intracellular Ca^{2+} homeostasis and their association with inositol polyphosphate metabolism.

Acknowledgements

Some of the work on the SH-SY5Y cell line described in this article was performed by Richard

Wojcikiewicz, John Baird and Stephen Safrany. The authors would like to thank the Wellcome Trust for financial support.

References

Adem, A., Mattsson, M.E.K., Nordberg, A. and Pahlman, S. (1987) Muscarinic receptors in human SH-SY5Y neuroblastoma cell line: regulation by phorbol ester and retinoic acid-induced differentiation. *Dev. Brain Res.*, 33: 235–242.

Akerman, K.E.O. (1989) Depolarization of human neuroblastoma cells as a result of muscarinic receptor-induced rise in cytosolic Ca^{2+}. *FEBS Lett.*, 242: 337–340.

Baird, J.G., Lambert, D.G., Mc Bain, J. and Nahorski, S.R. (1989) Muscarinic receptors coupled to phosphoinositide hydrolysis and elevated cytosolic calcium in a human neuroblastoma cell line SK-N-SH. *Br. J. Pharmacol.*, 98: 1328–1334.

Batty, I.H., Letcher, A.J. and Nahorski. (1989) Accumulation of inositol polyphosphate isomers in agonist stimulated cerebral-cortex slices, comparison with metabolic profiles in cell-free preparations. *Biochem. J.*, 258: 23–32.

Baumgold, J. and Fishman, P.H. (1988) Muscarinic receptor-mediated increase in cAMP levels in SK-N-SH human neuroblastoma cells. *Biochem. Biophys. Res. Commun.*, 154: 1137–1143.

Baumgold, J. and White, T. (1989) Pharmacological differences between muscarinic receptors coupled to phosphoinositide turnover and those coupled to adenylate cyclase inhibition. *Biochem. Pharmacol.*, 38: 1605–1616.

Barnard, E.A. (1988) Separating receptor subtypes from their shadows. *Nature*, 335: 301–302.

Benham, C.D and Tsien, R.W (1987) A novel receptor-operated Ca^{2+}-permeable channel activated by ATP in smooth muscle. *Nature*, 328: 275–278.

Berridge, M.J. (1987) Inositol trisphosphate and diacylglycerol: two interacting second mesengers. *Annu. Rev. Biochem.*, 56: 159–193.

Berridge, M.J. and Gallione, A. (1988) Cytosolic calcium oscillators. *FASEB J.*, 2: 3074–3082.

Biedler, J.L., Helson, L. and Spengler, R. (1973) Morphology and growth, tumorigenicity and cytogenetics of human neuroblastoma cells in continuous culture. *Cancer Res.*, 33: 2643–2652.

Blaustein, M.P. (1988) Calcium transport and buffering in neurons. *Trends NeuroSci.*, 11: 438–443.

Bonner, T.I., Buckley, N.J., Young, A.C. and Brann, M.R. (1987) Identification of a family of muscarinic acetylcholine receptor genes. *Science*, 237: 527–532.

Bonner, T.I., Young, A.C., Brann, M.R. and Buckley N.J. (1988) Cloning and expression of the human and rat m5 muscarinic receptor genes. *Neuron*, 1: 403–410.

Brown, E., Kendall, D.A. and Nahorski, S.R. (1984). Inositol phospholipid hydrolysis in rat cerebral cortical slices: 1. receptor characterisation. *J. Neurochem.*, 42: 1379–1387.

Buckley, N.J., Bonner, T.I., Buckley, C.M. and Brann, M.R. (1989) Antagonist binding properties of five cloned muscarinic receptors expressed in CHO-K1 cells. *J. Pharmacol. Exp. Ther.*, 35: 469–476.

Challiss, R.A.J., Batty, I.H. and Nahorski, S.R. (1988) Mass measurements of inositol(1,4,5)trisphosphate in rat cerebral cortex slices using a radioreceptor assay: effects of neurotransmitters and depolarisation. *Biochem. Biophys. Res. Commun.*, 157: 684–691.

Chilvers, E.R., Challiss, R.A.J., Barnes, P.J. and Nahorski, S.R. (1989) Mass changes of inositol(1,4,5)trisphosphate in trachealis muscle following agonist stimulation. *Eur. J. Pharmacol.*, 164: 587–590.

Christie, M.J. and North, R.A (1987) Control of ion conductances by muscarinic receptors. *Trends Pharmacol. Sci.*, (Suppl.) Subtypes of muscarinic receptors III: 30–34.

Clementi, F., Cabrini, D., Gotti, C. and Sher, E. (1986) Pharmacological characterisation of cholinergic receptors in a human neuroblastoma cell line. *J. Neurochem.*, 47: 291–297.

Cobbold, P.H. and Rink, T.J. (1987) Fluorescence and bioluminescence measurement of cytoplasmic free calcium. *Biochem. J.*, 248: 313–328.

Fasolato, C., Pandiella, A., Meldolesi, J. and Pozzan, T. (1988) Generation of inositolphosphates, cytosolic Ca^{2+} and ionic fluxes in PC12 cells treated with bradykinin. *J. Biol. Chem.*, 263: 17350–17359.

Fisher, S.K. (1985) Inositol lipids and signal transduction at CNS muscarinic receptors. *Trends Pharmacol. Sci.*, (Suppl.) Subtypes of muscarinic receptors 11: 61–65.

Fisher, S.K. (1988) Recognition of muscarinic cholinergic receptors in human SK-N-SH neuroblastoma cells by quaternary and tertiary ligands is dependent upon temperature, cell integrity, and the presence of agonists. *Mol. Pharmacol.*, 33: 414–422.

Fisher, S.K. and Heacock, A.M. (1988) A putative M_3 muscarinic cholinergic receptor of high molecular weight couples to phosphoinositide hydrolysis in human neuroblastoma cells. *J. Neurochem.*, 50: 984–987.

Fisher, S.K. and Snider, R.M. (1987) Differential receptor occupancy requirements for muscarinic cholinergic stimulation of inositol lipid hydrolysis in brain and in neuroblastomas. *Mol. Pharmacol.*, 32: 81–90.

Fisher, S.K., Domask, L.M. and Roland, R.M. (1989) Muscarinic receptor regulation of cytoplasmic Ca^{2+} concentrations in human SK-N-SH neuroblastoma cells: Ca^{2+} requirements for phospholipase C activation. *Mol. Pharmacol.*, 35: 195–204.

Fu, T., Okano, Y. and Nozawa, Y. (1988) Bradykinin-induced generation of inositol 1,4,5-trisphosphate in fibroblasts and neuroblastoma cells: effect of pertussis toxin, extracellular calcium, and down regulation of protein kinase C. *Biochem. Biophys. Res. Commun.*, 157: 1429–1435.

Fukuda, K., Higashida, H., Kubo, T., Maeda, A., Akiba, I., Bujo, H., Mishina, M. and Numa, S. (1988) Selective coupling of muscarinic acetylcholine receptor subtypes in NG108-15 cells. *Nature*, 335: 355–358.

Gallo, V., Ciotti, M.T., Coletti, A., Aloisi, F. and Levi, G. (1982) Selective release of glutamate from cerebellar granule cells differentiating in culture. *Proc. Natl. Acad. Sci. USA*, 79: 7919–7923.

Gatti, G., Madeddu, L., Pandiella, A., Pozzan, T. and Meldolesi, J. (1988) Second-messenger generation in PC12 cells. Interactions between cyclic AMP and Ca^{2+} signals. *Biochem. J.*,255: 753–760.

Gray, P.T.A. (1988) Oscillations of free cytosolic calcium evoked by cholinergic and catecholaminergic agonists in rat parotid acinar cells. *J. Physiol. (Lond.)*, 406: 35–53.

Grynkiewicz, G., Poenie, M. and Tsien, R.Y. (1985) A new generation of Ca^{2+} indicators with greatly improved fluorescence properties. *J. Biol. Chem.*, 260: 3440–3449.

Hallam, T.J. and Rink, T.J. (1985) Agonists stimulate divalent cation channels in the plasma membrane of human platelets. *FEBS Lett.*, 186: 175–179.

Harden, T.K., Tanner, L.I., Martin, M.W., Nakahata, N., Hughes, A.R., Helper, J.R., Evans, T., Masters, S.B. and Brown, J.H. (1985) Characteristics of two biochemical responses to stimulation of muscarinic cholinergic receptors. *Trends Pharmacol. Sci.*, (Suppl.) Subtypes of muscarinic receptors II: 14–18.

Heikkila, J.E., Scott, I.G., Suominen, L.A. and Akerman, K.E.O. (1987) Differentiation-associated decrease in muscarinic receptor sensitivity in human neuroblastoma cells. *J. Cell. Physiol.*, 130: 157–162.

Klinz, F.-J., Yu, V.C., Sadee, W. and Costa, T. (1987) Differential expression of α-subunits of G-proteins in human neuroblastoma-derived cell clones. *FEBS, Lett.*, 224: 43–48.

Lambert, D.G. and Nahorski, S.R. (1989a) Muscarinic receptors coupled to phosphoinositide hydrolysis and elevated cytosolic calcium in a human neuroblastoma cell SH-SY5Y. *Br. J. Pharmacol.*, 96: 132P.

Lambert, D.G. and Nahorski, S.R. (1989b) Muscarinic receptor linked Ca^{2+} entry in a human neuroblastoma cell line SH-SY5Y. *Br. J. Pharmacol.* 98: 913P.

Lambert, D.G. and Nahorski, S.R. (1990) Muscarinic receptor mediated changes in $[Ca^{2+}]_i$ and inositol (1,4,5)trisphosphate mass in a human neuroblastoma cell line, SH-SY5Y. *Biochem. J.*, 265: 555–562.

Lambert, D.G., Ghataorre, A.S. and Nahorski, S.R. (1989) Muscarinic receptor binding characteristics of a human neuroblastoma SK-N-SH and its clones SH-SY5Y and SH-EP1. *Eur. J. Pharmacol.*, 165: 71–77.

Lazareno, S., Kendall, D.A. and Nahorski, S.R. (1985) Pirenzepine indicates heterogeneity of muscarinic receptors linked to cerebral inositol phospholipid metabolism. *Neuropharmacology*, 24: 593–595.

McCarthy, K.D. and DeVellis, J. (1980) Preparation of separate astroglial and oligodendroglial cell cultures from rat cerebral tissue. *J. Cell. Biol.*, 85: 890–902.

McDonough, P., Eubanks, J.H. and Brown, J.H. (1988) Desensitization and recovery of muscarinic and histaminergic Ca^{2+} mobilization in 1321N1 astrocytoma cells. *Biochem. J.*, 249: 135–141.

Mei, L., Yamamura, H.I and Roeske, W.R. (1988) Muscarinic receptor-mediated hydrolysis of phosphatidylinositols in human neuroblastoma (SH-SY5Y) cells is sensitive to pertussis toxin. *Brain Res.*, 447: 360–363.

Meldolesi, J. and Pozzan, T. (1987) Pathways of Ca^{2+} influx at the plasma membrane: voltage-, receptor-, and second messenger-operated channels. *Exp. Cell Res.*, 171: 271–283.

Merritt, J.E. and Hallam, T.J. (1988) Platelets and parotid acinar cells have different mechanisms for agonist-stimulated divalent cation entry. *J. Biol. Chem.*, 263: 6161–6164.

Merritt, J.E. and Rink, T.J. (1987) Regulation of cytosolic free calcium in fura-2-loaded rat parotid acinar cells. *J. Biol. Chem.*, 262: 17362–17369.

Muallem, S., Pandol, S.J. and Beeker, T.G. (1988) Two components of hormone-evoked calcium release from intracellular stores of pancreatic acinar cells. *Biochem. J.*, 255: 301–307.

Nahorski, S.R. (1988) Inositol polyphosphates and neuronal calcium homeostasis. *Trends NeuroSci.*, 11: 449–452.

Nahorski, S.R. and Potter, B.V.L. (1989) Molecular recognition of inositol polyphosphates by intracellular receptors and metabolic enzymes. *Trends Pharmacol. Sci.*, 10:139–144.

Nahorski, S.R., Kendall, D.A. and Batty, I. (1986) Receptors and phosphoinositide metabolism in the central nervous system. *Biochem. Pharmacol.*, 35: 2447–2453.

Negulescu, P.A. and Machin, T.E. (1988) Release and reloading of intracellular Ca stores after cholinergic stimulation of the parietal cell. *Am. J. Physiol.*, 254: C498–C504.

Pandol, S.J., Schoeffield, M.S., Fimmel, C.J. and Muallem, S. (1987) The agonist-sensitive calcium pool in the pancreatic acinar cell. *J. Biol. Chem.*, 262: 16963–16968.

Peralta, E.G., Ashkenazi, A., Winslow, J.W., Ramachandran, J. and Capon, D.J. (1988) Differential regulation of PI hydrolysis and adenylyl cyclase by muscarinic receptor subtypes. *Nature*, 334: 434–437.

Prentki, M., Glennon, M.C., Thomas, A.P., Morris, R.L., Matschinsky, F.M. and Crrkey, B.E. (1988) Cell-specific patterns of oscillating free Ca^{2+} in carbomylcholine-stimulated insulinoma cells. *J. Biol. Chem.*, 263: 11044–11047.

Ross, R.A. and Biedler, J.L. (1985) Presence and regulation of tyrosinase activity in human neuroblastoma cell varients in vitro. *Cancer Res.*, 45: 1628–1632.

Schlegel, W., Wuarin, F., Zbaren, C. and Zahnd, G.R. (1985) Lowering of cytosolic free Ca^{2+} by carbachol, a muscarinic cholinergic agonist, in clonal pituitary cells (GH_3 cells). *Endocrinology*, 117: 976–981.

Scott, I.G., Akerman, K.E.O., Heikkila, J.E., Kaila, K. and Andersson, L.C. (1986) Development of a neural phenotype in differentiating ganglion cell-derived human neuroblastoma cells. *J. Cell. Physiol.*, 128: 285–292.

Serra, M., Mei, L., Roeske, W.R., Lui, G.K., Watson, M. and Yamamura, H.I. (1988) The intact human neuroblastoma cell (SH-SY5Y) exhibits high-affinity [^{3}H]pirenzepine binding associated with hydrolysis of phosphatidylinositols. *J. Neurochem.*, 50: 1513–1521.

Streb, H., Irvine, R.F., Berridge, M.J. and Schulz, I. (1983) Release of Ca^{2+} from a nonmitochondrial intracellular store in pancreatic acinar cells by inositol-1,4,5-trisphosphate. *Nature*, 306: 76–69.

Takemura, H. and Putney, J.W. Jr. (1989) Capacitative calcium entry in parotid acinar cells. *Biochem. J.*, 258: 409–412.

Volpe, P., Krause, K-H., Hashimoto, S., Zorzato, F., Pozzan,

T., Meldolesi, J. and Lew, D.P. (1988) Calciosome, a cytoplasmic organelle: the inositol 1,4,5-trisphosphate-sensitive Ca^{2+} store of nonmuscle cells? *Proc. Natl. Acad. Sci. USA*, 85: 1091–1095.

Waelbroeck, M., Camus, J., Tastenoy, M. and Christophe, J. (1988) 80% of muscarinic receptors expressed by the NB-OK1 human neuroblastoma cell line show high affinity for pirenzepine and are comparable to rat hippocampus M1 receptors. *FEBS Lett.*, 226: 287–290.

Wojcikiewicz, R.J.H. and Nahorski, S.R. (1989a) Guanine nucleotides modulate muscarinic stimulation of phosphoinositide metabolism in permeabilized neuroblastoma (SH-SY5Y) cells. *Br. J. Pharmacol.*, 96: 131P

Wojcikiewicz, R.J.H. and Nahorski, S.R. (1989b) Phosphoinositide hydrolysis in permeabilised SH-SY5Y human neuroblastoma cells is inhibited by mastoparan. *FEBS Lett.*, 247: 341–344.

S.-M. Aquilonius and P.-G. Gillberg (Eds.)
Progress in Brain Research, Vol. 84
© 1990 Elsevier Science Publishers B.V. (Biomedical Division)

CHAPTER 5

Function of nicotinic synapses

D. Colquhoun, A.B. Cachelin, C.G. Marshall, A. Mathie and D.C. Ogden

MRC Receptor Mechanisms Group, Department of Pharmacology, University College London, Gower Street, London, WC1E 6BT, U.K.

Introduction

There are at least three sorts of synapse at which the primary transmitter is acetylcholine (ACh) working on postsynaptic nicotinic receptors, and they differ considerably from one another. The most thoroughly investigated synapse is that between motor nerve and voluntary muscle fibres. A good deal of work has also been done on the neuro-neuronal synapses in autonomic ganglia. There is now reason to believe, e.g., from in situ hybridization studies and from nicotine binding studies, as well as from physiological work, that nicotinic synapses may be more common in the central nervous system (CNS) than had previously been supposed (see Clementi et al., 1988, for review); there is, however, relatively little known so far about central nicotinic synapses or about the nicotinic receptors in them.

In this paper we shall outline some of our recent work on synapses at the neuromuscular junction and in autonomic ganglia.

The neuromuscular synapse

The most detailed investigations of both synaptic transmission and the mechanism of activation of ion channels by ACh have been carried out at the frog neuromuscular junction, much of them by Katz and his colleagues. Indeed, the mechanism first proposed by del Castillo and Katz (1957) for channel activation is still used, essentially unchanged, except for the modification that is necessary to allow for the fact that two molecules of ACh, rather than one, are needed for efficient opening of the ion channel. This had long been suspected on the basis of electrophysiological measurements, and has been confirmed clearly by structural evidence which shows that each nicotinic receptor-channel contains two of the α subunits, each of which has an ACh binding site (see Karlin, 1980). This mechanism can be summarized as

$$R \underset{k_{-1}}{\overset{2k_{+1}}{\rightleftharpoons}} AR \underset{2k_{-2}}{\overset{k_{+2}}{\rightleftharpoons}} A_2R \underset{\alpha}{\overset{\beta}{\rightleftharpoons}} A_2R^* \qquad (1)$$

where A represents agonist, R is the shut receptor-channel and R* is the open channel, and k_{+1}, k_{+2} are association rate constants for ACh binding, k_{-1}, k_{-2} are dissociation rate constants, β is the rate constant for channel opening once it is fully liganded and α is the channel closing rate constant (so $1/\alpha$ is the mean channel open time). This mechanism can describe many of the phenomena that were discovered by means of noise analysis, voltage-jump analysis and subsequently single channel recording, all of which were invented long after the mechanism had been postulated. It cannot, however, explain such phenomena as the correlations between open times, and it does not include either channel block or desensitization, both of which are important in practice.

Neuromuscular transmission in mammals seems to be similar physiologically to that in frogs, and the recent use of single channel recording to investigate the equilibrium concentration-response relationship of rat endplate nicotinic receptors (Mulrine and Ogden, 1988) has shown them to be remarkably similar to those of the frog (Colquhoun and Ogden, 1988). Both seem to have a low affinity for ACh in the resting state ($K = 55$–80 μM) and, for both, the equilibrium between open and shut states for fully liganded channels is well over towards the open side (i.e. β/α is large, so ACh is a highly "efficacious" agonist). Thus most of the channels will be opened at high ACh concentrations (or, at least, they would be open if it were not for desensitization, and channel block by ACh molecules). For both species a concentration of ACh of 15–18μM is required to produce half-maximum channel opening (at negative membrane potentials).

The mechanism of activation of endplate nicotinic channels

Colquhoun and Sakmann (1981, 1985) interpreted the fine structure of individual channel activations (i.e. the brief channel closures within them), according to a suggestion of Colquhoun and Hawkes (1977), as representing re-openings of channels which had shut, but which still had one or both agonist molecules bound to them. This will be referred to as the *nachschlag* interpretation. It allows inferences about some of the details of mechanism (1) that cannot be obtained easily in other ways; for example, values for both the channel-opening rate constant, β and for the dissociation rate constant, k_{-2}, can be found. Such measurements have suggested that ACh, and most other agonists that have been tested too, are quite efficacious in the sense that β/α is quite large, and that the affinity of the agonist for the resting state, R, is quite low (i.e. $K = k_-/k_+$ is in the range tens or hundreds of micromolar). For example, it was inferred by Colquhoun and Sakmann (1985) that the reason that suberyldicholine is about 5-times more potent than ACh at equilibrium is a result of its higher affinity for the resting channel, its ability to open the channel once bound (as measured by β/α) being, if anything, slightly lower than that of ACh.

The interpretation of the fine structure of channel openings is potentially hazardous. Brief interruptions can occur for reasons other than those suggested above; for example, spontaneous brief shuttings that apparently have a quite different (but unknown) mechanism have been observed in the nicotinic receptors of the BC3H1 cell line (Sine and Steinbach, 1986). Channel blockages might also confuse the picture, though these should be distinguishable by their concentration dependence. One way to test the *nachschlag* interpretation is to obtain direct measurements of the maximum response with high agonist concentrations. For mechanism (1) this should correspond to a fraction of open channels equal to $(\beta/\alpha)/[1 + (\beta/\alpha)]$. The value found can be compared with that predicted from the separate values of β and α estimated from low-concentration measurements of the fine structure of channel activations. Colquhoun and Ogden (1988) measured the probability of a channel's being open (p_o, say) as a function of ACh concentration after elimination, as far as possible, of desensitized periods from the single channel record. This probability is simply the single channel equivalent of "the fraction of channels that are open" that would be measured on a large population of homogeneous channels. In fact the p_o curve did not reach a clear plateau, but after reaching a peak (at about $p_o = 0.9$) it fell again. This effect was shown to result from block of the open ion channel by ACh molecules themselves (Ogden and Colquhoun, 1985). This effect was corrected for by fitting to the data the following extension of mechanism (1);

$$\text{R} \underset{k_{-1}}{\overset{2k_{+1}}{\rightleftharpoons}} \text{AR} \underset{2k_{-2}}{\overset{k_{+2}}{\rightleftharpoons}} \text{A}_2\text{R} \underset{\alpha}{\overset{\beta}{\rightleftharpoons}} \text{A}_2\text{R}^* \underset{k_{-B}}{\overset{k_{+B}}{\rightleftharpoons}} \text{A}_2\text{R}^*\text{A} \quad (2)$$

in which $\text{A}_2\text{R}^*\text{A}$ represents an ion channel which is blocked (in this case by the agonist itself) and therefore non-conducting. Block becomes significant at ACh concentrations above 100 μM, the equilibrium constant for block ($K_B = k_{-B}/k_{+B}$)

being about 1.3 mM (at -120 mV). Correction for this effect indicated that ACh, in the absence of channel block, should be able to open about 97% of channels. This was in good agreement with predictions made from measurements of fine structure at low agonist concentrations. However, as a test of the *nachschlag* interpretation it is far from perfect. For example, values of the maximum p_o from 0.97 to 1.0 correspond to values of β/α from 32 up to infinity; thus if α were 1000 s^{-1} (i.e. a mean open time of 1 ms) then β would have values from 32 000 to infinity. Clearly it is not possible to infer precise values of β from the maximum p_0 when the latter is so close to 1.0. This fact was one motive for looking for a genuine partial agonist, i.e. an agonist that has a p_o of substantially less than 1.0 as a result of a low "efficacy" (low values of β/α). To this end p_o curves have been determined for a number of ACh analogues.

Activation of endplate nicotinic channels by ACh analogues

The following compounds have been tested: suxamethonium (succinyldicholine, SUX) (Marshall et al., 1990), carbachol (CCh), suberyldicholine (SubCh), the sulphonium analogue of ACh in which the quaternary nitrogen atom is replaced by a tertiary sulphonium atom (S-ACh), decamethonium, phenylpropyltrimethylammonium (PPTMA) and trimethylammonium (TMA) (Marshall et al., unpublished data). Two main conclusions derived from this work.

First, all of these agonists block the ion channel which they themselves open, especially at negative membrane potentials (as does *every* positively charged agonist and antagonist that has ever been tested by appropriate methods). The agonist with the least tendency to block channels, *relative* to its potency in opening them, is ACh itself, for which K_B is about 80-fold greater (at -120 mV) than the EC_{50} for channel opening in the absence of block. Although SubCh is substantially more potent than ACh (EC_{50} about 5–7-fold lower) its

tendency to block channels is much greater ($K_B \simeq$ 6 μM), so the ratio of K_B to EC_{50} is only about 2.7, and the maximum p_o that can actually be obtained (at -120 mV) is only about 0.47. The association rate constant for channel block, k_{+B}, was similar for all agonists, being around the usual value of 2–5×10^7 $M^{-1}s^{-1}$; the differences in potency result largely from differences in dissociation rate, k_{-B} (i.e. from differences in the mean duration of blockages).

The analysis of channel block by suxamethonium (SUX) provided a nice example of a problem that occurs in many single channel studies, namely the problem of errors that arise from failure to detect brief events. Experiments with modest SUX concentrations (10–50 μM) suggested that a component of the shut time distribution with a time constant of about 65 μs represented, predominantly, blockages of the ion channel by SUX. In so far as 65 μs is a good approximation to the mean lifetime of a blockage, it should be independent of concentration. However, this component appeared to become longer at higher SUX concentrations, being about 140 μs at 200 μM SUX. A simulation method was used to demonstrate that this was probably not a genuine lengthening, but resulted merely from the fact that openings get shorter at high SUX concentrations (as a result of channel block) so more of them were too short to be detected (Marshall et al., 1990). This conclusion was reached by estimating the rate constants for mechanism (2) from the results at the lowest SUX concentrations. A random-number generator was then used to generate exponentially distributed lifetimes for sojourns in each of the states, and to decide which state should be jumped to next. This produced simulated records, for a range of SUX concentrations, which resembled the experimental records except that they had perfect time resolution. A finite-time resolution was then imposed on the simulated record in exactly the same way as was done for the experimental records, and the distribution of shut times was fitted to it as though it had been a real experiment. The results mimicked closely the experimental observations despite the fact that the mean lifetime of the blockages ($1/k_{-B}$) was known to be constant in the simulated experiments.

The second major conclusion is that SUX, CCh, SubCh and S-ACh are all, like ACh itself, quite efficacious agonists at negative membrane potentials. Suxamethonium had the lowest value of β/α, viz., about 4.8 at -120 mV, which corresponds to a maximum p_o response of 83%. At low concentrations SUX is about 7.6-fold less potent than ACh; a 2.6-fold reduction of potency results from the lower "efficacy" of SUX, relative to ACh, and the remaining 2.9-fold lower potency is caused by the lower affinity of SUX for the resting receptor (Marshall et al., 1990). In fact the most convincing partial agonist found in these studies was ACh itself at positive membrane potentials (Colquhoun and Ogden, 1988). At $+100$ mV there is much less channel block than at negative potentials, and β/α is only about 0.7 so the p_o response reaches a clear plateau at a maximum value of 41%. The reduction in β/α in this case results mostly from an increase in α (i.e. a shortening of the mean open time) when the membrane is depolarized, rather than from any very pronounced reduction in β. The agonist "efficacy" is dependent on the membrane potential.

For the other agonists, decamethonium, PPTMA and TMA, the extent of channel block was so great, relative to ability to activate the channel, that it was impossible to make satisfactory estimates of β/α for them. In other words it is impossible to be sure whether their ineffectiveness in opening channels (maximum p_o of 1–4 percent) resulted from there being genuine partial agonists, or whether it resulted merely from powerful channel block.

In summary, all the agonists tested were quite efficacious in the sense that they would be capable of opening 83–98% of channels in the absence of desensitization and channel block. Under experimental conditions, however, the maximum response that could be obtained at negative membrane potentials (after correction for desensitization) was limited by their channel-blocking effects.

Desensitization at the neuromuscular synapse

Desensitization is a universal, and prominent, property of nicotinic receptors, but the mechanisms underlying it remain as obscure as they have always been (and as they are for most other receptor types). It is of dubious physiological significance, and from the experimental point of view it has usually been regarded as a great nuisance because, for example, it prevents one from obtaining useful concentration-response curves from whole cells. It is, therefore, ironic that without desensitization it would be very difficult to obtain stretches of single-channel record in which one can be sure that only one single channel is active, as is needed for the studies described above.

At one stage there was a good deal of speculation as to whether desensitization was some sort of metabolic phenomenon, or whether it was the manifestation of some discrete conformation of the receptor protein that was unresponsive to agonist. At present the evidence seems to favour the latter view. Structural studies by Unwin et al. (1988) have recently demonstrated directly that the shape of the desensitized receptor is different from that of the resting receptor. The fact that desensitization can occur with purified receptors reconstituted into lipid bilayers makes it most unlikely that metabolic factors are necessary (Nelson et al., 1980; Schindler and Quast, 1980; Popot et al., 1981). Furthermore many studies have shown that desensitization occurs in isolated membrane patches, and Cachelin and Colquhoun (1989) observed intense desensitization at the endplates of skeletal muscle fibres that had been filled with isosmotic potassium EGTA. It is clearly most unlikely that, for example, receptor phosphorylation could be the primary cause of desensitization. It is known that nicotinic receptors *can* be phosphorylated at a number of sites, and there is evidence that phosphorylation may *accelerate* desensitization in some species at least (Albuquerque et al., 1986; Huganir et al., 1986; Middleton et al., 1986). However, the role of phosphorylation, even as a modifier of pre-existing desensitization, is still rather controversial. Several studies have now shown that the effects of forskolin on "desensitization" rate is unlikely to be a result of cAMP-induced phosphorylation (e.g. McHugh and McGee, 1986; Wagoner and Pallotta, 1988), and Cachelin and Colquhoun (1989) were unable to detect any effects on desensitization (in frog endplate) of various procedures designed to alter receptor phosphorylation. One problem may be that "fade" of a response may result from phenomena other than desensitization (e.g. slow channel block). Another problem may well be that the putative phosphorylation effect can occur in some species and not others (see, for example, Steinbach and Zempel, 1987; Sumikawa and Miledi, 1989).

The complexities are increased by the finding that the onset and offset of desensitization show several exponential components with widely differing rates, and it is not always clear what component is being referred to in any particular study. The components with onset time constants of a few seconds and of a minute or two have been described (though not really explained) in some detail for nicotinic receptors (e.g. Feltz and Trautmann, 1982; Cachelin and Colquhoun, 1989). More recently, the use of rapidly perfused outside-out membrane patches has allowed much faster concentration changes than was possible previously. In this way Brett et al. (1986) found a much faster type of desensitization in nicotinic receptors of the BC3H1 cell line; the channel opening rate fell to a small fraction of its initial rate with a time constant of a few tens of milliseconds. It is not known how commonly this sort of ultra-fast desensitization occurs, but Cachelin and Colquhoun (1989) inferred, indirectly, that it is not a prominent feature of desensitization at frog endplates. They found that the peak response to a large (200 μM) ACh concentration was about 15 μA (measured in a vaseline gap voltage clamp which can pass such large currents); this corresponds to opening of essentially all the 10^7 or so channels in the endplate, despite the fact that it took about 260 ms for the peak response to develop. If a substantial fraction of channels had desensitized with a time constant measured in tens of milliseconds, such a large peak current could not have been observed.

Nicotinic receptors in autonomic ganglia

It has been known for a long time (e.g. Paton and Zaimis, 1951) that the nicotinic receptors in autonomic ganglia differ radically from those at the neuromuscular junction. More recently this was confirmed by studies showing that α-bungarotoxin is ineffective on most neuronal nicotinic receptors, though these receptors are blocked by a related toxin, now usually known as kappa-bungarotoxin (see, for example, Chiappinelli, 1985; Loring and Zigmond, 1988). The first cloning of a neuronal receptor subunit, by Boulter et al. (1986), showed the structural basis of these differences. The amino acid sequence of the α-subunit of the mammalian muscle receptor is far closer to the sequence of the α-subunit of the nicotinic receptor from the electric organ of *Torpedo* than it is to the sequence of mammalian neuronal receptors. Evidently the divergence of muscle and neuronal types is old in evolutionary terms. These and related questions have been reviewed at length in a recent book (Clementi et al., 1988), and more briefly by Colquhoun et al., (1987), Mathie et al. (1988) and Steinbach and Ifune (1989).

Several types of subunit have now been cloned which appear to be constituents of neuronal nicotinic receptors. It is, however, far from clear exactly which subunit types (with what stoichiometry) are combined to form the natural receptors found in autonomic ganglia and the central nervous system. This question may, in the future, be answered partially by comparison of the pharmacological properties of receptors in their natural environment with the pharmacological properties of receptors expressed in cells (such as *Xenopus* oocytes) from cloned cDNA for known subunit types. However, no drugs are known at present which distinguish between different subtypes of neuronal nicotinic receptor. The problem is further complicated by the fact that there seem to be substantial differences between species: for example, the actions of several antagonists in *frog* ganglionic receptors resemble more closely their actions on muscle receptors than is the case for *mammalian* ganglionic receptors (Lipscombe and Rang, 1988). It seems likely that the high resolution afforded by single channel measurements will be needed to discriminate between them. For this reason, among others, it is of interest to investigate the distinctive characteristics of the neuronal nicotinic receptor-channels.

Characteristics of neuronal nicotinic channels

At first sight single channel currents in rat sympathetic neurones look much like those in rat muscle, except that the mean open time is a little longer and the conductance is a little lower for the neuronal channels, and the neuronal channels are noisier when they are open, possibly as a result of rapid switching between closely spaced discrete conductance levels (Mathie et al., 1987; Derkach et al., 1987). Both types of channel show an increased single channel conductance when the extracellular concentration of calcium or magnesium is reduced (Mathie et al., 1987; Cachelin and Neuhaus, 1989), and for both types the individual activations of the channel are interrupted by brief channel closings. The sensitivity of the neuronal channels to ACh is probably not greatly different from that seen in muscle (A. Mathie, in preparation), and, as in muscle, the mean length of a single channel activation (the mean burst length) is similar to the time constant of decay of the excitatory postsynaptic current evoked by nerve stimulation (so the transmitter concentration in the synaptic cleft following release must fall rapidly at both sorts of synapse).

There is, however, one striking difference between the behaviour of the muscle and neuronal type of nicotinic receptor-channel. In whole-cell recordings sympathetic neurones pass very little outward current in response to agonists at positive membrane potentials, i.e. they show very strong inward rectification. In muscle the equilibrium current-voltage (I-V) relationship shows some inward rectification but it has a uniform curvature throughout the whole potential range (this curvature can be largely accounted for by the voltage-dependence of the mean channel open time). In contrast, the I-V curve for rat sympathetic neuronal channels is close to linear at potentials below zero, but virtually flat (no detectable current) at positive potentials (until extreme positive potentials, above $+80$ mV or so, are reached). (Once again frog ganglia are different from mammalian in that they show outward currents much like those in muscle; Lipscombe, 1986.) At first it was thought that lack of outward current might be an artefact resulting from block of outward current by the intracellular caesium ions that are used in most experiments (Hirano et al., 1987), but this is not the case. At the single channel level perfectly normal outwardly directed currents can be seen at positive potentials (Mathie et al., 1987). The reason for the lack of outward whole-cell currents is that channel openings become much less *frequent* at membrane potentials above zero (Marshall et al., 1990). In fact at positive membrane potentials it was found not only that channels open only rarely, but also that they desensitize only slowly. This behaviour is quite different from that seen with muscle-type nicotinic channels, and it should provide a useful tool for testing the characteristics of receptors expressed from the cloned cDNAs for known subunit types.

Conclusions

It seems that neuronal nicotinic receptors, like neuronal GABA and glutamate receptors, are, in many ways, more complex than muscle-type receptors. They have many subtypes and the subunit composition is not known with certainty for any of them, though many sorts of subunit have been cloned (though not yet for glutamate). They show multiple conductance states and/or excess open channel noise (which may result from oscillation between closely spaced discrete conductance states), which makes the measurement of records, and the drawing of conclusions about mechanism from them, much harder than is the case for the muscle nicotinic receptor.

References

Albuquerque, E.X., Deshpande, S.S., Aracava, Y., Alkondon, M. and Daly, J.W. (1986) A possible involvement of cyclic AMP in the expression of desensitization of the nicotinic acetylcholine receptor: A study with forskolin and its analogs. *FEBS Lett,* 199: 113–120.

Boulter, J., Evans, K., Goldman, D., Martin, G., Treco, D., Heinemann, S. and Patrick, J. (1986) Isolation of a cDNA clone coding for a possible neural nicotinic acetylcholine receptor alpha-subunit. *Nature,* 319: 368–374.

Brett, R.S., Dilger, J.P., Adams, P.R. and Lancaster, B. (1986) A method for the rapid exchange of solutions bathing excised membrane patches. *Biophys. J.,* 50: 987–992.

Cachelin, A.B. and Colquhoun, D. (1989) Desensitization of the acetylcholine receptor of frog end-plates measured in a vaseline-gap voltage clamp. *J. Physiol.,* 415: 159–188.

Cachelin, A.B. and Neuhaus, R. (1989) The effect of Mg^{2+} on currents through single acetylcholine channels of rat cultured phaeochromocytoma cells. *J. Physiol. (Proc.),* In press.

Chiappinelli, V.A. (1985) Actions of snake venom toxins on neuronal nicotinic receptors and other neuronal receptors. *Pharmacol. Ther.,* 31: 1–32.

Clementi, F., Gotti, C. and Sher, E. (Eds.) (1988) *Nicotinic Acetylcholine Receptors in the Nervous System.* NATO ASI series, Vol. H25, Springer-Verlag, Berlin.

Colquhoun, D. and Ogden, D.C. (1988) Activation of ion channels in the frog end-plate by high concentrations of acetylcholine. *J. Physiol.,* 395: 131–159.

Colquhoun, D. and Sakmann, B. (1981) Fluctuations in the microsecond time range of the current through single acetylcholine receptor ion channels. *Nature,* 294: 464–466.

Colquhoun, D. and Sakmann, B. (1985) Fast events in single-channel currents activated by acetylcholine and its analogues at the frog muscle end-plate. *J. Physiol.,* 369:501–557.

Colquhoun, D., Ogden, D.C. and Mathie, A. (1987) Nicotinic acetylcholine receptors of nerve and muscle: functional aspects. *Trends Pharmacol. Sci.,* 8: 465–472.

del Castillo, J. and Katz, B. (1957) Interaction at end-plate receptors between different choline derivatives. *Proc. R. Soc.* B146: 369–381.

Derkach, V.A., North, R.A., Selyanko, A.A. and Skok, V.I. (1987) Single channels activated by acetylcholine in rat superior cervical ganglion. *J. Physiol.,* 388: 141–151.

Feltz, A. and Trautmann, A. (1982) Desensitization at the frog neuromuscular junction: a biphasic process. *J. Physiol.,* 322: 257–272.

Hirano, T., Kidokoro, Y. and Ohmori, H. (1987) Acetylcholine dose-response relation and the effect of cesium ions in the rat adrenal chromaffin cell under voltage clamp. *Pflugers Arch.,* 408: 401–407.

Huganir, R.L., Delcour, A.H., Greengard, P. and Hess, G.P. (1986) Phosphorylation of the nicotinic acetylcholine receptor regulates its rate of desensitization. *Nature,* 321: 774–776.

Karlin, A. (1980) Molecular properties of nicotinic acetylcholine receptors. *Cell Surface Rev.,* 6: 191–260.

Lipscombe, D. (1986) Pharmacology of nicotinic receptors in frog neurones: electrophysiological studies on intact and dissociated ganglia. Ph.D. thesis, University of London.

Lipscombe, D. and Rang, H.P. (1988) Nicotinic receptors of frog ganglia resemble pharmacologically those of skeletal muscle. *J. Neurosci.,* 8: 3258–3265.

Loring, R.H. and Zigmond, R.E. (1988) Characterization of neuronal nicotinic receptors by snake venom toxins. *Trends Neurosci.,* 11: 73–78.

Marshall, C.G., Ogden, D.C. and Colquhoun, D. (1990) The actions of suxamethonium (succinyldicholine) as an agonist and channel blocker at the nicotine receptor of frog muscle. *J. Physiol.,* in press.

Mathie, A., Cull-Candy, S.G. and Colquhoun, D. (1987) Single-channel and whole cell currents evoked by acetylcholine in dissociated sympathetic neurons of the rat. *Proc. R. Soc. B,* 232: 239–248.

Mathie, A., Cull-Candy, S.G. and Colquhoun, D. (1988) The mammalian neuronal nicotinic receptor and its block by drugs. In G.G. Lunt (Ed.), *Neurotox "88: Molecular Basis of Drug and Pesticide Action,* Elsevier, Amsterdam, pp. 393–403.

Mathie, A., Colquhoun, D. and Cull-Candy, S.G. (1990) Rectification of currents activated by nicotine acetylcholine receptors in rat sympathetic ganglion neurones. *J. Physiol.,* 427, in press.

McHugh, E.M. and McGee, R. (1986) Direct anesthetic-like effects of forskolin on the nicotinic acetylcholine receptors of PC12 cells. *J. Biol. Chem.,* 261: 3103–3106.

Middleton, P., Jaramillo, F. and Schuetze, S.M. (1986) Forskolin increases the rate of acetylcholine receptor desensitization at rat soleus endplates. *Proc. Natl. Acad. Sci. USA.* 83: 4967–4971.

Mulrine, N.K. and Ogden, D.C. (1988) The equilibrium open probability of nicotinic ion channels at the rat neuromuscular junction. *J. Physiol.,* 401: 95P.

Nelson, N., Anholt, R., Lindstrom, J. and Montal, M. (1980) Reconstitution of purified acetylcholine receptors with functional ion channels in planar lipid bilayers. *Proc. Natl. Acad. Sci. USA,* 77: 3057–3061.

Ogden, D.C. and Colquhoun, D. (1985) Ion channel block by acetylcholine, carbachol and suberyldicholine at the frog neuromuscular junction. *Proc. R. Soc. B,* 225: 329–355.

Paton, W.D.M. and Zaimis, E.J. (1951) Paralysis of autonomic ganglia by methonium salts. *Br. J. Pharmacol.,* 6: 155–168.

Popot, J.-L., Cartaud, J. and Changeux, J.-P. (1981) Reconstitution of a functional acetylcholine receptor. Incorporation into artificial lipid vesicles and pharmacology of the agonist-controlled permeability changes. *Eur. J. Biochem.,* 118: 203–214.

Schindler, H. and Quast, U. (1980) Functional acetylcholine receptor from Torpedo marmorata in planar membranes. *Proc. Natl. Acad. Sci. USA,* 77: 3052–3056.

Sine, S.M. and Steinbach, J.H. (1986) Acetylcholine receptor activation by a site-selective ligand: nature of brief open and closed states in clonal BC3H-1 cells. *J. Physiol.,* 370: 357–379.

Steinbach, J.H. and Ifune, C. (1989) How many kinds of nicotinic acetylcholine receptor are there? *Trends Neurosci.,* 12: 3–6.

Steinbach, J.H. and Zempel, J. (1987) What does phosphorylation do for the nicotinic acetylcholine receptor? *Trends Neurosci.,* 10: 61–64.

Sumikawa, K. and Miledi, R. (1989) Change in desensitization of cat muscle acetylcholine receptor caused by coexpression of *Torpedo* acetylcholine receptor subunits in *Xenopus* oocytes. *Proc. Natl. Acad. Sci., USA,* 86 367–371.

Unwin, N., Toyoshima, C. and Kubalek, E. (1988) Arrangement of the acetylcholine receptor subunits in the resting and desensitized states, determined by cryoelectron microscopy of crystallized *Torpedo* postsynaptic membranes. *J. Cell Biol.,* 107: 1123–1138.

Wagoner, P.K. and Pallotta, B.S. (1988) Modulation of acetylcholine receptor desensitization by forskolin is independent of cAMP. *Science,* 240: 1655–1657.

S.-M. Aquilonius and P.-G. Gillberg (Eds.)
Progress in Brain Research, Vol. 84
© 1990 Elsevier Science Publishers B.V. (Biomedical Division)

CHAPTER 6

Expression and in vivo amplification of the human acetylcholinesterase and butyrylcholinesterase genes

Hermona Soreq [1] and Haim Zakut [2]

[1] *Department of Biological Chemistry, The Life Sciences Institute, The Hebrew University, Jerusalem (91904),*
and [2] Department of Obstetrics and Gynecology, The Edith Wolfson Medical Center,
The Sackler Faculty of Medicine of the Tel Aviv University, Holon (58100), Israel

Introduction

Cholinesterases are carboxylesterase type B enzymes capable of hydrolysing the neurotransmitter acetylcholine. The two principal members of this enzyme family are acetylcholinesterase (AChE) and butyrylcholinesterase (ChE). In addition to their well-known involvement in the termination of cholinergic neurotransmission (for comprehensive reviews see Toutant and Massoulie, 1987; Soreq and Gnatt, 1987; Brimijoin and Rackonzay, 1988), cholinesterases were implicated in several processes related to cellular differentiation and tissue reorganization. This was mainly because of their transiently coordinated expression in various embryonic tissues (see, for example, Layer and Sporns, 1987; Layer et al., 1987b; Zakut et al., 1985). In addition, acetylcholine analogues and cholinesterase inhibitors were found to induce promegakaryocytopoiesis and platelet production in the mouse (Paulus et al., 1981; Burstein et al., 1980). To deepen our understanding of these intriguing phenomena, we have used cloned cDNAs encoding both ChE (Prody et al., 1987) and AChE (Soreq and Prody, 1989) from man for various hybridization and expression experiments. Our findings demonstrate a multileveled regulation for the ChE and AChE genes in humans and are strongly indicative of their involvement in cellular growth and differentiation in multiple biosystems.

Results

In situ hybridization experiments using ChEcDNA and AChEcDNA probes revealed transcriptional activity and developmental alterations in the levels of cholinesterase mRNA transcripts in the non-cholinergic cerebellar neurons (Ayalon et al., 1990). Both AChEmRNA and ChEmRNA transcripts could be clearly observed in cell bodies of granular neurons. In contrast, cholinergic Golgi type I and II neurons in fetal basal nuclei expressed AChEmRNA transcripts alone, suggesting that preferential production of AChE occurs in cholinergic neurons early in their development and that the coordinated synthesis of both ChE and AChE in the developing cerebellum reflects a developmental role for these proteins (Ayalon et al., 1990). Furthermore, transcriptional activity of the cholinesterase genes was also observed in developing human oocytes (Soreq et al., 1987a; Malinger et al., 1989). Fig. 1 demonstrates the high levels of ChEmRNA transcripts in pre-antral human oocytes, found by in situ hybridization with ChEcDNA and dark-field photography. Together with previous findings of cholinesterase activities and acetylcholine receptors in oocytes from various species (reviewed in Malinger et al., 1989), these findings indicate that oocyte maturation is affected by cholinergic mechanisms, and may therefore imply that oocyte development could be sensitive to blockers of cholinesterase activities.

When microinjected into *Xenopus* oocytes, synthetic recombinant ChEmRNA induced the pro-

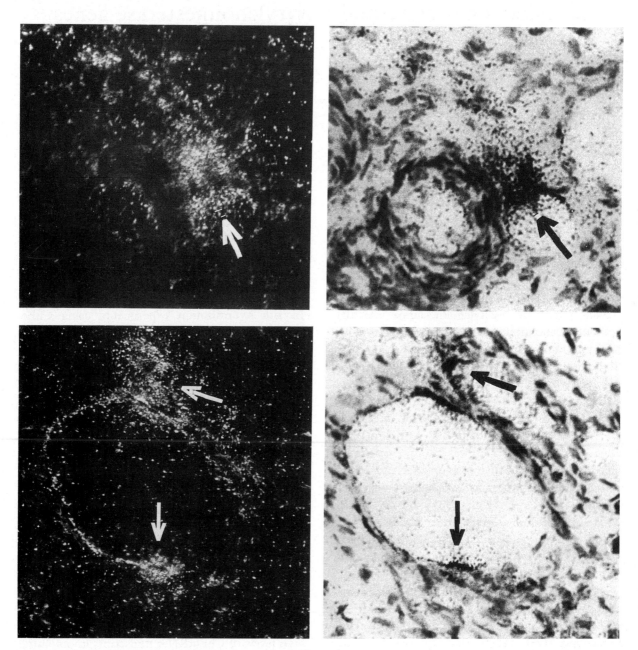

Fig. 1. In situ hybridization of frozen ovarian sections with [^{35}S]ChEcDNA. Frozen ovarian sections were hybridized with cloned ChEcDNA labeled with ^{35}S by nick translation, as detailed elsewhere (Malinger et al., 1989). High magnification dark-field (left) and bright-field (right) photography is presented for primordial (top) and pre-antral oocytes (bottom), which were intensely labeled with silver grains. Exposure was for 3 weeks.

duction of catalytically active ChE which mostly remained attached to the external oocyte surface (Soreq et al., 1989; Dreyfus et al., 1989). Both the substrate preference and the sensitivity to selective inhibitors of this recombinant enzyme were very similar to those reported for the native enzyme (reviewed by Seidman and Soreq, 1990). This implied that the biochemical properties of ChE and AChE were mostly inherent to the primary amino acid sequence of these enzymes. It also demonstrated that ChE can serve as a potential scavenger of cholinesterase inhibitors, for example organophosphorous poisons. This may become crucial under conditions where ChE and/or AChE activities are essential for undefined developmental processes: one may postulate a situation where a developing cell producing sufficient quantities of active cholinesterases will survive under exposure to such poisons, while cells or organisms with defects in the expression of cholinesterases may not.

Exposure to metabolically poisonous materials which are primarily aimed to destroy developing or rapidly dividing cells is a common paradigm in chemotherapy. A well-known example is the use of methotrexate, an inhibitor of the enzyme dihydrofolate reductase, DHFR, in the treatment of leukemia. The cytotoxic effect of methotrexate depends, however, on the ability of the drug to block DHFR activity completely. Under conditions of overproduction of DHFR cells may therefore divide even in the presence of high methotrexate concentrations. One way in which cells become overproducers of DHFR and resistant to methotrexate cytotoxicity is by amplification of the DHFR gene (Schimke, 1984).

The discovery of DHFR gene amplification led to many further studies of controlled exposure to cytotoxic inhibitors, and it was found that in many such cases the genes encoding the target proteins of these inhibitors amplified, creating resistance to the toxic effects. It is generally assumed that gene amplification occurs spontaneously, with higher frequency in transcriptionally active genes and dividing cells. Under conditions where the amplification of a particular gene will provide the cell in which it occurred with a survival advantage over other cells, the amplified DNA will become inheritable. Thus drug-resistant cell lines were developed with progressive increases in DHFR (or other genes) copy numbers (Stark, 1986; reviewed by Soreq and Zakut, 1990a,b).

As stated above, we believe that cholinesterase activities are essential for the well-being of various developing cells. Under exposure to cholinesterase inhibitors, such cells may become analogous to leukemic cells treated with methotrexate, and it is conceivable that the cholinesterase genes amplify in these cells and provide them with a survival advantage over cells with non-amplified cholinesterase genes.

The commonly used organophosphorous (OP) agricultural insecticides are effective cholinesterase inhibitors, which are toxic to the human enzymes as well (Koelle, 1972). Particularly vulnerable to these poisons are individuals with genetic ChE defects, a relatively common trait in Israel (Szeinberg et al., 1972). The serum ChE in these individuals displays low or abnormal catalytic activities and insensitivity to specific ChE inhibitors, for example Dibucaine (Whittaker, 1986). When exposed to OP poisons, such people fulfil both prerequisites for the appearance of ChE gene amplification: acute ChE inhibition on one hand and its requirement for growth on the other. Fig. 2 presents an example for a family pedigree of such individuals and the ChE activities measured in them (see also Prody et al., 1989; Soreq and Zakut, 1990a). Two members in this family presented ChE gene amplifications: one of the sons, M.I., and one of his own sons, O.F. In contrast, the parents (M.O. and R.U.) had normal copy numbers of ChE genes. Gene mapping by in situ hybridization has further demonstrated that the amplified ChE sequences were localized in the 3q26-ter position, either indicating that the amplification occurred in loco, where we have previously mapped the original site of this gene (Soreq et al., 1987b; Zakut et al., 1989) or suggesting that it was inserted therein. Fig. 3 presents a

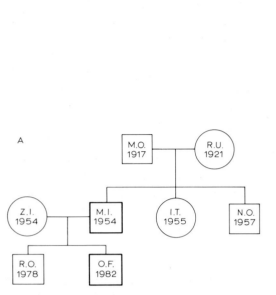

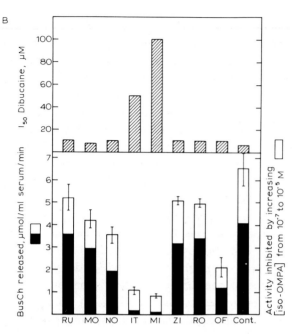

Fig. 2. A: the H family pedigree and birth dates. B: butyrylcholinesterase catalytic activities were measured spectrophotometrically by following butyrylthiocholine (Busch) hydrolysis as described (Prody et al., 1989), in the absence or presence of iso-OMPA (tetraisopropyl pyrophosphoramide) or Dibucaine (2-butyoxy-N-(2-diethylaminoethyl)-4-quinoline carboxamide).

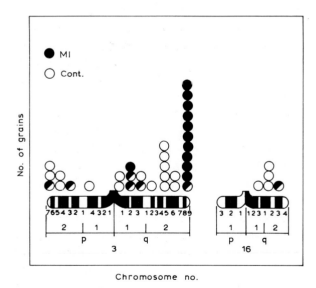

Fig. 3. In situ hybridization with M.I. and control chromosomes was done as described (Soreq et al., 1987b). Cumulative number of silver grains for 21 chromosome spreads from each sample is presented.

schematic distribution of the gene mapping results.

To initiate structural analysis of the amplified ChE genes DNA blot hybridization was employed. Fig. 4 presents a representative DNA blot with M.I.'s and M.O.'s DNAs. Enzymatic restriction followed by blot hybridization reproducibly revealed irregular positions for EcoRI sites spanning the amplified fragment in M.I.'s DNA, resulting in hybridizable bands of variable sizes. In contrast, HindIII restriction yielded a single 2.7 kb long amplified band. Finally, a 1.4 kb TaqI fragment from the central part of the coding region was considerably more amplified than the external, smaller TaqI fragments. Altogether, this analysis indicated an initial onion-skin amplification event (Schimke, 1984), creating a tandemly repeated core amplification unit which contains HindIII and TaqI sites and with EcoRI sites being external to this core unit.

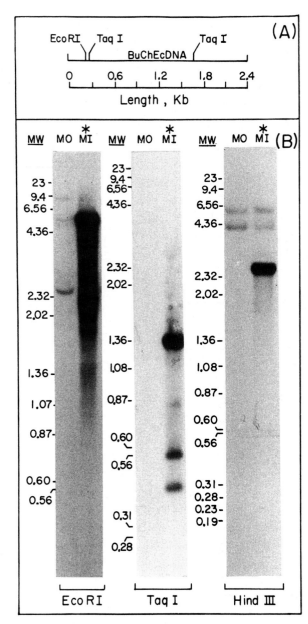

Fig. 4. A: BuChEcDNA contains one and two EcoRI and TaqI restriction sites, respectively. B: DNA blot hybridization was performed as described (Prody et al., 1987). Exposure was for 1 week.

on the origin of this unprecedented phenomenon in humans, and it remains to be proved whether OP exposure can be implicated in it. In addition, the first finding of amplified ChE genes in humans raised the question whether this is a unique, exceptional event or whether it reflects a recurrent phenomenon. Also, we postulated that the AChE genes should be subject to the same survival pressures under OP exposure, and wished to find out whether these genes amplify as well. Finally, we knew that both genes are transiently expressed in embryonic development and display particularly high levels of expression in various malignant tumors. Therefore, further amplification cases were pursued in tumors in which the Chr. 3q26-ter position, where the ChE gene resides, tends to break frequently. This survey was based on the assumption that gene amplification could be a putative origin for such breakage (see, for example, reports on breaks in Chr. 7 at the position of the amplified EGFR-erb2 oncogene in glioblastomas (Libermann et al., 1985)).

Breaks in the long arm of chromosome No. 3 appear repeatedly in leukemias (Pintado et al., 1985). This happens in patients with rapid progress of the disease and abnormal platelet counts, which implies defects in promegakaryocytopoiesis (Bernstein et al., 1985). Because of the previous publications implicating cholinesterases in this hemocytopoietic process (Paulus et al., 1981), we examined DNA from patients with leukemias and/or platelet disorders for ChE and AChE gene amplification. Four out of 16 samples of leukemic DNAs and 3 out of 5 from patients with platelet disorders were found to have 10–200 copies of both these genes (Lapidot-Lifson et al., 1989). This raised the question whether the co-amplification of cholinesterase genes in hemopoietic cells could be linked with enhanced production of their protein products and be involved in the etiology of hemocytopoietic disorders (Soreq and Zakut, 1990b).

In order to pursue further the putative correlation between cholinesterase gene amplification and overexpression, we searched for parallel phenom-

To become inheritable, the amplification of ChE genes should occur in germ cells. Logical candidates are developing sperm cells, where ChE activities are known to be expressed (Sastri and Sadavongviad, 1979). However, one can only speculate

Chromosomal Aberrations in Ovarian Carcinoma

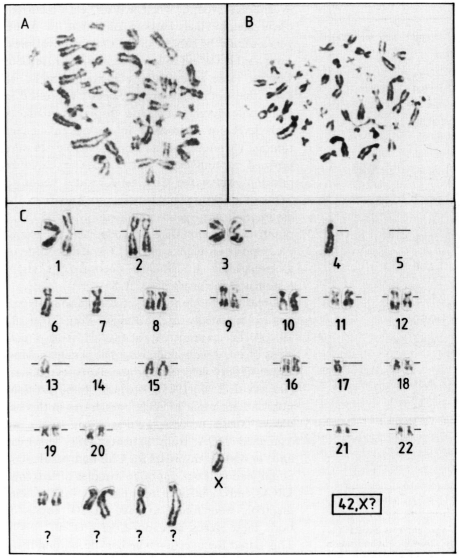

Fig. 5. Chromosome spreads and a representative partial karyotype from an ovarian papillary adenocarcinoma tumor. Chromosomes were prepared from a papillary adenocarcinoma tumor essentially as described elsewhere (Zakut et al., 1989a,b). Briefly, tissue samples were treated immediately following operation with 10 ml/50 mg tissue of RPMI 1640 medium (Gibco) containing 10 IU/ml of Heparin as well as penicillin, streptomycin and neomycin (Biolabs, 1:1000). Minced tissue was transferred into 3 ml of fresh RPMI medium containing 20% fetal calf serum and 4 mg/ml colcemid for 60 min at 37°C with 5% CO_2. Medium was replaced by 0.8% sodium citrate for 15 min at 37°C for hypotonic treatment. Chromosomes were fixed by two successive 10-min incubations in methanol:acetic acid mixture (3:1, V/V). Cells were dissociated in 60% glacial acetic acid and spreads were manually dropped onto glass slides. Chromosomes were then G-banded, photographed and cut for karyotype analysis. A, B: two unrelated spreads showing prominent chromosomal aberrations. C: Karyotype analysis of A. Note that either one or two of the chromosomes 4–7, 13, 14, X and 17 are missing, whereas six unidentifiable chromosomes appeared, probably the results of translocations and deletions.

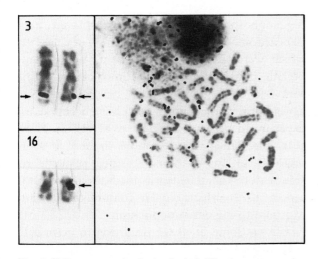

Fig. 6. ChE gene mapping by in situ hybridization onto ovarian carcinoma chromosomes. Chromosome spreads were prepared as in Fig. 5 and subjected to in situ hybridization with [^{35}S]ChEcDNA as detailed previously (Soreq et al., 1987b; Zakut et al., 1989b). Exposure was for 12 days. Note labeling of both chromosomes No. 3 and on one chromosome No. 16 (left) and abnormalities in karyotype.

ena in ovarian carcinomas. It has long been known that cholinesterases are intensively expressed in these tumors (Drews, 1975). Using in situ and blot hybridization, we could show that co-amplification of the ChE and AChE genes was correlated with their overexpression in ovarian carcinomas (Malinger, 1986; Zakut et al., 1990).

Localization of specific genes in chromosomes from malignant tumors is generally rather difficult due to the appearance of multiple chromosomal aberrations in tumor cells. When cells from ovarian tumors were grown in culture, we repeatedly detected missing chromosomes as well as abnormally sized and banded tumor-specific chromosomes (Fig. 5). However, the use of in situ hybridization with ChEcDNA permitted the direct localization of the ChE genes in chromosomes 3 and 16 in tumor chromosomes (Fig. 6), in agreement with our previous gene-mapping studies in adult (Soreq

TABLE I

Altered cholinesterases in various human tissues

Source	Alterations in ChE protein	Detected by	Ref.
1. Glioblastoma primary tumors	Overexpression of ChE tetramers	Sucrose gradient centrifugation and biochemical measurements	Razon et al., 1984
2. Meningioma primary tumors	Overexpression of ChE monomers	Sucrose gradient centrifugation and biochemical measurements	Razon et al., 1984
3. Ovarian carcinomas	Overexpression of ChE	Cytochemical staining	Malinger, 1986
4. Serum from patients with various carcinomas	Enzyme dimers sensitive to both BW284C51 and iso-OMPA, selective inhibitors of AChE and ChE, respectively	Sucrose gradient centrifugation and biochemical measurements	Zakut et al., 1988
5. Individuals with postanesthetic apnea	Low catalytic activity, insensitivity to Dibucaine, ChE gene amplification	Biochemical measurements in serum, DNA blot hybridization	Prody et al., 1989
6. cDNA libraries from glioblastoma and neuroblastoma	Asp70 → Gly Ser425 → Pro	cDNA sequencing	Gnatt et al., 1990
7. Ovarian carcinomas	Focal intense sites of production	1) Immunocytochemical 2) Cytochemical 3) In situ hybridization	Zakut et al., 1989b; Drews, 1975
8. Leukemias and platelet disorders	Potential overproduction from amplified genes	DNA blot hybridization	Lapidot–Lifson et al., 1989

et al., 1987b) and fetal chromosomes (Zakut et al., 1989).

ChE/AChE gene amplification was observed in each ovarian tumor sample where the RAF1 or SIS oncogenes were amplified. Moreover, several of these primary tumors displayed amplified ChE/AChE genes although none of the examined oncogene probes detected an amplified signal (Zakut et al., 1990). Further experiments will be required to determine whether cholinesterase gene amplification occurs earlier than that of oncogenes in the course of tumor progression.

Discussion

Variable modes of expression and gene amplification were observed for cholinesterases in multiple types of human developing and tumor tissue. Table 1 presents examples of such alterations. Altogether, these studies indicate an involvement of this family of proteins in cell division and/or growth mechanisms. In view of parallel studies on the amplification of genes producing target proteins to cytotoxic inhibitors, this raises the question whether organophosphorous poisons could induce selection pressure for cholinesterase gene amplifications.

A considerable body of information, accumulated over the years, demonstrates the cytotoxic and mitogenic effects of organophosphorous poisons. Pesticide-induced DNA damage and repair processes were shown by several research groups in cultured human cells (Ahmed et al., 1977; Alam et al., 1976; Belvins et al., 1976). Sister chromatid exchange and cell cycle delay were further demonstrated in cultured mammalian cells treated with eight different organophosphorous insecticides (Chen et al., 1981), including the common agricultural insecticide malathion (Nicholas et al., 1979). Animal studies have, in parallel, shown similar effects in vivo, in the mouse (Degraeve and Moutschen, 1983), guinea pig (Dikshith, 1973) and rat (Martson and Voronina, 1976). Damaging effects of organophosphorous poisons were also found in humans: workers producing

organophosphorous insecticides displayed transient chromosome aberrations (Kiraly et al., 1979), which were also found in patients under acute organic phosphate insecticide intoxication (Trinh Van Bao et al., 1974) and in lymphocytes from agricultural workers during extensive occupational exposure to pesticides (Yoder et al., 1973). However, the damage may not be limited to these high-risk groups of humans, since pesticide residues were found in basic food products (FAO report, 1979), which implies continuous subacute exposure to the entire population.

Chromosome breakage occurring in germ cells may induce hereditary changes in the affected genes. Organophosphorous insecticides have been shown to inhibit testicular DNA synthesis (Seiler, 1977) and induce sperm abnormalities in mice (Wyrobek and Bruce, 1975), findings which may explain the hereditary ChE gene amplification in the organophosphorous-exposed H family (Prody et al., 1989). Animal studies have demonstrated that methyl parathion administration suppressed growth and induced ossification in both mice and rats, as well as high mortality and cleft palate in the mouse (reviewed by Soreq and Zakut, 1990a). In humans, malformations of the extremities and fetal death were correlated with exposure to methyl parathion in 18 cases (Ogi et al., 1965). In addition, a neonatal lethal syndrome of multiple malformations was reported in women exposed to unspecified insecticides during early pregnancy (Hall et al., 1980). All of these findings most probably reflect the impairment of developmental function(s) of cholinesterases by these poisons, and may be related to ChE and AChE gene amplifications and chromosome breakage in these individuals.

The molecular mechanism leading to cholinesterase gene amplifications is not yet clear. It is possible that the ChE and AChE genes contain internal origins of replication, making them appropriate subjects for gene amplification, and that this explains the overexpression of these genes in brain tumors as well (Razon et al., 1984) and the modified ChE properties which we have found in carcinomas (Zakut et al., 1988). Further studies should be performed to examine whether such alterations are correlated with the occurrence of the "silent" or the "atypical" cholinesterase phenotypes and with the appearance of ChE/AChE gene co-amplification, to determine the scope and abundance of this phenomenon in various tumors and to examine whether exposure to additional ecological poisons induces similar amplifications in other human genes.

Assuming a relationship between the exposure to organophosphorous insecticides and cholinesterase gene amplifications implies a fundamental importance for cholinergic responses in cell division and growth, as well as in reproduction and embryogenesis. This assumption is strongly supported by recent findings demonstrating the stimulation of DNA synthesis in brain-derived cells exposed to acetylcholine analogues (Ashkenazi et al., 1989). In this system, the response occurred in fetal and neonate astrocytes and depended on the expression of specific muscarinic receptor subtypes and the hydrolysis of phosphatidyl inositol. Similar induction of DNA synthesis may occur in other cell types under exposure to organophosphorous insecticides. These block acetylcholine hydrolysis by covalently intereacting with cholinesterases and thus induce increased concentrations of the G-protein-linked neurotransmitter. It has previously been shown that acetylcholine analogues induce phosphatidyl inostol hydrolysis in *Xenopus* oocytes (reviewed by Seidman and Soreq, 1990) and promegakaryocytopoiesis in mouse bone marrow cultures (reviewed by Soreq and Zakut, 1990b). The findings presented in this report suggest that cholinergic intercellular communication may play a pivotal role in developing cells, in addition to its important function in communicating between cholinergic neurons and in neuromuscular junctions.

Acknowledgements

Supported by Contract DAMD 17-87-C-7169 (to H.S.) and by the Research Fund at the Edith Wolfson Medical Center (to H.Z.). Thanks to L. Milner for the secretarial work.

References

Ahmed, F., Hart, R. and Lewis, N. (1977) Pesticide induced DNA damage and its repair in cultured human cells. *Mutat. Res.*, 42: 161–174.

Alan, M. and Kasatiya, S. (1976) Cytological effects of an organic phosphate pesticide on human cells in vitro. *Can. J. Cytol.*, 18: 665–671.

Ashkenazi, A., Ramachandran, J. and Capon, D.J. (1989) Acetylcholine analogue stimulates DNA synthesis in brain-derived cells via specific muscarinic receptor subtypes. *Nature*, 340: 146–150.

Ayalon, A., Zakut, H., Prody, C.A. and Soreq, H. (1990) Preferential transcription of acetylcholinesterase over butyrylcholinesterase mRNAs in fetal human cholinergic neurons. In A.M. Giuffrida-Stella (Ed.), *Gene Expression in the Nervous System*. Alan R. Liss, New York, in press.

Bernstein, R., Pinto, M.R., Behr, A.S. and Mendelow, B. (1982) Chromosome abnormalities in acute nonlymphocytic leukemia (ANLL) with abnormal thrombopoiesis: Report of three patients with a "new" inversion anomaly and a further case of homologous translocation. *Blood*, 60: 613–617.

Blevins, R., Lijinsky, W. and Regan, J.M. (1977) Nitrosated methylcarbamate insecticides: effect on the DNA of human cells. *Mutat. Res.*, 44: 1–7.

Burstein, S.A., Adamson J.W. and Harker, L.A. (1980) Megakaryocytopoiesis in culture: Modulation by cholinergic mechanisms. *J. Cell Physiol.*, 103: 201–208.

Chen, H., Hsueh, J., Sirianni, S. and Huang, C. (1981) Induction of sister chromatid exchanges and cell cycle delay in cultured mammalian cells treated with eight organophosphorous insecticides. *Mutat. Res.*, 88: 307–316.

Degraeve, N. and Moutschen, J. (1983) Genotoxicity of an organophosphorous insecticide, dimethoate, in the mouse. *Mutat. Res.*, 119: 331–337.

Dikshith, T. (1973) In vivo effects of Parathion on Guinea pig chromosomes. *Environ. Physiol. Biochem.*, 3: 161–168.

Drews, U. (1985) Cholinesterase in embryonic development. *Prog. Histochem. Cytochem.*, 7: 1–52.

Dreyfus, P.A., Seidman, S., Pincon-Raymond, M., Murawsky, M., Rieger, F., Schejter, E., Zakut, H. and Soreq, H. (1989) Tissue-specific processing and polarized compartmentalization of clone-produced cholinesterase in microinjected *Xenopus* oocytes. *Mol. Cell Neurobiol.*, 9: 323–341.

Food and Agriculture Organization of the United States (F.A.O.). (1979) Pesticide residues in food. FAO Plant production and protection paper. *IS Rev.*, 27: 379–392.

Gnatt, A., Prody, C.A., Zamir, R., Liemann-Hurwitz, J., Zakut, H. and Soreq, H. (1990) Expression of alternatively terminated unusual CHEmRNA transcripts mapping to chromosomal 3q26-ter in nervous system tumors. *Cancer Res.*, 50: 1983–1987.

Hall, J.G., Pallister, P.D., Clarren, S.K., Beckwith, J.B., Wiglesworth, F.W., Fraser, F.C., Cho, S., Benke, P.J., Reed,

S.D. (1980) Congenital hypothalamic hamartoblastoma, hypopituitarism, imperforate anus, and postaxial polydactly–a new syndrome? Part I: Clinical, causal and pathogenetic considerations. *Am. J. Med. Genet.,* 7: 47–74.

Kiraly, J., Szentesi, I., Ruzicska, M. and Czeizel, A. (1979) Chromosome studies in workers producing organophosphate insecticides. *Arch. Environ. Contamin. Toxicol.,* 8: 309–319.

Koelle, G.B. (1972) In L.S. Goodman and A. Gilman (Eds.), *Anticholinesterase agents.* MacMillan, New York, pp. 445–466.

Layer, P.G and Sporns, O. (1987) Spatiotemporal relationship of embryonic cholinesterases with cell proliferation in chicken brain and eye. *Proc. Natl. Acad. Sci. USA,* 84: 284–288.

Layer, P.G., Alber, R. and Sporns, O. (1987) Quantitative development and molecular forms of acetyl- and butyrylcholinesterase during morphogenesis and synaptogenesis of chicken brain and retina. *J. Neurochem.,* 49: 175–182.

Lapidot-Lifson, Y., Prody, C.A., Ginzberg, D., Meytes, D., Zakut, H. and Soreq, H. (1989) Co-amplification of human acetylcholinesterase and butyrylcholinesterase genes in blood cells: correlation with various leukemias and abnormal megakaryocytopoiesis. *Proc. Natl. Acad. Sci. USA,* 86: 4715–4719, 1989.

Libermann, T.A., Nusbaum, H.R., Razon, N., Kris, R., Lax, I., Soreq, H., Whittle, N., Waterfield, M.D., Ullrich, A., Schlessinger, J. (1985) Amplification, enhanced expression and possible rearrangement of EGF-receptor gene in primary human brain tumors of glial origin. *Nature (Lond.),* 313: 144–147.

Malinger, G., Zakut, H. and Soreq, H. (1989) Cholinoceptive properties of human primordial, pre-antral and antral oocytes: In situ hybridization and biochemical evidence for expression of cholinesterase genes. *J. Mol. Neurosci.,* 1: 77–84.

Malinger, G. (1986) Basic Science Thesis: Expression of human cholinesterase genes in normal and malignant ovary. Weizmann Institute of Science, Rehovot, Israel.

Martson, L. and Voronina, V. (1976) Experimental study of the effect of a series of phosphoroorganic pesticides (Dipterex and Imidan) on embryogenesis. *Environ. Health Perspect.,* 13: 121–125.

Nicholas, A., Vienne, M. and Van Den Berghe, H. (1979) Induction of sister chromatid exchanges in cultured human cells by an organophosphorus insecticide: malathion. *Mutat. Res.,* 67: 167–172.

Ogi, D. and Hamada, A. (1965) Case reports on fetal deaths and malformations of extremities probably related to insecticide poisoning. *J. Jpn. Obstet. Gynecol. Soc.,* 17: 569.

Paulus, J.P., Maigen, J. and Keyhani, E. (1981) Mouse megakaryocytes secrete acetylcholinesterase. *Blood,* 58: 1100–1106.

Prody, C.A., Gnatt, A., Zevin-Sonkin, D., Goldberg, O., Soreq, H. (1987) Isolation and characterization of full-length cDNA clones coding for cholinesterase from fetal human tissues. *Proc. Natl. Acad. Sci. USA,* 84: 3555–3559.

Prody, C.A., Dreyfus, P., Zamir, R., Zakut, H. and Soreq, H.

(1989) De novo amplification within a "silent" human cholinesterase gene in a family subjected to prolonged exposure to organophosphorous insecticides. *Proc. Natl. Acad. Sci. USA,* 86: 690–694.

Pintado, T., Ferro, M.T., San Roman, C., Mayayo, M. and Larana, J.G. (1985) Clinical correlations of the 3q21;q26 cytogenetic anomaly: a leukemic or myelodysplastic syndrome with preserved or increased platelet production and lack of response to cytotoxic drug therapy. *Cancer,* 55: 535–541.

Rakonczay, Z. and Brimijoin S. (1988) Biochemistry and pathophysiology of the molecular forms of cholinesterases. In J.R. Harris (Ed.), *Subcellular Biochemistry, Vol. 12,* Plenum Press, New York, pp. 378.

Razon, N., Soreq, H., Roth, E., Bartal, A., Silman, I. (1984) Characterization of levels and forms of cholinesterases in human primary brain tumors. *Exp. Neurol.,* 84: 681–695.

Sastry, B.V.R., Sadavongviad, C. (1979) Cholinergic systems in non-nervous tissues. *Pharmacol. Rev.,* 39: 65–132.

Schimke, R.T. (1984) Gene amplification in cultured animal cells. *Cell,* 37: 705–713.

Seidman, S. and Soreq., H. (1990) Co-injection of Xenopus oocytes with cDNA-produced and native mRNAs: a Molecular Biological approach to the tissue specific processing of human cholinesterases. *Int. Rev. Neurobiol.,* in press.

Seiler, J. (1977) Inhibition of testicular DNA synthesis by chemical mutagens and carcinogens. *Mutat. Res.,* 46: 305–310.

Soreq, H. and Gnatt, A. (1987) Molecular biological search for human genes encoding cholinesterases. *Mol. Neurobiol.,* 1:47–80.

Soreq, H. and Prody, C. (1989) Sequence similarities between human acetylcholinesterase and related proteins: Putative implications for therapy of anticholinesterase intoxication. In A. Golombek and T. Rein (Eds.), *Computer-Assisted Modeling of Receptor-Ligand Interactions, Theoretical Aspects and Applications to Drug Design.* Alan R Liss, New York, pp. 347–359.

Soreq, H. and Zakut, H. (1990a) Amplification of acetylcholinesterase and butyrylcholinesterase genes in normal and tumor tissues: Putative relationship to organophosphorous poisoning. *Pharm. Res.,* 7: 1–7.

Soreq, H. and Zakut, H. (1990b) *Cholinesterase genes: multileveled regulation. Monographs in Human Genetics, Vol. 13,* Karger, Basel.

Soreq, H., Malinger, G. and Zakut, H. (1987a) Expression of cholinesterase genes in developing human oocytes revealed by in situ hybridization. *Hum. Reprod.,* 2: 689–693.

Soreq, H., Zamir, R., Zevin-Sonkin, D. and Zakut, H. (1987b) Human cholinesterase genes localized by hybridization to chromosomes 3 and 16. *Hum. Genet.,* 77: 325–328.

Soreq, H., Seidman, S., Dreyfus, P.A., Zevin-Sonkin, D. and Zakut, H. (1989) Expression and tissue-specific assembly of human butyrylcholinesterase in microinjected *Xenopus* oocytes. *J. Biol. Chem.,* 264: 10608–10613.

Stark, G.R. (1986) DNA amplification in drug resistant cells and tumors. *Cancer Surv.,* 5: 1–23.

Szeinberg, A., Pipano, S., Assa, M., Medalie, J.H. and Neufeld,

H.N. (1972) High frequency of atypical pseudo-cholinesterase gene among Iraqi and Iranian Jews. *Clin. Genet.,* 3: 123–127.

Toutant, J.P. and Massoulie, J. (1987) Acetylcholinesterase. In A.J. Kenny and A.J. Turner (Eds.), *Mammalian Ectoenzymes,* Elsevier, Amsterdam, pp. 298–328.

Trinh Van Bao, Szabo, I., Ruzicska, P. and Czeizel, A. (1974) Chromosome aberrations in patients suffering acute organic phosphate insecticide intoxication. *Hum. Genet.,* 24: 33–57.

Whittaker, M. (1986) *Cholinesterase: Monographs in Human Genetics, Vol. 11,* Basel, Karger.

Wyrobek, A. and Bruce, W. (1975) Chemical induction of sperm abnormalities in mice. *Proc. Natl. Acad. Sci. USA,* 72: 4425–4429.

Yoder, J., Watson, M. and Benson, W. (1973) Lymphocyte chromosome analysis of agricultural workers during extensive occupational exposure to pesticides. *Mutat. Res.,* 21: 335–340.

Zakut, H., Matzkel, A., Schejter, E., Avni, A. and Soreq, H. (1985) Polymorphism of acetylcholinesterase in discrete regions of the developing fetal brain. *J. Neurochem.,* 45: 382–389.

Zakut, H., Even, L., Birkenfeld, S., Malinger, G., Zisling, R. and Soreq, H. (1988) Modified properties of serum cholinesterase in carcinoma patients. *Cancer,* 61: 727–739.

Zakut, H., Ehrlich, G., Ayalon, A., Prody, C.A., Malinger, G., Seidman, S., Kehlenbach, R. and Soreq, H. (1990) Acetylcholinesterase and butyrylcholinesterase genes co-amplify in primary ovarian carcinomas. *J. Clin. Invest.,* in press.

Zakut, H., Zamir, R., Sindel, L. and Soreq, H. (1989) Gene mapping on chorionic villi chromosomes by hybridization in situ: localization of cholinesterase cDNA binding sites to chromosomes 3q21, 3q26-ter and 16q21. *Hum. Reprod.,* 4: 941–946.

SECTION II

Cholinergic Mechanisms in the Peripheral Nervous System

A: Neuromuscular Transmission

S.-M. Aquilonius and P.-G. Gillberg (Eds.)
Progress in Brain Research, Vol. 84
© 1990 Elsevier Science Publishers B.V. (Biomedical Division)

CHAPTER 7

Spontaneous synaptic activity at developing neuromuscular junctions

Nacira Tabti and Mu-ming Poo *

Department of Biological Sciences, Columbia University, New York, NY 10027, U.S.A.

Introduction

Spontaneous synaptic activity occurs early in development. In *Xenopus* embryo, spontaneous synaptic potential can be detected in the muscle cell within hours after the motor axon leaves the spinal cord (Blackshaw and Warner, 1976; Kullberg et al., 1977). This early synaptic activity is responsible for the early embryonic motility which characterizes many vertebrate embryos (Hamburger and Balaban, 1963). Several lines of evidence suggest that early synaptic activity plays an important role in the maturation of synaptic connections and the differentiation of muscle fibers. Elimination of poly-neuronal innervation is delayed by blocking synaptic activity (Thompson et al., 1979). Muscle-fiber-type transformation is strongly influenced by the pattern of neuronal activity impinging upon it (Salmons and Sreter, 1976). Metabolism of muscle cell and the expression of synaptic components, including acetylcholine (ACh) receptors and acetylcholinesterases, are regulated by the electrical activity of the muscle cells (Schutze and Role, 1987). In this paper we summarize results from recent work on the physiological and morphological basis of the early synaptic activity, with a focus on the spontaneous transmitter secretion, which is the predominant

activity during the first few days of nerve–muscle contact. Cultured *Xenopus* nerve and muscle cells were used in these studies.

Synaptic transmission during the early phase of synaptogenesis

Recent studies in cell culture have shown that cholinergic neurons are capable of secreting transmitter prior to their contact with the target cell (Hume et al., 1983; Young and Poo, 1983; Sun and Poo, 1987). Growth cone secretion of ACh is similar to evoked ACh release at mature neuromuscular junctions in many aspects: the nerve-evoked release is abolished in the absence of external Ca^{2+} or by addition of 10 mM Co^{2+} and it exhibits post-tetanic potentiation (Sun and Poo, 1987). The existence of an efficient mechanism for transmitter secretion at the growth cone implies that embryonic spinal neurons are ready for immediate establishment of synaptic transmission with the skeletal muscle cell. By manipulating a whole-cell clamped spherical myocyte into contact with the growth cone of a neuron and supplying suprathreshold stimuli to the soma, evoked synaptic currents could be elicited as soon as the nerve–muscle contact was made. Fig. 1 illustrates the early synaptic activity observed in a 1-d-old culture. The evoked transmitter release was completely abolished in the absence of external Ca^{2+}, while spontaneous release still persisted.

---

* To whom correspondence should be addressed.

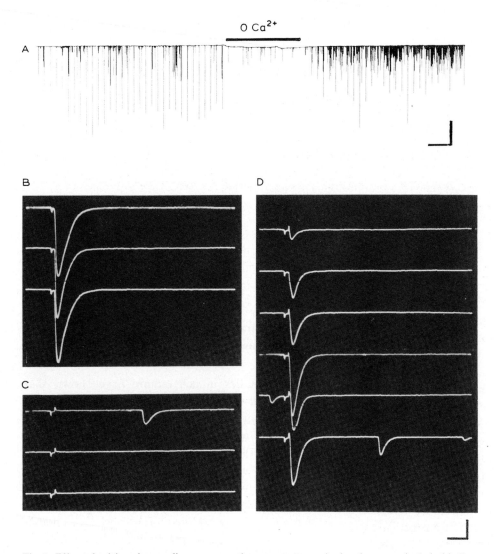

Fig. 1. Effect of calcium-free medium on synaptic currents at manipulated synapse in 1-d-old *Xenopus* nerve muscle co-culture. The soma was stimulated at 0.10 Hz and evoked as well as spontaneous end-plate activity was recorded from the myoball with the whole-cell voltage clamp technique (holding potential −70 mV). (A) Note the reduction in synaptic currents during perfusion with calcium-free medium. Scale: 40 s and 500 pA. (B–D) Samples of synaptic currents before, during and after the perfusion, respectively. Note the total absence of evoked response in Ca^{2+}-free medium, but the persistence of spontaneous activity. Scale: 10 ms, 500 pA. (Adapted from Evers et al., 1989.)

Despite the demonstration of efficient evoked synaptic transmission at early phase of synaptogenesis in culture, it is still unknown whether or how much neuronal activity occurs at this early stage of development in vivo. Studies in cell culture, however, have demonstrated the presence of spontaneous synaptic activity at the developing nerve–muscle synapses. Because of the high input resistance of developing muscle cell, early spontaneous potentials (miniature endplate potentials, MEPPs) are relatively large in amplitude, and many of them lead to firing of action potentials and muscle contraction. Thus propagated electrical activity in the developing muscle fiber does not require the presence of neuronal activity and spontaneous transmitter release from the neuron

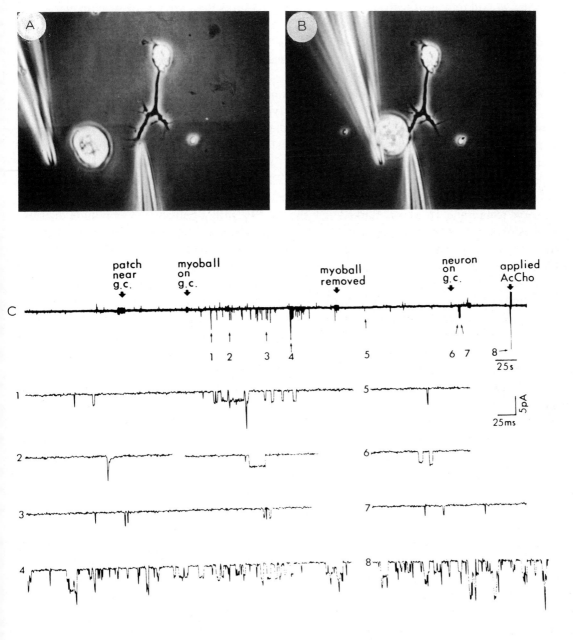

Fig. 2. Induction of ACh release from *Xenopus* growth cone by myoball contact. (A) An excised patch of muscle membrane (ACh probe) was used to detect ACh release by the appearance of single channel currents. The phase-contrast photograph shows the ACh probe positioned near the growth cone. (B) The myoball was manipulated into contact with the growth cone while the ACh probe remained at the same site. (C) Tracings of the patch membrane current (inward current downward) recorded at a holding potential of −80 mV. The first tracing represents continuous recordings (at low sweep speed) showing the entire course of the experiment. Tracings 1 to 8 show samples of single channel events recorded at higher time resolution. Notice that (i) little channel activity was observed before myoball contact, (ii) the myoball but not the neuron was effective in triggering ACh release, (iii) at the end of the experiment (tracing 8), a test of ACh sensitivity of the myoball was performed by exogenous application of ACh. (Adapted from Xie and Poo, 1986.)

may exert a dominant influence on muscle activity. In the following we will only deal with spontaneous transmitter release, with a focus on the cellular mechanisms responsible for the induction and regulation of ACh release.

Induction of spontaneous acetylcholine secretion

Before the contact with the muscle cell, spontaneous secretion of ACh from the growth cone is a rare event. Excised, outside-out muscle membrane patch (ACh probe) detected little extracellular ACh if care was taken to avoid contact of the probe with the nerve membrane. However, marked ACh secretion was observed as soon as the probe touched the nerve membrane. This ACh secretion was induced specifically by muscle contact, since contact with a clean glass pipet or a neuronal surface is not effective (Xie and Poo, 1986). As shown in Fig. 2, when a muscle cell was manipulated into contact with the growth cone, there was an immediate appearance of spontaneous release of ACh from the growth cone. Persistent spontaneous ACh release during the initial period of the contact apparently depends upon the constant presence of the muscle surface, since the release ceased as soon as the muscle cell was removed. It seems that the ACh release was triggered by the physical contact with some muscle surface specific component, since contact with the neuron was much less effective. Ultrastructural studies (see below) showed that the spacing between the nerve and muscle cells at the initial contact site is extremely narrow (< 10 nm): direct molecular interaction between components on the opposing surfaces is thus likely. Such interaction could trigger opening of Ca^{2+} channels in the nerve membrane, leading to spontaneous secretion. During the first day of contact, however, the synaptic cleft is formed and the basal lamina is deposited between the nerve and muscle membranes, preventing direct molecular interactions between membrane-bound components. At this more mature state of the synapse, the muscle's inductive role may be replaced by basal lamina material; or

alternatively, the spontaneous ACh release no longer requires the presence of specific extracellular interaction.

Regulation of spontaneous transmitter secretion

It is now well established that at least two different types of spontaneous quantal release co-exist at the adult vertebrate neuromuscular junction (Thesleff and Molgo, 1983). Both types of release give rise to discrete end-plate depolarizations (MEPPs), which can be distinguished by their rise time and their amplitude distribution. The fast-rising MEPPs with a bell-shaped amplitude distribution represent the main population of spontaneous events. These MEPPs are modulated by intraterminal Ca^{2+}. The slow-rising MEPPs, so called slow MEPPs (or giant MEPPs), show a skewed amplitude distribution with a large variability. They represent 4–20% of the total spontaneous events recorded at the vertebrate neuromuscular junctions, and are characterized by their calcium-insensitivity. Slow MEPPs are prominent in botulinum-poisoned neuromuscular preparations and during the early stages of skeletal muscle reinnervation. They have been suggested to reflect an embryonic type of transmitter release (Colmeus et al., 1982; Lupa et al., 1986; Thesleff, 1989). Miniature end-plate currents recorded at *Xenopus* neuromuscular synapse during the first few days of synaptogenesis in culture showed a skewed amplitude distribution with a large variability (Xie and Poo, 1986; Fig. 3). It is of interest to determine whether these release events are related to the Ca-insensitive type observed at adult synapses.

The calcium sensitivity of the early spontaneous activity was tested by three different experiments: (1) Changing external Ca^{2+} concentration, (2) depolarizing nerve membrane with high external K^+, and (3) increasing intraterminal Ca^{2+} concentration by the use of a mitochondrial uncoupler of oxidative phosphorylation (carbonyl cyanide *m*-chlorophenylhydrazone, CCCP) which releases Ca^{2+} from the mitochondrial calcium store (Benz and McLaughlin, 1983; Nachsen, 1985;

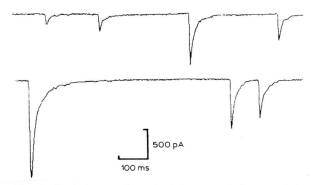

Fig. 3. Typical examples of miniature end-plate currents (MEPCs) recorded with the whole-cell voltage clamp technique from a naturally occurring synapse in a 1-d-old *Xenopus* nerve-muscle culture. Note the variability in the amplitude of these synaptic events.

Molgo and Pecot-Dechavassine, 1988). In the first experiment, media of differing Ca concentrations were introduced into the culture during whole-cell voltage-clamp recording of synaptic activity at an innervated muscle cell (Fig. 4). The mean MEPC frequency ($\pm$ SEM) was calculated for each experimental condition and compared with the respective control by the unpaired Student t-test. We found that raising the Ca^{2+} concentration in the medium from 1.5 to 5.5 mM led to a small but significant increase in the MEPC frequency from 0.099 ± 0.013 to 0.147 ± 0.013 Hz ($p < 0.05$). A further increase to 9.5 mM external Ca^{2+} gave rise to a marked elevation of the MEPC frequency to 1.49 ± 0.17 ($p < 0.001$). However, the elevated release was not sustained and dropped within 15

Fig. 4. Changes in the MEPC frequency induced at *Xenopus* developing synapses by procedures known to increase the intraterminal calcium concentration. MEPCs were recorded with the whole-cell voltage clamp technique (holding potential -80 mV) from 1–2-d-old cultures. Each point corresponds to the MEPC frequency recorded for one minute. (A) Effect of external Ca^{2+} on the frequency of MEPCs recorded from one synapse. C stands for control (1.5 mM Ca^{2+}); the two arrows mark the time at which the concentration of Ca^{2+} was increased to 5.5 and 9.5 mM successively. (B) Effect of high external K^+ (24 mM) on MEPC frequency. (C) Effect of 2 μM carbonyl cyanide *m*-chlorophenylhydrazone (CCCP). Note that in this case recordings started 10 min after the application of CCCP.

min to a level slightly higher than the control level. In the second experiment, K^+ was added to the culture medium for a final concentration of 24 mM during the course of recording. Exposure to

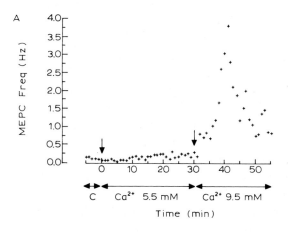

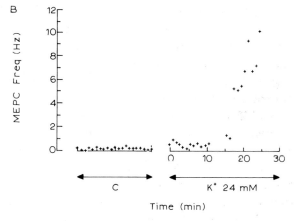

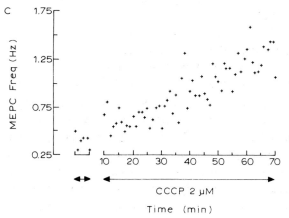

24 mM K^+, which presumably causes a depolarization of the membrane potential of about 45 mV and the opening of voltage-sensitive Ca channels in the plasma membrane, led to a significant increase in the MEPC frequency from 0.205 ± 0.015 to 0.542 ± 0.052 ($p < 0.001$) during the first 10 min and to a marked elevation after 15 min. Similarly, exposure of the culture to CCCP ($2 \mu M$) significantly increased the MEPC frequency from a mean value of 0.393 ± 0.032 to 0.887 ± 0.039 Hz. Moreover, examination of the amplitude distribution of the MEPPs before and after experimental treatments indicated that there was no selective increase of one particular population of the MEPPs. The different procedures used to elevate intraterminal calcium were able to stimulate the spontaneous ACh release responsible for MEPCs at this early synapse. Similar observations were made in 1-h-old synapses, which were made by manipulating muscle cells into contact with the neurons. Taken together, these results suggest that spontaneous secretion in this developing system is predominantly of the Ca-sensitive type. However, quantitative differences are noticed when comparing these results with those reported at the adult neuromuscular junction. In particular, the effect of CCCP was relatively small compared to the tremendous increase (over 100-times the control values) in MEPP frequency induced by this drug at the adult frog NMJ (Molgo and Pecot-Dechavassine, 1988). Finally, we note that the existence of a small population of Ca-insensitive MEPCs at this early *Xenopus* synapse cannot be ruled out.

Besides changing intraterminal Ca^{2+} concentration, the spontaneous secretion of ACh could also be regulated by changing the sensitivity of the secretion mechanism to the Ca^{2+}. This may be illustrated by the action of phorbol ester, which is a potent activator of protein kinase C. Addition of phorbol ester TPA (12-*O*-tetradecanoylphorbol 13-acetate) at a concentration of 20 nM rapidly increases both the frequency and the average amplitudes of the early MEPCs. As shown in Fig. 5A, the elevated secretion after the TPA treatment

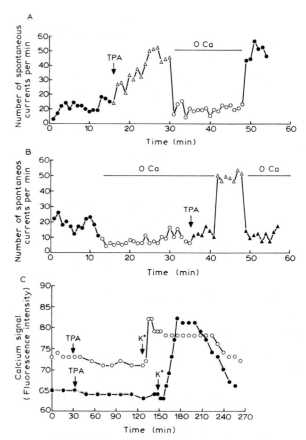

Fig. 5. Potentiation of synaptic activity by phorbol ester TPA. (A) The frequency of MEPCs was increased by addition of 20 mM TPA. The elevated secretion, however, requires the presence of external Ca^{2+}, since Ca^{2+} removal led to immediate reduction of the secretion to control level. (B) In the absence of external Ca^{2+}, TPA treatment produced little enhancement of secretion. However, the drug action was revealed by the marked secretion immediately following return of normal external Ca^{2+} concentration. (C) TPA treatment did not significantly change the cytoplasmic Ca^{2+} level, as indicated by the fluorescent Ca^{2+} indicator Fluo-3/AM. Data are from two separate *Xenopus* neurons loaded with the dye. As a control of the dye sensitivity, high external K^+ (70 mM) was introduced into the culture, and the resulting Ca^{2+} influx was clearly seen.

depends on external Ca^{2+}. When the external Ca^{2+} was removed, the frequency of MEPPs quickly reduced to a level equal to or below that before the TPA treatment. Moreover, when the culture was treated with TPA briefly in the absence of external Ca^{2+}, no significant elevation of secretion was observed until normal Ca^{2+} was restored in the external medium. The simplest interpretation of the potentiation effect of TPA is that activation of C-kinase increases the sensitivity of the Ca^{2+}-dependent secretion mechanism, rather than elevating cytoplasmic Ca^{2+}. Direct measurement of Ca^{2+} signals within the neuron, using the Ca^{2+}-sensitive fluorescence dye Fluo-3/AM (Molecular Probes), also indicated that TPA does not alter the Ca level within the neuron (see Fig. 5C).

In summary, experimental manipulations have revealed that there are at least two direct means of regulating the spontaneous ACh secretion: changing the level of intraterminal Ca^{2+} or changing the Ca^{2+}-sensitivity of the secretion machinery, through modulation of C-kinase activity. The cellular signals involved in triggering these changes during synaptic development and the way in which these signals are developmentally regulated are subjects for future investigation.

Morphology of early synaptic contacts

To delineate cellular processes underlying early synaptic activity, the morphology of the nerve–muscle contact during the first day of synaptogenesis in *Xenopus* culture has been examined with electron microscopy. The precise timing of nerve–muscle contact was achieved by manipulating isolated spherical myocytes into contact with the growth cones of neurites of co-cultured spinal neurons. The contacts were shown to be functional by the recording of nerve-evoked synaptic currents in the muscle cell. A umber of prominent features of the contact area were identified, as summarized in the following, in the sequence of their appearance.

Immediately following the nerve–muscle contact, points of focal contacts were observed between the nerve and muscle cells. These focal contacts are similar in appearance to the focal adhesion sites observed frequently between cultured cells and the substratum. Within tens of minutes, extensive membrane-membrane apposition between the nerve and muscle cell was observed. The apposition shows regular and narrow

spacing of less than 10 nm, suggesting the formation of intercellular bonds between the cells. A few hours after the contact, prominent thickening of muscle membrane appeared at the contact area and patches of extracellular material were found in the synaptic cleft. The latter events seem to correlate with a widening of intercellular spacing between the cells. Despite an extensive search, we were unable to find any sign of presynaptic differentiation during the first few hours of synaptic contact, when stable synaptic transmission has been well established. Fig. 6A shows an example of a 3-h-old nerve–muscle contact. However, presynaptic differentiation, as shown by the clustering of clear vesicles near the presynaptic membrane and formation of distinct basal lamina, was found at contacts which had existed for 12 h or more in these cultures, as shown in Fig. 6B.

Developmental relevance of early spontaneous activity

Two types of postsynaptic effect are expected from the presence of spontaneous synaptic activity at the early phase of synaptogenesis. Many of the spontaneous synaptic potentials are suprathreshold and capable of eliciting propagating action potentials in the muscle cell. The frequency and pattern of action potentials and/or the resulting muscle contractile responses are likely to have an important influence on the muscle metabolism, including differential gene expression and protein synthesis. Kidokoro and Saito (1988) has found that neurite-contacted myocytes, which frequently show spontaneous twitching, developed cross-striations earlier than neighboring non-twitching cells. Electrical and/or contractile activity of the muscle cell has also been shown to regulate the level of AChR mRNA, the synthesis and surface expression of AChR, acetylcholinesterases, and N-CAM (see Schuetze and Role, 1987).

Besides the 'global' influence of the propagation action potentials, there are local effects of subthreshold synaptic potentials. A few percent of the ACh-induced synaptic current is carried by

70

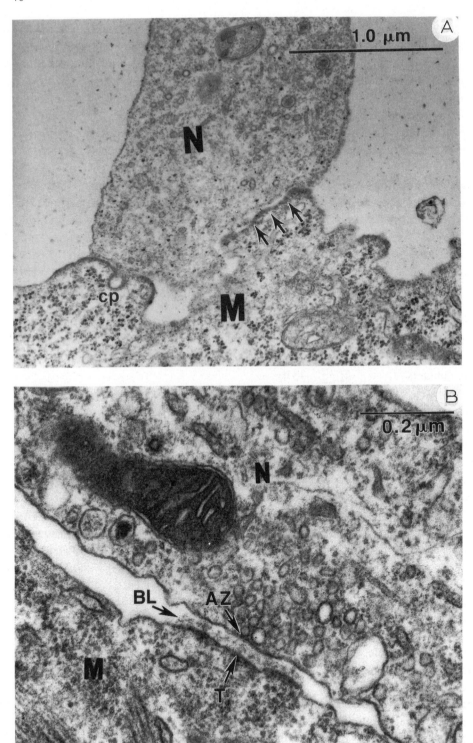

Fig. 6. Ultrastructure of early synapses. (A) A 3-h manipulated neurite-myoball contact, showing the thickening of postsynaptic muscle membrane at contact area and beyond. M, myoball; N, neurite; cp, coated pit. (B) A naturally occurring contact in a 1-d-old culture, showing synaptic differentiation. AZ, active zone. Note clustering of presynaptic vesicles, marked thickening (T) and infolding of the muscle membrane, the widening of the cleft, and the presence of basal lamina (BL). (Adapted from Buchanan et al., 1989.)

Ca^{2+}. Influx of Ca^{2+} at the subsynaptic region of the muscle could trigger a number of Ca^{2+} -dependent enzymatic processes that are important in subsynaptic differentiation, e.g., local gene expression (Merlie and Sanes, 1986), in modulating the properties of synaptic receptors and ion channels, and in regulating the cytoskeletal organization, which may change the synaptic efficacy (Baudry et al., 1988). While direct evidence is lacking, it is likely that neurotrophic molecules are co-released with the spontaneous secretion of ACh. The factors may act locally for differentiation of synaptic structure, e.g., formation of AChR clusters (Nitkin et al., 1987), or globally as a general hormone. Finally, studies of the diffusional and electrokinetic mobilities of cellular components suggest that localized synaptic currents may cause electrokinetic migration of the membrane receptors or cytoplasmic components toward or away from the synaptic site (Fraser and Poo, 1982; Poo and Young, 1989). Such migration may play a role in the activity-dependent synaptic stabilization and synaptic competition.

In conclusion, synaptogenesis begins with the appearance of spontaneous synaptic activity, and the diverse cellular effects that accompany this activity must play important roles during the course of synaptic differentiation and muscle maturation.

Acknowledgements

This work is supported by grants from the National Institute of Health (NS 22764) and the National Science Foundation (BNS 13306).

References

Baudry, M., Larson, J. and Lynch, G. (1988) Long-term changes in synaptic efficacy: potential mechanisms and implications. In P.W. Landfield and S.A. Deadwyler, (Eds.), *Long-Term Potentiation: From Biophysics to Behavior,* Alan R. Liss, New York, pp. 109–138.

Benz, R. and MacLaughlin, S. (1983), The molecular mechanism of action of the proton ionophore FCCP (carbonylcyanide p-trifluoromethoxyphenylhydrazone). *Biophys. J.,* 41: 381–398.

Blackshaw, S.E. and Warner, A.E. (1976) Low resistance junctions between mesoderm cells during development of truck muscles. J. Physiol., 255: 209–230.

Buchanan, J., Sun, Y. and Poo, M.-m. (1989) Studies of nerve-muscle interactions in *Xenopus* cell culture: Morphology of early functional contacts. *J. Nuerosci.,* 9: 1540–1554.

Colmus, C., Gomez, S., Molgo, J. and Thesleff, S. (1982) Discrepancies between spontaneous and evoked potentials at normal, regenerating and botulinum poisoned mammalian neuromuscular junctions. *Proc. R. Soc. B,* 215: 63–74.

Evers, J., Laser, M., Sun, Y., Xie, Z. and Poo, M.-m. (1989) Studies of nerve-muscle interactions in *Xenopus* cell culture: Analysis of early synaptic currents. *J. Neurosci.,* 9: 1523–1539.

Fraser, S. and Poo, M.-m. (1982) Development, maintenance, and modulation of patterned membrane topography. Models based on acetylcholine receptors. *Curr. Top. Dev. Biol.,* 17: 77–100.

Hamburger, V. and Balaban, M. (1963) Observations and experiments on spontaneous rhythmical behavior in the chick embryo. *Dev. Biol.,* 7: 533–545.

Hume, R.I., Role, L.W. and Fischbach, G.D. (1983) Acetylcholine release from growth cones detected with patches of acetylcholine receptor-rich membranes. *Nature,* 305: 632–634.

Kidokoro, Y. and Saito, M. (1988) Early cross-striation formation in twitching *Xenopus* myocytes in culture. *Proc. Natl. Acad. Sci. USA,* 85: 1978–1982.

Lupa, M.T., Tabti, N., Thesleff, S., Vyskocil, F. and Yu, S.P. (1986). The nature and origin of calcium-insensitive miniature end-plate potentials at rodent neuromuscular junction. *J. Physiol (Lond.),* 381: 607–618.

Merlie, J.P. and Sanes, J.R. (1986) Regulation of synapse specific genes. In E. Kandel and R. Levi-Montalcini (Eds.), *Molecular Aspects of Neurobiology,* Springer-Verlag, Berlin/Heidelberg, pp. 72–80.

Molgo, J. and Pecot-Dechavassine, M. (1988) Effect of carbonyl cyanide m-chlorophenylhydrazone (CCCP) on quantal transmitter release and ultrastructure of frog motor nerve terminals. *Neuroscience,* 24: 695–708.

Nachsen, D.A. (1985) Regulation of cytosolic calcium concentration in presynaptic nerve endings isolated from rat brain. *J. Physiol. (Lond.),* 363: 87–101.

Nitkin, R.M., Smith, M.A., Magill, C., Fallon, J.R., Yao, U., Wallace, B.G. and McMahan, U.J. (1987) Identification of agrin, a synaptic organizing protein from Torpedo electric organ, *J. Cell Biol.,* 105: 2471–2478.

Poo, M. and Young, S. (1990) Diffusional and electrokinetic redistribution at the synapse: a physicochemical basis of synaptic competition. *J. Neurobiol.,* 21: 157–168.

Salmons, S. and Sreter, F.A. (1976) Significance of impulse activity in the transformation of skeletal muscle type. *Nature,* 263: 30–34.

Schuetze, S.M. and Role, L.W. (1987) Developmental regulation of nicotinic acetylcholine receptors, *Annu. Rev. Neurosci.* 10: 403–457.

Sun, Y. and Poo, M.-m. (1987) Evoked release of acetylcholine from the growing embryonic neuron. *Proc. Natl. Acad. Sci. USA,* 84: 2540–2544.

Thesleff, S. (1989) Calcium insensitive quantal transmitter release. In L.C. Sellin, R. Libelius, and S. Thesleff (Eds.), *Neuromuscular Junction,* Elsevier, Amsterdam, pp. 189–195.

Thesleff, S. and Molgo (1983) Commentary: a new type of transmitter release at the neuromuscular junction. *Neuroscience,* 9: 1–8.

Thompson, W., Kuffler, D.P. and Jansen, J.K.S. (1979) The effect of prolonged, reversible block of nerve impulses on the elimination of polyneuronal innervation of new-born rat skeletal muscle fibers. *Neuroscience,* 2: 271–281.

Young, S.H. and Poo, M.-m. (1983) Spontaneous release of transmitter from growth cones of embryonic neurons. *Nature,* 305: 634–637.

Xie, Z. and Poo, M.-m. (1986) Initial events in the formation of neuromuscular synapse. *Proc. Natl. Acad. Sci. USA,* 83: 7069–7073.

S.-M. Aquilonius and P.-G. Gillberg (Eds.)
Progress in Brain Research, Vol. 84
© 1990 Elsevier Science Publishers B.V. (Biomedical Division)

CHAPTER 8

The basal lamina and stability of the mammalian neuromuscular junction

Clarke R. Slater

Division of Neurobiology, University of Newcastle upon Tyne, U.K.

Introduction

At the neuromuscular junction (NMJ), vertebrate skeletal muscle fibres are highly specialized to allow an effective response to the acetylcholine (ACh) released from the motor axon terminal by the nerve impulse. The most important molecular feature of this postsynaptic specialization is the accumulation of ACh receptors (AChRs) present in the muscle fibre membrane. The density of AChRs is highest at the tops of the deep infoldings of sarcolemma opposite the sites of ACh release from the nerve (Salpeter, 1987) but falls steeply at the edges of the region of contact with the nerve and within the depths of the folds. So far, it is unclear at a molecular level how this very precise localization of AChRs is brought about and maintained.

Changes in AChR distribution during development

In immature mammalian muscle fibres, AChRs are present over most of the cell surface. Soon after contact with the nerve, AChRs accumulate at the site of nerve-muscle contact (Bevan and Steinbach, 1977). In rats and mice, the diffuse distribution of AChRs within the immature synaptic zone changes during the first 2–3 weeks after birth, and comes to follow closely the contours of the developing motor axon terminal (Steinbach, 1981; Slater, 1982a; Matthews-Bellinger and Salpeter, 1983). During the same period, the

AChRs are lost from the extrajunctional region (Diamond and Miledi, 1962; Bevan and Steinbach, 1977), where their synthesis is suppressed by the activity of the muscle fibre (Scheutze and Role, 1987).

The changes in AChR distribution during development depend on a continuing interaction between the nerve and the muscle. In rats and mice, denervation at birth leads to a dispersal of the synaptic AChR cluster and a failure of further maturation of the postsynaptic specializations (Slater, 1982b). Denervation 2–3 weeks after birth, when the distribution of AChRs is qualitatively mature, results in little change. Thus, during early maturation of the NMJ, the factors governing AChR distribution lose their dependence on the nerve and come to be situated in the muscle fibre.

This nerve-independent positional stability of the AChRs at the mature NMJ is accompanied by a similarly nerve-independent resistance of the junctional AChRs to activity. If a mature muscle is denervated, AChRs are synthesized all along the muscle fibres and appear throughout the extrajunctional membrane. If such a denervated muscle is electrically stimulated, AChRs disappear from the extrajunctional region (Lømo and Rosenthal, 1972), but persist at the site of the NMJ (Frank et al., 1975a).

It thus seems that the maintenance of a high concentration of AChRs at the NMJ involves two important mechanisms: one for the continued, local, synthesis of AChRs by active muscle fibres, in which synthesis in the non-junctional region is suppressed, the other for the precise localization of AChRs after synthesis. In mature muscles, neither of these mechanisms requires the integrity of the motor nerve terminal.

The basal lamina as a determinant of AChR distribution on regenerating frog muscle

A number of cellular and molecular components may play a role in ensuring the long-term stability of the junctional AChR cluster. Many cytoskeletal proteins are present in the postsynaptic cytoplasm and it is likely that they link AChRs to the cytoskeleton (reviewed by Bloch and Pumplin, 1988). At present, however, the role of the cytoskeleton in AChR localization is not understood in any detail.

There is strong and direct evidence that components of the extracellular basal lamina can influence AChR distribution on regenerating muscle fibres of the frog (Burden et al., 1979; McMahan and Slater, 1984). When frog muscle fibres are damaged in ways that leave the basal lamina intact, AChRs at the NMJ are first lost as the muscle fibre degenerates and are then replaced when new muscle fibres regenerate within the surviving basal lamina sheath. This reaccumulation of AChRs occurs even if the nerve and Schwann cells are destroyed at the time of muscle damage, leaving the basal lamina as the only component of the original NMJ to provide the local cues required for AChR accumulation. Good progress is now being made in identifying the molecular basis of those cues (Nitkin et al., 1987).

In the rest of this paper, I will describe experiments which confirm that AChR clusters are also present at original synaptic sites on regenerating mammalian muscles, and that many of these clusters are relatively resistant to muscle activity.

AChR distribution on regenerating rat soleus muscle

The original experiments defining the ability of synaptic basal lamina to cause AChR accumula-

tion on regenerating muscle fibres were carried out in the frog. We have extended this analysis to the rat, where previous studies of the formation and maintenance of NMJs, in both developing and adult animals, provide opportunities for further analysis of the properties of the AChR clusters induced by synaptic basal lamina.

Response to notexin

Rat soleus muscle fibres can be effectively destroyed by a single injection of notexin, a myotoxin isolated from the venom of the Australian tiger snake (Harris et al., 1975; Harris and Johnson, 1978). Within the space of 3 days, the original muscle fibres are destroyed and their contents are removed by phagocytes. At the same time, the surviving myosatellite cells proliferate to produce a new population of presumptive muscle fibre nuclei and then fuse to generate new myotubes. If the original innervation is left intact, the myotubes are rapidly innervated and go on to form muscle fibres of normal size and appearance, with the exception of the persistence of central nuclei. If the original innervation is cut at the time of notexin injection, as in all the experiments described below, the new muscle fibres form normally but show little increase in girth.

AChRs at original synaptic sites

As in the frog, the original synaptic sites in regenerated rat muscle can be identified by virtue of the acetylcholinesterase (AChE), much of which is normally concentrated in the synaptic basal lamina (McMahan et al., 1978). The AChE survives muscle fibre degeneration and regeneration and can be labelled with an appropriate antibody.

After notexin treatment, AChRs can be clearly seen at the original synaptic sites on the regenerated muscle fibres after labeling with rhodamine-α-bungarotoxin (R-BgTx) (Slater and Allen, 1985). The distribution of AChRs is very similar to that of AChE, but both are different from that seen at comparable normal or denervated endplates (Fig. 1). Instead of the clearly outlined region of synaptic contact, the labelling is more diffuse and

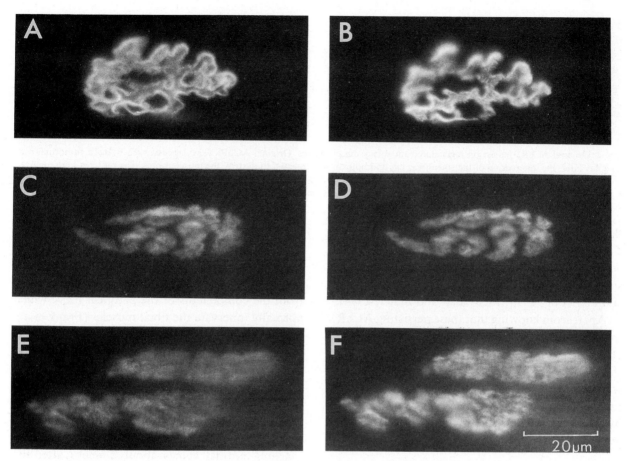

Fig. 1. AChRs and AChE at synaptic sites on normal, denervated and denervated-regenerated rat soleus muscles. Teased bundles of muscle fibres were labelled with R-BgTx to reveal AChRs (A,C,E), and an antibody to rat brain AChE (gift of Dr. M. Vigny) with an FITC-labelled second antibody to reveal AChE (B,D,F). A,B: normal muscle. C,D: denervated muscle 6 days after cutting the nerve. E,F: denervated-regenerated muscle, 6 days after denervation and exposure to notexin to damage the muscle.

"speckled', suggesting that the synaptic molecules are limited to many tiny patches within the original zone. A similar distribution of AChRs persists for at least 2 months after notexin damage.

Persistence of original AChRs

When muscles were examined during the first few days after notexin treatment, prior to new myotube formation, AChRs were seen at many junctional sites on the degenerating muscle fibres (Slater and Allen, 1985). This suggested that some of the AChRs from the original muscle fibre might survive and contribute to the labelling seen in the regenerated muscles. To test this idea, AChRs were labelled in the animal with R-BgTx 1 day before the muscle was damaged. When the muscles were examined a week after notexin injection, and exposed to fluorescein-BgTx (F-BgTx), most of the synaptic sites were found to be doubly labelled (Fig. 2), indicating that some of the original AChRs, together with their R-BgTx label, had survived.

To estimate the number of surviving AChRs, muscles were prelabelled with ^{125}I-BgTx, in conditions in which at least 80% of the AChRs were saturated. When these muscles were examined 6 days later, approximately 35% of the radioactivity original bound at the NMJs was still present in

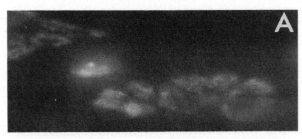
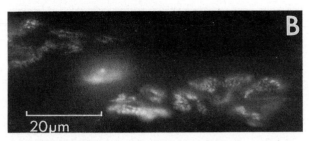

Fig. 2. Original AChRs persist on regenerated rat soleus muscle fibres. Original AChRs were labelled with R-BgTx in normal rats. One day later, the innervation of the soleus was cut and notexin was injected to destroy the muscle fibres. The muscles were removed after a further 6 days and stained with F-BgTx to indicate the position of the original synaptic site. A: junctional AChRs on regenerated muscle fibre labelled with F-BgTx. B: original AChRs stained with R-BgTx.

the junctional region of the muscle (Slater, 1987). This is in contrast to the situation in the frog, where no more than 5–10% of the BgTx binding sites survive acute necrosis of the muscle fibres (Burden et al., 1979; McMahan and Slater, 1984).

Apart from knowing that these persisting AChR molecules can still bind BgTx, we know little about their physical state. One possibility is that they survive as a result of some direct interaction with the basal lamina and that they are incorporated into the growing membrane of the new muscle fibre when it makes contact with the synaptic basal lamina.

AChRs on muscles innervated at ectopic sites

In all the experiments described so far, both in the frog and in the rat, the observations of AChRs at original synaptic sites were on regenerated muscles that were inactive as a result of denervation. In such muscles, AChRs are present and are presumably synthesized all along the muscle fibre. It is thus possible that the AChRs at the original synaptic sites are synthesized in the extrajunctional regions and become trapped at the original synaptic sites, as seems to happen during normal development (Anderson et al., 1977; Ziskind-Conhaim et al., 1984). The question then arises whether AChRs would remain at the original synaptic sites on regenerated muscles if the generalized synthesis of AChRs was shut off by making the muscle fibres active. To test this possibility, I have allowed notexin-treated muscles, whose own nerve

had been cut and prevented from regenerating, to be innervated by a "foreign" nerve at ectopic sites, remote from the original NMJs. As in earlier experiments, the foreign innervation was derived from the components of the peroneal nerve which normally innervate the tibial muscles (Frank et al., 1975b; Lømo and Slater, 1978).

Intact muscles

When undamaged soleus muscles are ectopically reinnervated in this way, extrajunctional ACh sensitivity initially increases to a level characteristic of fully denervated muscles and then declines, reaching normal values about 2 weeks after the new ectopic junctions become able to elicit contraction (Lømo and Slater, 1978). In contrast, the sensitivity at the still denervated original NMJs persists (Frank et al., 1975b). When viewed after R-BgTx labelling, AChRs are still highly concentrated at these sites (Fig. 3A) and their distribution is similar to that on fully denervated muscles (Fig. 3B).

Regenerated muscles

When a "foreign" nerve was presented to soleus muscles at the time of notexin treatment and section of the soleus innervation, many of the muscle fibres that regenerated became innervated at ectopic sites, leaving the original NMJs still denervated. Up to 8 weeks later, the longest time we have studied, these muscle fibres could still be recognized by their central nuclei, indicating that they had regenerated, and by their large cross-sec-

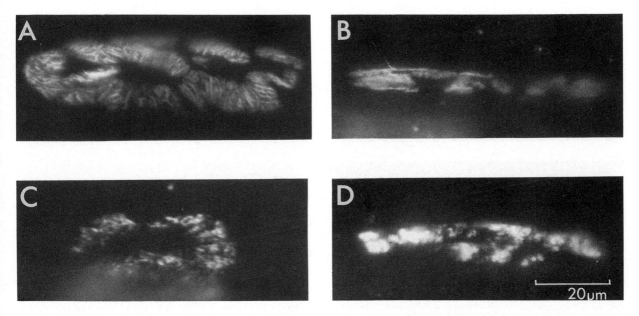

Fig. 3. AChRs are present at original synaptic sites on denervated-regenerated muscle fibres that are kept active by innervation at ectopic sites. All frames show original synaptic sites 2 months after denervation. Regenerated muscles were treated with notexin at the time of denervation. Teased bundles were labelled with R-BgTx to reveal AChRs. A: undamaged muscle, ectopically innervated. B: undamaged muscle, no ectopic innervation (note atrophy of muscle fibres). C: regenerated muscle, ectopically innervated. D: regenerated muscle, no ectopic innervation.

tional area, indicating that they were innervated and active.

The original synaptic sites in these muscle fibres could be easily identified using the AChE labelling technique. Many of the AChE-positive sites also had clear labelling with R-BgTx, indicating that AChRs were still present, up to 6 weeks after they would have disappeared from the extrajunctional region. The distribution of R-BgTx labelling at the junctional sites (Fig. 3C) was qualitatively similar to that seen on regenerated muscle fibres which are fully denervated but the labelled zones were larger, owing to the greater diameter of the reinnervated fibres. The appearance of this labelling was in marked contrast to that at original synaptic sites on ectopically innervated muscle fibres which had not been damaged or to that at the newly formed ectopic junctions on the same muscle fibres (Fig. 3D). The intensity of junctional R-BgTx labelling was variable, ranging from barely detec-

table to as intense as that on fully denervated fibres.

AChRs clusters at extrajunctional sites

An important distinction between AChRs at normal NMJs and those present generally on immature or denervated muscle fibres is that junctional AChRs are present in high-density clusters. Such clusters might have an inherent stability, quite apart from any special influence of the nerve, which could account for the persistence of AChRs we have observed at denervated synaptic sites on degenerated muscles.

It is well known that AChR clusters form on non-innervated muscle fibres in a variety of situations, both in animals and in cultured muscle cells (Fischbach and Cohen, 1973; Sytkowski et al., 1973; Ko et al., 1977). These clusters are similar in many ways to those at immature NMJs (Bloch and Pumplin, 1988). Many such clusters are pre-

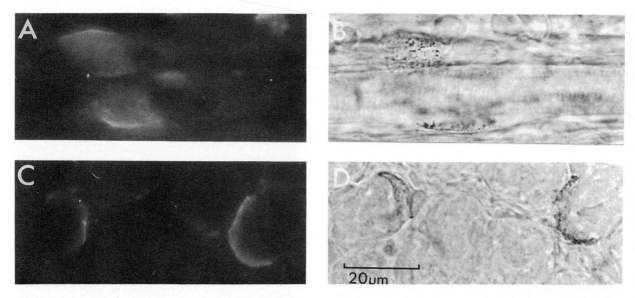

Fig. 4. Extrajunctional AChR clusters. AChRs were labelled with R-BgTx, on muscle 1 week after denervation and exposure to notexin; AChE activity labelled by the method of Karnovsky and Roots (1964). A,B: teased fibre bundles. C,D: transverse frozen section. A,C: AChRs. B,D: AChE activity.

sent on newly regenerated soleus muscle fibres (Fig. 4), where they generally appear as uniformly labelled, oval regions ranging from 5 to 15 μm in length (Fig. 4). Most of these clusters have associated with them a concentration of AChE and of cytoskeletal proteins in the muscle fibre.

Instability

The number of these extrajunctional clusters is greatest within a day or two after the first regenerated muscle fibres have formed. During the following week, the number of clusters falls to about 25% of its peak value. This is true whether the muscle becomes reinnervated, and is therefore active, or not. A similar loss of extrajunctional AChR clusters has been reported in rat muscles regenerating after ischaemic damage (Womble, 1986). The instability of these extrajunctional clusters, which contain a number of components associated with normal NMJs, is in marked contrast to the stability of AChRs at the original synaptic sites.

Discussion

It is clear from much previous work that the presence of a high density of AChRs precisely aligned with the sites of transmitter release involves both the local synthesis of AChRs by active muscle fibres and a mechanism for localizing the molecules after their synthesis. Together with the earlier work on the frog, the studies reviewed here and several other studies on the rat (Bader, 1981; Hansen-Smith, 1986; Womble, 1986) strongly support the view that the synaptic basal lamina is able to regulate the distribution of AChRs on regenerating muscle fibres.

Efforts to elucidate the molecular basis for this effect have revealed that agrin, a glycoprotein from the basal lamina of *Torpedo* electric organ which causes aggregation of AChRs in cultured myotubes (Nitkin et al., 1987), is concentrated at the frog NMJ (Reist et al., 1987). While various members of a library of 13 monoclonal antibodies to *Torpedo* agrin label NMJs in fish, birds and amphibia, none of them labels rat NMJs (Reist et al., 1987). It remains to be seen whether this reflects variations in agrin structure between the vertebrate classes or a more substantial difference in the molecular basis for AChR localization in mammals.

A striking feature of the results from notexin-treated rat soleus muscle is the persistence on the regenerated muscles of a substantial fraction of the BgTx initially bound to junctional AChRs in the undamaged muscle. In grafted sternohyoid muscles of the rat, which degenerate fully, but more slowly than notexin-treated soleus muscle, AChRs were reported to be undectable at the time of maximum muscle degeneration (Hansen-Smith, 1986). Whether this reflects a difference in the muscles studied, the means of inducing degeneration, or the sensitivity of the method of detection is not clear.

One possible explanation for the survival of some AChR molecules, in spite of the complete breakdown of the muscle fibres, is stabilization by some form of attachment to the synaptic basal lamina. This might protect the AChRs from ingestion by phagocytes or breakdown by soluble enzymes. It may be that a fraction of AChR molecules at normal NMJs is normally linked to components of the basal lamina, such as agrin, and that lateral interactions with other AChR molecules together with cross-linking by cytoskeletal components serve to stabilize the whole cluster.

In contrast to the persistance of AChR clusters at the original synaptic site, most newly formed AChR clusters in extrajunctional regions of regenerating rat soleus muscle fibres survive only a few days (Womble, 1986). The instability of these extrajunctional clusters, particularly in muscle fibres in the process of becoming innervated, has been noted by others (e.g., Moody-Corbett and Cohen, 1982; Kuromi and Kidokoro, 1984; Smith and Slater, 1985). In regenerating rat muscles, the loss occurs in the absence of innervation. The local differences which allow the persistence of one form of cluster and not the other are not known.

A number of accessory molecules found at junctional AChR clusters are also found at extrajunctional clusters, including components of the basal lamina (Anderson and Fambrough, 1983; Bayne et al., 1984) and the cytoskeleton (cf. Bloch and Pumplin, 1988). It is clear that those molecules do not in themselves confer long-term stability on AChR clusters.

Of particular interest is the finding that AChR clusters can survive at original synaptic sites on regenerating muscles when the fibres are kept active by ectopic innervation. In these fibres, AChRs are present at the junctional sites well after they disappear from the extrajunctional region. It seems likely that the presence of a high density of AChRs on regenerated muscle fibres 1 month after their formation would require the continuing synthesis of new AChRs. If so, information associated with the synaptic basal lamina must be able not only to regulate the distribution of AChRs, but also to ensure continued AChR synthesis by active muscle fibres.

So far, little is known about the factors that control the expression of genes in the myonuclei in the immediate vicinity of the NMJ, apart from the important fact that they produce more mRNA coding for the alpha subunit of the AChR than nuclei in the extrajunctional region of the muscle fibre (Merlie and Sanes, 1985; Fontaine and Changeux, 1989). The experiments on ectopically innervated regenerating muscles raise the possibility that factors associated with the synaptic basal lamina may somehow enable the underlying myonuclei to produce mRNA for AChR subunits in the face of activity.

Acknowledgements

The original work reported here was supported by the Wellcome Trust, the Muscular Dystrophy Group of Great Britain and the SmithKline (1982) Foundation. I thank Carol Young for her excellent technical assistance in all aspects of this work.

References

Anderson, M.J., Cohen, M.W. and Zorychta, E. (1977) Effects of innervation on the distribution of acetylcholine receptors on cultured amphibian muscle cells. *J. Physiol. (Lond.),* 268: 731–756.

Anderson, M.J. and Fambrough, D.M. (1983) Aggregates of acetylcholine receptors are associated with plaques of a basal lamina heparan sulfate proteoglycan on the surface of skeletal muscle fibres. *J. Cell Biol.,* 97: 1396–1411.

Bader, D. (1981) Density and distribution of α-bungarotoxin binding sites in postsynaptic structures of regenerated rat skeletal muscle. *J. Cell Biol.,* 88: 338–345.

Bayne, E.K., Anderson, M.J. and Fambrough, D.M. (1984) Extracellular matrix organization in developing muscle: correlation with acetylcholine receptor aggregates. *J. Cell Biol.,* 99: 1486–1501.

Bevan, S. and Steinbach, J.H. (1977) The distribution of α-bungarotoxin binding sites on mammalian skeletal muscle developing in vivo. *J. Physiol. (Lond.),* 267: 195–213.

Bloch, R.S. and Pumplin, D.W. (1988) Molecular events in synaptogenesis: nerve-muscle adhesion and postsynaptic differentiation. *Am. J. Physiol.,* 254: C345–C364.

Burden, S.J., Sargent, P.B. and McMahan, U.J. (1979) Acetylcholine receptors in regenerating muscle accumulate at original synaptic sites in the absence of nerve. *J. Cell Biol.,* 82: 412–425.

Diamond, J. and Miledi, R. (1962) A study of foetal and new-born rat muscle fibres. *J. Physiol. (Lond.),* 162: 393–408.

Fischbach, G.D. and Cohen, S.A. (1973) The distribution of acetylcholine sensitivity over uninnervated and innervated muscle fibers grown in cell culture. *Dev. Biol.,* 31: 147–162.

Fontaine, B. and Changeux, J.-P. (1989) Localization of nicotinic acetylcholine receptor α-subunit transcripts during myogenesis and motor endplate development in the chick. *J. Cell Biol.,* 108: 1025–1037.

Frank, E., Gautvik, K. and Sommerschild, H. (1975a) Cholinergic receptors at denervated mammalian motor end-plates. *Acta Physiol. Scand.,* 95: 66–76.

Frank, E., Jansen, J.K.S., Lømo, T. and Westgaard, R.H. (1975b) The interaction between foreign and original motor nerves innervating the soleus muscle of rat. *J. Physiol. (Lond.),* 247: 725–743.

Hansen-Smith, F.M. (1986) Formation of acetylcholine receptor clusters in mammalian sternohyoid muscle regenerating in the absence of nerves. *Dev. Biol.,* 118: 129–140.

Harris, J.B. and Johnson, M.A. (1978) Further observations on the pathological responses of rat skeletal muscle to toxins isolated from the venom of the Australian tiger snake, *Notechus scutatus scutatus. Clin. Exp. Pharmacol. Physiol.,* 5: 587–600.

Harris, J.B., Johnson. M.A. and Karlsson, E. (1975) Pathological responses of rat skeletal muscle to a single subcutaneous injection of a toxin isolated from the venom of the Australian tiger snake, *Notechus scutatus scutatus. Clin. Exp. Pharmacol. Physiol.,* 2: 383–404.

Karnovsky, M.J. and Roots, L. (1964). A "direct coloring"

thiocholine method for cholinesterase. *J. Histochem. Cytochem.,* 12: 219–221.

Ko, P.K., Anderson, M.J. and Cohen, M.W. (1977) Denervated skeletal muscle fibres develop patches of high acetylcholine receptor density. *Science (Wash. DC),* 196: 540–542.

Kuromi, H. and Kidokoro, Y. (1984) Nerve disperses preexisting acetylcholine receptor clusters prior to induction or receptor accumulation in *Xenopus* muscle cultures. *Dev. Biol.,* 103: 53–61.

Lømo, T. and Rosenthal, J. (1972) Control of ACh sensitivity by muscle activity in the rat. *J. Physiol. (Lond.),* 252: 603–626.

Lømo, T. and Slater, C.R. (1978) Control of acetylcholine sensitivity and synapse formation by muscle activity. *J. Physiol. (Lond.),* 275: 391–402.

Matthews-Bellinger, J.A. and Salpeter, M.M. (1983) Fine structural distribution of acetylcholine receptors at developing mouse neuromuscular junctions. *J. Neurosci.,* 3: 644–657.

McMahan, U.J. and Slater, C.R. (1984) The influence of basal lamina on the accumulation of acetylcholine receptors at synaptic sites in regenerating muscle. *J. Cell Biol.,* 98: 1453–1473.

McMahan, U.J., Sanes, J.R. and Marshall, L.M. (1978) Cholinesterase is associated with the basal lamina at the neuromuscular junction. *Nature (Lond.),* 193: 281–282.

Merlie, J.P. and Sanes, J.R. (1985) Concentration of acetylcholine receptor mRNA in synaptic regions of adult muscle fibres. *Nature (Lond.),* 317: 66–68.

Moody-Corbett, F. and Cohen, M.W. (1982) Influence of nerve on the formation and survival of acetylcholine receptor and acetylcholinesterase patches on embryonic *Xenopus* muscle cells in culture. *J. Neurosci.,* 2: 633–646.

Nitkin, R.M., Smith, M.A., Magill, C., Fallon, J.R., Yao, Y.-M. M., Wallace B.G. and McMahan, U.J. (1987) Identification of agrin, a synaptic organizing protein from *Torpedo* electric organ. *J. Cell Biol.,* 105: 2471–2478.

Reist, N.E., Magill, C. and McMahan, U.J. (1987) Agrin-like molecules at synaptic sites in normal, denervated and damaged skeletal muscles. *J. Cell Biol.,* 105: 2457–2469.

Salpeter, M.M. (1987) Vertebrate neuromuscular junctions: general morphology, molecular organization, and functional consequences. In M.M. Salpeter (Ed.), *The Vertebrate Neuromuscular Junction,* Alan R. Liss, New York, pp. 1–54.

Scheutze, S.M. and Role, L.W. (1987) Developmental regulation of nicotinic acetylcholine receptors. *Annu. Rev. Neurosci.,* 10: 403–457.

Slater, C.R. (1982a) Postnatal maturation of nerve-muscle junctions in hindlimb muscles of the mouse. *Dev. Biol.,* 94: 11–22.

Slater, C.R. (1982b) Neural influence on the postnatal changes in acetylcholine receptor distribution at nerve-muscle junctions in the mouse. *Dev. Biol.,* 94: 23–30.

Slater, C.R. (1987) Persistence of acetylcholine receptors following degeneration of rat soleus muscle fibres. *J. Physiol. (Lond.),* 391: 60P.

Slater, C.R. and Allen, E.G. (1985) Acetylcholine receptor distribution on regenerating mammalian muscle fibres at sites of mature and developing nerve-muscle junctions. *J. Physiol. (Paris),* 80: 238–246.

Smith, M.A. and Slater, C.R. (1983) Spatial distribution of acetylcholine receptors at developing chick neuromuscular junctions. *J. Neurocytol.,* 12: 993–1005.

Steinbach, J.H. (1981) Developmental changes in acetylcholine receptor aggregates at rat skeletal neuromuscular junctions. *Dev. Biol.,* 84: 267–276.

Sytkowski, A.J., Vogel, Z. and Nirenberg, M.W. (1973) Devel-

opment of acetylcholine receptor clusters on cultured muscle cells. *Proc. Natl. Acad. Sci. USA,* 70: 270–274.

Womble, M.D. (1986) The clustering of acetylcholine receptors and formation of neuromuscular junctions in regenerating mammalian muscle grafts. *Am. J. Anat.,* 176: 191–205.

Ziskind-Conhaim, L., Geffen, I. and Hall, Z.W. (1984) Redistribution of acetylcholine receptors on developing rat myotubes. *J. Neurosci.,* 4: 2346–2349.

S.-M. Aquilonius and P.-G. Gillberg (Eds.)
Progress in Brain Research, Vol. 84
© 1990 Elsevier Science Publishers B.V. (Biomedical Division)

CHAPTER 9

Functional morphology of the nerve terminal at the frog neuromuscular junction: recent insights using immunocytochemistry

F. Torri Tarelli, F. Valtorta, A. Villa and J. Meldolesi

Department of Medical Pharmacology, "B. Ceccarelli" Center for the Study of Peripheral Neuropathies and Neuromuscular Diseases, CNR Center of Cytopharmacology, University of Milan, via Vanvitelli 32, 20129 Milan, Italy

Introduction

Acetylcholine (ACh) is secreted from motor nerve terminals by two means: (a) by release of multi-molecular packages or quanta (Fatt and Katz, 1952; Del Castillo and Katz, 1954) and (b) by molecular leakage across the presynaptic membrane (Katz and Miledi, 1977; Gorio et al., 1978; Vyskocil and Illes, 1979; Edwards et al., 1985). The spontaneous or neurally evoked release of quanta generates the discrete, transient miniature end-plate potentials (mepps) as well as the end-plate potentials that mediate neuromuscular transmission. As far as molecular leakage is concerned, this process can be the predominant way in which neurotransmitter is released under resting conditions. However, the physiological significance and the factor(s) of its regulation have not been defined yet.

As long as 30 years ago, the identification within the nerve terminals of a rich population of synaptic vesicles filled with neurotransmitter (de Robertis and Bennet, 1955; Whittaker et al., 1964) led to the interpretation that synaptic vesicles are the anatomical correlates of quanta. Indeed, the most widely accepted hypothesis to explain the quantal nature of transmitter release holds that the molecular packets are preformed in the nerve terminal, each quantum being confined within one

synaptic vesicle and released by exocytosis (del Castillo and Katz, 1956). Though this view is still challenged by some workers (Tauc, 1982; Israel and Manaranche, 1985), strong evidence from electrophysiological and electron microscopy studies has been accumulated in support of its validity (for reviews see Zimmermann, 1979; Ceccarelli and Hurlbut, 1980b; Reichardt and Kelly, 1983; Valtorta et al., 1990).

Recent evidence supporting the vesicle hypothesis of quantal secretion

A conclusive proof of the validity of the vesicle hypothesis of quantal secretion requires the demonstration that vesicle fusion and release of quanta are coincident events. The temporal correlation between these phenomena has been investigated by the application of the quick-freezing technique to the study of synaptic function. In this technique neuromuscular preparations are dropped against a copper block held at a temperature close to $4°K$ at known time intervals after a single suprathreshold electrical stimulus to the nerve. Cryofixation of the most superficial layer ($\approx 10 \ \mu m$ thick) of the muscle is achieved within ≈ 1 ms. The structural and chemical changes occurring in this layer are therefore arrested within the same time and can be preserved for later examination. Under physiological conditions, the quantal content (i.e. the number of quanta released at the frog neuromuscular junction in response to a single shock) is of the order of 200. The expected density of images of vesicle fusions with the presynaptic membrane of the terminal, which is about 600 μm long, is therefore very low. This low density has precluded the possibility of quantitative correlative analyses of electrophysiological records with freeze-fracture replicas, which are usually only a few microns in length (Heuser et al., 1979). Quantal content can be strongly increased by prolonging the duration of the presynaptic action potential with K^+-channel blockers such as 4-aminopyridine (Katz and Miledi, 1979). Under these conditions Heuser and coworkers (Heuser et al., 1979; Heuser and Reese, 1981) demonstrated the occurrence of vesicle fusions in the appropriate time scale (few milliseconds) after the delivery of a single shock to the nerve. However, the observed delay exceeded that expected from the sum of the nerve conduction time and the presynaptic delay. Such a result was not due to a dissociation between vesicle fusion and quantal release. In fact, by using an improved

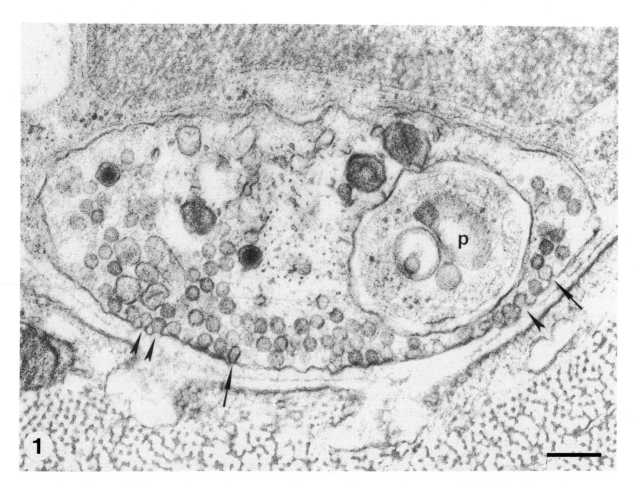

Fig. 1. Electron micrograph of a frog neuromuscular junction, quick-frozen 2.5 ms after a single electrical stimulus in 1 mM 4-aminopyridine and cryosubstituted. In this cross-section different degrees of association between synaptic vesicles and the prejunctional membrane are evident at the level of an active zone. Arrowheads indicate clear openings, and arrows indicate images that suggest intermediate states between the fusion and fission steps as proposed by Palade (1975). p, invagination of a Schwann cell process. Scale marker: 0.2 μm (from Torri-Tarelli et al., 1985).

apparatus, we successively demonstrated that fusions can be seen in thin-sectioned terminals from preparations quick-frozen as soon as 2.5 ms after the shock. In order for these experiments to be successful, precooling of the preparation during its travelling toward the copper block was minimized and care was taken to examine terminals located only in the very superficial layer of the tissue (Torri-Tarelli et al., 1985; see Fig. 1). 2.5 ms was exactly the time one would have expected vesicle fusion to occur, since under the experimental conditions employed conduction time was known to be close to 2 ms, and about 0.5 ms is needed for calcium to enter the nerve terminal and to stimulate transmitter release (Llinas et al., 1981).

Additional evidence for the validity of the vesicle hypothesis came from studies of morphofunctional correlation between quantal secretion and vesicle population. Intense synchronous secretion evoked by electrical stimulation of the nerve can be measured from the amplitude of end-plate potentials in nerve–muscle preparations treated with curare (Ceccarelli et al., 1973). To measure the high rates of asynchronous quantal secretion, an original statistical analysis procedure was developed and applied to electrophysiological recordings obtained from end-plates exposed to a variety of treatments that vigorously activate this process (Haimann et al., 1985; Segal et al., 1985; Fesce et al., 1986a,b). This procedure, based on the principles of noise analysis, allows derivation of the mepp rate, amplitude and time course from the variance, skew and power spectrum of the fluctuations in the muscle membrane potential recorded at the end-plate region (Segal et al., 1985; Fesce et al., 1986b).

Measurements of total ACh quantal release during intense secretion combined with the morphometric analysis of the concomitant changes in nerve-terminal ultrastructure supported the general conclusion that, whenever secretion is stimulated under conditions which block vesicle recycling, the average number of vesicles lost corresponds closely to the average number of quanta secreted. Moreover, in these cases the maximum number of quanta secreted was found to approach the number of synaptic vesicles present in resting nerve terminals (Haimann et al., 1985; Fesce et al., 1986b; Ceccarelli et al., 1988; Valtorta et al., 1988a). In contrast, when vesicle recycling was not impaired, the number of quanta secreted was found to greatly exceed both the number of vesicles lost and the number of vesicles in resting terminals (Segal et al., 1985; Valtorta et al., 1988a).

Movements of the vesicle membrane during quantal secretion

Under physiological conditions the fusion process is balanced by a reverse process of vesicle membrane removal from the axolemma, so that the population of synaptic vesicles is maintained constant in the face of vigorous and prolonged secretion. Vesicle recycling appears therefore to be an important aspect of synaptic function. However, the mechanism by which the membrane of the vesicle is recovered from the axolemma after exocytosis remains poorly defined. At the frog neuromuscular junction two possible mechanisms have been proposed to be operating. The first implies the collapse of the fused vesicle membrane into the axolemma with intermixing of the two membrane components, followed by reassembly of the vesicle membrane components into coated pits and recycling by endocytosis via coated vesicles (Heuser and Reese, 1973; Lentz and Chester, 1982; Miller and Heuser, 1984); the second implies the rapid direct removal of the vesicle membrane without its flattening into and intermixing with the presynaptic membrane (Ceccarelli et al., 1973; Torri-Tarelli et al., 1985). It has been suggested that at actively secreting synapses these two mechanisms can coexist, the latter being predominant in those conditions of stimulation which allow the balance between exocytosis and endocytosis to be maintained. When, on the other hand, the endocytotic process is outstripped by exhaustive rates of secretion, the vesicle membrane would accumulate into the axolemma, thereby increasing its surface area, and this would in turn activate the coated-

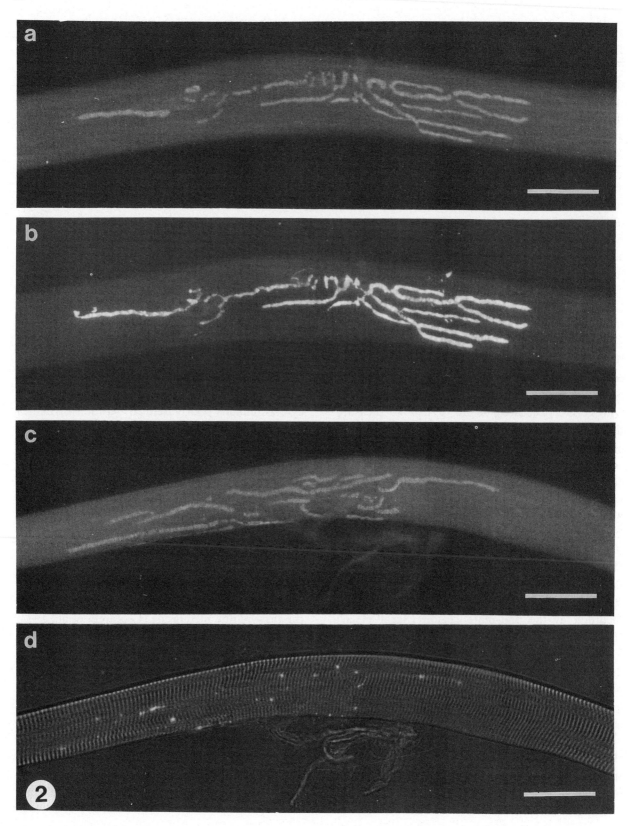

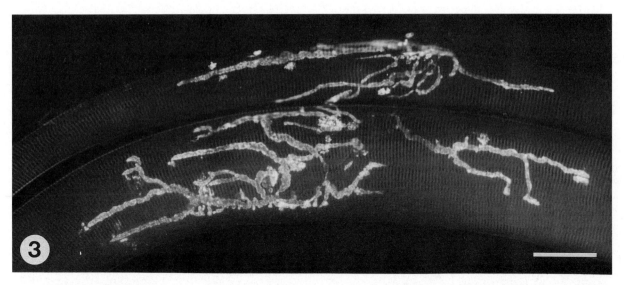

Fig. 3. Fluorescence micrographs of neuromuscular junctions on intact fibers stained for synaptophysin immunoreactivity after 1 h exposure to 0.2 μg/ml α-LTx in Ca^{2+}-free solution. No detergent was used. In this condition no permeabilization was necessary to reveal synaptophysin immunoreactivity. The nerve terminal branches show a marked increase in their transverse dimension. Scale marker: 50 μm (from Valtorta et al., 1988a).

vesicle-mediated mechanism (Meldolesi and Ceccarelli, 1981; Haimann et al., 1985; Torri-Tarelli et al., 1987).

Detailed information on the mechanism of retrieval of the vesicle membrane from the axolemma can be obtained by tracing the fate of vesicle membrane components during intense secretion. The movements of synaptic vesicle membranes during intense quantal secretion induced by α-latrotoxin (α-LTx) have been investigated by immunocytochemistry using antisera against synaptophysin, an integral glycoprotein of the synaptic vesicle membrane (Jahn et al., 1985; Wiedenmann and Franke, 1985). α-LTx, the purified active component of the black widow spider venom (Meldolesi et al., 1986), represents a useful tool for studying the redistribution of vesicular proteins upon exocytosis. In fact, low doses of this toxin exert different effects on the exo-endocytotic process when applied in the absence or in the presence of extracellular Ca^{2+} (Ceccarelli and Hurlbut, 1980a; Valtorta et al., 1988a). In Ca^{2+}-free solution, 0.2 μg/ml α-LTx induces very high initial rates of quantal secretion that subside to very low levels within 20 min. Under these conditions the recycling of both vesicles and quanta is blocked: the terminals stop secreting after they have released their initial store of quanta ($\approx$ 800 000). Ultrastructurally these terminals appear swollen and totally depleted of synaptic vesicles.

Fig. 2. Fluorescence micrographs of neuromuscular junctions exposed for 1 h to 0.2 μg/ml α-LTx in Ca^{2+}-containing solution. The preparation shown in a and b was treated with 0.1% Triton X-100 after fixation and double stained with fluoresceinated α-bungarotoxin (a) and with anti-synaptophysin antiserum followed by rhodamine-conjugated goat anti-rabbit IgGs (b). Similar patterns of nerve terminal branches are revealed by the post-synaptic (a) and presynaptic (b) markers. The nerve terminal shown in c and d is from a preparation double stained as in a and in b (c = α-bungarotoxin; d = synaptophysin), except that no detergent was used. In this condition, synaptophysin labelling is undetectable and the nerve terminal region can be identified only by the distribution of α-bungarotoxin labelling. Scale markers: 50 μm (from Valtorta et al., 1988a).

88

When the same concentration of α-LTx is applied in the presence of extracellular Ca^{2+}, quantal secretion rates remain high and constant for at least 1 h, and about two million quanta are secreted during that time. Neither depletion of vesicles nor swelling of the terminal is observed, and when the

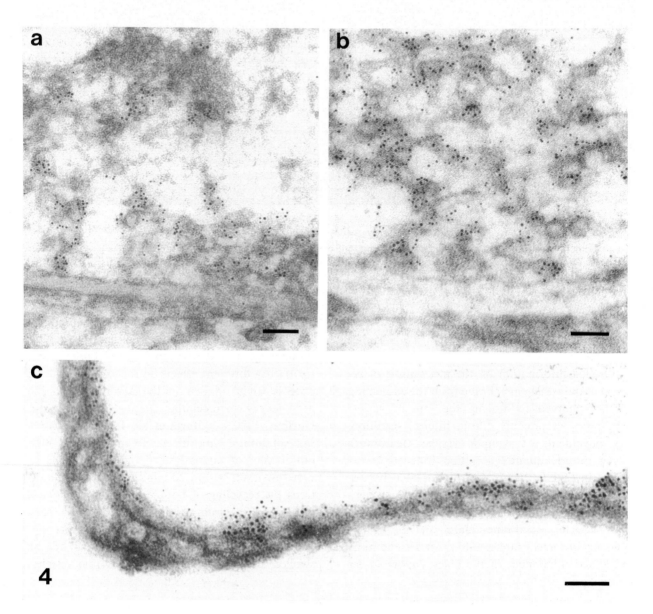

Fig. 4. Electron micrographs of ultra-cryosections of neuromuscular junctions exposed to rabbit antibodies against frog synaptophysin and colloidal gold-labelled goat anti-rabbit IgGs. Only high-magnification images of portions of the terminals are presented to make the small gold particles more evident. (a) Portion of a nerve terminal from a resting preparation. Gold particles are present in regions where synaptic vesicles are concentrated. The post-junctional region is not labelled. (b) Portion of a terminal treated for 1 h with 0.2 μg/ml α-LTx in Ca^{2+}-containing solution. The distribution of immunolabelling is similar to that shown in a. Only synaptic vesicles are labelled and the region of the axolemma is virtually free of gold particles. (c) Portion of a nerve terminal swollen and depleted of synaptic vesicles after 1 h exposure to the same concentration of α-LTx in Ca^{2+}-free solution. The gold particles are associated with the axolemma. Scale markers 0.1 μm (original from F. Torri-Tarelli, A. Villa and F. Valtorta).

experiments are carried out in the presence of extracellular tracers most of the synaptic vesicles appear tracer-positive, indicating that the vesicle population is maintained by active membrane recycling (Ceccarelli and Hurlbut, 1980a; Valtorta et al., 1988a).

The recycling of synaptophysin was first investigated by immunofluorescence. In this study, bright fluorescent staining of terminals from resting preparations was observed only when membranes were permeabilized by detergents to allow for penetration of the antibodies into the cytoplasm. A similar result was obtained with preparations exposed to α-LTx in the Ca^{2+}-containing medium (Valtorta et al., 1988a; see Fig. 2). In contrast, preparations depleted of synaptic vesicles by treatment with α-LTx in Ca^{2+}-free medium showed immunoreactivity for synaptophysin even without previous permeabilization (Valtorta et al., 1988a; see Fig. 3). These results support the validity of the vesicle hypothesis of quantal release, indicating that, when the endocytotic wing of the cycle is impaired, exocytosis leads to the permanent incorporation of the vesicular proteins into the axolemma. In addition, the results obtained in the Ca^{2+}-containing medium indicate that, in spite of the active vesicle and neurotransmitter turnover triggered by α-LTx under this condition, no extensive intermixing occurs between vesicle and axolemma components.

In order to extend at the molecular level the study of the different steps of the exo-endocytotic pathway, high-resolution immunocytochemistry appeared particularly appropriate. The immunofluorescence observations were therefore extended at the electron microscope level by applying an immunogold labelling technique to frozen sections from both control and α-LTx-stimulated nerve-muscle preparations (Torri-Tarelli et al., 1989). After secretion induced by α-LTx applied in Ca^{2+}-containing medium, the immunoreactivity pattern resembled that observed in resting preparations. Immunogold particles were selectively associated with the membrane of synaptic vesicles, whereas the axolemma was unlabelled (see Fig.

4a,b). When the toxin was applied in Ca^{2+}-free solution, the gold particles were uniformly distributed along the axolemma of the swollen terminals (see Fig. 4c). These findings corroborate the results of the immunofluorescence studies. The failure to detect the vesicular membrane protein in the axolemma under conditions of active recycling indicates that the retrieval of components of the synaptic vesicle membrane is an efficient process. It appears therefore that, when exocytosis and endocytosis are kept in balance, the mean residence time of the synaptic vesicle membrane on the surface of the nerve terminal is very short, possibly because most vesicles are directly recycled after fusion, without completely collapsing into and intermixing with the axolemma.

An additional interesting result of the electron microscopy analysis was the demonstration that in the preparation depleted of synaptic vesicles the distribution of synaptophysin is not limited to the region facing the synaptic cleft, where exocytosis has been shown to occur, but it is associated with the entire nerve-terminal plasma membrane. This result indicates that, when recycling is blocked, the vesicle membrane components are capable of diffusing away from the sites of fusion and probably of intermixing with the molecular components specific to the terminal plasma membrane (Torri-Tarelli et al., 1989).

Synapsin I at the frog neuromuscular junction

The neuron-specific phosphoprotein synapsin I is present in high concentration within nerve terminals, where it is localized on the cytoplasmic surface of small synaptic vesicles (for review see De Camilli and Greengard, 1986; Greengard, 1987). This protein seems to play a crucial role in the regulation of neurotransmitter release. Because of its ability to interact with both the vesicle surface (Schiebler et al., 1986) and actin filaments (Bähler and Greengard 1987; Petrucci and Morrow 1987), synapsin I has been hypothesized to connect synaptic vesicles with the nerve terminal cytoskeleton, keeping the vesicles away from the presynaptic discharge sites. Any increase in the intraterminal free Ca^{2+} concentration induces the activation of Ca^{2+}/calmodulin-dependent protein kinase II and the phosphorylation of synapsin I, with ensuing marked decrease of its affinity for the vesicle membrane. This could increase the number of vesicles available for exocytosis and therefore positively modulate the secretory re-

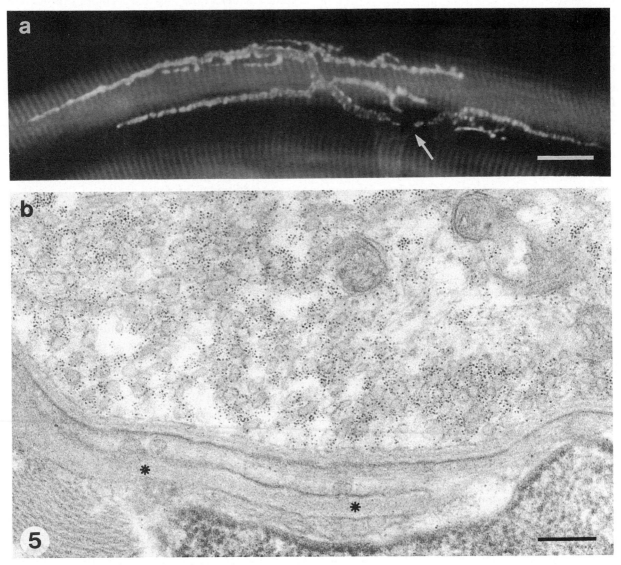

Fig. 5. (a) Immunofluorescence micrograph showing the distribution of immunoreactivity for synapsin I at a resting neuromuscular junction. Immunoreactivity is highly concentrated in the nerve terminal region and virtually no fluorescence is associated with the muscle fiber or with the unmyelinated preterminal axon (arrow). The regions of intense fluorescence are arranged in the branching pattern characteristic of frog motor nerve endings. (b) Electron micrograph showing the distribution of synapsin I immunoreactivity at a resting neuromuscular junction as revealed by immunoferritin labelling. Agarose-embedded 25-μm-thick sections from cutaneus pectoris muscle were processed for immunoelectron microscopy using anti-synapsin I antibodies and ferritin-conjugated goat anti rabbit F(ab)₂s. Most of the ferritin particles are located in regions where synaptic vesicles are highly concentrated. The synaptic cleft, the postjunctional folds (asterisks) and the muscle fiber are virtually devoid of ferritin particles. Scale markers: (a) 25 μm, (b) 0.2 μm (from Valtorta et al., 1988b).

sponse which occurs during stimulation. Indeed, it has been recently demonstrated that microinjection of mammalian synapsin I into the squid giant presynaptic terminal modulates transmitter release, and that this modulation is dependent on the state of phosphorylation of the protein (Llinas et al., 1985).

Using biochemical and immunocytochemical techniques, we have recently characterized and localized synapsin I at the frog neuromuscular junction both at the light and the electron microscope level (Valtorta et al., 1988b; see Fig. 5).

The study of synapsin I and of the regulation of its state of phosphorylation at the neuromuscular junction may provide important information on its role in synaptic function, since at present this is one of the few systems in which a correlation can be made between biochemical, morphological and electrophysiological data.

Immunocytochemical studies of the fate of synapsin I upon exocytosis were carried out in terminals fixed under the same conditions of stimulation used for the study of synaptophysin (Torri-Tarelli et al., 1989). Synapsin I immunoreactivity was found to remain associated with synaptic vesicles even in terminals intensely stimulated by α-LTx in Ca^{2+}-containing medium. These results indicate that rapidly recycled vesicles still have the bulk of synapsin I associated with their membrane. In contrast, in terminals exhaustively stimulated by α-LTx in Ca^{2+}-free medium, synapsin I immunoreactivity was found to be associated with the axolemma, a situation similar to that observed for synaptophysin. This indicates that synaptic vesicles which have permanently fused with the axolemma still retain synapsin I associated with their membrane (Torri-Tarelli et al., 1989). Thus, the dissociation of this protein from the vesicles does not appear to be a prerequisite for fusion, as previously hypothesized. It should be acknowledged, however, that the mechanism by which α-LTx induces neurotransmitter release in Ca^{2+}-free medium is different from those triggered by action potential and depolarizing agents, since under this condition no increase in the in-

traterminal Ca^{2+} concentration nor phosphorylation of synapsin I is observed (Meldolesi et al., 1984). Whether or not synapsin I remains bound to the fused vesicle membrane when terminals are exposed to other stimulatory agents which increase the intraterminal Ca^{2+} concentration remains to be established.

References

Bähler, M. and Greengard, P. (1987) Synapsin I bundles F-actin in a phosphorylation-dependent manner. *Nature,* 326: 704–707.

Ceccarelli, B. and Hurlbut, W.P. (1980a) Ca^{2+}-dependent recycling of synaptic vesicles at the frog neuromuscular junction. *J. Cell Biol.,* 87: 297–303.

Ceccarelli, B. and Hurlbut, W.P. (1980b) Vesicle hypothesis of the release of quanta of acetylcholine. *Physiol. Rev.,* 60: 396–441.

Ceccarelli, B., Hurlbut, W.P. and Mauro, A. (1973) Turnover of transmitter and synaptic vesicles at the frog neuromuscular junction. *J. Cell Biol.,* 57: 499–524.

Ceccarelli, B., Hurlbut, W.P. and Iezzi, N. (1988) Effect of α-latrotoxin on the frog neuromuscular junction at low temperature. *J. Physiol. (Lond.),* 402: 195–217.

De Camilli, P. and Greengard, P. (1986) Synapsin I: a synaptic vesicle-associated neuronal phosphoprotein. *Biochem. Pharmacol.,* 35: 4349–4357.

del Castillo, J. and Katz, B.(1954) Quantal components of the end plate potential. *J. Physiol. (Lond.),* 124: 560–573.

del Castillo, J. and Katz, B. (1956) Biophysical aspects of neuromuscular transmission. *Prog. Biophys. Chem.,* 6: 121–170.

de Robertis, E.D.P. and Bennet, H.S. (1955) Some features of submicroscopic morphology of synapses in frog and earthworm. *J. Biophys. Biochem. Cytol.,* 1: 47–58.

Edwards, C., Dolezal, V., Tucek, S., Zemkova, H. and Vyskocil, R. (1985) Is an acetylocholine transport system responsible for nonquantal release of acetylcholine at the rodent myoneural junction? *Proc. Natl. Acad. Sci. USA,* 82: 3514–3518.

Fatt, P. and Katz, B. (1952) Spontaneous subthreshold activity at motor nerve endings. *J. Physiol. (Lond.),* 117: 109–128.

Fesce, R., Segal, J.R., Ceccarelli, B. and Hurlbut, W.P. (1986a) Effects of Black Widow Spider Venom and Ca^{2+} on quantal secretion at the frog neuromuscular junction. *J. Gen. Physiol.,* 88: 59–81.

Fesce, R., Segal, J.R. and Hurlbut, W.P. (1986b) Fluctuation analysis of nonideal shot noise. Application to the neuromuscular junction. *J. Gen. Physiol.,* 88: 25–57.

Gorio, A., Hurlbut, W.P. and Ceccarelli, B. (1978) Acetylcholine compartments in mouse diaphragm. Comparison of the effects of Black Widow Spider venom, electrical stimulation, and high concentrations of potassium. *J. Cell Biol.,* 78: 716–733

Greengard, P. (1987) Neuronal phosphoproteins. Mediators of signal transduction. *Mol. Neurobiol.,* 1: 81–119.

Haimann, C., Torri-Tarelli, F., Fesce, R. and Ceccarelli, B. (1985) Measurement of quantal secretion induced by ouabain and its correlation with depletion of synaptic vesicles. *J. Cell Biol.,* 101: 1953–1965.

Heuser, J.E. and Reese, T.S. (1973) Evidence for recycling of synaptic vesicle membrane during transmitter release at the frog neuromuscular junction. *J. Cell Biol.,* 57: 315–344.

Heuser, J.E. and Reese, T.S. (1981) Structural changes following transmitter release at the frog neuromuscular junction. *J. Cell Biol.,* 88: 564–580.

Heuser, J.E., Reese, T., Dennis, M.J., Jan, Y. and Evans, L. (1979) Synaptic vesicle exocytosis captured by quick-freezing and correlated with quantal transmitter release. *J. Cell Biol.,* 81: 275–300.

Israel, M. and Manaranche, R. (1985) The release of acetylcholine: from a cellular towards a molecular mechanism. *Biol. Cell,* 55: 1–14.

Jahn, R., Schiebler, W., Ouimet, C. and Greengard, P. (1985) A 38,000-dalton membrane protein (p38) present in synaptic vesicles. *Proc. Natl. Acad. Sci. USA,* 82: 4137–4141.

Katz, B. and Miledi, R. (1977) Transmitter leakage from motor nerve endings. *Proc. R. Soc. Lond. B,* 196: 59–72.

Katz, B. and Miledi, R. (1979) Estimates of quantal content during chemical potentiation of transmitter release. *Proc. R. Soc. Lond. B,* 205: 369–378.

Lentz, T.L. and Chester, J.(1982) Synaptic vesicle recycling at the neuromuscular junction in the presence of a presynaptic membrane marker. *Neuroscience,* 7: 9–20.

Llinas, R., Steinberg, Z. and Walton, K. (1981) Relationship between calcium current and post-synaptic potential in squid giant synapse. *Biophys. J.,* 33: 323–352.

Llinas, R., McGuinness, T.L., Leonard, C.S., Sugimori, M. and Greengard, P. (1985) Intraterminal injection of synapsin I or calcium/calmodulin dependent protein kinase II alters neurotransmitter release at the squid giant synapse. *Proc. Natl. Acad. Sci. USA,* 82: 3035–3039.

Meldolesi, J. and Ceccarelli, B. (1981) Exocytosis and membrane recycling *Phyl. Trans. R. Soc. Lond. Ser. B,* 296: 55–65.

Meldolesi J., Huttner, W.P., Tsien, R.Y. and Pozzan, T. (1984) Free cytoplasmic Ca^{2+} and neuratransmitter release: Studies on PC12 cells and synaptosomes exposed to α-latrotoxin. *Proc. Natl. Acad. Sci. USA,* 81: 620–624.

Meldolesi, J., Scheer, H., Madeddu, L. and Wanke, E. (1986) Mechanism of action of α-Latrotoxin: the presynaptic stimulatory toxin of the black widow spider venom. *Trends Pharmacol. Sci.,* 7: 685–698.

Miller, T.M. and Heuser, J.E. (1984) Endocytosis of synaptic vesicle membrane at the frog neuromuscular junction. *J. Cell Biol.,* 98: 685–698.

Palade, G.E. (1975) Intracellular aspects of the process of protein synthesis. *Science (Wash. DC),* 189: 347–358.

Petrucci, T.C and Morrow, J.S. (1987) Synapsin I: an actin-bundling protein under phosphorylation control. *J. Cell Biol.,* 105: 1355–1363.

Reichardt, L.F. and Kelly, R.B. (1983) A molecular description of nerve terminal function. *Annu. Rev. Biochem.,* 52: 871–926.

Schiebler, W., Jahn, R., Doucet, J.-P., Rothlein, J. and Greengard, P. (1986) Characterization of synapsin I binding to small synaptic vesicles. *J. Biol. Chem.,* 261: 8383–8390.

Segal, J.R., Ceccarelli, B., Fesce, R. and Hurlbut, W.P. (1985) Miniature endplate potential frequency and amplitude determined by an extension of Campbell's theorem. *Biophys. J.,* 47: 183–202.

Tauc, L. (1982) Non-vesicular release of neurotransmitter. *Physiol. Rev.,* 62: 857–893.

Torri-Tarelli, F., Grohovaz, F., Fesce, R. and Ceccarelli, B. (1985) Temporal coincidence between synaptic vesicle fusion and quantal secretion of acetylcholine. *J. Cell Biol.,* 81: 1386–1399.

Torri-Tarelli, F., Haimann, C. and Ceccarelli, B. (1987) Coated vesicles and pits during enhanced quantal release of acetylcholine at the neuromuscular junction. *J. Neurocytol.,* 16: 205–214.

Torri-Tarelli, F., Villa, A., Valtorta, F., De Camilli, P., Greengard, P. and Ceccarelli, B. (1989) Redistribution of synaptophysin and synapsin I during intense release of neurotransmitter at the neuromuscular junction. *J. Cell Biol.,* submitted.

Valtorta, F., Jahn, R., Fesce, R., Greengard, P. and Ceccarelli, B. (1988a) Synaptophysin (p38) at the frog neuromuscular junction: its incorporation into the axolemma and recycling after intense quantal secretion. *J. Cell Biol.,* 107: 2719–2730.

Valtorta, F., Villa, A., Jahn, R., De Camilli, P., Greengard, P. and Ceccarelli, B. (1988b) Localization of synapsin I at the frog neuromuscular junction. *Neuroscience,* 24: 593–603.

Valtorta, F., Fesce, R., Grohovaz, F., Haimann, C., Hurlbut, W.P., Iezzi, N., Torri-Tarelli, F., Villa A. and Ceccarelli, B. (1990) Neurotransmitter release and synaptic vesicle recycling. *Neuroscience,* in press.

Vyskocil, R. and Illes, P. (1979) Non-quantal release of transmitter at mouse neuromuscular junction and its dependence on the activity of Na^+-K^+-ATPase. *Pfluegers Arch.,* 370: 295–297.

Whittaker, V.P., Michaelson, I.A. and Kirkland, R.J. (1964) The separation of synaptic vesicles from nerve ending particles (synaptosomes). *Biochem. J.,* 90: 293–303.

Wiedenmann, B. and Franke, W. (1985) Identification and localization of synaptophysin, an integral membrane glycoprotein of M_r 38,000 characteristic of presynaptic vesicles. *Cell,* 41: 1017–1028.

Zimmermann, H. (1979) Vesicle recycling and transmitter release. *Neuroscience,* 4: 1773–1804.

S.-M. Aquilonius and P.-G. Gillberg (Eds.)
Progress in Brain Research, Vol. 84
© 1990 Elsevier Science Publishers B.V. (Biomedical Division)

CHAPTER 10

Functional aspects of quantal and non-quantal release of acetylcholine at the neuromuscular junction

Stephen Thesleff

Department of Pharmacology, University of Lund, Sölvegetaan 10, S-223 62, Lund, Sweden

There is general agreement that the physiological function of the motor nerve is (1) to induce voluntary contractile activity in the muscle and (2) to control a number of long-term muscle properties in synapse formation, the contractile apparatus and the excitability of the muscle membrane. These latter influences are usually referred to as neurotrophic and involve the control of gene expressions in the muscle.

The motor nerve has at least four different types of acetylcholine (ACh) secretion and the purpose of this presentation is to outline and to speculate upon their possible physiological role within the framework of these two kinds of nervous control of skeletal muscle.

The best known type of ACh secretion is nerve-impulse-evoked phasic quantal release, extensively characterized by Katz and coworkers (see review by Katz, 1969). The synchronous release of transmitter quanta from the motor nerve gives rise in the muscle to the end-plate potential (epp) and thereby to a propagated action potential and a muscle twitch (Fig. 1A). The obvious physiological role of this type of ACh release is to permit low- and high-frequency nerve impulse propagation across the synaptic cleft and thereby to ensure nervous control of muscle activity and muscle tone. Since the pattern of mechanical muscle activity is a major trophic mechanism, as elegantly demonstrated by Lömo and Rosenthal (1972), Lömo and Westgaard (1975) and in recent reviews by Pette and Vrbová (1985) and Lömo

and Gundersen (1988), it is obvious that this type of ACh release serves both neurotransmission and long-term trophic control of muscle.

A closely related kind of transmitter secretion is the spontaneous quantal release of ACh which in the muscle fibre is recorded as small, intermittent electric potential changes (0.5–1 mV) of rather uniform time course. These potentials are similar to, but much smaller than, the nerve-impulse-evoked epp (Fig. 1B) and were therefore called miniature end-plate potentials (mepps) by Fatt and Katz (1952).

Subsequently del Castillo and Katz (1955) suggested that each quantum of ACh, whether released spontaneously or by a nerve impulse, was preformed within synaptic vesicles in the nerve terminal. Calcium ions inside the nerve terminal

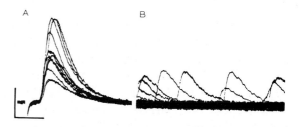

Fig. 1. A. Superimposed quantal end-plate potentials (epps) recorded in a single fibre of a normal rat extensor digitorum longus muscle. The phasic release of transmitter was reduced by high Mg^{2+} in the Ringer solution. B. Spontaneous miniature end-plate potentials (mepps) in the same fibre as in A. Note the similarity of the potentials caused by spontaneous and nerve-impulse-evoked quantal release of ACh. Calibrations 1 mV and 2 ms.

were suggested to induce fusion between synaptic vesicles and the nerve terminal membrane and thereby the exocytic release of the transmitter quanta (Katz and Miledi, 1965; and reviews by Llinas and Heuser, 1977; Silinsky, 1985).

Despite the fact that spontaneous quantal ACh release recorded as mepps was detected more than 35 years ago no one has been able to ascribe to it a physiological function. The potentials are far too small to trigger action potentials and thereby mechanical activity in the muscle. It has been speculated that mepps might have a trophic influence on muscle (Thesleff, 1960a) but experimental evidence for such an action is lacking.

A third type of ACh secretion was described by Liley (1957). It was a spontaneous release of large amounts of ACh which postsynaptically gave rise to large mepps, which were called giant mepps. Typically such mepps have a prolonged time-to-peak (up to 10 ms), the mean more than twice as long as that of ordinary mepps (Kim et al., 1984). Fig. 2 illustrates such slow-rising, large-amplitude mepps. Their frequency is unaltered by nerve stimulation, by nerve terminal depolarization and by changes in the extra- or intraterminal concentration of calcium ions (Thesleff and Molgó, 1983). Consequently, this type of spontaneous ACh release, in contrast to that causing the normal type of quantal mepps, is calcium-insensitive. Furthermore, this type of ACh secretion is selectively stimulated by certain drugs such as 4 amino quinoline (Molgó and Thesleff, 1982), vinblastine, cytochalasin B (Tabti et al., 1986) and emetine (Alkadhi, 1989). The slow, large-sized mepps are increased in frequency by temperature with a Q_{10} of about 12, while normal mepps are increased by a Q_{10} of 2–3 (Thesleff et al., 1983). The ACh responsible for these potentials comes from the same pool of transmitter as that released by nerve impulses (Lupa et al., 1986). It is apparently also of synaptic vesicular origin (Lupa et al., 1986). Electronmicroscopic studies have not revealed unusually large synaptic vesicles or clustering of vesicles which might explain exocytic release of such huge amounts of ACh (Pécot-Dechavassine

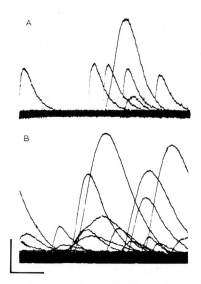

Fig. 2. A. Spontaneous mepps in a normal rat extensor digitorum longus muscle. Note the appearance of one giant, slow-rising mepp. B. The frequency of spontaneous giant, slow-rising mepps is greatly increased following prolonged blockade of neuromuscular transmission. The record is from a rat extensor digitorum longus muscle paralysed for 16 days by the use of botulinum neurotoxin type A. Calibrations 1 mV and 4 ms.

and Molgó, 1982). However, the nerve terminals contain so-called large, dense-core synaptic vesicles with a volume of about 10-times that of normal clear synaptic vesicles. These vesicles are believed to contain neuropeptides such as the calcitonin gene-related peptide (CGRP), and the ACh-receptor aggregating peptides agrin and aria. CGRP has been shown to be exocytically released by a mechanism unaffected by nerve stimulation and calcium ions (Matteoli et al., 1988). If those vesicles in addition to neuropeptides contained ACh, the release of their content might well induce postsynaptically slow and large-sized potentials (Thesleff, 1989).

At the normal adult rat neuromuscular junction large, slow-rising mepps constitute, on average, a few percent of all mepps recorded (Liley, 1957; Heinonen et al., 1982; Colméus et al., 1982; Kim et al., 1984) but their number is greatly increased following long-term block of neuromuscular transmission by botulinum toxin (Thesleff et al., 1983), curare (Ding et al., 1983) or tetrodotoxin (Gundersen, 1987). At reinnervated end-plates giant, slow potentials are common (Bennett et al., 1973; Colméus et al., 1982) and growth cones of embryonic neurons in culture secrete ACh by a similar mechanism (Hume et al., 1983; Young and Poo, 1983).

Since this kind of ACh secretion is unaffected by nerve impulses it has no role in impulse transmission across the synaptic gap. Its prevalence during embryogenesis, synapse formation and various kinds of transmission blockade indicates that it is in some way related to synapse formation and maintenance.

The neuropeptide CGRP is believed to have a regulatory influence on the appearance and number of postsynaptic nicotinic ACh receptors and thereby to be a part of neurotrophism (Laufer and Changeux, 1987; Fontaine et al., 1986). The neuropeptides agrin and aria have been shown to regulate the aggregation of ACh receptors and cholinesterase at the end-plate region (see review by Fischbach et al., 1989). If ACh is co-released with those neuropeptides one might ask whether its role is to facilitate the uptake or to modulate the action of neuropeptides in the muscle cell.

In addition to the three types of quantal discharge of ACh described, there is biochemical (Mitchell and Silver, 1963; Fletcher and Forrester, 1975) and electrophysiological (Katz and Miledi, 1977; Vyskocil and Illés, 1977) evidence that ACh is secreted from the nerve by a continuous non-quantal process. At the frog and mammalian neuromuscular junction one observes a steady release of ACh which, when cholinesterase is inhibited, builds up an ACh concentration in the synaptic cleft of the order of 10^{-8} to 10^{-7} M. Since the release is continuous the total amount of ACh secreted exceeds the spontaneous quantal release causing mepps by about two orders of magnitude and therefore accounts for by far the largest part of ACh secreted during resting conditions. One way to detect this spontaneous leakage of ACh from the nerve is to apply curare to a nerve–muscle preparation in which cholinesterase activity is in-

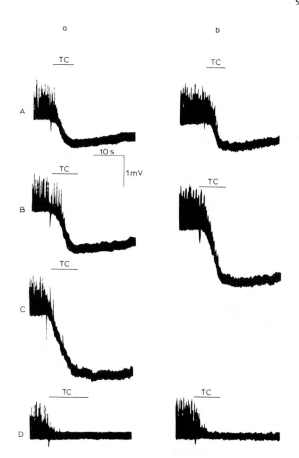

Fig. 3. Local curarization of the end-plate region of a mouse diaphragm causes, in the presence of cholinesterase inhibition by 6×10^{-6} M prostigmine (a) or by pretreatment with soman (b), a hyperpolarizing response (A). Inhibition of Na^+-K^+-activated ATPase by 2×10^{-5} M ouabain (B) or a K^+-free solution (C) enhances the hyperpolarizing response, while activation of ATPase by re-admission of K^+ (D) blocks the response. Horizontal bars indicate the time of tubocurarine (TC) diffusion from a pipette located in the end-plate area. From Vyskocil and Illés (1978).

hibited. The block of postsynaptic ACh receptors, stimulated by the released ACh, causes repolarization of the end-plate region as illustrated in Fig. 3. The continuous non-quantal release of ACh is not affected by nerve impulses but is somehow regulated by the sodium, potassium-activated membrane ATPase, since inhibition of that enzyme greatly increases this type of ACh secretion, as is also shown in Fig. 3 (Paton et al., 1971; Vizi, 1973, 1977; 1978; Vizi and Vyskocil, 1979).

Again very little is known about the physiological role of this type of ACh secretion. Growth cones of cholinergic neurones have this type of ACh secretion (Poo and Robinson, 1977; Poo, 1984; Sun and Poo, 1985). Poo et al. (1978, 1979) and Lin-Liu et al. (1984) have demonstrated that a uniform electric field across the surface of myotubes results in the accumulation of lectin- and ACh-receptor proteins towards the cathodal pole of the cell. Thus, it is possible that the depolarization caused by the continuous leakage of ACh contributes to the aggregation of nicotinic ACh receptors and of sodium channel proteins at the neuromuscular junction (Thesleff et al., 1974; Betz et al., 1984; Ziskind-Conhaim et al., 1984; Stollberg and Frazer, 1988).

Desensitization of the nicotinic ACh receptor has been proposed to be a form of short-term regulation of synaptic efficacy (Thesleff, 1960b; Heidmann and Changeux, 1982; Changeux et al., 1983; Changeux, 1986). It is therefore possible that the continuous leakage of ACh, by causing a varying degree of desensitization, exerts a modulatory influence on the sensitivity level of postjunctional nicotinic ACh receptors (Miles and Huganir, 1988). CGRP enhances the rate of desensitization of the nicotinic ACh receptor (Mulle et al., 1988) and therefore the release of this neuropeptide together with ACh might be an important mechanism in the regulation of synaptic efficacy.

Discussion

From the aforementioned brief presentation of the different kinds of ACh release at the neuromuscular junction it is obvious that only one kind, i.e. nerve-impulse-evoked quantal transmitter release, has a documented physiological function. It is responsible for synaptic transmission of the nerve impulse and thereby not only for nervous control of muscle activity but also for the variety of trophic influences which depend upon the activity pattern of the muscle.

The embarrassing question therefore arises, do the other three kinds of ACh release (spontaneous quantal release giving rise to either normal mepps or giant mepps and non-quantal continuous secretion of ACh) lack a physiological function? Are they simply leftovers or rudimentary processes from previous evolutionary stages? I refuse to believe that for the following reasons.

Spontaneous quantal secretion of transmitter is apparently a property of all chemical synapses irrespective of the type of transmitter substance involved and that seems to apply both to the calcium-sensitive and to the calcium-insensitive type of secretion (Thesleff, 1986). The same apparently applies to non-quantal molecular release of transmitter, which has been demonstrated at a variety of chemical synapses (Antonov and Magazanik, 1988). That such generalized and metabolically expensive processes could survive during evolution, if they were of no functional value, is in my opinion unlikely.

Since several kinds of ACh release are not involved in neuronal control of muscle activity I assume that they are part of trophic interactions between nerve and muscle. In that connection it is interesting that Fontaine et al. (1987) and Horovitz et al. (1989) have shown that distinct messengers are involved in the regulation of nicotinic ACh receptors at junctional and extrajunctional areas of the muscle fibre. According to Fontaine et al. (1987) CGRP exerts a regulatory influence on the level of mRNA for ACh receptors in nuclei of the end-plate, whereas muscle activity, possibly with calcium ions as second messengers, controls gene expression in nuclei of the extrajunctional part of the muscle fibre. Apparently the nuclei at junctional areas differ from those in the extrajunctional part of the fibre, as was also suggested by Harris et al. (1989). It is worth remembering that a muscle fibre is formed by the fusion of a number of myoblasts. Maybe two classes of myoblasts exist, as suggested by Tågerud et al. (1989); some myoblasts may be predestined to form the junctional and others the extrajunctional part of the muscle fibre.

Obviously the mechanisms by which innervation controls gene expressions in the muscle fibre are complex and at present little understood. The great variety of changes induced in muscle by denervation suggests multiple controls involving several neuronal messengers. We already know that the motor nerve in addition to ACh secretes a number of putative messengers such as neuropeptides and ATP. To that I should like to add that the nerve may use the same chemical substance but different kinds of release mechanisms, intermittent or continuous and calcium-dependent or -independent ones, as exemplified here for ACh, to convey various messages to its target cell.

References

Alkadhi, K.A. (1989) Giant miniature end-plate potentials at the untreated and emetine-treated frog neuromuscular junction. J. Physiol. (Lond), 412: 475–491.

Antonov, S M. and Magazanik, L G. (1988) Intense non-quantal release of glutamate in an insect neuromuscular junction. Neurosci Lett, 93: 204–208.

Bennett, M.R., McLachlan, E.M. and Taylor, R.S. (1973) The formation of synapses in reinnervated mammalian striated muscle. J. Physiol. (Lond), 233: 481–500.

Betz, W.J., Caldwell, J.H. and Kinnamon, S.C. (1984) Increased sodium conductance in the synaptic region of rat skeletal muscle fibers. J. Physiol. (Lond), 352: 189–202.

Changeux, J.P. (1986) Coexistence of neuronal messenger and molecular selection. Prog. Brain Res., 68: 373–403.

Changeux, J.P., Bon, F., Cartaud, J., Devillers-Thiéry, A., Giraudet, J., Heidmann, T., Holton, B., Nghiem, H.O. and Popot, J.L., van Rapenbusch, R. and Tzartos, S. (1983) Allosteric properties of the acetylcholine receptor protein from Torpedo marmorata. Cold Spring Harbor Symp. Quant. Biol., 48–35.

Colméus, C., Gomez, S., Molgó, J. and Thesleff, S. (1982) Discrepancies between spontaneous and evoked potentials at normal, regenerating and botulinum toxin poisoned mammalian neuromuscular junctions. Proc. R. Soc. Lond. B, Biol. Sci., 215: 63–74.

del Castillo, J. and Katz, B. (1955) Local activity at a depolarized nerve-muscle junction. J. Physiol. (Lond), 128: 396–411.

Ding, R., Jansen, J.K.S., Laing, N.G. and Tönnesen, H. (1983) The innervation of skeletal muscle in chicken curarized during early development. J. Neurocytol., 12: 887–919.

Fatt, P. and Katz, B. (1952) Spontaneous subthreshold activity at motor nerve endings. J. Physiol. (Lond.), 117: 109–128.

Fischbach, G.D., Harris, D.A., Falls, D.I., Dubinsky, J.M., Morgan, K., Engish, K.L. and Johnson, F.A. (1989) The accumulation of acetylcholine receptors at developing chick nerve-muscle synapses. In L.C. Sellin, R. Libelius and S. Thesleff (Eds.), Neuromuscular Junction, Elsevier, Amsterdam, pp. 515–532.

Fletcher, P. and Forrester, T. (1975) The effect of curare on the release of acetylcholine from mammalian motor nerve terminals and an estimate of quantal content. J. Physiol. (Lond.), 251: 131–144.

Fontaine, B., Klarsfeld, A., Hökfelt, T. and Changeux, J.P. (1986) Calcitonin gene-related peptide, a peptide present in spinal cord motoneurons, increase the number of acetylcholine receptors in primary cultures of chick embryo myotubes. Neurosci. Lett., 71: 59–65.

Fontaine, B., Klarsfeld, A. and Changeux, J.P. (1987) Calcitonin gene-related peptide and muscle activity regulate acetylcholine receptor α-subunit mRNA levels by distinct intracellular pathways. J. Cell Biol., 105: 1337–1342.

Gundersen, K. (1987) Giant "miniature" endplate potentials appear in nerve endings chronically deprived of impulse activity. Neuroscience, 22: Suppl. 701.

Harris, D.A., Falls, D.L. and Fischbach, G.D. (1989) Differential activation of myotube nuclei following exposure to an acetylcholine receptor-inducing factor. Nature, 337: 173–176.

Heidmann, T. and Changeux, J.P. (1982) Un modéle moléculaire de régulation d'efficacité d'un synapse chimique au niveau postsynaptique. C. R. Acad. Sci. (Paris), 295: 665–670.

Heinonen, E., Jansson, S.-E. and Tolppanen, E.-M. (1982) Independent release of supranormal acetylcholine quanta at the rat neuromuscular junction. Neuroscience, 7: 21–24.

Horovitz, O., Knaack, D., Podleski, T.R. and Salpeter, M.M. (1989) Acetylcholine receptor α-subunit mRNA is increased by ascorbic acid in cloned L_5 muscle cells: Northern blot analysis and in situ hybridization. J. Cell Biol., 108: 1823–1832.

Hume, R.I., Role, L.W. and Fischbach, G.D. (1983) Acetylcholine release from growth cones detected with patches of acetylcholine receptor-rich membrane. Nature, 305: 632–634.

Katz, B. (1969) The release of neural transmitter substances. In The Sherrington Lectures X, Vol. 10, Liverpool Univ. Press, Liverpool.

Katz, B. and Miledi, R. (1965) The effect of calcium on acetylcholine release from motor nerve terminals. Proc. R. Soc. Lond. B, Biol. Sci., 161: 496–503.

Katz, B. and Miledi, R. (1977) Transmitter leakage from motor nerve endings. Proc. R. Soc. Lond. B, Biol. Sci., 196: 59–72.

Kim, Y.I., Lömo, T., Lupa, M.T. and Thesleff, S. (1984) Miniature endplate potentials in rat skeletal muscle poisoned with botulinum toxin. J. Physiol. (Lond.), 356: 587–599.

Laufer, R. and Changeux J.P. (1987) Calcitonin gene-related peptide elevates cyclic AMP levels in chick skeletal muscle: possible neurotrophic role for a coexisting neuronal messenger. EMBO J, 6: 901–906.

Liley, A.W. (1957) Spontaneous release of transmitter substance in multiquantal units. J. Physiol. (Lond.), 136: 595–605.

Lin-Liu, S., Adey, W.R. and Poo, M. (1984) Migration of cell surface concanavalin A receptors in pulsed electric fields. *Biophys. J.,* 45: 1211–1217.

Llinas, R. and Heuser, J.R. (1977) Depolarization-release coupling systems in neurons. *Neurosci. Res. Prog. Bull.,* 15: 557–687.

Lömo, T. and Gundersen, K. (1988) Trophic control of skeletal muscle membrane properties. In H.L. Fernandez (Ed.), *Nerve – Muscle Cell Trophic Communication,* CRC Press, Boca Raton, Fl. pp. 61–79.

Lömo, T. and Rosenthal, J. (1972) Control of acetylcholine sensitivity by muscle activity in the rat. *J. Physiol. (Lond.),* 221: 493–513.

Lömo, T. and Westgaard, R.H. (1975) Further studies on the control of ACh sensitivity by muscle activity in the rat. *J. Physiol. (Lond.),* 258: 603–626.

Lupa. M.T., and Tabti, N., Thesleff, S., Vyskocil, F. and Yu, S.P. (1986) The nature and origin of calcium-insensitive miniature end-plate potentials at rodent neuromuscular junction. *J. Physiol. (Lond.).* 381: 607–618.

Matteoli, M., Haimann, C., Torri-Tarelli, F., Polak, J.M., Ceccarelli, B. and De Camilli, P. (1988) Differential effect of latrotoxin on exocytosis from small synaptic vesicles and from large dense-core vesicles containing calcitonin gene-related peptide at the frog neuro-muscular junction. *Proc. Natl. Acad. Sci. USA,* 85: 7366–7370.

Miles, K. and Huganir, R.L. (1988) Regulation of nicotinic acetylcholine receptors by protein phosphorylation. *Mol. Neurobiol.,* 2: 91–124.

Mitchell, J.F. and Silver, A. (1963) The spontaneous release of acetylcholine from the denervated hemidiaphragm of the rat. *J. Physiol. (Lond.),* 165: 117–129

Molgó, J. and Thesleff, S. (1982) 4-Aminoquinoline induced giant miniature endplate potentials at mammalian neuro-muscular juctions. *Proc. R. Soc. Lond. B, Biol. Sci.,* 214: 229–247.

Mulle, C., Benoit, P., Pinset, C., Roa, M. and Changeux, J.-P. (1988) Calcitonin gene-related peptide enhances the rate of desensitization of the nicotinic acetylcholine receptor in cultured mouse muscle cells. *Proc. Natl. Acad. Sci. USA,* 85: 5728–5732.

Paton, W.D.M., Vizi, E.S. and Zar, M.A. (1971) The mechanism of acetylcholine release from parasympathetic nerves. *J. Physiol. (Lond.),* 215: 819–848.

Pécot-Dechavassine, M. and Molgó, J. (1982) Attempt to detect a morphological correlate for the giant miniature endplate potentials induced by 4-aminoquinoline. *Biol. Cell.,* 46: 93–96.

Pette, D. and Vrbová, G. (1985) Invited review: Neural control of phenotypic expression in mammalian muscle fibers. *Muscle Nerve,* 8: 676–689.

Poo, M. (1984) Transmitter secretion from embryonic Xenopus neurons. In: *Conf. Neurobiol. Gif Aspects Mol. Differ. Neuron.,* 9th Abstract.

Poo, M. and Robinson, K.R. (1977) Electrophoresis of concanavalin A receptors along embryonic muscle cell membrane. *Nature (Lond.),* 265: 602–605.

Poo, M., Poo, W.H. and Lam, J.W. (1978) Lateral electrophoresis and diffusion of concanavalin A receptors in the membrane of embryonic muscle cells. *J. Cell. Biol.,* 76: 483–501.

Poo, M., Lam, J.W. and Orida, N. (1979) Electrophoresis and diffusion in the plane of the cell membrane. *Biophysics,* 26: 1–22.

Silinsky, E.M. (1985) The biophysical pharmacology of calcium-dependent acetylcholine secretion. *Pharmacol. Rev.,* 37: 81–132.

Stollberg, J. and Fraser, S.E. (1988) Acetylcholine receptors and Concanavalin A-binding sites on cultured *Xenopus* muscle cells: Electrophoresis, diffusion, and aggregation. *J. Cell. Biol.,* 107: 1397–1408.

Sun, Y. and Poo, M. (1985) Non-quantal release of acetylcholine at a developing neuromuscular synapse in culture. *J. Neurosci.,* 5: 634–642.

Tabti, N., Lupa, M.T. and Thesleff, S. (1986) Pharmacological characterization of the calcium-insensitive, intermittent acetylcholine release at the rat neuromuscular junction. *Acta Physiol. Scand.,* 128: 4239–436.

Tågerud, S., Libelius, R. and Shainberg, A. (1990) Rat myotubes differentiated in vitro have segments with high endocytic and lysosomal activities. *Cell Tissue Res.,* 259: 225–232.

Thesleff, S. (1960a) Supersensitivity of skeletal muscle produced by botulinum toxin. *J. Physiol. (Lond.),* 151: 598–607.

Thesleff, S. (1960b) Effects of motor innervation on the chemical sensitivity of skeletal muscle. *Physiol. Rev.,* 40: 734–752.

Thesleff, S. (1986) Different kinds of acetylcholine release from the motor nerve. *Int. Rev. Neurobiol.,* 28: 59–88.

Thesleff, S. (1989) Botulinal neurotoxins as tools in studies of synaptic mechanisms. *Q. J. Exp. Physiol.,* 74: 1003–1017.

Thesleff, S. and Molgó, J. (1983) A new type of transmitter release at the neuromuscular junction. *Neuroscience,* 9: 1–8.

Thesleff, S., Vyskocil, F. and Ward, M.R. (1974) The action potential in endplate and extra-junctional regions of rat skeletal muscle. *Acta Physiol. Scand.,* 91: 196–202.

Thesleff, S., Molgó, J. and Lundh, H. (1983) Botulinum toxin and 4-aminoquinoline induce a similar abnormal type of spontaneous transmitter release at the rat neuromuscular junction. *Brain Res.,* 264: 89–97.

Vizi, E.S. (1973) Does stimulation of Na^+-K^+-Mg^{2+}-activated ATPase inhibit acetylcholine release from nerve terminals?. *Br. J. Pharmacol. Chemother.,* 48: 346–347.

Vizi, E.S. (1977) Termination of transmitter release by stimulation of sodium-potassium activated ATPase. *J. Physiol. (Lond.),* 267: 261–280.

Vizi, E.S. (1978) Commentary. Na^+-K^+-activated adenosinetriphosphatase as a trigger in transmitter release. *Neuroscience,* 3: 367–384.

Vizi, E.S. and Vyskocil, F. (1979) Changes in total and quantal release of acetylcholine in the mouse diaphragm during activation and inhibition of membrane ATPase. *J. Physiol. (Lond.),* 286: 1–14.

Vyskocil, F. and Illés, P. (1977) Non-quantal release of transmitter at mouse neuromuscular junction and its dependence of the activity of Na^+-K^+ ATPase. *Pflügers Arch.,* 370: 295–297.

Vyskocil, F. and Illés, P. (1978) Electrophysiological examination of transmitter release in non-quantal form in the mouse diaphragm and the activity of membrane ATPase. *Physiol. Bohemoslov.,* 27: 449–455.

Young, S.H. and Poo, M. (1983) Spontaneous release of transmitter from growth cones of embryonic neurons. *Nature,* 305: 634–637.

Ziskind-Conhaim, L., Geffen, I. and Hall, Z.W. (1984) Redistribution of acetylcholine receptors on developing rat myotubes. *J. Neurosci.,* 4: 2346–2349.

S.-M. Aquilonius and P.-G. Gillberg (Eds.)
Progress in Brain Research, Vol. 84
© 1990 Elsevier Science Publishers B.V. (Biomedical Division)

CHAPTER 11

Mediatophore: a nerve terminal membrane protein supporting the final step of the acetylcholine release process

M. Israël and N. Morel

*Département de Neurochimie, Laboratoire de Neurobiologie Cellulaire et Moléculaire,
Centre National de la Recherche Scientifique, 91190 Gif sur Yvette, France*

Introduction

The pioneering works of King and Marchbanks (1982) and Meyer and Cooper (1983) have opened the field of protein reconstitution applied to nerve terminal membrane proteins such as the choline carrier or proteins involved in transmitter release. Working with *Torpedo* electric organ synaptosomes Vyas and O'Regan (1985) and Ducis and Whittaker (1985) have obtained good incorporations of the choline carrier activity into liposomal membranes. In these experiments, ionic effects and pharmacological actions were studied in exceptionally favorable conditions. In parallel experiments we have been able to reconstitute the acetylcholine (ACh) release mechanism, since we showed that proteoliposomal membranes became able to translocate ACh in a strictly calcium-dependent manner when they inherited from synaptosomal membranes a material sensitive to proteolysis (Israël et al., 1983, 1984; Birman et al., 1986). We knew from previous work that cytoplasmic ACh decreased upon stimulation and that in the course of release, integral membrane particles became more numerous, pointing towards a membrane mechanism for the final steps of transmitter efflux (Dunant and Israël, 1985). An initial series of experiments showed that nerve terminal membrane sacs filled with ACh released the trans-

mitter in response to an influx of calcium (Israël et al., 1981). Following the same line of research, we showed that the material which endowed artificial membranes with ACh release properties could be solubilized in detergents and several steps of purification were achieved (Birman et al., 1986). The following year we found that an alkaline disruption of the synaptosomal membranes similar to the procedure of Steck and Yu (1973) combined with an organic solvent extraction of proteolipids similar to the procedures of Folch and Lees (1951) led to the purification of a protein which had the ACh-releasing properties. This protein was named mediatophore (Israël et al., 1986). We shall in the present study compare some essential properties of the release mechanism studied on isolated synaptosomes or on reconstituted mediatophore.

Materials and Methods

Preparation of synaptosomes

Torpedo electric organ synaptosomes were prepared as described by Israël et al. (1976) and Morel et al. (1977). Synaptosomes were purified from 20–30 g of tissue and were recovered in 40 ml of a fraction containing (in mM) 280 NaCl, 3 KCl, 1.8 $MgCl_2$, 3.4 $CaCl_2$, 400 sucrose, 5.5 glucose, 1.2 sodium phosphate buffer (pH 6.8) and 5

NaHCO₃. For some experiments, synaptosomes were prepared in the absence of calcium in the gradient solutions.

ACh release from synaptosomes

The choline oxidase chemiluminescent procedure described by Israël and Lesbats (1981a,b, 1982, 1985, 1986) was used for monitoring the release of ACh. A reaction mixture consisting of acetylcholinesterase, choline oxidase, horseradish peroxidase and luminol is added to an alkaline (pH 8.4) physiological solution containing the synaptosomes. The released ACh gives rise to a light emission measured with a luminometer (Israël and Lesbats, 1981a,b, 1985). The release of ACh was measured using an amount of synaptosomes containing 0.2 nmol ACh. The release was calibrated by injecting ACh standards in the reaction mixture.

Purification of the mediatophore

This presynaptic membrane protein was purified by the procedure described by Israël et al. (1986). The purification consists of three steps. First, the large-scale preparation of presynaptic membranes (Morel et al., 1985) allows the isolation of 75 mg of presynaptic membrane protein from 0.5 kg of frozen tissue. Second, the alkaline extraction of the mediatophore from these membranes was performed as described by Birman et al. (1986) and Israël et al. (1986). About half the mediatophore and 15% of the total proteins were recovered in the alkaline extract after centrifugation. Third, the selective extraction of the mediatophore with organic solvents was performed by treating the lyophilized alkaline extract with chloroform/methanol (1:1 v/v). The lyophilized alkaline extract derived from 250 g of tissue was moistened with 200 μl of water before addition of 4 ml of the chloroform/methanol mixture. Most proteins precipitate, whereas the mediatophore remains in solution. After centrifugation, the solvent was evaporated, and 125 μg of pure mediatophore were recovered. It was found that its association with lipids was essential for preserving its activity (Israël et al., 1988a).

ACh release from proteoliposomes equipped with mediatophore

The proteoliposomes were prepared as described by Israël et al. (1984, 1986). Mediatophore (15–20 μg) was mixed with 4 mg of lecithin (dipalmitoyl-L-α-phosphatidylcholine) dissolved in 1 ml of 1-butanol. After evaporation of the organic solvent, the preparation was sonicated in an internal solution containing 50 mM ACh, 100 mM potassium succinate, 10 mM Tris buffer (pH 7.2) and 90 μM phospholine. The proteoliposomes were then gel-filtered on Sephadex G50 columns and collected in an external solution (50 mM NaCl and 180 mM Tris buffer, pH 8.4) devoid of ACh. The release of ACh from the proteoliposomes was measured as from synaptosomes with the choline oxidase chemiluminescent procedure. In this case, an amount of proteoliposomes corresponding to 1 nmol of entrapped ACh was used per assay. Release was measured in a solution consisting of 100 mM potassium succinate and 100 mM Tris buffer (pH 8.4). When the background light returned to baseline after addition of proteoliposomes, the calcium ionophore A23187 (Boehringer) was added (7 μM) and then ACh release was elicited by calcium (0.5–10 mM).

Large-scale purification of mediatophore

A simplified method leading to 100 μg of essentially lipid-free protein has been developed. The electric organ (500 g) is cut into 2–3-g fragments, and washed for 90 min at 4°C in 2.5 l of a solution consisting of 300 mM NaCl, 1 mM EDTA, 20 mM Tris buffer, pH 7.4. The solution is renewed once, and then the tissue is dried on filter paper and stored at − 80°C as described in Morel et al. (1985). When needed, 500 g of tissue are allowed to thaw in 1 litre of a hypotonic solution (10 mM Tris buffer, pH 8, 1 mM EDTA). The tissue is stirred for 20 min in the solution, which is renewed once, after collecting the tissue on a rigid

gauze. Homogenization is carried out at 4°C in 1.2
l final volume of the hypotonic solution, using
first a blender with a 5 cm propeller for two
periods of 45 s, and then a Potter (glass-Teflon) 3
up-and-down strokes. The homogenate is mixed
with 120 ml of sucrose (2 M) and the volume is
made up to 1.5 l with the hypotonic Tris-EDTA
solution. The crude membranes are pelleted in
6 × 250 ml buckets of the GSA rotor of a Sorvall
RC2B centrifuge at 1400 × g for 15 or 20 min.
The supernatant is collected and centrifuged once
more at the same speed. The supernatant, about
800 ml, is carefully collected below the foam, half
diluted with the hypotonic Tris-EDTA solution
and centrifuged at 25 500 × g for 1 h in the same
GSA rotor. Six membrane pellets are obtained;
they are alkaline-extracted by resuspending each
of them in 15 ml of 50 mM Tris buffer, pH 11, 10
mM NaCl. The final pH should be close to 9.5.
After 30 min at 16°C the material is centrifuged at
41 000 × g for 70 min and the supernatant is collected. After 4–5 h of dialysis against 2 × 10 l of
H_2O using dialysis membranes of 14 000 Da
molecular mass cut off, the supernatant is partitioned into six batches and lyophilized. Each of
the six dry powders is then moistened with 600 μl
H_2O and extracted with 12 ml chloroform-
methanol (1/1). The material is well resuspended
and extracted for 30 min. After centrifugation at
41 000 × g for 1 h, six clear supernatants are collected. Each is shaken with 2 vol. of H_2O (24 ml)
before centrifugation at 31 000 × g for 15 min in a
Sorvall SS34 rotor. The six interfaces (I_1) are
separated from the lipid-containing organic phase
(L) and the aqueous supernatant (A). Each interface is dried in a glass vial under a stream of N_2
and then suspended in 50 μl H_2O and 4 ml
chloroform-methanol (1/1). The samples are
pooled and partitioned into two 12 ml samples
which are centrifuged at 41 000 × g for 30 min to
get rid of any undissolved protein. The clear supernatants are shaken with 2 vol. of H_2O and the
second interfaces (I_2) formed again by centrifugation at 12 000 × g for 10 min. I_2 contains a total
amount of 100 μg of mediatophore.

Results

Acetylcholine release from synaptosomes and from reconstituted mediatophore shows similar pharmacological properties

The release of ACh from synaptosomes or proteoliposomes made with mediatophore was monitored using the choline oxidase procedure (Israël
and Lesbats, 1981a,b, 1986). The synaptosomes
were incubated in a physiological solution containing the reaction mixture (choline oxidase, peroxidase, luminol) and stimulated with the calcium

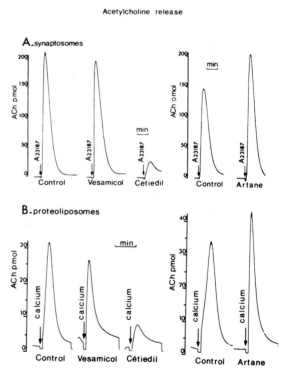

Fig. 1. Comparison of pharmacological actions in ACh release from synaptosomes and from proteoliposomes. A: The release of ACh from synaptosomes was monitored using the choline oxidase procedure. Release was triggered by the addition of the calcium ionophore A23187 in the presence of calcium. Vesamicol had no effect, while cetiedil strongly reduced the release (left traces). Artane induced a slight stimulation of release (right traces). B: The release of ACh from proteolipo-somes made with pure mediatophore reconstituted in lecithin vesicles was triggered by the addition of calcium in the pres-ence of calcium ionophore A23187. As above, vesamicol had no effect, while cetiedil reduced release (left traces); artane provoked a stimulation of release (right traces).

ionophore A23187 plus calcium. The release of ACh was measured by recording continuously the light emitted by the chemiluminescent reaction as previously described. A typical example is shown in Fig. 1A. Three compounds were compared in the present work for their effects on synaptosomal ACh release. Cetiedil blocked release (Morot Gaudry-Talarmain et al., 1987) while artane increased it. Vesamicol (AH5183) was inactive on the release of endogenous ACh, as previously reported by Michaelson and Burstein (1985), Michaelson et al. (1986) and Morot Gaudry-Talarmain et al. (1989a). The same compounds were tested on the release of ACh from proteoliposomes which had incorporated in their membrane the ACh translocating protein, mediatophore isolated from *Torpedo* synaptosomes (Israël et al., 1986). Fig. 1B shows that the pattern of drug action is similar to that obtained for synaptosomes. This indicated that these drugs, which affect release after the calcium entry step, interfere most probably with the properties of the mediatophore.

The pharmacological profile of drug actions on ACh release from synaptosomes and proteoliposomes is given in Fig. 2. In both preparations, cetiedil and its analogue MR4148 were potent inhibitors, whereas two other analogues of cetiedil, MR4172 and MR520, had little effect or even

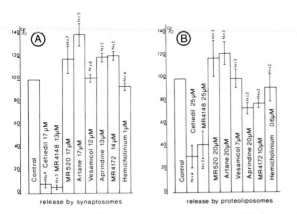

Fig. 2. Pattern of pharmacological actions on acetylcholine and choline fluxes. Panels A and B show the effect of different drugs on ACh release from synaptosomes and from proteoliposomes. Release was measured as in Fig. 1. The two patterns of ACh release (A and B) are very close.

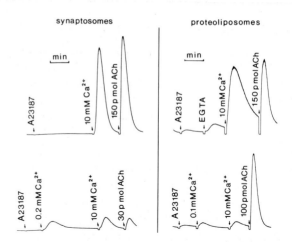

Fig. 3. Calcium-induced activation and desensitization of ACh release from synaptosomes (left) or from proteoliposomes made with pure mediatophore (right). The top traces show the test release triggered by A23187 at 10 mM calcium. The bottom traces show that if a conditioning calcium influx of 0.2 mM in the presence of A23187 is first given, then a subsequent 10 mM calcium addition fails to release ACh (0.2 mM EGTA was added in the left trace to remove traces of external calcium).

potentiated release. As for the other drugs tested, artane increased release in both preparations and vesamicol, aprindine and hemicholinium-3 had a small or no effect. These drugs have a completely different pattern of action on the uptake of ACh by synaptic vesicle and on the choline carrier (Morot Gaudry-Talarmain et al., 1989b).

As far as we are concerned here, we may conclude that ACh release from synaptosomes and that from reconstituted mediatophore show clear pharmacological similarities.

Fatigue of acetylcholine release from synaptosomes or reconstituted mediatophore

A typical characteristic of the release mechanism is the dual effect of calcium on its activation and desensitization (Israël et al., 1987b). The phenomenon is demonstrated in Fig. 3, left. A test stimulation of synaptosomes with the ionophore A23187 plus calcium is delivered alone, or a couple of minutes after a small conditioning stimulation at low external calcium. The conditioning stimulus releases very small ACh amounts but blocks the release of the second test stimulation at high external calcium. This phenomenon was also observed on proteoliposomes made with mediatophore (Fig. 3, right). The activation of ACh release by calcium took place rapidly in the millimolar range of external calcium concentration while desensitization or fatigue developed slowly but for micromolar external calcium concentrations. From these observations one may postulate that the opening of a calcium channel will result in the synchronous activation of neighbouring mediatophore molecules via a rapid and local increase in internal calcium concentration; at some distance mediatophore molecules will desensitize owing to internal calcium buffers which lower the calcium concentration. This would result in the quantification of ACh release by a finite number of activated mediatophore molecules (Israël et al., 1987b).

Mediatophore: an integral membrane protein

The active mediatophore protein was found to be associated with lipids which were essential for preserving the functional integrity of the protein, the ether-precipitated lipid-free mediatophore being irreversibly denatured. A procedure to remove most of the lipids without denaturation of the protein was found. In this technique the mediatophore is collected at the interface between an organic and an aqueous phase (Israël et al., 1988a). Fig. 4 illustrates this observation, which indicates that mediatophore behaves as one expects for integral membrane proteins. We also know from cryofracture studies with intact synaptosomes (Israël et al., 1980; Egea et al., 1987) or with whole membrane proteoliposomes (Israël et al., 1986) that integral membrane proteins are

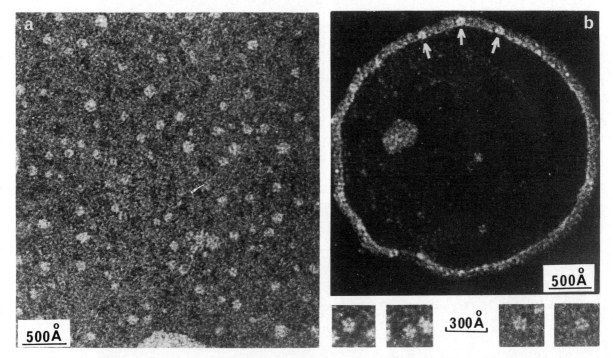

Fig. 4. Electron microscopic observation of the mediatophore in the interface fraction. Most of the mediatophore in the I_2 interface was found as free molecules in the background (a) but some could be seen in the lipidic membrane structures still present at the interface (b) (arrows). The insets on the right are large magnifications of the mediatophore of the interface I_2, which is comparable to the delipidified mediatophore obtained by the standard ether precipitation method (left insets). Negative staining with 2% neutral phosphotungstic sodium salt.

involved in the final steps of the release process: the number of large intramembrane particles increases in the course of release, an observation also reported for stimulated electric organ prisms (Muller et al., 1987). It is possible that the mediatophore is a constituent of these large particles, the release blocker cetiedil being able to inhibit their formation (Israël et al., 1987a).

Presence of mediatophore in rat brain

With minor modifications, the method described by Whittaker (1959) was applied to rat cerebral cortex and used to purify pinched-off nerve endings from that tissue. A negatively stained synaptosome is shown (inset, Fig. 5) for comparison with presynaptic membrane ghosts purified from the osmotically disrupted synaptosomes (Fig. 5).

The purified presynaptic membranes were submitted to the mediatophore extraction procedure previously developed for *Torpedo* electric organ presynaptic membranes. The rat membrane extract was mixed with synthetic lecithin to prepare proteoliposomes containing ACh. The release of transmitter from these particles was tested in response to a calcium influx generated by the successive additions of calcium ionophore A23187 and calcium (Israël et al., 1988a). ACh release was monitored using the choline-oxidase chemiluminescent procedure and a typical curve is shown in Fig. 6. This calcium-dependent ACh release was blocked in the presence of the drug cetiedil, which has been shown to inhibit the translocation of ACh in *Torpedo* electric organ (Morot Gaudry-Talarmain et al., 1987) and from rat brain synaptosomes. Inhibition of rat brain mediato-

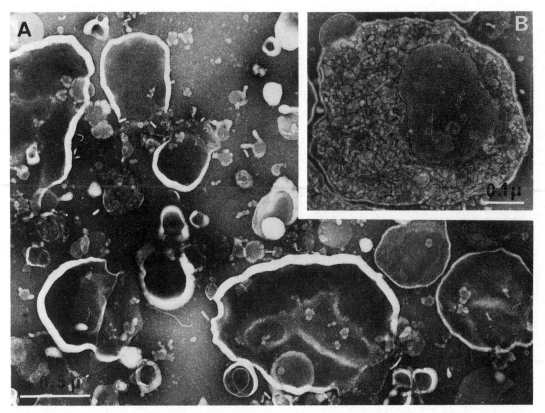

Fig. 5. Electron micrograph of synaptosomal membrane ghosts negatively stained. The inset (B) shows a negatively stained synaptosome before the water shock necessary to isolate the presynaptic membrane.

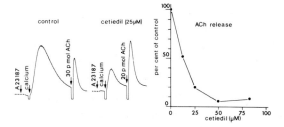

Fig. 6. Acetylcholine release from proteoliposomes made with rat presynaptic membrane proteins. (Left trace) ACh release from proteoliposomes made with a mediatophore extract prepared from purified presynaptic membranes and reconstituted into artificial liposomal membranes. When release subsides, an ACh standard is injected for calibration. (Middle trace) Inhibition of ACh release from proteoliposomes by cetiedil (25 µM). The graph plots the inhibition of ACh release from these proteoliposomes for increasing cetiedil concentration. In all cases the entrapped ACh in the liposomes was 1 nmol per assay. The incubation medium contained 6 µM EGTA. The release was monitored with the choline oxidase chemiluminescent method, after addition of ionophore A23187 (6.6 µM) and calcium (5 mM).

phore activity was half maximum at about 12 µM.

ACh release from proteoliposomes was then used to evaluate the mediatophore content of different brain areas. Three regions were chosen: the caudate plus putamen nuclei, the brain cortex and the cerebellum. We checked that choline acetyltransferase activities in P_2 fractions obtained from these regions were markedly different: 430, 119 and 6 nmol/h per g tissue, respectively. These P_2 fractions were extracted and tested for mediatophore activity as described in Methods. Mediatophore activity was maximal in caudate nuclei and lowest in cerebellum (Israël et al., 1988b).

The protein patterns of the mediatophore-containing extracts obtained from these brain areas were determined after sodium dodecyl sulfate gel electrophoresis and compared to the pattern of extracts prepared from presynaptic plasma membranes purified from cortex synaptosomes (Fig. 7). Four bands were stained from purified synaptosomal membrane extract in the 10–15 kDa region, which is to be compared to the 15 kDa *Torpedo* mediatophore monomer. When P_2 fractions are extracted, rather than purified presynaptic membranes, the protein pattern is more complex and a

12 kDa band becomes dominant. Nevertheless the four bands of purified presynaptic membrane extract are present and the intensity of the 15 kDa band seems to follow mediatophore activity.

Discussion

In the description of the quantal ACh release (see Katz, 1969) an intermediate membrane element is supposed to interact with the synaptic vesicle before exocytosis. In more recent works on exocytosis in mast cells a transient fusion pore has been characterized by Breckenridge and Almers (1981).

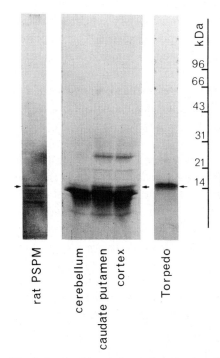

Fig. 7. Acrylamide gel electrophoresis of mediatophore extracts of various membrane preparations. Lane 1: four bands are stained by Coomassie blue after gel electrophoresis of a mediatophore extract prepared from presynaptic membranes purified from rat cortex synaptosomes. Lanes 2–4: mediatophore extracted from P_2 membranes of different brain regions. The pattern is more complex but a 15 kDa band seems to be faint in cerebellum, and stronger in caudate and cortex areas, which showed more mediatophore activity. Lane 5: purified *Torpedo* mediatophore showing the characteristic 15 kDa monomer. In all cases fractions were boiled in 5% SDS in the presence of 5% β-mercaptoethanol.

The membrane element which would serve as a docking protein for synaptic vesicles might indeed be the mediatophore. Such a view should not, however, rule out a possible direct release of cytoplasmic ACh through the mediatophore. It is also possible that both mechanisms coexist. As far as the final steps of release are concerned, we think that the properties of the mediatophore explain most aspects of quantal release.

If some 20 mediatophore molecules close to a calcium channel are simultaneously activated by the sudden rise of calcium at the cytoplasmic opening of this calcium channel, then a quantum of transmitter will be released giving a miniature end-plate potential similar to the one originally observed by Fatt and Katz (1952). The mediatophore molecules are functionally synchronized by the calcium concentration gradient. The mediatophore molecules situated at some distance from the calcium channel in a diluted region of the calcium gradient are desensitized, and do not release transmitter. Hence the mediatophore molecules which are within a given range of calcium diffusion will open together, giving the normal miniature end-plate potential. If stimulation synchronizes the opening of calcium channels then an additive response – the end-plate potential – will necessarily represent a sum of miniature end-plate potentials. Now if some experimental condition (heat challenge) disorganizes the calcium concentration gradient found at the opening of the calcium channel, then one might record the smallest events due to the activation of single mediatophore molecules giving sub-miniature end-plate potentials such as those found by Kriebel and Gross (1974) and Kriebel et al. (1982). This also implies that the normal miniature is itself the necessary addition of sub-miniatures. It should also be said that in some experimental conditions the boundary between activated and desensitized mediatophores can be changed, giving giant miniature end-plate potentials. Some of these very big miniatures might also result from an occasional exocytotic event similar to the exocytosis found for some glandular tissues.

In conclusion we shall summarize some properties of the mediatophore.

(1) It is a protein purified from the nerve terminal membrane of cholinergic synaptosomes; it is not found in post-synaptic membranes.

(2) It is an integral membrane protein purified in association with lipids, which are essential for maintaining its activity.

(3) The effects of calcium on a category of intramembrane particles more numerous during transmitter release might well be related to the calcium-binding properties of the mediatophore.

(4) Mediatophore endows artificial membranes with an ACh-release mechanism which is strictly calcium-dependent, antagonized by Mg.

(5) Like the normal release mechanisms, mediatophore-supported release shows a dual effect of calcium. Activation takes place at high calcium concentrations, while desensitization or fatigue is observed in low calcium conditions. A predicted consequence is that mediatophore molecules close to the calcium channel will be synchronously activated by the high local calcium concentration while at some distance desensitization takes place.

(6) Cetiedil analogues and drugs which affect ACh release after the calcium entry step show similar actions on the mediatophore-supported release. A completely different pattern of actions was observed on other cholinergic processes such as vesicular ACh uptake or choline pumping activity.

(7) Mediatophore activity was also found in rat brain synaptosomes, particularly in cholinergic areas.

References

Birman, S., Israël, M., Lesbats, B. and Morel, N. (1986) Solubilization and partial purification of a presynaptic membrane protein ensuring calcium-dependent acetylcholine release from proteoliposomes. *J. Neurochem.*, 47: 433–444.

Breckenridge, L.J. and Almers, W. (1987) Currents through the fusion pore that forms during exocytoses of a secretory vesicle. *Nature*, 328: 814–817.

Ducis, I. and Whittaker, V.P. (1985) High-affinity, sodium-gradient-dependent transport of choline into vesiculated presynaptic plasma membrane fragments from the electric organ of *Torpedo marmorata* and reconstitution of the solubilized transporter into liposomes. *Biochim. Biophys. Acta*, 815: 109–127.

Dunant, Y. and Israël, M. (1985) The release of acetylcholine. *Sci. Am.*, 252: 58–66.

Egea, G., Esquerda, J.E., Calvet, R., Solsona, C. and Marsal, J. (1987) Structural changes at pure cholinergic synaptosomes during the transmitter release induced by A 23187 in *Torpedo marmorata*. A freeze fracture study. *Cell Tissue Res.*, 248: 207–214.

Fatt, P. and Katz, B. (1952) Spontaneous subthreshold activity at motor nerve endings. *J. Physiol. (Lond.)*, 117: 109–128.

Folch, J. and Lees, M. (1951) Proteolipids, a new type of tissue lipoproteins. Their isolation from brain. *J. Biol. Chem.*, 191: 807–817.

Israël, M. and Lesbats, B. (1981a) Chemiluminescent determination of acetylcholine and continuous detection of its release from Torpedo electric organ synapses and synaptosomes. *Neurochem. Int.*, 3: 81–90.

Israël, M. and Lesbats, B. (1981b) Continuous determination by a chemiluninescent method of acetylcholine release and compartmentation in Torpedo electric organ synaptosomes. *J. Neurochem.*, 37: 1475–1483.

Israël, M. and Lesbats, B. (1982) Application to mammalian tissues of the chemiluminescent method for detecting acetylcholine. *J. Neurochem.*, 39: 248–250.

Israël, M. and Lesbats, B. (1985) Chemiluminescent determination of acetylcholine and continuous detection of its release from tissues. In K. Van Dyke (Ed.), *Bioluminescence and Chemiluminescence. Instruments and Applications, Vol. 2*, CRC Press, Boca Raton, FL, pp. 1–12.

Israël, M. and Lesbats, B. (1986) The use of bioluminescence techniques in neurobiology, with emphasis on the cholinergic system. In A.J. Turner and H.S. Bachelard (Eds.), *Neurochemistry, A Practical Approach*, IRL Press, Oxford, pp. 113–135.

Israël, M., Manaranche, R., Mastour, P. and Morel, N. (1976) Isolation of pure cholinergic nerve endings from the electric organ of *Torpedo marmorata*. *Biochem. J.*, 160: 113–115.

Israël, M., Manaranche, R., Morel, N., Dedieu, J.C., Gulik-Krzywicki, T. and Lesbats, B. (1980) Redistribution of intramembrane particles related to acetylcholine release by cholinergic synaptosomes. *J. Ultrastruct. Res.*, 75: 162–178.

Israël, M., Lesbats, B. and Manaranche, R. (1981) ACh release from osmotically shocked synaptosomes refilled with transmitter. *Nature*, 294: 474–475.

Israël, M., Lesbats, B., Manaranche, R. and Morel, N. (1983) Acetylcholine release from proteoliposomes equipped with synaptosomal membrane constituents. *Biochim. Biophys. Acta*, 728: 438–448.

Israël, M., Lesbats, B., Morel, N., Manaranche, R., Gulik-Krzywicki, T. and Dedieu, J.C. (1984) Reconstitution of a functional synaptosomal membrane possessing the protein constituents involved in acetylcholine translocation. *Proc. Natl. Acad. Sci. USA*, 81: 277–281.

Israël, M., Morel, N., Lesbats, B., Birman, S. and Manaranche, R. (1986) Purification of a presynaptic membrane protein

which mediates a calcium-dependent translocation of acetylcholine. *Proc. Natl. Acad. Sci. USA*, 83: 9226–9230.

Israël, M., Manaranche, R., Morot Gaudry-Talarmain, Y., Lesbats, B., Gulik-Krzywicki, T. and Dedieu, JC. (1987a) Effect of cetiedil on acetylcholine release and intramembrane particles in cholinergic synaptosomes. *Biol. Cell*, 61: 59–63.

Israël, M., Meunier, F.M., Morel, N. and Lesbats, B. (1987b) Calcium-induced desensitization of acetylcholine release from synaptosomes of proteoliposomes equipped with mediatophore, a presynaptic membrane protein. *J. Neurochem.*, 49: 975–982.

Israël, M., Lesbats, B., Morel, N., Manaranche, R. and Birman, S. (1988a) The lipid requirements of mediatophore for acetylcholine release activity. Large-scale purification of this protein in a reactive form. *Neurochem. Int.*, 13: 199–205.

Israël, M., Lesbats, B., Morel, N., Manaranche, R. and Le Gal la Salle, G. (1988b) Is the acetylcholine releasing protein mediatophore present in rat brain? *FEBS Lett.*, 233: 421–426.

Katz, B. (1969) The release of neural transmitter substances. In *The Sherrington Lectures*, Liverpool University Press, Liverpool.

King, R.G. and Marchbanks, R.M. (1982) The incorporation of solubilized choline-transport activity into liposomes. *Biochem. J.*, 204: 565–576.

Kriebel, M.E. and Gross, C.E. (1974) Multimodal distribution of frog miniature endplate potentials in adult denervated and tadpole leg muscle. *J. Gen. Physiol.*, 64: 85–103.

Kriebel, M.E., Llados, F. and Matteson, D.R. (1982) Histograms of the unitary evoked potential of the mouse diaphragm show multiple peaks. *J. Physiol. (Lond.)*, 322: 211–222.

Meyer, E.M. and Cooper, J.R. (1983) High affinity choline uptake and calcium-dependent acetylcholine release in proteoliposomes derived from rat cortical synaptosomes. *J. Neurosci.*, 3: 987–994.

Michaelson, D.M. and Burstein, M. (1985) Biochemical evidence that acetylcholine release from cholinergic nerve terminals is mostly vesicular. *FEBS Lett.*, 188: 389.

Michaelson, D.M., Burstein, M. and Licht, R. (1986) Translocation of cytosolic acetylcholine into synaptic vesicles and demonstration of vesicular release. *J. Biol. Chem.*, 261: 6831.

Morel, N., Israël, M., Manaranche, R. and Mastour, P. (1977) Isolation of pure cholinergic nerve endings from *Torpedo* electric organ. Evaluation of their metabolic properties. *J. Cell Biol.*, 75: 43–55.

Morel, N., Marsal, J., Manaranche, R., Lazereg, S., Mazie, J.C. and Israël, M. (1985) Large scale purification of presynaptic plasma membranes from Torpedo marmorata electric organ. *J. Cell Biol.*, 101: 1757–1762.

Morot Gaudry-Talarmain, Y., Israël, M., Lesbats, B. and Morel, N. (1987) Cetiedil, a drug that inhibits acetylcholine release in *Torpedo* electric organ. *J. Neurochem.*, 49: 548–554.

Morot Gaudry-Talarmain, Y., Diebler, M.F. and O'Regan, S. (1989a) Compared effects of two vesicular acetylcholine uptake blockers, AH5183 and cetiedil, on cholinergic functions in *Torpedo* synaptosomes: acetylcholine synthesis, choline transport, vesicular uptake and evoked acetylcholine release. *J. Neurochem.,* 52: (in press).

Morot Gaudry-Talarmain, Y., Diebler, M.F., Robba, M., Lancelot, J.C., Lesbats, B. and Israël, M. (1989b) Pharmacological differentiation of evoked acetylcholine release, vesicular acetylcholine uptake and choline transport effects of cetiedil analogs and some other compounds. *Eur. J. Pharmacol.,* in press.

Muller, D., Garcia-Segura, L.M., Parducz, A. and Dunant, Y. (1987) Brief occurence of a population of presynaptic intramembrane particles coincides with transmission of a nerve impulse. *Proc. Natl. Acad. Sci. USA,* 84: 590–594.

Steck, T.L. and Yu, J. (1973) Selective solubilization of proteins from red blood cell membranes by protein pertubants. *J. Supramol. Struct.,* 1: 220–232.

Vyas, S. and O'Regan, S. (1985) Reconstitution of carrier mediated choline transport in proteoliposomes prepared from presynaptic membranes of *Torpedo* electric organ and its internal and external ionic requirements. *J. Membrane Biol.,* 85: 111–119.

Whittaker, V.P. (1959) The isolation and characterization of acetylcholine-containing particles from brain. *Biochem. J.,* 72: 694–706.

S.-M. Aquilonius and P.-G. Gillberg (Eds.)
Progress in Brain Research, Vol. 84
© 1990 Elsevier Science Publishers B.V. (Biomedical Division)

CHAPTER 12

Cell surface ATP (P2y) purinoceptors trigger and modulate multiple calcium fluxes in skeletal muscle cells

J. Häggblad *, H. Eriksson and E. Heilbronn

Unit of Neurochemistry and Neurotoxicology, University of Stockholm, S-106 91 Stockholm, Sweden

Introduction

It is accepted today that adenosine 5′-triphosphate (ATP) takes part in transmission events in many neuronal systems by a variety of actions. Both transmitter and modulator-like effects are documented; some are elicited by the dephosphorylation product adenosine.

Interestingly, both pre- and postsynaptic release of ATP, as well as effects elicited by the released compound, have been observed.

This paper discusses some recent results, obtained in the authors' laboratory, on the biochemical effects of extracellular ATP in skeletal muscle cells and the role extracellular ATP might play in neuromuscular transmission, and in events following that.

ATP release and salvage

In the *Torpedo* electric organ it has been known for some time that there is, besides the well known cholinergic mechanism, a presynaptic release/salvage system for ATP and adenosine (Zimmermann, 1982). In this model for cholinergic neurotransmission, depolarization-induced release of ATP from the postsynaptic cells has also been

observed (Israel et al., 1980). This latter source of extracellular ATP is larger, and probably more diffuse in its release pattern, than the presynaptically released ATP, which due to its origin is released into the synaptic cleft. Furthermore, due to the fact that postsynaptic ATP release is induced by depolarization, there is a delay as compared to the presynaptic transmitter release.

The existence of ATP within the synaptic vesicles of motor nerve endings was only recently proven (Volknandt and Zimmermann, 1986), while release of ATP, seemingly of presynaptic origin, was shown in the early seventies (Silinsky and Hubbard, 1973). Release of ATP from depolarized skeletal muscle cells has been shown by several laboratories (Abood et al., 1962; Häggblad, 1987). However, the precise postsynaptic location of this latter release in relation to, for example, the nerve terminals has never been shown. In addition, the effective lifetime and thereby the range of action of released ATP in relation to its source is unknown.

Physiological effects of extracellular ATP in skeletal muscle and its site of action

As discussed above, it is well known that there is a release of ATP during and following neurotransmission. The released nucleotide is degraded to adenosine, which, at the motor nerve ending as in many neuronal systems, acts presynaptically

---

* To whom correspondence should be addressed.

through adenosine receptors (P1 purinoceptors) to inhibit continued release of the neurotransmitter, in this case acetylcholine (ACh). The presynaptic P1-purinoceptor on motor nerve endings has been suggested to modulate depolarization-induced calcium entry into the nerve terminal. Cell surface P1 purinoceptors are generally categorized into A1 and A2 subtypes, depending on their coupling to adenylate cyclase (the former negatively and the latter positively coupled) and on the pharmacology of the tissue response. As the effect of adenosine on transmitter release does not seem to be mediated through a cyclic AMP-triggered mechanism a third subtype, defined as A3, has (mainly on a physico-pharmacological basis) been suggested to exert the feed-back in this case (for a discussion see Ribeiro and Sebastiao, 1986). The basis for this nomenclature is, however, controversial.

The postsynaptic action of ATP, as suggested by our results, is mediated by the action of the parent nucleotide ATP rather than by adenosine. Reported postsynaptic effects in skeletal muscle preparations of extracellular ATP are a potentiation of ACh-induced contractions (Buchtahl and Folkow, 1948) and an increase in ACh-triggered ion currents (Akasu et al., 1983). The latter report suggested a direct allosteric interaction with the nicotinic acetylcholine receptor (nAChR). Criticism has been aimed at the use of high concentrations of ATP, which may have reversible detergent-like effects and which may also contain contaminants that might have evoked the observed physiological effects. However, as will be discussed below, there are clear-cut effects on phosphatidylinositol (PI) turnover and cytosolic calcium levels caused by extracellular ATP acting on ATP receptors (P2 purinoceptors) localized on the cell surface of cultured skeletal muscle cells.

The precise localization of the P2 purinoceptors in skeletal muscle is not known yet as neither antibodies to the receptor nor specific receptor ligands exist. Thus, it is not known today whether P2 purinoceptors are localized in synaptic or extrasynaptic regions, or both.

Calcium transients in cultured myotubes induced by activation of P2y purinoceptors

It was shown by us that ATP when applied to cultured myotubes obtained from chick, rat and mouse skeletal muscle induced a rapid increase in PI turnover (Fig. 1) through the action on the P2y subtype of purinoceptors (Häggblad, 1987; and Häggblad and Heilbronn, 1987). The subclassification of P2 receptors into the P2x and P2y subtypes is based on the effects of a series of agonists in which methylene-substituted ATP derivatives are more potent than ATP when acting on P2x than on P2y receptors (Burnstock, 1987) (Fig. 2). Using fura 2-loaded chick myotubes, we found that extracellular ATP triggered a biphasic change in cytosolic calcium levels. A rapid initial peak, caused by release of calcium from internal stores, was followed by a more sustained peak of calcium influx (Häggblad and Heilbronn, 1988; Eriksson and Heilbronn, 1989) (Fig. 3). The dose dependencies for ATP triggering either PI turnover or calcium transients (in this case measured as peak calcium levels in quin 2 experiments) in the myotubes were closely parallel (Fig. 4); both processes had EC_{50} values of approximately 10 μM. In preliminary experiments, using fura 2, we also found that the late peak was partially sensi-

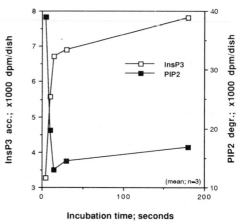

Fig. 1. Inositol trisphosphate ($InsP_3$) accumulation and phosphatidylinositol 4,5-bisphosphate (PIP_2) degradation in chick myotubes following addition of external ATP (300 μM).

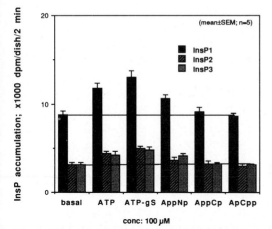

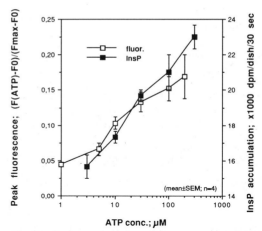

Fig. 2. Effect of ATP derivatives on inositol phosphate accumulation in chick myotubes. ATP-γS, adenosine (3-thio) triphosphate; AppNp, β,γ-imido ATP; ApCpp, α,β-methylene ATP; AppCp, β,γ-methylene ATP.

Fig. 4. Concentration dependence of ATP-induced inositol phosphate (InsP) accumulation and quin 2 fluorescence in chick myotubes.

tive to submicromolar concentrations of dihydropyridines (such as PN 200-110), in that they decrease it. This effect of the dihydropyridines indicates that ATP may open voltage-dependent calcium channels.

As the late peak in the biphasic change in cytosolic calcium in response to extracellular ATP might be composite, it is possible that part of it is due to the opening of a second-messenger-operated calcium channel triggered, for example, by metabolites of inositol 1,4,5-trisphosphate. Thus, what we observe are multiple effects on the cytosolic calcium levels following activation of P2y purinoceptors on skeletal muscle cells; one initial

rapid peak of sarcoplasmic reticulum (SR) origin followed by at least one event that is dependent on extracellular calcium.

It is also interesting to note that in myotubes cultured from dysgenic mice the effect of ATP on PI turnover remains but the subsequent changes in cytosolic calcium are diminished or completely absent. This may indicate that the excitation-contraction coupling process in the dysgenic mutants is non-functional at the level of the SR and/or may be due to a lack of voltage-operated calcium channels (Tassin et al., 1989).

The effect of P2y purinoceptor activation on depolarization-induced changes in cytosolic calcium

An obvious issue to study in skeletal muscle in order to investigate *one* possible physiological role for the observed effects on PI turnover elicited by extracellular ATP are the different steps comprising excitation-contraction coupling, a process which is strictly dependent on precise control of calcium homeostasis.

Similarly to the effects induced by ATP, we found that depolarization of cultured chick myotubes with either carbachol or high levels of potassium caused a biphasic change in cytosolic calcium as measured using the fluorescent probe

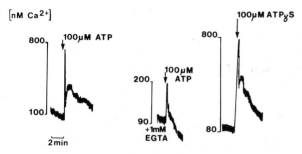

Fig. 3. Calcium transients in fura 2-loaded chick myotubes following external ATP; effect of EGTA. ATPγS, adenosine (3-thio) triphosphate.

114

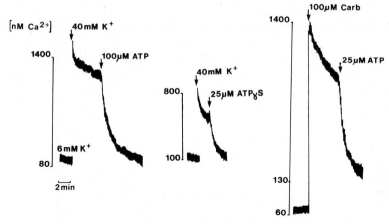

Fig. 5. Effects of ATP on calcium transients induced by depolarization of fura 2-loaded chick myotubes. ATPγS, adenosine (3-thio) triphosphate; Carb, carbachol.

fura 2 (Eriksson and Heilbronn, 1989). These changes were, however, of greater amplitude than those elicited by ATP. On tonic depolarization a very rapid peak is followed by a decline towards baseline levels. But instead of having a bulge-like shape with a duration of less than 10 min, as in the case of the P2y purinoceptor activation, this second phase starts mid-height on the first rapid peak and declines steadily during the course of 20–30 min. (Fig. 5). The second phase is also dependent on extracellular calcium and is inhibited by dihydropyridines, suggesting that it is due to influx of calcium through voltage-dependent calcium channels (Fig. 6).

When ATP was added to depolarized myotubes during the slowly declining phase a rapid decrease in cytosolic calcium to baseline levels was observed (Fig. 5). This effect of ATP had, interestingly enough, the same dose-response relationship as the P2y purinoceptor-triggered PI turnover and the subsequent calcium transients, which suggests that they are related phenomena. When ATP was added to the cells before depolarization only the first rapid peak was observed after depolarization of the cells (Fig. 6). These two latter effects of ATP could in most cases be mimicked by addition of phorbol esters (unpublished results).

In summary, these results may be interpreted as

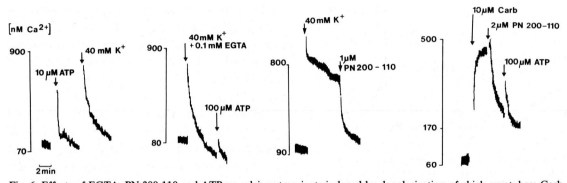

Fig. 6. Effects of EGTA, PN 200-110 and ATP on calcium transients induced by depolarization of chick myotubes; Carb, carbachol.

an ATP-induced formation of diacylglycerol that activates PKC, which modulates the conductance of voltage-operated calcium channels.

Other possible effects of extracellular ATP and the physiological role of P2y purinoceptors on skeletal muscle cells

The phenomenon of ATP-induced PI turnover and events following it is not restricted to skeletal muscle cells. Many different cell types respond to ATP in a similar manner, though the physiological results differ with the specialization of the given cell type. The effects exerted by extracellular ATP acting on P2y purinoceptors range from triggering of secretory (cf. Forsberg et al., 1987; Okajima et al., 1988) and mitotic processes (Gonzales et al., 1988) to initiation of glycogenolysis (Keppens and DeWulf, 1986). In some cases (e.g. neuroblastoma and glioma cells and astrocytes; Häggblad, unpublished results) only the triggering of PI turnover and calcium transients have so far been described. Thus, it is quite possible that, depending on where and when ATP triggers PI turnover in skeletal muscle in a physiological situation, not only an action on depolarization-induced calcium transients may be evoked, as reported in this paper, but also, for example, glycogenolysis to replenish intracellular pools of ATP that have been consumed following contraction. Still other effects may include modulation of the excitability of the skeletal muscle cells through the opening of calcium activated potassium and/or chloride channels by the increased levels of intracellular calcium; and of increased protein kinase C- or calcium/calmodulin-dependent protein kinase activities leading to phosphorylation of ion channels, including the nAChR, which are involved in the excitation. Furthermore, ATP released from the skeletal muscle cells may also have effects on other cells in the tissue, such as increasing the blood flow through the action on blood vessels.

There are many gaps in our knowledge of how ATP modulates skeletal muscle function. It is, however, clear that there exist release/degrada-

tion/salvage mechanisms as well as activation of intracellular messenger systems of physiological importance in skeletal muscle tissue. Future investigations in the very active field of purinergic mechanisms will help us fill the gaps and probably also tie cholinergic and purinergic research closer together.

References

Abood, L.G., Koketsu, K. and Miyamoto, S. (1962) Outflux of various phosphates during membrane depolarization of excitable membranes. *Am. J. Physiol.*, 202: 469–474.

Akasu, T., Hirai, K. and Koketsu, K. (1981) Increase in acetylcholine-receptor sensitivity by adenosine triphosphate: a novel action of ATP on ACh-sensitivity. *Br. J. Pharmacol.*, 74: 505–507.

Buchthal, F. and Folkow, B. (1948) Interaction between acetylcholine and adenosine triphosphate in normal, curarized and denervated muscle. *Acta Physiol. Scand.*, 15: 150–160.

Burnstock, G. (1987) A basis for distinguishing two types of purinergic receptors. In Bolis and Straub (Eds.), *Cell membrane receptors for drugs and hormones*, Raven Press, New York, pp. 107–115.

Eriksson, H. and Heilbronn, E. (1989) Extracellularly applied ATP alters the calcium flux through dihydropyridine-sensitive channels in cultured chick myotubes. *Biochem. Biophys. Res. Commun.*, 159: 878–885.

Forsberg, E.J., Feuerstein, G., Shomami, E. and Pollard, H.B. (1987) Adenosine triphosphate stimulates inositol phospholipid metabolism and prostacyclin formation in adrenal medullary endothelial cells by means of P2-purinoceptors. *Proc. Natl. Acad. Sci. USA* 84: 5630–5634.

Gonzales, F.A., Heppel, L.A., Gross, D.J., Webb, W.W. and Parries G. (1988) The rapid desensitization of receptors for platelet derived growth factor, bradykinin and ATP: Studies on individual cells using quantitative digital video fluorescence microscopy. *Biochem. Biophys. Res. Commun.*, 151: 1205–1212.

Häggblad, J. (1987) Neuromuscular junction revisited. Biochemical studies on mechanisms involved in transmission events. Dissertation, University of Stockholm, Sweden.

Häggblad, J. and Heilbronn E. (1987) Externally applied adenosine-5′-triphosphate causes inositol trisphosphate accumulation in cultured chick myotubes. *Neurosci. Lett.*, 74: 199–204.

Häggblad, J. and Heilbronn E. (1988) P2-purinoceptor-stimulated phosphoinositide turnover in chick myotubes. Calcium mobilization and the role of guanyl nucleotide-binding proteins. *FEBS Lett.*, 1,2: 133–136.

Israel, M., Lesbats, B., Manaranche, R., Meunier, F.M. and Frachon, P. (1980) Retrograde inhibition of transmitter release by ATP. *J. Neurochem.*, 34: 923–932.

Keppens, S. and DeWulf, H. (1986) Characterization of the liver P2-purinoceptor involved in the activation of glycogen phosphorylase. *Biochem. J.,* 240: 367–371.

Okajima, F., Sho, K. and Kondo, Y. (1988) Inhibition by islet-activating protein, pertussis toxin, of P2-purinergic receptor-mediated iodide efflux and phosphoinositide turnover in FRTL-5 cells. *Endocrinology,* 123: 1035–1043.

Ribeiro, J.A. and Sebastiao, A.M. (1986) Adenosine receptors and calcium: Basis for proposing a third (A3) adenosine receptor. *Prog. Neurobiol.,* 26: 179–209.

Silinsky, E.M. and Hubbard, J.I. (1973) Release of ATP from rat motor nerve terminals. *Nature,* 234: 404–405.

Tassin, A.-M., Häggblad, J. and Heilbronn, E. (1989) Receptor triggered polyphosphoinositide turnover produces less cytosolic free calcium in cultured dysgenic myotubes than in normal. *Muscle Nerve,* in press.

Volknandt, W. and Zimmermann, H. (1986) Acetylcholine, ATP and proteoglycan are common to presynaptic vesicles isolated from electric organs of electric eel and electric catfish as well as from rat diaphragm. *J. Neurochem.,* 47: 1449–1462.

Zimmermann, H. (1982) Coexistence of adenosine-5′-triphosphate in the electromotor synapse. In Cuello (Ed.), *Cotransmission,* MacMillan Press, London, pp. 243–259.

S.-M. Aquilonius and P.-G. Gillberg (Eds.)
Progress in Brain Research, Vol. 84
© 1990 Elsevier Science Publishers B.V. (Biomedical Division)

CHAPTER 13

Immunogenetic mechanisms in myasthenia gravis

Lawrence Steinman

Departments of Neurology, Pediatrics and Genetics, Stanford University, Stanford CA 94305, U.S.A.

Introduction

T cells can recognize fragments of self-constituents, such as acetylcholine receptor, and provide specific stimulatory signals for the activation of B cells which differentiate into autoantibody-secreting plasma cells. Myasthenia gravis (MG) results from an antibody-mediated autoimmune response to the nicotinic acetylcholine receptor (AChR). Individuals with MG have a higher frequency of certain major histocompatibility complex (MHC) antigens, particularly HLA-B8, DR3 and DQw2 (Säfwenberg et al., 1978). Since the target antigen is known, MG will be one of the first human autoimmune diseases to be fully characterized at the molecular level. HLA-DR, DQ and DP antigens have already been sequenced in MG patients (Todd et al., 1988; Mantegazza et al., 1989), some T and B cell epitopes have been characterized (Brocke et al., 1988; Harcourt et al., 1988; Hohlfeld et al., 1989), and T cell receptor (TcR) gene polymorphisms associated with the disease have been described (Oksenberg et al., 1989).

The ternary interaction of class II major histocompatibility molecules, the T cell receptor, and AChR peptides

This subject has been recently reviewed by us (Wraith et al., 1989). The minimal requirement for activation of helper T (T_H) cells is the occupation of their TcR by a complex formed between fragments of antigen and class II MHC molecules. Class II molecules are encoded by I-A and I-E genes of the H-2 complex in mice and DP, DQ and DR genes of the HLA complex in man. In addition to this molecular triad, accessory (cell differentiation) molecules on the surface of the T cell (CD4 for T_H and CD8 for cytotoxic T (T_C) cells) interact with MHC molecules on the surface of the antigen-presenting cell (APC), increase the overall affinity of cell-cell contact, and permit recognition of the antigen-MHC complex by low affinity TcR.

The majority of antigens for T cells are recognized in a denatured or fragmented form (Möller et al., 1987). This requirement presumably allows for association of fragments with the antigen-binding "cleft" of class I (Bjorkman et al., 1987) and the predicted "cleft" of class II MHC molecules (Brown et al., 1988). The majority of polymorphic MHC residues are clustered around this "cleft', and this indicates how these residues directly influence antigen binding and interaction with TcR (Bjorkman et al., 1987).

The immune system can respond to a wide variety of different protein antigens, and this implies that any one MHC molecule can associate with a vast assortment of antigenic structures. MHC molecules are highly polymorphic, and products of separate alleles can associate with different sets of peptide antigenic structures. In spite of the promiscuous nature of MHC-antigen associations, it has proved difficult to measure peptide binding. This can be explained by the relatively low-affinity constant for association between MHC and peptide (Babbit et al., 1985; Buus et al., 1986) or by the premise that MHC proteins are normally occupied by endogenous self-peptides, as suggested by recent studies (Buus et al., 1988). This information, combined with the demonstration that APC from normal tissues constitutively present self-antigens, such as hemoglobin (Lorenz and Allen, 1988), is evidence that the recognition of self-antigen-MHC complexes may be involved in immunoregulation (Kourilsky and Claverie, 1986). However, the overall significance of endogenous peptides to immune responsiveness and tolerance to self-antigens awaits further experimentation.

It is now quite clear that there is a single antigen binding site on class II molecules, since cross-linking of class II MHC with radiolabeled peptide probes produces complexes of the appropriate size for a 1:1 ratio of binding (Luescher et al., 1988; Wraith et al., unpublished data). Furthermore, peptides can compete with one another for MHC binding and T cell activation (Guillet et al., 1987). The furthest extension of this observation has been the demonstration that a mouse lysozyme peptide can competitively inhibit priming with a foreign lysozyme peptide on co-injection into a mouse strain normally responsive to the foreign peptide (Adorini et al., 1988). The mouse lysozyme peptide binds to one of the two responder MHC molecules (I-A^k), thus specifically blocking binding of and preventing an immune response to the foreign peptide. This experiment was successful since, even though the peptide bound to the I-A^k molecule, the responder mouse was tolerant to the self-lysozyme peptide.

Ideally, an effective immune system would be able to respond to any foreign antigen and yet would remain unresponsive to, or tolerant of, its own self-antigens throughout life. To a large extent the immune system of higher animals has evolved to achieve this end. Immunological tolerance is believed to be induced during a perinatal period when immature lymphocytes are exposed to self-antigens. In humans this period terminates before birth, while in rodents the process is complete shortly after birth.

Recent studies have clarified the role of the thymus in preparing T lymphocytes for life in an effective immune system. Studies in normal and transgenic mice have revealed how interaction of TcRs with an appropriate MHC molecule can lead to increased cell numbers in the periphery (positive selection) (reviewed by Von Boehmer et al., 1989). Conversely, analysis of the distribution of either MLS (mouse lymphocyte stimulating) locus reactive or MHC class II antigen (I-E) specific T cells in normal mice has shown how developing T cells can be deleted from the repertoire following interaction of TcR with the self-antigen-MHC complex in the thymus (negative selection) (reviewed by Marrack and Kappler, 1988). By subjecting T cells to such education, the system selects for cells that are "obsessed" with self-MHC and yet are unable to react with self-MHC combined with any self-antigen that the T cell encountered during the later stages of ontogeny. How the thymus manages to turn MHC recognition from providing a positive signal at one stage to a negative signal at another is not clear at this time. One explanation relies on the differential recognition of, or different affinities for, MHC molecules on epithelial as opposed to bone marrow-derived macrophages and dendritic cells by the maturing T lymphocytes (Sprent et al., 1988).

T cell-dependent autoimmune diseases arise from a breakdown in self-tolerance. There are essentially four ways in which tolerance to self-antigens can be viewed. First, an individual can be unresponsive to self if the antigen, or fragment thereof, is unable to bind to self-MHC. Secondly, potentially self-antigen-reactive T cells can be deleted from the T cell repertoire by clonal deletion in the thymus. Unfortunately, neither of the first two possibilities would explain why autoreactive T cells, specific for myelin basic protein (MBP) for example, can readily be isolated from the mature T cell repertoire and yet do not normally cause disease (Schluesner and Wekerle, 1984). A third possibility, which would account for this paradox, is that self-antigens, such as MBP, are sequestered from the immune system either physically, by the blood-brain barrier, or by being presented in a nonimmunogenic fashion. According to this theory, self-antigens associated with class II negative cells may never be immunogenic unless they are reprocessed by class II positive cells such as B lymphocytes, macrophages, dendritic or interdigitating cells. However, it should be noted that some cells can be induced to express class II molecules when treated with lymphokines (e.g., γ-interferon). Ectopic MHC expression is believed to contribute to the presentation of "sequestered" antigens in autoimmune disease (Bottazzo et al., 1986). Finally, in cases where clonal deletion does not eliminate potentially autoreactive T_H cells, autoimmune attack may be guarded against by the action of T suppressor (T_S) cells. In certain mouse strains, T_H cells specific for autoantigens are functional and remain quiescent because of the action of such antigen-specific T_S cells (Jensen and Kapp, 1985). If homeostasis in the system is seen as a "balance" between T cell help and suppression, and self-antigen-specific T cells are present in the normal individual, one can imagine how the "balance" could be tipped by stimulation with cross-reactive antigen contained in an infectious bacterium or virus.

MHC and MG

Recent molecular studies of several autoimmune conditions reveal that MHC class II genes play a major role. In patients with rheumatoid arthritis, 80–90% are either HLA-DR1 or HLA-DR4 (Dw4, Dw14 or Dw15). The HLA-DR4 Dw10 variant is associated with resistance to rheumatoid arthritis. HLA-DR1 and HLA-DR4 (Dw4, Dw14 or Dw15) have a very similar sequence in the third hypervariable region of HLA-DR, while HLA-DR4 Dw10 is strikingly different (Todd et al., 1988). A similar analysis of HLA class II genes in insulin-dependent diabetes mellitus localizes susceptibility to residue 57 in the DQ beta chain (Todd et al., 1988).

In pemphigus vulgaris (PV), a severe autoimmune disease of the skin mediated by autoantibodies to an epidermal cell surface protein, there is a striking association of disease with MHC class II genes. Thus, nearly 100% of individuals with PV are HLA-DR4, DRw6, or DR4/DRw6 heterozygotes. The DR4 susceptibility is highly associated with the Dw10, DRβ1 allele, implicating polymorphic residues in the third hypervariable region, while the DRw6 susceptibility is strongly associated with a rare DQβ allele (DQβ1.9). This allele differs from a common DQβ allele (DQβ1.1) only by a valine to aspartic acid substitution at position 57 (Scharf et al., 1988; Sinha et al., 1988).

Susceptibility to MG correlates with HLA-DR3, DQw2. Serological techniques have established a relative risk of 3.5 for MG if HLA-DR3 is present (Säfwenberg et al., 1978). RFLP studies on German and Northern California caucasoid MG patients revealed a closer association of HLA-DQ and MG. An HLA-DQ beta polymorphism in MG patients revealed a relative risk of 36 (Bell et al., 1986). This polymorphism may be closely linked to a genetic locus encoding a binding site for an AChR epitope.

Susceptibility to experimental allergic myasthenia gravis (EAMG), like susceptibility to MG, is linked to the MHC (Berman and Patrick, 1980a,b). The immune response to AChR has been mapped to the I-A genes of H-2 (the murine homologue of the human DQ region)(Christadoss et al., 1979). Studies with B6[bm12] and B6 mice have shown that particular I-A alleles play an essential role in the development of an antibody response to AChR and clinical EAMG. The bm12 mouse differs from the B6 mouse only in the I-A beta chain at amino acid residues 68, 71 and 72 (Waldor et al., 1986). These three amino acid changes result in the conversion of a strain which is susceptible to the induction of EAMG, B6, to one that is resistant to EAMG, bm12. Since I-A molecules exert an essential role in the development of an immune response to AChR, we investigated whether in vivo administration of monoclonal anti-I-A antibodies could suppress the immune response to AChR.

Reduction of anti-AChR antibody titers

C57BL/6 (H-2^b) and SJL/J (H-2^s) are both high responders to AChR and susceptible to EAMG (Berman and Patrick, 1980a). Monoclonal anti-I-A antibody was administered in vivo to these high-responder mice before immunization with soluble AChR or AChR in complete Freund's adjuvant. Four mg of monoclonal antibody (0.5 ml ascites fluid) were injected intraperitoneally, 1 day before and 1 day after immunization with AChR. This injection regimen was repeated at the time of secondary immunization. In vivo treatment with anti-I-A antibody prevented the secondary antibody response to soluble AChR (Table I). Anti-I-A antibody treatment only prevented the anti-AChR antibody response in the appropriate strain of mice. Thus, anti-I-A^b antibody had no effect on the anti-AChR antibody response in SJL/J (H-2^s) mice, and likewise, anti-I-A^s antibody did not alter the anti-AChR antibody response in C57BL/6 (H-2^b) mice (Table I). Anti-I-A injection also reduced anti-AChR antibody titers in mice immunized with AChR in complete Freund's adjuvant (Table II).

Prevention of clinical EAMG

The effect of in vivo anti-I-A treatment on clinical EAMG in SJL/J mice was assessed. Myasthenia symptoms included a characteristic hunched posture with drooping of the head and

TABLE I

Anti-I-A antibody treatment prevents the secondary antibody response to soluble AChR

Treatment **	Anti-AChR antibody levels (μl $\times 10^{-3}$) *	
	SJL/J(H-2^s)	C57BL/6(H-2^b)
None	22.3 ± 5.9	7.5 ± 7.6
Anti-I-A^s	0.2 ± 0.4	6.2 ± 4.8
Anti-I-A^b	18.6 ± 17.7	1.6 ± 3.9

* Mean ± standard deviation of the anti-AChR antibody levels determined by ELISA 1 week after secondary immunization with soluble AChR.

** 4 mg of the monoclonal antibody in ascites fluid were injected intraperitoneally on the day before and the day after primary and secondary immunization with 50 μg of soluble AChR.

TABLE II

Anti-I-A treatement reduces the secondary antibody response to AChR in complete Freund's adjuvant

Treatment *	Anti-AChR antibody levels in C57BL/6 mice (H-2^b) ** (μl $\times 10^{-2}$)
None	5.4 ± 0.5
Anti-I-A^b	1.0 ± 0.4
Anti-I-A^s	4.6 ± 0.6

* Mice were immunized with 15 μg of AChR in CFA in the hind footpads and at the base of the tail. One week later a booster injection of 50 μg of soluble AChR was given intraperitoneally. Antibody treatments were as in Table I.

** Mean ± standard deviation of anti-AChR antibody levels determined by ELISA 1 week after secondary immunization.

neck, exaggerated arching of the back, splayed limbs, abnormal walking, and difficulty in righting. Weakness was alleviated with 5–10 min of administration of neostigmine bromide and atropine sulfate intraperitoneally. Clinical disease was apparent in 11 of 19 control animals and only 2 of 10 anti-I-A^s treated mice.

TcR and MG

To investigate which parts of the AChR are involved in the initiation and development of MG, peptides representing different sequences of the human AChR α-subunit were synthesized. These peptides were tested for their ability to stimulate T cells of myasthenic patients and healthy control patients in proliferation assays and to bind to sera antibodies. Three of eight peptides discriminated significantly between the two groups in the proliferation assay, as well as in their ability to bind to serum antibodies. HLA-DR3 and DR5 were associated with proliferative responses to specific AChR peptides in the group of myasthenics. Acetylcholine receptor epitopes which might play a specific role in myasthenia gravis were thus demonstrated.

Proliferative responses of PBL of MG patients to peptides representing sequences of the human AChR

PBL of MG patients and of healthy controls were tested for their ability to proliferate in the

TABLE III

Synthetic peptides of the AChR α-subunit

Peptides	Species	Sequence
p195–212	Human	Asp Thr Pro Tyr Leu Asp Ile Ile Tyr His Phe Val Met Gln Arg Leu Pro Leu
p257–269	Human	Leu Leu Val Ile Val Glu Leu Ile Pro Ser Thr Ser Ser
p310–327	Human	Asn Trp Val Arg Lys Ile Phe Ile Asp Thr Ile Pro Asn Ile Met Phe Phe Ser
p169–181	Human	Asn Phe Met Glu Ser Gly Glu Trp Val Ile Lys Glu Ser
p183–196	Human	Gly Trp Lys His Ser Val Thr Tyr Ser Cys Cys Pro Asp Thr
p185–196	Human	Lys His Ser Val Thr Tyr Ser Cys Cys Pro Asp Thr
p351–368	Human	Ile Ser Gly Lys Pro Gly Pro Pro Pro Met Gly Phe His Ser Pro Leu Ile Lys
p394–409	Human	Asn Ala Ala Glu Glu Trp Lys Tyr Val Ala Met Val Ile Asn His Ile

presence of an in vitro stimulus with the various peptides representing regions of the AChR α-subunit listed in Table III.

Table IV summarizes the results of the proliferative assays specific to eight sequences of the AChR performed with PBL of MG patients and healthy controls. As shown in the table, the myasthenic patients responded better to all the peptides. However, only three peptides (p195–212, p257–269 and p310–327) could discriminate significantly between MG patients and controls on the basis of the proliferative responses of PBL. The differences between MG patients and controls were the most significant when the responses to p195–212 were measured (Table IV).

Antibody levels specific to synthetic peptides representing AChR in sera of MG patients

It was of interest whether sera of patients with myasthenia gravis possess antibodies that react with the different peptides representing the AChR α-subunit.

Table V summarizes the percentages of positive antibody titers specific to the seven peptides in sera of MG patients and controls. It can be seen in the table that the percentages of sera with antibody titers specific to p195–212, p257–269, and p310–327 are significantly higher than those determined in sera of controls.

HLA typing of MG patients

The HLA-A, B, C, DR and DQ phenotypes of 45 MG patients were tested. Fifteen patients (33%) possessed HLA-B8. Fourteen of the 45 patients (31%) possessed HLA-DR3. In 12 cases of the latter, DR3 occurred jointly with HLA-B8. Note that both HLA-B8 and DR3 are present in relatively low frequencies of 9.4 and 10.4%, respectively, in the Israeli population. Moreover, the joint occurrence of B8 and DR3 in the healthy

TABLE IV

Percentages of positive proliferative PBL responses of MG patients and healthy controls to peptides representing different sequences of the human AChR

Peptides	MG patients	Healthy controls
p195–212	72.5% (20/28)	21.2% (7/33) $p < 0.001$
p257–269	56 % (14/25)	16 % (4/25) $p < 0.01$
p310–327	44.4% (12/27)	15.6% (5/32) $p < 0.01$
p169–181	26.9% (7/26)	9.5% (2/21)
p183–196	26.9% (7/26)	19.2% (5/26)
p185–196	5.4% (4/26)	3.8% (1/26)
p351–368	35.7% (10/28)	26.9% (7/26)
p394–409	26.9% (7/26)	19.2% (5/26)

TABLE V

Percentages of positive serum antibody levels of MG patients and healthy controls to peptides representing different sequences of the human AChR

Peptides	MG patients	Healthy controls
p195–212	79.5% (31/39)	6.5% (2/31) $p < 0.0001$
p257–269	47.5% (19/40)	3.3% (1/30) $p < 0.001$
p310–327	49% (21/43)	6.5% (2/31) $p < 0.001$
p169–181	14% (6/43)	6.5% (2/31)
p185–196	5% (2/40)	3.3% (1/30)
p351–368	5% (2/40)	3.3% (1/30)
p394–409	16% (7/43)	6.5% (2/31)

TABLE VI

Correlation between HLA-DR3 and proliferative responses to p257–269

	Responder	Nonresponder
HLA-DR3 myasthenic	7/7 [a/b] (100%)	0/7 [a] (0%)
Not HLA-DR3 myasthenic	6/16 [b] (38%)	10/16 (62%)
HLA-DR healthy	1/1 (100%)	0/0 (0%)
Not HLA-DR3 healthy	3/17 (18%)	14/17 (82%)

[a] $p < 0.0003$, Fisher's exact test.
[b] $p < 0.006$, Fisher's exact test.

Israeli population is rather low (5.7%) but significantly higher ($\chi^2 = 11.3$, $p < 0.001$) in the Israeli MG patients. The relative risk for B8, DR3 carriers is 6.1.

A possible correlation was sought between the proliferative capacity of PBL of MG patients and control individuals to the various peptides of the AChR and HLA. Table VI demonstrates that all seven HLA-DR3-type patients responded to p257–269 ($p < 0.0003$). The one HLA-DR3 healthy individual also responded to p257–269. Non-HLA-DR3 patients also responded to p257–269, but less frequently (7 of 7 vs. 6 of 16; $p < 0.006$). Table VII demonstrates that 10 of 12 (83%) of the HLA-DR5 myasthenic patients responded to p195–212 by proliferation, compared with 2 of 12 (17%) of myasthenic DR5 carriers who did not respond. In the group of HLA-DR5 healthy controls, the distribution was different, with 3 of 14 (21%) responding and 11 of 14 not responding to p195–212 ($p < 0.007$). Non-HLA-DR5 myasthenics also responded frequently to p195–212 (9 of 15 vs. 10 of 12, $P = NS$). No

TABLE VII

Correlation between HLA-DR5 and proliferative responses to p195–212

	Responder	Nonresponder
HLA-DR5 myasthenic	10/12 [a] (83%)	2/12 (17%)
Not HLA-DR5 myasthenic	9/15 (60%)	6/15 (40%)
HLA-DR5 healthy	3/14 [a] (21%)	11/14 (79%)
Not HLA-DR5 healthy	3/15 (20%)	12/15 (80%)

[a] $\chi^2 = 7.6$, $p < 0.01$.

correlation could be observed between proliferative responses to p310–327 and any HLA-DR antigen. Antibody reactivity to p195–212, p257–269 and p310–327 in the sera of MG patients was not associated with any particular HLA type.

This study suggests that peptides of AChR are particularly immunogenic for certain HLA-DR types. HLA-DR5 individuals responded better than healthy controls to p195–212. Moreover, all HLA-DR3 respond to p257–269. It has been demonstrated that immunogenic peptides bind directly to class II MHC products (Babbitt et al., 1985). In this context, it is possible that p195–212 binds more readily with an MG-associated class II HLA product, whereas p257–269 binds preferentially to HLA-DR3. The fact that HLA-DR3 class II molecules have identical sequences in MG patients and controls may underlie the observation that some healthy individuals respond to some AChR peptides (Todd et al., 1988). This may account for the fact that individuals with different HLA-class II genotypes can respond to a given AChR peptide.

These studies represent one of the first attempts to analyse the determinants of the AChR molecule involved in the aberrant immune response in MG in humans. Hohlfeld and others have reported responses to three NH_2-terminal AChR peptides in T cell lines from two MG patients that react with *Torpedo* AChR (Hohlfeld et al., 1988). Atassi and colleagues have studied the response in inbred mouse strains to various AChR peptides from the α subunit of *Torpedo* AChR (Atassi et al., 1987). Our studies demonstrate significant differences between MG patients and healthy controls in the immune response potential to various sequences of the human AChR and its association with HLA. Other epitopes of AChR, when tested, may also be shown to play a critical role in the pathogenesis of MG.

Polymorphic markers in genes encoding the α chain of the human TcR have been detected by Southern blot analysis in *Pss*I digests. Polymorphic bands were observed at 6.3 and 2.0 kilobases (kb) with frequencies of 0.30 and 0.44, respectively, in the general population. Using the poly-

TABLE VIII

Distribution of TcR V^α and C^α in MG patients

	6.3 kb		2.0 kb	
	+	−	+	−
MG Stanford	14	3	17	0
Control Stanford	21	49	31	39

merase chain reaction (PCR) method, we amplified selected sequences derived from the full-length TcR α cDNA probe. These PCR products were used as specific probes to demonstrate that the 6.3-kb polymorphic fragment hybridizes to the variable (V) region probe and the 2.0-kb fragment hybridizes to the constant (C) region probe. Segregation of the polymorphic bands was analysed in family studies. To look for associations between these markers and autoimmune diseases, we have studied the restriction fragment length polymorphism (RFLP) distribution of the *Pss*I markers in patients with multiple sclerosis, myasthenia gravis and Graves disease. Significant differences in the frequency of the polymorphic V_α and C_α markers were identified between MG patients and healthy controls.

For MG patients, the 6.3-kb positive phenotype is significantly more common than in controls and confers a relative risk of 11 ($\chi^2 = 15.6$), while the 2.0-kb positive phenotype is also significantly more common than in controls (17 of 17 MG patients versus 31 of 70 controls; $\chi^2 = 17.2$) (Table VIII).

Conclusion

Autoimmune disease results from a breakdown in self-tolerance. The root cause of many serious human diseases is the aberrant activation of self-reactive T cells. Two striking features are emerging. First, individuals expressing certain class II MHC genes are more likely to be affected. Furthermore, there appears to be a common thread between the susceptible MHC genes in that, as shown for RA and IDDM, susceptibility alleles share regions of allelic hypervariability. We be-

lieve that the similarity between susceptible alleles reflects the role of MHC molecules in the maintenance of T cell tolerance. However, it is not yet clear whether this lies at the level of self-antigen binding to MHC, thymic T cell education, or immunoregulation via T suppressor cells. We need to know much more about the molecular nature of T cell recognition in human diseases to identify the antigens recognized and to correlate MHC restriction of disease-associated T cells with known susceptibility alleles. Even so, the striking association between disease and MHC class II alleles holds promise for immunotherapy. Second, a common finding in many experimental models is the oligoclonality in some human autoimmune conditions, though it is not certain that the T cell populations studied were the primary effectors of disease. When this can be established, specific TcR-targeted immunotherapy may also be feasible for human autoimmune diseases (Acha-Orbea et al., 1988).

References

Acha-Orbea, H., Mitchell, D.J., Timmerman, L., Wraith, D.C., Waldor, M.K., Tausch, G.S., Zamvil, S.S., McDevitt, H.O. and Steinman, L. (1988) Limited heterogeneity of T cell receptors from lymphocytes mediating autoimmune encephalomyelitis allows specific immune intervention. *Cell*, 54: 263–273.

Adorini, L., Muller, S., Cardinaux, F., Lehmann, P.V., Falcioni, F. and Nagy, Z.A. (1988) In vivo competition between self peptides and foreign antigens in T-cell activation. *Nature*, 334: 623–625.

Atassi, M.I., Mulac-Jericevic, B., Yokoi, T. and Manshour, T. (1987) Localization of the functional sites on the α chain of acetylcholine receptor. *Fed. Proc.*, 46: 2538–2547.

Babbit, D.P., Allen, P.M., Matsueda, G., Heber, E. and Unanue, E.R. (1985) Binding of immunogenic peptides to Ia histocompatibility molecules. *Nature*, 317: 359–361.

Bell, J., Smoot, S., Newby, C., Toyka, K., Rassenti, L., Smith, K., Hohlfeld, R., McDevitt, H.O. and Steinman, L. (1986) HLA-DQ beta chain polymorphism linked to myasthenia gravis. *Lancet*, ii: 1058–1060.

Berman, P. and Patrick, J. (1980a) Linkage between the frequency of muscular weakness and loci that regulate responsiveness in EAMG. *J. Exp. Med.*, 152: 507–520.

Berman, P. and Patrick, J. (1980b) Experimental myasthenia gravis. *J. Exp. Med.*, 151: 204–223.

Bjorkman, P.J., Saper, M.A., Samraoui, B., Bennett, W.S., Strominger, J.L. and Wiley, D.C. (1987a) Structure of the

124

human class I histocompatibility antigen, HLA-A2. *Nature,* 329: 506–512.

Bjorkman, P.J., Saper, M.A., Samraoui, B., Bennett, W.S., Strominger, J.L. and Wiley, D.C. (1987b) The foreign antigen binding site and T cell recognition regions of class I histocompatibility antigens. *Nature,* 329: 512–518.

Bottazzo, G.F., Todd, I., Mirakian, R., Belfiore, A. and Pujol-Borrell, R. (1986) Organ-specific autoimmunity. *Immunol. Rev.,* 94: 137–169.

Brocke, S., Brautbar, L., Steinman, L., Abromsky, O., Rothbard, J. and Mozes, E. (1988) In vitro proliferative responses and antibody titres specific to human acetylcholine receptor synthetic peptides in patients with myasthenia gravis and relation to MHC class II genes. *J. Clin. Invest.,* 82: 1894–1900.

Brown, J.H., Jardetzky, T., Saper, M.A., Samraoui, B., Bjorkman, P.J. and Wiley, D.C. (1988) A hypothetical model of the foreign antigen binding site of class II histocompatibility molecules. *Nature,* 332: 845–850.

Buus, S., Colon, S., Smith, C., Freed, J.H., Miles, C. and Grey, H.M. (1986) Interaction between a "processed" ovalbumin peptide and Ia molecules. *Proc. Natl. Acad. Sci. USA,* 83: 3968–3971.

Buus, S., Sette, A., Colon, S.M. and Grey, H.M. (1988) Autologous peptides constitutively occupy the antigen binding site on Ia. *Science,* 242: 1045–1047.

Christadoss, P., Lennon, V. and David, C. (1979) Genetic control of experimental allergic myasthenia gravis. *J. Immunol.,* 123: 2540–2545.

Guillet, J.-G., Lai, M.Z., Briner, T.J., Buus, S., Sette, A., Grey, H.M., Smith, J.A. and Gefter, M.L. (1987) Immunological self non-self discrimination. *Science,* 235: 865–870.

Harcourt, G.C., Sommer, N., Rothbard, J., Willcox, H.N.A. and Newsom-Davis, J. (1988) A juxta-membrane epitope on the human acetylcholine receptor recognized by T cells in myasthenia gravis. *J. Clin. Invest.,* 82: 1295–1300.

Hohlfeld, R., Toyka, K., Miner, L., Walgrave, S. and Conti-Tronconi, B. (1988) Amphipathic segment of the nicotinic AChR α-subunit contains epitopes recognized by T-lymphocytes in myasthenia gravis *J. Clin. Invest.,* 81: 657–660.

Jensen, P.E. and Kapp, J.A. (1985) Genetics of insulin-specific helper and suppressor T cells in non-responder mice. *J. Immunol.,* 135: 2990–2995.

Kourilsky, P. and Claverie, J.M. (1986) The peptidic self model: a hypothesis on the molecular nature of the immunological self. *Ann. Inst. Pasteur,* 137D: 3–21.

Lorenz, R.G. and Allen, P.M. (1988) Direct evidence for functional self protein/La-molecule complexes in vivo. *Proc. Natl. Acad. Sci. USA,* 85: 5220–5223.

Luescher, I.F., Allen, P.M. and Unanue, E.R. (1988) Binding of photo-reactive lysozyme peptides to murine histocompatibility class II molecules. *Proc. Natl. Acad. Sci. USA,* 85: 871–876.

Mantegazza, R., Cornelia, F., Begovich, A., Erlich, H., Oksenberg, J. and Steinman, L. (1989) Genetic loci linked to myasthenia gravis susceptibility. *Proceedings of the 2nd European Myasthenia Gravis Conference,* in press.

Marrack, P. and Kappler, J. (1988) The T-cell repertoire for antigen and MHC. *Immunol. Today,* 9: 308–315.

Möller, G. (1987) Antigenic requirements for activation of MHC restricted responses. *Immunol. Rev.,* 98: 1–187.

Oksenberg, J.R., Sherritt, M., Begovich, A.B., Erlich, H.A., Bernard, C.C., Cavalli-Sforza, L.L. and Steinman, L. (1989) T cell receptor V alpha and C alpha alleles associated with multiple sclerosis and myasthenia gravis. *Proc. Natl. Acad. Sci. USA,* 86: 988–992.

Scharf, S.J., Friedmann, A., Brautbar, C., Szafer, F., Steinman, L., Horn, G., Gyllenstein, U. and Erlich, H.A. (1988) HLA class II allelic variation and susceptibility to pemphigus vulgaris. *Proc. Natl. Acad. Sci. USA,* 85: 3504–3508.

Schluesener, H.J. and Wekerle, H. (1984) In vitro selection of permanent T lymphocyte lines with receptors for myelin basic protein (MBP). *Prog. Clin. Biol. Res.,* 146: 285–290.

Sinha, A.A., Brautbar, C., Szafer, F., Friedman, A., Tzfoni, E., Todd, J.A. and Steinman, L. (1988) A newly characterized HLA-DQ β allele associated with pemphigus vulgaris. *Science,* 239: 1026–1029.

Sprent, J., Lo, D., Gao, E.-K., and Ron, Y. (1988) T cell selection in the thymus. *Immunol. Rev.,* 101: 172–189.

Säfwenberg J., Hammerstrom, J., Lindblom, B., et al. (1978) HLA-A, B, C and D antigens in male patients with myasthenia gravis. *Tissue Antigens,* 12: 136–141.

Todd, J.A., Acha-Orbea, H., Bell, J.I., Chao, N., Fronek, Z., Jacob, C.O., McDermott, M., Sinha, A., Timmerman, K., Steinman, L. and McDevitt, H.O. (1988) A molecular basis for MHC class II-associated autoimmunity. *Science,* 240: 1003–1009.

Von Boehmer, H., Teh, H.S. and Kisielow, P. (1989) The thymus selects the useful, neglects the useless and destroys the harmful. *Immunol. Today,* 10: 57–61.

Waldor, M.K., O'Hearn, M., Sriram, S., and Steinman, L. (1986) Treatment of experimental autoimmune myasthenia gravis with monoclonal antibodies to immune response gene products. *Ann. N. Y. Acad. Sci.,* 505: 655–668.

S.-M. Aquilonius and P.-G. Gillberg (Eds.)
Progress in Brain Research, Vol. 84
© 1990 Elsevier Science Publishers B.V. (Biomedical Division)

CHAPTER 14

Newly recognized congenital myasthenic syndromes:
I. Congenital paucity of synaptic vesicles and reduced quantal release
II. High-conductance fast-channel syndrome
III. Abnormal acetylcholine receptor (AChR) interaction with acetylcholine
IV. AChR deficiency and short channel-open time

Andrew G. Engel, Timothy J. Walls [a], Alexandre Nagel and Osvaldo Uchitel [b]

Neuromuscular Research Laboratory, Mayo Clinic and Mayo Foundation, Rochester, MN 55905, U.S.A.

Introduction

In the congenital myasthenic syndromes the safety margin of neuromuscular transmission is compromised by one or more specific mechanisms. The recognition and characterization of these diseases requires the combined use of clinical, electromyographic (EMG), in vitro electrophysiological and morphological data. Those syndromes which have been adequately characterized to date include congenital neuromuscular junction (NMJ) acetylcholinesterase (AChE) deficiency (Engel et al., 1977; Walls et al., 1989), the slow-channel syndrome (Engel et al., 1982, Oosterhuis et al., 1987), familial infantile myasthenia (Hart et al., 1979; Engel and Lambert, 1987; Mora et al., 1987), and various forms of congenital NMJ acetylcholine receptor (AChR) deficiency (Vincent et al., 1981; Lecky et al., 1986; Smit et al., 1988; Wokke et al., 1989) (Table I). The clinical and laboratory features of these diseases have been recently reviewed (Engel, 1988). At this symposium, we would like to present data from our laboratory on four previously uncharacterized congenital myasthenic syndromes.

---

[a] Present address: Newcastle General Hospital, Newcastle upon Tyne, U.K.
[b] Present address: Faculty of Medicine, University of Buenos Aires, Buenos Aires, Argentina.

TABLE I

Previously recognized congenital myasthenic syndromes

Syndrome	Factors reducing the safety margin of neuromuscular transmission
Congenital AChE deficiency	Small nerve terminals; small m due to small n. Also mild AChR deficiency from focal degeneration of junctional folds: relatively small MEPP.
Slow-channel myasthenic syndrome	Long open time of AChR ion channel; focal postsynaptic calcium excess. In clinically affected muscles focal degeneration of junctional folds with loss of AChR and small MEPP.
Familial infantile myasthenia	Reduced ACh resynthesis; abnormal decrease of the MEPP during stimulation.
Congenital AChR deficiency	Decreased AChR on simplified junctional folds; small MEPP.

Abbreviations: AChE, acetylcholinesterase; AChR, acetylcholine receptor; MEPP, miniature end-plate potential; EPP, end-plate potential; m, quantal content of the end-plate potential; n, number of readily releasable quanta.

Congenital paucity of synaptic vesicles and reduced quantal release

A female, now 23 years of age, had had fatigable weakness and intermittent bulbar symptoms since infancy. Her symptoms were partially improved by small doses of anticholinesterase drugs. An older brother and the parents were unaffected. The patient had a small stature, slender muscle bulk, hypernasal voice, fluctuating ophthalmoparesis, and moderately severe weakness of the facial, tongue, neck flexor and extremity muscles. The arm abduction time was only 12 seconds, and she could not rise from squatting without help. The EMG showed a decremental response at 2 Hz stimulation which was improved by pretreatment with neostigmine. There was no significant facilitation of the evoked compound muscle action potential (CMAP) at 50 Hz stimulation.

An external intercostal muscle specimen was obtained for in vitro microelectrode and morphological studies. The relevant data are summarized in Table II. The MEPP and miniature end-plate current (MEPC) were normal in amplitude and time course. The MEPP frequency was normal, and increased normally when the extracellular potassium concentration was increased. The quantal content of the EPP at 1 Hz stimulation was markedly reduced owing to a reduction in the number of readily releasable quanta. The prob-

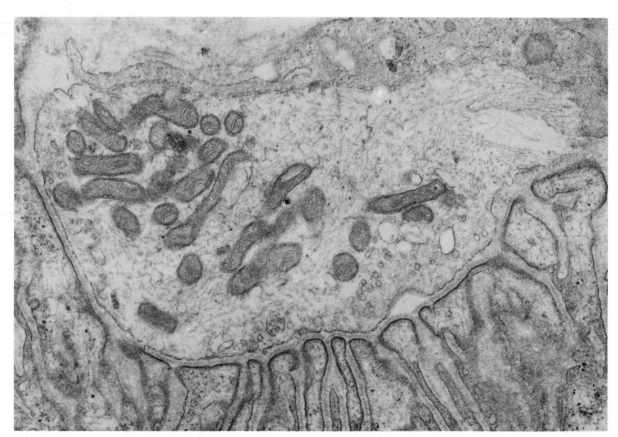

Fig. 1. Congenital paucity of synaptic vesicles and reduced quantal release. The nerve terminal contains very few synaptic vesicles; most of these are close to the presynaptic membrane. The junctional folds are intact. ×31 000.

TABLE II

Congenital paucity of synaptic vesicles and reduced quantal release [a]

	Controls	Patient
^{125}I-BGT/NMJ ($\times 10^{-6}$)	13.23 ± 0.85 [b] (n = 11)	11.58 [c] (n = 198)
MEPP (mV)	1.02 ± 0.10 [b] (n = 11)	0.79 ± 0.05 [d] (n = 15)
EPP quantal content at 1 Hz	41.1 ± 3.5 [b] (n = 11)	8.05 ± 0.75 [d] (n = 17)
Probability of quantal release (p)	0.155 ± 0.015 [e] (n = 8)	0.235 [f] (n = 12)
Number of readily releasable quanta (n)	326 ± 32 [e] (n = 8)	77 [f] (n = 12)
Synaptic vesicles (No./μm^2)	50.3 ± 3.6 [g] (n = 59)	15.1 ± 1.8 [h] (n = 23)

[a] The electrophysiological measurements were at 29°C by conventional intracellular microelectrode methods. Potential amplitudes were corrected for a resting membrane potential of −80 mV and for nonlinear summation. The quantal content of the EPP was determined by the variance method. Estimates of n and p were obtained as described by Kamenskaya et al. (1975).
[b] Mean ± SE of individual control means and number of control subjects (in parentheses).
[c] Pooled data for number of NMJ (in parenthesis).
[d] Mean ± SE and number of NMJ (in parentheses) analysed in the patient.
[e] Mean ± SE and number of subjects (in parentheses) are listed. Each control value was obtained by pooling the results at 8–12 NMJ.
[f] Pooled value for 12 NMJ.
[g] Mean ± SE for 59 nerve terminals in 13 control muscles.
[h] Mean ± SE for 23 nerve terminals in the patient.

ability of quantal release was normal. Increasing the extracellular calcium concentration from 2 mM to 5 mM increased the quantal content of the EPP approximately 2-fold, as in normal subjects. Analysis of the ACh-induced current noise revealed no abnormality in the conductance or open time of the AChR ion channel. The number of ^{125}I-α-bungarotoxin (^{125}I-BGT) binding sites per NMJ was normal.

Quantitative electron microscopic study of the NMJ demonstrated a significant decrease in synaptic vesicle density (number/μm^2) (Fig. 1 and Table II). The nerve terminals were of normal size. There were no postsynaptic abnormalities, and the density and distribution of peroxidase-labeled α-bungarotoxin (P-BGT) on the junctional folds were normal.

In this new syndrome the safety margin of neuromuscular transmission is compromised by the decreased quantal content of the EPP, and this can be attributed to a marked decrease in the number of readily releasable quanta. The basis of this alteration is an approximately proportionate decrease in the density of synaptic vesicles in the nerve terminal. Synaptic vesicles are transported by fast axonal flow from the anterior horn cell perikaryon to the motor nerve terminal (Llinas et al., 1989; Kiene and Stadler, 1987; Booj et al., 1986; Schroer et al., 1985), where they undergo exocytosis and recycling (Ceccarelli and Hurlbut, 1980; Heuser and Reese, 1977). The paucity of synaptic vesicles in this syndrome could be due to an impaired axonal transport of preformed vesicles to the nerve terminal, or to impaired vesicle recycling in the nerve terminal after activity. The fact that the synaptic vesicles were depleted even in the rested state implicates the axonal vesicle transport mechanism.

High-conductance fast-channel syndrome

A girl, now 9 years of age, had poor suck and cry in the neonatal period and delayed motor milestones. Since infancy, she had intermittent weakness of selected bulbar and limb muscles. The symptoms were provoked or worsened by exertion and by exposure to heat. Examination revealed only mild weakness in facial, cervical, and selected limb muscles. There was no clear improvement with anticholinesterase drugs. The EMG showed a mild decrement of the femoral CMAP after 3 min of exercise. Two sisters and the parents were unaffected.

An intercostal muscle specimen was obtained for electrophysiological (Table III) and morphological studies. The quantal content of the EPP at 1 Hz stimulation was normal. The MEPP and MEPC amplitudes were abnormally large and the MEPP and MEPC decay time constants were abnormally short. AChR channel kinetics were investigated by analysis of the end-plate current noise induced by iontophoretically applied ACh. The mean single channel conductance was determined by regression of the variance of conductance fluctuations on the induced conductance change (i.e., from the "conductance plot") (Fig. 2), and from the noise power spectrum (Fig. 3). The two different methods showed a 1.64-fold and a 1.67-fold increase of the channel conductance over the corresponding mean control values (Table III). The mean channel-open time was evaluated from the decay time constant of the MEPC, and from the power spectrum (Fig. 3). The two methods indicated a 39% and a 29% decrease from the corresponding mean control values, respectively (Table III). The voltage dependence of channel closure and the reversal potential fell in the normal range.

TABLE III

High-conductance fast-channel syndrome [a]

	Controls [b]	Patient [c]
EPP quantal content	41.1 ± 3.5	36.3 ± 4.7
at 1 Hz	(n = 11)	(n = 10)
MEPP (mV)	1.02 ± 0.10	1.56 ± 0.09
	(n = 11)	(n = 13)
MEPC at 80 mV (nA)	3.80 ± 0.21	7.72 ± 0.50
	(n = 7)	(n = 4)
MEPC decay time constant	3.27 ± 0.12	2.02 ± 0.24
(ms)	(n = 7)	(n = 4)
Channel open time (ms)	2.27 ± 0.05	1.62 ± 0.07
(from power spectrum)	(n = 5)	(n = 5)
Channel conductance (pS)	32.86 ± 1.23	54.06 ± 4.39
(from conductance plot)	(n = 5)	(n = 5)
Channel conductance (pS)	31.51 ± 0.67	52.47 ± 4.91
(from power spectrum)	(n = 5)	(n = 5)

[a] The EPP quantal content and the MEPP amplitude were determined at 29°C as described in the footnote to Table II. MEPC were recorded with a two-electrode voltage clamp at 21°C. Analysis of the ACh-induced current noise was at 21°C as described by Anderson and Stevens (1973).
[b] Means ± SE of individual control means and numbers of control subjects (in parentheses). In the noise analysis studies, 5–6 NMJ were studied in each subject.
[c] Means ± SE and numbers of NMJ (in parentheses) analysed in the patient.

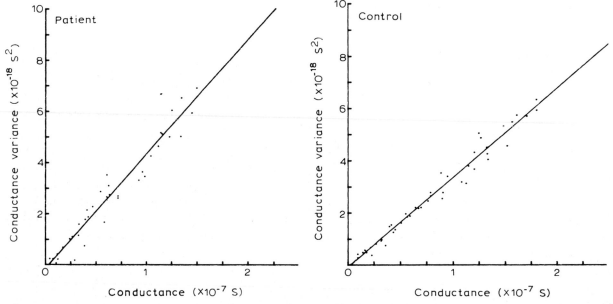

Fig. 2. High-conductance fast-channel syndrome. Plot of the variance of conductance fluctuations against the ACh-induced conductance change at a NMJ in the patient (left) and in a control (right). In both patient and control, data were pooled from 4 consecutive ACh applications; −80 mV membrane potential, 22°C. The current signals were filtered to produce a bandwidth of 1–300 Hz and digitized at 1000 Hz. The slope of each line was corrected for loss of fluctuations above 300 Hz by dividing by $(2/3.14)\tan^{-1}(300/f_c)$, where f_c is the half-power frequency of the corresponding power spectrum (Colquhoun et al., 1977). The corresponding power spectra are shown in Fig. 3. The corrected mean channel conductance is 55.9 pS for the patient and 39 pS for the control.

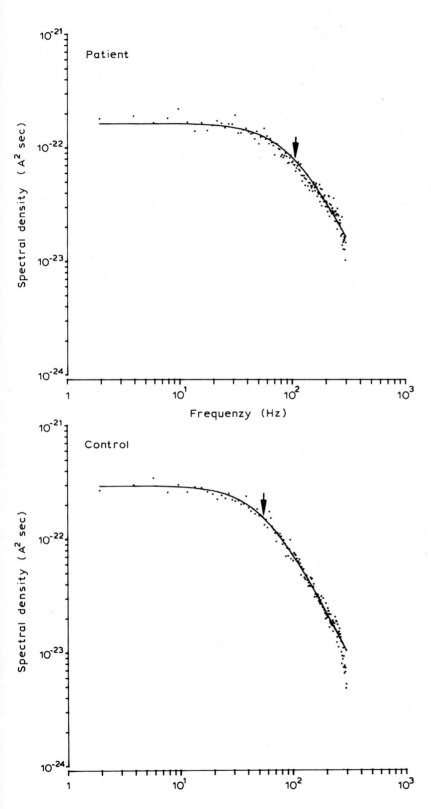

Fig. 3. High-conductance fast-channel syndrome. ACh induced current fluctuations at an NMJ in the patient (top) and in a control (bottom). For both patient and control, the data were obtained under the same conditions, from the same NMJ, and during the same four consecutive ACh applications as the data shown in Fig. 2. The lines represent single Lorentzian functions. For the patient and the control, the mean induced currents were 5.58 and 9.48 nA, respectively. The respective half-power frequencies (arrows) are 99.8 and 56.5 Hz; the channel open times are therefore 1.59 and 2.82 ms. The single channel conductances, calculated from the fitted curves, are 57.5 pS for the patient and 34.8 pS for the control. The channel conductance values are only slightly different from those derived from the conductance plots in Fig. 2.

130

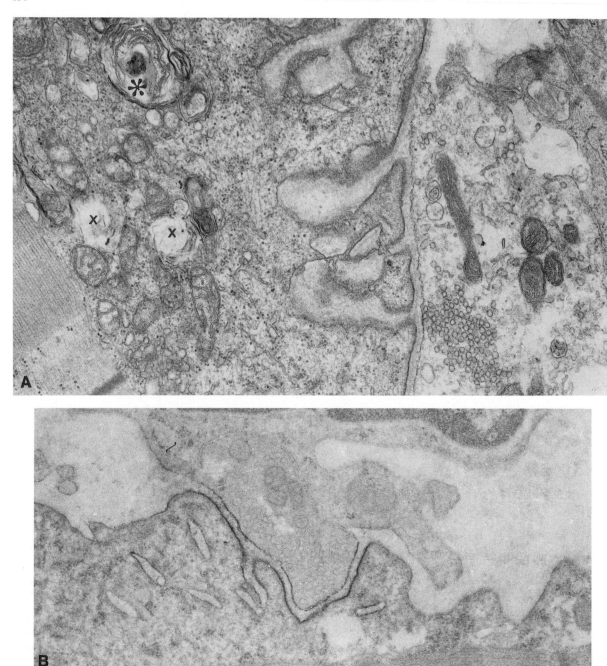

Fig. 4. Electron micrographs of abnormal NMJ in the high-conductance fast-channel syndrome. In A, the junctional sarcoplasm contains myeloid structures (asterisk), degenerating mitochondria and small abnormal spaces (×). NMJ imaged in B has been reacted with P-BGT for the localization of AChR; the section is unstained. Here the simplified postsynaptic region contains only one junctional fold and the primary synaptic cleft opens into a single secondary cleft. A, ×29 400; B, ×27 600.

The number of ^{125}I-BGT binding sites per NMJ was normal. Electron microscopy of the NMJ demonstrated no abnormality of the nerve terminals. The synaptic vesicles were of normal size. Most postsynaptic regions were normal, but a few showed degenerative changes in the junctional sarcoplasm (Fig. 4A), and a few were simplified (Fig. 4B), suggesting previous degeneration of the junctional folds or remodeling of the NMJ.

The findings are consistent with a functionally abnormal AChR ion channel due to a mutation in an AChR subunit. Site-directed mutagenesis studies indicate that single amino acid substitutions in any subunit which alter the distribution of negative or positive charges close to the external or cytoplasmic vestibule of the ion channel affect the cation flux through the channel (Dani, 1989; Imoto et al., 1988; Leonard et al., 1988). An increase in a negative charge near the external vestibule would increase the channel current and could account for the high channel conductance in this syndrome. The fact that the high channel conductance is associated with a shorter than normal channel life-time indicates that the mutation has a dual affect on the kinetic properties of the ion channel.

The manner in which the physiological defect produces clinical symptoms is unclear, but it may be due to the development of an end-plate myopathy in severely affected muscles, as occurs in the slow-channel syndrome.

Congenital myasthenic syndrome with abnormal ACh–AChR interaction

A 21-year-old female had had severe generalized weakness and abnormal fatigability of all muscles since birth. Her symptoms were partially improved by anticholinesterase drugs. Two younger sisters and the parents were unaffected. The EMG showed a decremental response at 2 Hz stimulation.

An intercostal muscle specimen was obtained for further studies (Table IV). The quantal content

of the EPP was normal. The MEPP and MEPC amplitudes were markedly reduced. Despite the small MEPP and MEPC, the number of ^{125}I-BGT binding sites per NMJ was in the high normal range. The kinetic properties of the AChR ion channel were investigated by analysis of ACh-induced end-plate current fluctuations. The mean single channel conductance, determined from regression of the variance of conductance fluctuations on the induced conductance change, was normal. The noise power spectrum was abnormal; it was best fitted by the sum of two Lorentzian functions, consistent with biexponential kinetics (Fig. 5). The recorded MEPC were too small for

TABLE IV

Syndrome with abnormal ACh-AChR interaction [a]

	Controls [b]	Patient [c]
^{125}I-BGT/NMJ ($\times 10^{-6}$)	13.23 ± 0.85 (n = 11)	17.49 (n = 237)
EPP quantal content at 1 Hz	41.1 ± 3.5 (n = 11)	34.4 ± 3.5 (n = 17)
MEPP (mV)	1.02 ± 0.10 (n = 11)	0.17 ± 0.02 [d] (n = 17) 0.29 ± 0.08 [e] (n = 4)
MEPC at 80 mV (nA)	3.80 ± 0.21 (n = 7)	< 1.5 (n = 5)
Channel conductance (pS) (from conductance plot)	32.86 ± 1.23 (n = 5)	33.69 ± 1.92 (n = 7)
Channel open time (ms) (from power spectrum)	2.27 ± 0.05 (n = 5)	4.97 ± 0.49 and 0.44 ± 0.02 (n = 6)

[a] The electrophysiological methods are described in the footnote to Table III.
[b] Means $\pm$ SE of individual control means and numbers of control subjects (in parentheses). In the noise analysis studies, 5–6 NMJ were studied in each subject.
[c] Means $\pm$ SE and numbers of NMJ (in parentheses) analysed in the patient.
[d] Indirect estimates based on m/mean EPP amplitude ratios.
[e] Measured in the presence of 1 μg/ml neostigmine.
[f] The power spectrum was fitted as the sum of two Lorentzians. The two open times were calculated from the cutoff frequencies of the separate Lorentzians. If the double exponential relaxation results from an altered affinity of ACh for AChR, then the derived values could reflect ACh occupancy time rather than channel open time (Colquhoun and Hawkes, 1977).

132

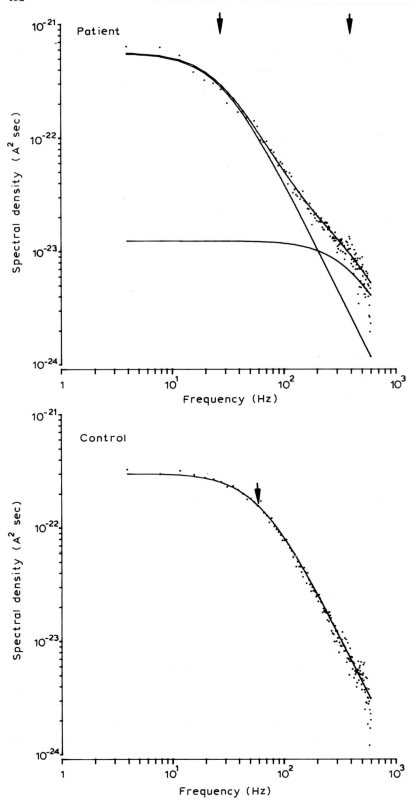

Fig. 5. Myasthenic syndrome with abnormal ACh–AChR interaction. Power density spectra of ACh current noise at a NMJ in the patient (top) and in a control subject (bottom); membrane potential −80 mV, 22°C. The current signals were filtered to produce a bandwidth of 2–600 Hz and digitized at 2000 Hz. The results shown are the average of three applications in the patient and four in the control. At the patient's NMJ, the mean induced current was 13.57 nA. This spectrum is best fitted by two Lorentzian curves with half-power frequencies of approximately 25.5 and 396 Hz; apparent channel open times, 6.24 and 0.4 ms. At the control NMJ, the induced current was 9.87 nA. The spectrum is fitted with a single Lorentzian curve: half-power frequency, 59 Hz (arrow); channel open time, 2.70 ms; channel conductance, 36.5 pS.

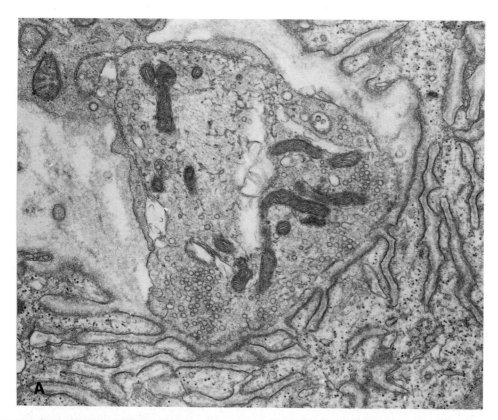

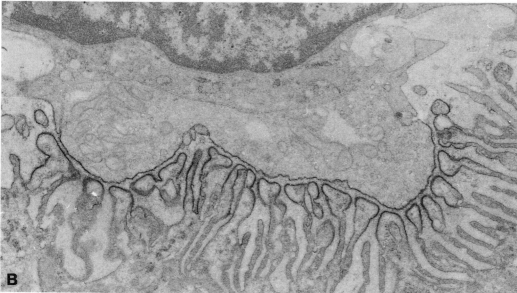

Fig. 6. Myasthenic syndrome with abnormal ACh–AChR interaction: electron micrographs of NMJ. A shows a typical end-plate region. The density and dimensions of the synaptic vesicles are normal and the junctional folds are intact. The NMJ imaged in B has been reacted with P-BGT for the the localization of AChR; the section is unstained. The density and distribution of AChR on the junctional folds is normal. A, ×21 300; B, ×15 700.

determining whether their decay phase was biexponential.

Electron microscopic examinations of the NMJ showed no pre- or postsynaptic abnormality. In particular, the synaptic vesicles were of normal size and there was no degeneration of the junctional folds (Fig. 6). The density and distribution of P-BGT binding sites on the junctional folds were also normal (Fig. 6B).

The small MEPP and MEPC in the presence of a normal number of AChR per NMJ and a normal distribution and density of AChR on the junctional folds could be explained by (1) a decrease in the ACh content of the synaptic vesicles, or (2) an abnormality of AChR. The fact that the synaptic vesicle size was not reduced points away from a reduced synaptic vesicle ACh content (Jones and Kwanbunbumpen, 1970; Nagel and Engel, 1989). On the other hand, the abnormal kinetics of the AChR ion channel would be consistent with an abnormal interaction of ACh with AChR.

Biexponential AChR ion channel kinetics could result from (1) a dual population of AChR, as in the immature NMJ (Fischbach and Schuetze, 1980); (2) blocking of the AChR ion channel (Ruff, 1977; Ogden and Colquhoun, 1985; Adams, 1987); (3) a decrease in the rate constant for agonist dissociation (k_{-2}) from diliganded closed AChR (Colquhoun and Hawkes, 1977), or another abnormality of ACh–AChR interaction, so that the closure of the diliganded channel is no longer rate-limiting (Adams, 1987).

A dual population of AChRs with different rate constants of closure is an unlikely explanation because both types of receptor would have to have a low conductance to also explain the small MEPC. However, the effective conductance of the population of channels that did open was normal.

If the abnormal power spectrum resulted from an abnormal channel blocking effect of ACh, then this effect would have to occur before channel opening so as to also account for the small MEPC; i.e., ACh would be acting as a closed channel blocker (Masukawa and Albuquerque, 1978). This explanation, however, appears to be inconsistent with the clinical improvement seen with some anticholinesterase medications, and the fact that neostigmine slightly increased the MEPP amplitude in vitro (Table IV).

A reduced affinity of AChR for ACh could explain the small MEPC, the normal channel conductance, the responsiveness to anticholinesterases, and may also account for the biexponential channel kinetics. Single channel recordings will be required to characterize further the AChR abnormality in this syndrome.

Congenital AChR deficiency and short channel-open time

A girl, now 27 months of age, was born by forceps delivery and required assisted ventilation for the first 3 weeks of life. During infancy, she was hypotonic, had facial diplegia and ophthalmoplegia, fed poorly, and had frequent bouts of respiratory insufficiency. Weakness of other muscles and abnormal fatigability became apparent during the first year of life. Motor milestones were delayed. Her symptoms were improved by anticholinesterase drugs. The EMG showed a decremental response in the facial muscles at 2 Hz stimulation. There were no other siblings. The parents were unaffected.

An intercostal muscle specimen was obtained for further studies (Table V). The quantal content of EPP was normal. The MEPP amplitude was abnormally small but increased with neostigmine. The number of ^{125}I-BGT binding sites per NMJ was only 7% of the mean control value. The reduced number of bungarotoxin binding sites could not be attributed to smallness of the patient's NMJ. The mean NMJ length on cholinesterase-reacted muscle fibers was 25.2 μm for the patient and 25.8–26.6 μm in three adult controls.

The kinetic properties of the AChR ion channel were investigated by analysis of the ACh-induced current fluctuations. The mean single channel con-

TABLE V

AChR deficiency and short channel-open time [a]

	Controls [b]	Patient [c]
^{125}I-BGT/NMJ ($\times 10^{-6}$)	13.23 ± 0.85	0.97
	(n = 11)	(n = 335)
EPP quantal content at 1 Hz	41.1 ± 3.5	38.5 ± 5.0
	(n = 11)	(n = 12)
MEPP (mV)	1.02 ± 0.10	0.22 ± 0.09 [d]
	(n = 11)	(n = 16)
MEPC at 80 mV (nA)	3.80 ± 0.21	2.1 ± 0.24 [e]
	(n = 7)	(n = 9)
Channel conductance (pS)	32.86 ± 1.23	36.33 ± 4.07
(from conductance plot)	(n = 5)	(n = 6)
Channel open time (ms)	2.27 ± 0.05	1.61 ± 0.04
(from power spectrum)	(n = 5)	(n = 6)

[a] The electrophysiological methods are described in the footnote to Table III.
[b] Means ± SE of individual control means and numbers of control subjects (in parentheses). In the noise analysis studies, 5–6 NMJ were studied in each subject.
[c] Means ± SE and numbers of NMJ (in parentheses) analysed in the patient.
[d] Normalized for a fiber diameter of 60 μm. Uncorrected value = 0.56 ± 0.03.
[e] Measured in the presence of 1 μg/ml neostigmine.

ductance was normal, but the mean channel-open time was abnormally short (Table V).

Electron microscopy of the NMJ using P-BGT to localize AChR confirmed the AChR deficiency (Fig. 7). The junctional folds were abundant and there were no signs of postsynaptic degeneration.

This syndrome is characterized by a kinetic abnormality as well as a deficiency of NMJ AChR. The functional abnormality is likely to stem from a mutation in an AChR subunit. The reduced number of NMJ AChR may be due to reduced synthesis, impaired membrane incorporation, or decreased metabolic stability of the mutant AChR.

Acknowledgements

This work was supported by NIH Grant NS 6277, a Research Center Grant from the Muscular Dystrophy Association, and the Mogg Fund.

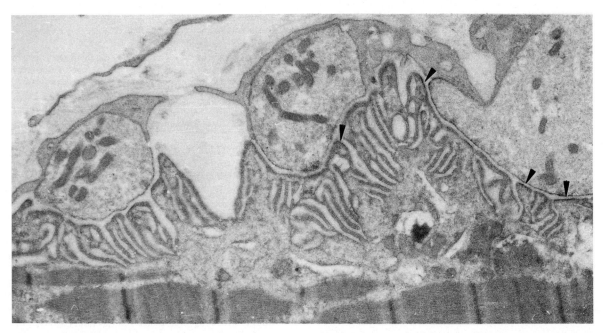

Fig. 7. Electron micrograph of NMJ in patient with congenital AChR deficiency and short channel-open time. The specimen has been reacted with P-BGT for the localization of AChR; the section is unstained. The junctional folds are numerous and well developed, but display barely any reaction for AChR; arrowheads indicate the few sites where faint black reaction product can be detected. Compare with the localization of AChR in Fig. 6B. ×12 200.

References

Adams, P.R. (1987) Transmitter action at endplate membrane. In M.M. Salpeter (ED.) *The Vertebrate Neuromuscular Junction,* Alan Liss, New York, pp. 317–359.

Anderson, C.R. and Stevens, C.F. (1973) Voltage clamp analysis of acetylcholine produced end-plate current fluctuations at frog neuromuscular junctions. *J. Physiol. (Lond.),* 235: 655–691.

Booj, S. (1986) Axonal transport of synapsin I and cholinergic synaptic vesicle-like material. Further immunohistochemical evidence for transport of axonal cholinergic transmitter vesicles in motor neurons. *Acta Physiol. Scand.,* 128: 155–165.

Ceccarelli, B. and Hurlbut, W.P. (1980) Vesicle hypothesis of the release of quanta of acetylcholine. *Physiol. Rev.,* 60: 396–441.

Colquhoun, D. and Hawkes, A.G. (1977) Relaxation and fluctuations of membrane currents that flow through drug-operated ion channels. *Proc. R. Soc. Lond. B.,* 199: 231–262.

Colquhoun, D., Large, W.A. and Rang, H.P. (1977) An analysis of the action of a false transmitter at the neuromuscular junction. *J. Physiol. (Lond.),* 266: 361–395.

Dani, J.A. (1989) Site-directed mutagenesis and single-channel currents define the ionic channel of the nicotinic acetylcholine receptor. *Trends Neurosci.,* 12: 125–128.

Engel, A.G. (1988) Congenital myasthenic syndromes. *J. Child Neurol.,* 3: 233–246.

Engel, A.G. and Lambert, E.H. (1987) Congenital myasthenic syndromes. *Electroencephalogr. Clin. Neurophysiol., Suppl* 39: 91–102.

Engel, A.G., Lambert, E.H. and Gomez, M.R. (1977) A new myasthenic syndrome with end-plate cholinesterase deficiency, small nerve terminals and reduced acetylcholine release. *Ann. Neurol.,* 1: 315–330.

Engel, A.G., Lambert, E.H., Mulder, D.M., Torres, C.F., Sahashi, K., Bertorini, T.E. and Whitaker, J.N. (1982) A newly recognized congenital myasthenic syndrome attributed to a prolonged open time of the acetylcholine-induced ion channel. *Ann. Neurol.,* 11: 553–569.

Fischbach, G.D. and Schuetze, S.M. (1980) A post-natal decrease in acetylcholine channel open time at rat end-plates. *J. Physiol. (Lond.),* 303: 125–137.

Hart, Z., Sahashi, K., Lambert, E.H., Engel, A.G. and Lindstrom, J. (1979) A congenital, familial myasthenic syndrome caused by a presynaptic defect of transmitter resynthesis or mobilization (Abstract). *Neurology,* 29: 559.

Heuser J.E. and Reese T.S. (1977) Structure of the synapse. In *Handbook of Physiology – The Nervous System, Vol. 1,* American Physiological Society, Bethesda, MD, pp. 261–294.

Imoto, K., Busch, C., Sakmann, B., Mishina M., Konno, T., Nakai, J., Bujo, H., Mori, Y., Fukuda, K. and Numa, S. (1988) Rings of negatively charged amino acids determine the acetylcholine receptor channel conductance. *Nature,* 335: 645–648.

Jones, S.F. and Kwanbunbumpen, S. (1970) The effects of nerve stimulation and hemicholinium on synaptic vesicles at the mammalian neuromuscular junction. *J. Physiol. (Lond.),* 207: 31–50.

Kamenskaya, M.A., Elmqvist, D. and Thesleff, S. (1975) Guanidine and neuromuscular transmission. II. Effect on transmitter release in response to repetitive nerve stimulation. *Arch. Neurol.,* 32: 510–518.

Kiene, M.L. and Stadler, H. (1987) Synaptic vesicles in electromotoneurons. I. Axonal transport, site of transmitter uptake and processing of a core proteoglycan during maturation. *EMBO J.,* 6: 2209–2215.

Lecky, B.R.F., Morgan-Hughes, J.A., Murray, N.M.F., Landon, D.N., Wray, D. and Prior, C. (1986) Congenital myasthenia: further evidence of disease heterogeneity. *Muscle Nerve,* 9: 233–242.

Leonard, R.J., Labarca, C.G., Charnet, P., Davidson, N. and Lester, H.A. (1988) Evidence that the M2 membrane spanning region lines the ion channel pore of the nicotinic receptor. *Science,* 242: 1578–1581.

Llinas, R., Sugimori, M., Lin, J.W., Leopold, P.L. and Brady, S.T. (1989) ATP-dependent directional movement of rat synaptic vesicles injected into the presynaptic terminal of squid giant synapse. *Proc. Natl. Acad. Sci. USA,* 86: 5656–5660.

Masukawa, L.M. and Albuquerque, E.X. (1978) Voltage- and time-dependent action of histrionicotoxin on the endplate current of the frog muscle. *J. Gen. Physiol.,* 72: 351–367.

Mora, M., Lambert, E.H. and Engel, A.G. (1987) Synaptic vesicle abnormality in familial infantile myasthenia. *Neurology,* 37: 206–214.

Nagel, A. and Engel, A.G. (1989) Vesamicol decreases both quantal and synaptic vesicle size at the neuromuscular junction (Abstract.) *Soc. Neurosci., Abstracts,* 15:814.

Ogden, D.C. and Colquhoun, D. (1985) Ion channel block by acetylcholine, carbachol and suberidylcholine at the frog neuromuscular junction. *Proc. R. Soc. Lond. B,* 225: 329–355.

Oosterhuis, H.J.G.H., Newsom-Davis, J., Wokke, J.H.J., Molenaar, P.C., Weerden, T.V., Oen, B.S., Jennekens, F.G.I., Veldman, H., Vincent, A., Wray, D.W., Prior, C. and Murray, N.M.F. (1987) The slow channel syndrome. Two new cases. *Brain,* 110: 1061–1079.

Ruff, R.L. (1977) A quantitative analysis of local anaesthetic alteration of miniature end-plate currents and end-plate current fluctuations. *J. Physiol. (Lond.),* 264: 89–124.

Schroer, T.A., Brady, S.T. and Kelly, R.B. (1985) Fast axonal transport of foreign synaptic vesicles in squid axoplasm. *J. Cell Biol.,* 101: 568–572.

Smit, L.M.E., Hageman, G., Veldman, H., Molenaar, P.C., Oen, B.S. and Jennekens, F.G.I. (1988) A myasthenic syndrome with congenital paucity of secondary synaptic clefts: CPSC syndrome. *Muscle Nerve,* 11: 337–348.

Vincent, A., Cull-Candy, S.G., Newsom-Davis, J., Trautmann A., Molenaar, P.C. and Polak, R.L. (1981) Congenital myasthenia: end-plate acetylcholine receptors and electrophysiology in five cases. *Muscle Nerve,* 4: 303–318.

Walls, T.J., Engel, A.G., Harper, C.M., Groover, R.V. and Peterson, H.A. (1989) Congenital neuromuscular junction acetylcholinesterase deficiency (Abstract). *Ann. Neurol.,* 26: 147.

Wokke, J.H.J, Jennekens, F.G.I., Molenaar, P.C., Van den Oord, C.J.M., Oen, B.S and Busch, H.F.M. (1989) Congenital paucity of secondary synaptic clefts (CPSC) syndrome in 2 adult sibs. *Neurology,* 39: 648–654.

S.-M. Aquilonius and P.-G. Gillberg (Eds.)
Progress in Brain Research, Vol. 84
© 1990 Elsevier Science Publishers B.V. (Biomedical Division)

CHAPTER 15

Clinical pharmacokinetics of acetylcholinesterase inhibitors

Per Hartvig, Lars Wiklund, Sten-Magnus Aquilonius and Björn Lindström

Hospital Pharmacy, Departments of Anesthesiology and Neurology, University hospital, S-751 85 Uppsala, and Department of Drugs, National Board of Health and Welfare, Uppsala, Sweden

Introduction

Clinical pharmacokinetics in the present context means the study of absorption, distribution and elimination of drugs in patients. Clinical pharmacokinetics also includes studies on the relationship between any clinical effect and the measured plasma concentrations of the drug. The clinical pharmacokinetics of acetylcholinesterase inhibitors has only been established over the last ten years, although these drugs have been in clinical use for more than a century for the enhancement of acetylcholine activity. The development of selective and sensitive analytical methods for the assay of biological samples of acetylcholinesterase inhibitors is an important step forwards towards understanding their pharmacokinetic properties and hence their mode of action and the interindividual variation of clinical response, as well as providing a guide for dosage strategies aimed at optimal effect without side-effects.

This report surveys the clinical pharmacokinetic information available on the reversible acetylcholinesterase inhibitors and particularly results emanating from our own studies. This means that irreversible inhibitors such as metrifonate will not be dealt with.

Bioanalysis of acetylcholinesterase inhibitors

Analysis of acetylcholinesterase inhibitors in biological samples presents a particular challenge to the analytical chemist, since the plasma concentrations of these drugs are usually in the low ng/ml range. Furthermore, acetylcholinesterase inhibi-

tors are rapidly degraded in blood and plasma by esterases, which puts certain demands on sample handling and storage. Several studies on the pharmacokinetics of acetylcholinesterase inhibitors provide very poor information, since the problems of in vitro degradation in blood and plasma samples have been overlooked. Rapid cooling and separation of plasma together with the addition of internal standard to the frozen sample will minimize this problem in the case of neostigmine (Aquilonius et al., 1979) and pyridostigmine (Aquilonius et al., 1980). In the case of physostigmine it was necessary to add a large amount of neostigmine to the sampling tube together with rapid centrifugation of blood and cooling of plasma to be able to determine plasma concentrations accurately (Hartvig et al., 1986).

Early methods of analysis based on paper chromatography, spectrometry and radioisotope studies suffer from poor sensitivity and selectivity regarding the accurate measurement of plasma concentrations following therapeutic doses. Recent advances in gas and liquid chromatography and improvement of detection principles have made possible the analysis of these drugs in biological samples (for review, see Aquilonius and Hartvig, 1986).

Acetylcholinesterase inhibitors with a peripheral site of action

Pharmacokinetics

The plasma clearances of peripheral cholinesterase inhibitors are high, with a volume of

TABLE I

Clinical pharmacokinetics of acetylcholinesterase inhibitors with peripheral site of action: mean values

Drug	Pat.	Clearance (l/min)	Volume of distribution (l)	Half-life of distribution (min)	Half-life of elimination (min)	Oral bioavail-ability (%)
Neostigmine	S	1.23	70	0.9	54	1– 2
Pyridostigmine	M,H	0.66	84	0.8	84	10–20
Edrophonium	S	0.43	77	0.8	108	

S = surgical patients; M = myasthenia gravis patients; H = healthy volunteers.

distribution in the range 0.5–1.7 l/kg. The plasma elimination half-lives are in the range 60–90 min, being somewhat longer for pyridostigmine (Table I) (Aquilonius et al., 1979, 1980).

One to two hours after oral administration peak plasma concentrations are measured with both pyridostigmine and neostigmine (Aquilonius et al., 1979, 1980). The oral bioavailability of these quaternary ammonium compounds is low. Pyridostigmine oral bioavailability is 10–20% (Breyer-Pfaff et al., 1985) and the figure for neostigmine is only 1–2%. In spite of the short elimination half-life of pyridostigmine, intraindividual variations in the plasma concentrations during a dose interval are small in patients with myasthenia gravis on oral maintenance therapy, probably as a result of slow absorption from the gastrointestinal tract (Aquilonius et al., 1980).

The higher oral bioavailability and slightly longer plasma elimination half-life favour the use of pyridostigmine in monotherapy of myasthenia gravis (Aquilonius and Hartvig, 1986)

Effect studies

Several studies have been conducted to find a relationship between the plasma concentrations of peripheral cholinesterase inhibitors and the effect on muscle strength in patients with myasthenia gravis. Some studies have indicated a positive relationship (Cohan et al., 1976; Aquilonius et al., 1980), whereas others have not found any such correlation (Davison et al., 1981). Thus, in previously untreated myasthenic patients a relationship exists between the effect on muscle response and plasma concentration in the range 5–30 ng/ml

(Aquilonius et al., 1980) following intravenous pyridostigmine and 1–10 ng/ml after oral and intravenous neostigmine (Aquilonius et al., 1983). In fact a "bell-shaped" dose-response curve was shown, with maximum effects with plasma concentrations in the range 30–60 and 5–15 ng/ml of pyridostigmine and neostigmine, respectively. There is, however, a large difference between these low plasma concentrations having an effect on muscle response and the much higher steady-state concentrations measured in myasthenic patients on long-term treatment. This indicates that higher concentrations are required to restore neuromuscular transmission at the end-plates in more advanced disease.

It was reported very recently that good control of myasthenic symptoms was obtained within a narrow range of plasma pyridostigmine concentrations (Breyer-Pfaff et al., 1989). A plasma concentration above 100 ng/ml gave a poorer clinical effect, thus supporting the previous concept of a "bell-shaped" relationship between clinical effect measured as improvement of muscle function and plasma concentration of pyridostigmine in patients with myasthenia gravis (Aquilonius et al., 1983).

Centrally active acetylcholinesterase inhibitors

Pharmacokinetics

Physostigmine. The pharmacokinetics of physostigmine has mainly been studied in surgical patients in the early postoperative period (Hartvig et al., 1986, 1990a). The pharmacokinetics following the intravenous administration of physostigmine

TABLE II

Clinical pharmacokinetics of acetylcholinesterase inhibitors with central site of action: mean values

Drug	Pat.	Clearance (l/min)	Volume of distribution (l)	Half-life of distribution (min)	Half-life of elimination (min)	Oral bioavail-ability (%)
Physostigmine	S	1.55	47	2.3	22	–
	S	2.83			(20–30)	25.3
9-Aminotetrahydroacridine	ALS	2.42	349	1.8	98	17.4
	S	2.70	477	2.1	133	–

S = surgical patients; ALS = patients with amyotrophic lateral sclerosis.

was characterized by a high plasma clearance and a comparative small volume of distribution (Table II). The resulting distribution and elimination half-lives were 2.3 and 22 min, respectively. After both intramuscular and subcutaneous administration the systemic availability was almost complete and the plasma terminal half-lives were only somewhat longer than that following intravenous administration (Hartvig et al., 1986). The rapid elimination of physostigmine was paralleled by a short effect duration (Peterson et al., 1986).

A two-rate infusion of physostigmine in surgical patients aiming at plasma concentrations in the range 1–10 ng/ml resulted in highly variable concentrations (Hartvig et al., 1989). Steady-state plasma concentrations were generally lower than those predicted. Plasma clearance was very high, 40.8 ± 21.0 ml/min per kg, with an 8-fold variation.

Oral bioavailability is low, with large interindividual variations, at $25.3 \pm 11.1\%$ (Hartvig et al., 1989) (Table II).

THA. The reversible cholinesterase inhibitor 9-amino-1,2,3,4-tetrahydroacridine (THA) has been used in clinical anesthesiology for more than 40 years for the reversal of postoperative sedation, prolongation of muscle relaxation by succinyl choline (Hunter, 1965) and antagonism of overdoses of barbiturates (Gordh, 1962). The advantage of THA compared to another centrally active cholinesterase inhibitor, physostigmine, was its claimed longer duration of action due to its longer elimination half-life. Recently, two pharmacokinetic studies on THA have been conducted in

our hospital, one in patients with amyotrophic lateral sclerosis, ALS (Hartvig et al., 1990a) and one in surgical patients for the reversal of postoperative sedation (Hartvig et al., 1990b). There was no significant difference in the pharmacokinetics between these two patient groups following an intravenous dose of THA (Table II). Plasma clearance was almost identical, but a higher volume of distribution was found in the surgical patients (Hartvig et al., 1990b). A larger volume of distribution has previously been connected to anesthesia and surgery. Volume of distribution of THA was 5-times that of physostigmine. The resulting plasma elimination half-life of THA is also 5-fold that of physostigmine since they have a similar plasma clearance.

Following oral doses of THA to patients with ALS a low and highly variable oral bioavailability was measured (Hartvig et al., 1990a). Mean oral bioavailability was $17.4 \pm 13.1\%$. The large interindividual variation in oral bioavailability is supported by other studies in patients with Alzheimer's disease (Nybäck et al., 1988).

The main plasma metabolite, 1-hydroxy-9-amino-1,2,3,4-tetrahydroacridine, appeared rapidly following both intravenous (Hartvig et al., 1990b) and oral THA (Hartvig et al., 1990a). The elimination rate of THA and its metabolite are similar, indicating that the metabolite formation rate determines its pharmacokinetics. After 7 weeks of continuous oral treatment with THA the plasma concentration of the metabolite exceeded the THA plasma concentration 3–10-fold (Hartvig et al., 1990a).

Effect studies

Physostigmine. Studies on the relationship between plasma concentrations of physostigmine and effects have only been done for the antagonistic postoperative sedation. It has been shown that a physostigmine plasma concentration in the range 3–5 ng/ml was required to antagonize an effect on postoperative sedation (Hartvig et al., 1986). The effect was of short duration and a two-rate constant infusion of physostigmine was suggested for the prolongation of the antagonistic effect on postoperative somnolence. Effects on somnolence were, however, poorly correlated to steady-state concentrations of physostigmine measured (Hartvig et al., 1989). The magnitude and duration of the arousal effect were considered to be not better than that resulting from an intravenous bolus dose of physostigmine (Hartvig et al., 1989).

THA. Various different pharmacological effects of THA have been reported. Besides being a well-known cholinesterase inhibitor with central effects (Shaw and Bentley, 1953), some nicotine receptor agonist activity has also been suggested (Nilsson et al., 1987). THA has recently been reported to antagonize the normethyl-D-aspartate receptor complex (Davenport et al., 1988), which is of special interest since it has been suggested that neurotoxic amino acids are implicated in the pathogenesis of ALS (Spencer et al., 1987) and even Alzheimer's disease. Following intravenous administration an immediate but short-lived beneficial effect on muscle strength was seen in some patients with ALS. This was not seen, however, following a single oral dose or after 7 weeks of continuous oral THA treatment (Askmark et al., 1990). Furthermore, adverse reactions such as dizziness, nausea and tiredness were reported following intravenous THA. Besides nausea and tiredness, elevated transaminases were reported following oral medication. As a result of these findings, it was concluded that THA probably has no place in the treatment of ALS (Askmark et al., 1990).

THA has also been given intravenously to surgical patients to antagonize postoperative sedation probably caused by large doses of anticholinergic drugs given during anesthesia (Hartvig et al., 1990b). Arousal occurred rapidly after administration and had a duration of 60–90 min. The duration of effect of THA in antagonizing sedation was thus only about double that seen after intravenous physostigmine even though the THA plasma elimination half-life is 5-times that of physostigmine. Resedation occurred at a plasma concentration varying from 17 to 75 ng/ml between patients, although most patients resedated at plasma concentrations of 40–50 ng/ml (Hartvig et al., 1990b). Furthermore, large interindividual variations, 0–80 ng/ml, in plasma concentrations of the metabolite 1-hydroxy-9-aminotetrahydroacridine were measured at the same point in time (Hartvig et al., 1990b). Since the metabolite also has some cholinergic activity (Puri et al., 1988), it may have contributed to the effect of THA.

Conclusion

The clinical pharmacokinetics of acetylcholinesterase inhibitors is characterized by a high plasma clearance and short plasma elimination half-lives (Aquilonius and Hartvig, 1986). Furthermore, oral bioavailability is low and shows large interindividual differences. This knowledge is of importance in the understanding of the large fluctuations in clinical effect and also the large interindividual differences in response in patients given these drugs. Furthermore, the relationship between effect on muscle strength and plasma concentration found in myasthenic patients indicates a therapeutic window for pyridostigmine and neostigmine plasma concentrations. Even for acetylcholinesterase inhibitors with a central site of action some relationship between clinical effect and pharmacokinetics may exist. For safer drug therapy using these compounds this relationship must be determined.

References

Aquilonius, S.M. and Hartvig, P. (1986) Clinical pharmacokinetics of cholinesterase inhibitors. *Clin. Pharmacokinet.,* 11: 236–249.

Aquilonius, S.M., Eckernäs, S.Å., Hartvig, P., Hultman, J., Lindström, B. and Osterman, P.O. (1979) A pharmacokinetic study of neostigmine in man using gas chromatography-mass spectrometry. *Eur. J. Clin. Pharmacol.,* 15: 367–371.

Aquilonius, S.M., Eckernäs, S.Å., Hartvig, P., Lindström, B. and Osterman, P.O. (1980) Pharmacokinetics and oral bioavailability of pyridostigmine in man. *Eur. J. Clin. Pharmacol.,* 18: 423–428.

Aquilonius, S.M., Eckernäs, S.Å., Hartvig, P., Lindström, B., Osterman, P.O. and Stålberg, E. (1983) Clinical pharmacology of pyridostigmine and neostigmine in patients with myasthenia gravis. *J. Neurol. Neurosurg. Psychiatr.,* 46: 929–935.

Askmark, H., Aquilonius, S.M., Gillberg, P.G., Hartvig, P., Hilton-Brown, P., Lindström, B., Nilsson, D., Stålberg E. and Winkler, T. (1990) Functional and pharmacokinetic studies of tetrahydroaminoacridine in patients with amyotrophic lateral sclerosis. *Acta Neurol. Scand.,* in press.

Breyer-Pfaff, U., Maier, U., Brinkmann, A.M. and Schumm, F. (1985) Pyridostigmine kinetics in healthy subjects and in patients with myasthenia gravis. *Clin. Pharmacol. Ther.,* 367: 495–501.

Breyer-Pfaff, U., Schmezer, A., Maier, U., Brinkmann, A.M. and Schumm, F. (1989) Pyridostigmine plasma levels and neurological symptoms in patients with myasthenia gravis. *Eur. J. Clin. Pharmacol.,* 36: Suppl. 1, A294.

Cohan, S.L., Pohlman, J.L.W., Mikszewski, J. and O'Doherty D.S. (1976) The pharmacokinetics of pyridostigmine. *Neurology,* 26: 536–539.

Davenport, C.J., Monyer, H. and Choi, D.W. (1988) Tetrahydroacridine selectively attenuates NMDA receptor-mediated neuro-toxicity. *Eur. J. Pharmacol.,* 154: 73–78.

Davison, S.C., Hyman, N.M., Delighan, A. and Chan, K. (1981) The relationship of plasma levels of pyridostigmine to clinical effect in patients with myasthenia gravis. *J. Neurol. Neurosurg. Psychiatr.,* 44: 1141–1145.

Gordh, T. (1962) Behandling av sömnmedelsförgiftningar. (Swe) *Nord. Med.,* 68: 132.

Hartvig, P., Wiklund, L. and Lindström, B. (1986) Pharmacokinetics of physostigmine after intravenous, intramuscular and subcutaneous administration in surgical patients. *Acta Anaesthesiol. Scand.,* 30: 177–182.

Hartvig, P., Lindström, B., Pettersson, E. and Wiklund, L (1989) Reversal of postoperative somnolence using a two-rate infusion of physostigmine. *Acta Anaesthesiol. Scand.,* 33: 681–685.

Hartvig, P., Askmark, H., Aquilonius, S.M., Wiklund, L. and Lindström, B. (1990a) Clinical pharmacokinetics of intravenous and oral 9-aminotetrahydroacridine, Tacrine. *Eur. J. Clin. Pharmacol.,* 38: 259–263.

Hartvig, P., Pettersson, E., Wiklund, L. and Lindström, B. (1990b) Pharmacokinetics and effects of 9-amino-1,2,3,4-tetrahydroacridine, Tacrine, in the immediate postoperative period in neurosurgical patients. *J. Clin. Anesthes.,* in press.

Hunter, A.R. (1965) Tetrahydroacridine in anesthesia. *Br. J. Anaesthesiol.,* 37: 505–513.

Nilsson, L., Adem, A., Hardy, J., Winblad, B. and Nordberg, A. (1987) Do tetrahydroaminoacridine (THA) and physostigmine restore acetyl choline release in Alzheimer brain via nicotinic receptors? *J. Neural Transm.,* 70: 357–368.

Nybäck, H., Nyman, H., Öhman, G., Nordgren, I. and Lindström, B. (1988) Preliminary experiences and results with THA for the amelioration of symptoms of Alzheimer's disease. In E. Giacobini and R. Becker (Eds.), *Current Research on Alzheimer Therapy.* Taylor and Francis, London, pp. 231–236.

Petersson, J., Gordh, T.E., Hartvig, P. and Wiklund, L. (1986). A double-blind trial of the analgesic properties of physostigmine in postoperative patients. *Acta Anaesthesiol. Scand.,* 30: 283–288.

Puri, S.K., Hsu, R., Ho, I. and Lassman, H.B. (1988) Single-dose safety, tolerance and pharmacokinetics of HP 029 in elderly men: A potent Alzheimer agent. *Curr. Ther. Res.,* 44: 766–780.

Shaw, F.H. and Bentley, G.A. (1953) The pharmacology of some new anticholinesterases. *Aust. J. Exp. Biol.,* 31: 573–576.

Spencer, P., Nunn, P.B., Hugon, J., et al. (1987) Guam amyotrophic lateral sclerosis-Parkinsonism-dementia linked to a plant excitant neurotoxin. *Science,* 237: 517–522.

S.-M. Aquilonius and P.-G. Gillberg (Eds.)
Progress in Brain Research, Vol. 84
© 1990 Elsevier Science Publishers B.V. (Biomedical Division)

CHAPTER 16

Synaptic adaptation in diseases of the neuromuscular junction

P.C. Molenaar

Department of Physiology of the University of Leiden, Wassenaarseweg 72, 2333 AL Leiden, The Netherlands

Introduction

More than 35 years ago MacIntosh and Oborin (1953) observed that atropine, which was known as an antagonist of the action of acetylcholine (ACh) on muscarinic receptors, enhanced the release of ACh from the cerebral cortex of the cat. Other workers, using similar techniques, confirmed this observation for the cortex and extended it to the hippocampus and the caudate nucleus (see for review Molenaar and Polak, 1980). Some degree of activity is required in the cholinergic nerves from which the ACh is released for atropine to exert its stimulating action: for instance, atropine has no effect on spontaneous ACh release from the cerebral cortex under halothane anaesthesia, but when the release of ACh is stimulated by electrical stimulation of the reticular formation, atropine causes a 4-fold further increase in the release.

At this stage the problem was taken up by Polak, who with in vitro methods began to analyse the paradoxical effect of atropine on ACh release using cortex slices from rat brain. The results of this work led Polak (1971) eventually to propose that there is a mechanism locally regulating ACh release in central cholinergic neurones. According to his hypothesis the released ACh stimulates inhibitory presynaptic muscarinic receptors and thus depresses its own release, an effect which is counteracted by atropine through its effect on the same presynaptic receptors. Later a similar effect of

atropine was discovered in the muscarinic synapses of the guinea-pig ileum (Kilbinger, 1977).

In 1975 I discovered that in skeletal muscle from myasthenia gravis (MG) patients the transmitter release was much higher than that in muscle biopsied from people without a muscular disease. Since the main defect in MG is characterized by a considerable reduction of nicotinic ACh receptors the question arose whether in skeletal muscle there is a regulatory mechanism for ACh release resembling that in muscarinic synapses of the brain. To this end we set out to study synaptic parameters in neuromuscular diseases, in particular MG and the Lambert-Eaton myasthenic syndrome (LEMS), and in animal models for these diseases, in the hope, taking advantage of the pathology, of learning more about the mechanism of the neuromuscular synapse. This article summarizes what we have found.

Methods

The outline of the procedure is given in Fig. 1. In brief the general procedure was as follows. A biopsy was taken of intercostal muscle under general anaesthesia: for MG from a parasternal site during operative removal of the thymus and for LEMS from a lateral site during thoracotomy. Control muscle was also taken laterally during thoracotomy (often from patients with lung cancer, without signs of muscular disease). Subsequently,

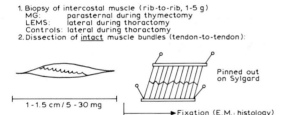

PROCEDURE

1. Biopsy of intercostal muscle (rib-to-rib, 1-5 g)
   MG: parasternal during thymectomy
   LEMS: lateral during thoracotomy
   Controls: lateral during thoracotomy
2. Dissection of <u>intact</u> muscle bundles (tendon-to-tendon):

Pinned out on Sylgard

1 - 1.5 cm / 5 - 30 mg

→ Fixation (E.M.; histology)

<u>Intact</u>
- Electrophysiology
  (MEPPS, quantal content)
- Biochemistry
  (AChR; ACh release)

<u>Homogenization</u>
- Biochemistry
  (ACh content; ChAT; ACHE)

Fig. 1. Procedure for assays on human skeletal muscle.

muscle bundles were dissected from tendon-to-tendon and pinned out so that the endplates were aligned in the middle. In this way the muscle could be divided into a portion without and a portion containing the endplates. The muscle segments were then homogenized. Subsequently choline acetyltransferase and sometimes also cholinesterase were measured. Other bundles were left intact and incubated in Ringer for electrophysiological studies, the biochemical measurements of ACh release, and the determination of ACh receptors (AChRs).

As an animal model for MG we used rats injected with AChR from electric eel (see for review Vincent, 1979) and as a non-immunogenic model we injected rats every 48 h with 15–30 μg/kg α-bungarotoxin. For LEMS we used a passive immunization model described by Lang et al. (1983).

Results

Choline acetyltransferase

In human myasthenic muscle ChAT was increased nearly 3-fold compared to control muscle (Molenaar et al., 1981). In experimental autoimmune MG (EAMG) an increase of ChAT in rabbit skeletal muscle has been reported by others (Clementi et al., 1976). However, in the α-toxin MG model (ETMG) there was no change in ChAT.

In human LEMS and in mouse LEMS the ChAT was unchanged in skeletal muscle (Molenaar et al., 1982; Lang et al., 1984).

ACh content

In human myasthenic muscle the ACh content was roughly twice as high as in controls (Ito et al., 1976). On the other hand, no changes in ACh content were observed in EAMG and ETMG (Molenaar et al., 1979).

In human and mice LEMS no changes in ACh were observed (Molenaar et al., 1982; Lang et al., 1984).

ACh release

Resting release. In all cases spontaneous transmitter release was normal except in human and mouse LEMS muscle, in which reduced ACh release was observed (Molenaar et al., 1982; Lang et al., 1984).

Evoked release. In human myasthenic muscle the ACh release evoked by 50 mM KCl was about three times the ACh release from controls. Upon continued stimulation the ACh release of myasthenic muscle, but not that of controls, subsided (Molenaar et al., 1979). Increased evoked ACh release was confirmed by electrophysiological measurements of the quantal content (Cull-Candy et al., 1980). ACh release was also increased in both the immunological (EAMG) and nonimmunological (ETMG) model for MG (Molenaar et al., 1979; unpublished observations).

Acute receptor blockade in vitro is known to cause increased evoked release, although spontaneous release remains unaffected (Miledi et al., 1978) and the question arose whether the effect seen under chronic blockade in myasthenic muscle is due to the same mechanism as under the condition of acute blockade. However, it was found that the ACh release from myasthenic muscle from ETMG rats was higher than controls in the presence of excess α-toxin in the incubation medium, suggesting different mechanisms for acute and chronic blockade of ACh receptors.

In both human and mouse LEMS evoked ACh release was decreased (Molenaar et al., 1982; Lang et al., 1984) in accordance with electrophysiological measurements of the quantal content (Lambert and Elmqvist 1971; Cull-Candy et al., 1980).

ACh receptors

On the basis of the reduction of amplitude of miniature endplate potentials (MEPPS) and the reduction of radiolabelled α-bungarotoxin binding there is now ample evidence that the number of AChRs per endplate is much decreased in MG, roughly to 25% of control values (see for review Vincent, 1980). In EAMG the reduction observed in rats is usually less (about 40% of controls). In ETMG the reduction of AChRs was about 30% of controls: if AChRs decreased below this value the animals were in immediate danger of suffocation. In acute experiments, using a single dose of α-toxin, I found that rats could not tolerate such a

loss of AChRs: a reduction to 40% was already in the lethal range. (This indicates that synaptic adaptation of ACh release in the chronic experiments with the α-toxin is effective in the living animal.)

In human and mouse LEMS muscle, there is no evidence that the number of AChRs is altered (Lambert and Elmqvist, 1971; Cull-Candy et al., 1980; Lindstrom and Lambert, 1978; Lang et al., 1983).

Discussion

Table I, summarizing our data together with some results taken from the literature, has as a "leitmotiv" how the neuromuscular junction reacts towards a disturbance of its function. In general such a disturbance can be caused by a disease (as discussed in this article) or by a pharmacological tool. It appears that synaptic adaptation is *asym-*

TABLE I

Synaptic adaptation in the neuromuscular junction

Disease/pharmacological tool	ChAT	ACh release	AChR
Postsynaptic			
MG/EAMG [a]	up (1)	up (2)	down (3)
ETMG	± (4)	up (4)	down (4)
Congenital MG [a]	?	?	down (5)
Presynaptic			
LEMS man/mouse	± (6,7)	down (8,9)	± (9,10)
Botulinum [a]; TTX	?	down	up (11,12) [c]
Denervation	down	down	up
Long ACh potentials			
Slow-channel syndrome [b]	?	?	down (13,14)
AChE deficiency [b]	?	?	down (15)
Neostigmine [b]	± (4)	down (16,17)	down (16,17)

[a] Enlarged endplates, sprouting of nerve terminals;
[b] postsynaptic damage;
[c] "upregulation" of AChRs occurs only outside the junctions;
?, not investigated; ±, unchanged. The numbers between parentheses refer to publications (for some effects no reference is given): 1, Molenaar et al. (1981); 2, Molenaar et al. (1979); 3, Vincent (1979); 4, P.C. Molenaar, unpublished; 5, Smit, L.M.E., et al. (1988) *Muscle Nerve*, 11: 337–348; 6, Molenaar et al. (1982); 7, Lang et al. (1984); 8, Lambert and Elmqvist (1971); 9, Lang et al. (1983); 10, Lindstrom and Lambert (1978); 11, Simpson, L.L. (1977) *J. Pharmacol. Exp. Ther.*, 200: 343–350; 12, Pestronk, A., et al. (1976) *Nature*, 264: 787–787; 13, Engel, A.G. (1982) *Ann. Neurol.*, 11: 553–569; 14, Oosterhuis, H.J.G.H., et al. (1987) *Brain*, 110: 1061–1079; 15, Engel, A.G., et al. (1977) *Ann. Neurol.*, 1: 315–330; 16, Roberts, D.V. and Thesleff, S. (1969) *Eur. J. Pharmacol.*, 6: 281–285; 17, Chang et al. (1973).

metric. By this I mean that a postsynaptic defect leads to increased presynaptic function, but not the other way round: a presynaptic defect as found in LEMS does not lead to increased sensitivity of the postsynaptic membrane. Furthermore, though a great increase in the number of AChRs is found after denervation and botulinum toxin, it is important to bear in mind that the corresponding synthesis of AChRs takes place at extrajunctional sites. In fact the number of AChRs at the junction itself does not change at all and it would be thus misleading to speak in these examples of a truly adaptive increase of AChRs.

As far as ChAT is concerned there is an interesting difference between MG and EAMG on the one hand and ETMG on the other hand. It is possible that the increases of ChAT are associated with some outgrowth of nerve terminals. Apparently this does not take place in our ETMG model. It would be interesting to know whether the *duration* of the animal experiment is an important factor or whether the autoimmune reactions per se are responsible for outgrowth of nerve terminals.

Another way to influence neuromuscular transmission is to potentiate and prolong the synaptic potentials with cholinesterase inhibitors. As a result there is some down regulation of AChRs, whereas ChAT remains unchanged (Chang et al., 1973; Van Kempen and Molenaar, unpublished observation). There are two diseases which are comparable to anti-esterase treatment, namely the slow-channel syndrome and the disease in which the synaptic esterase is absent (see Table 1 for references). In both cases there seems to be down regulation of AChRs.

What is the moral of this story? Clearly the mature neuromuscular junction has the capacity for synaptic adaptation. On the other hand, one might argue that this synapse, characterized by a "crude" all-or-none propagation of impulses, has nothing to win with a subtle modulation of transmitter release. However, it is conceivable that adaptation is important for the tuning of presynaptic elements to the postsynaptic membrane when synapse formation takes place at the embryonic stage or when synapses are repaired after injury to the motor nerve.

Acknowledgement

This work has been supported by the Prinses Beatrix Fonds.

References

Chang, C.C., Chen, T.F. and Chuang, S.-T. (1973) Influence of chronic neostigmine treatment on the number of acetylcholine receptors and the release of acetylcholine from the rat diaphragm. *J. Physiol.,* 230: 613–618.

Clementi, F., Conti-Tronconi, B., Berti, F. and Folco, B. (1976) Immunization of rabbits with specific components of postsynaptic membrane. Acetylcholinesterase and cholinergic receptor. *J. Neuropath. Exp. Neurol.,* 35: 665–678.

Cull-Candy, S.G., Miledi, R. Trautmann, A. and Uchitel, O.D. (1980) On the release of transmitter at normal, myasthenia gravis and myasthenic syndrome affected human endplates. *J. Physiol.,* 299: 621–638.

Kilbinger, H. (1977) Modulation by oxotremorine and atropine of acetylcholine release evoked by electrical sytimulation of the myenteric plexus of the guinea-pig ileum. *Naunyn-Schmiedebergs's Arch. Pharmacol.,* 300: 145–151.

Lambert, E.H. and Elmqvist, D. (1971) Quantal components of endplate potentials in the myasthenic syndrome *Ann. N.Y. Acad. Sci.,* 183: 183–199.

Lindstrom, J. and Lambert, E.H. (1978) Content of acetylcholine receptor in myasthenia gravis, experimental autoimmune myasthenia gravis and Eaton-Lambert syndrome. *Neurology,* 228: 130–138.

Ito, Y., Miledi, R., Molenaar, P.C., Vincent, A., Polak, R.L., Van Gelder, M. and Newsom-Davis, J. (1976) Acetylcholine in human muscle. *Proc. R. Soc. Lond. B,* 192: 475–480.

Lang, B., Newsom-Davis, J., Prior, C. and Wray D. (1983) Antibodies to motor nerve terminals: an electrophysiological study of a human myasthenic syndrome transferred to mouse. *J. Physiol. Lond.,* 344: 335–345.

Lang, B., Molenaar P.C., Newsom-Davis, J. and Vincent, A. (1984) Passive transfer of Lambert-Eaton myasthenic syndrome in mice: decreased rates of resting and evoked release of acetylcholine from skeletal muscle. *J. Neurochem.,* 42: 658–662.

MacIntosh, F.C. and Oborin, P.E. (1953) Release of acetylcholine in nervous tissue. *Abstr. XIX Physiol. Congr.,* pp. 580–581.

Miledi, R., Molenaar, P.C. and Polak, R.L. (1978) α-Bungarotoxin enhances transmitter "released" at the neuromuscular junction. *Nature,* 272: 641–643.

Molenaar, P.C. and Polak, R.L. (1980) Inhibition of acetylcholine release by activation of acetylcholine receptors. *Prog. Pharmacol.,* 3/4: 39–44.

Molenaar, P.C., Polak, R.L., Miledi, R., Alema, S., Vincent, A. and Newsom-Davis, J. (1979) Acetylcholine in intercostal muscle from myasthenia gravis patients and in rat diaphragm after blockade of acetylcholine receptors. *Prog. Brain Res.,* 49: 449–458.

Molenaar, P.C., Newsom-Davis J., Polak, R.L. and Vincent, A. (1981) Choline acetyltransferase in skeletal muscle from patients with myasthenia gravis. *J. Neurochem.,* 37: 1081–1088.

Molenaar, P.C., Newsom-Davis, J., Polak, R.L. and Vincent, A. (1982) Eaton-Lambert syndrome: acetylcholine and choline acetyltransferase in skeletal muscle. *Neurology,* 32: 1062–1065.

Polak, R.L. (1971) The stimulating action of atropine on the release of acetylcholine by rat cerebral cortex in vitro. *Br. J. Pharmacol.,* 41: 600–606.

Vincent, A. (1979) Experimental autoimmune myasthenia gravis. In F.C. Rose (Ed.), *Neuroimmunology,* Blackwells, Oxford, pp. 115–127.

Vincent, A. (1980) Immunology of acetylcholine receptors in relation to myasthenia gravis. *Physiol. Rev.,* 60: 756–824.

S.-M. Aquilonius and P.-G. Gillberg (Eds.)
Progress in Brain Research, Vol. 84
© 1990 Elsevier Science Publishers B.V. (Biomedical Division)

CHAPTER 17

Current treatment of myasthenia gravis

Per Olof Osterman

Department of Neurology, Uppsala University, Akademiska sjukhuset, S-751 85 Uppsala, Sweden

Introduction

Modern therapy for severe myasthenia gravis (MG), based on increasing knowledge of the auto-immune background and pathogenetic mechanisms, and advances in intensive care, has improved the management of these patients during the last 25 years, with a dramatic decrease in mortality. Unfortunately, most treatments are still non-specific and associated with side-effects. Continued search for more specific forms of therapy is therefore important.

Muscular weakness and fatigue in MG typically vary considerably in severity and location between different patients, and in the same patient during different periods of time. Because of the varying natural course of MG, it is difficult to evaluate the effect of individual treatments in uncontrolled studies, especially when, as is often the case, multiple therapeutic approaches are used simultaneously. Unfortunately, there has been a remarkable lack of controlled prospective studies concerning what is now considered to be established treatment. The main reason for this is that controlled studies comprising an adequate number of patients, followed up for an appropriate length of time, are difficult to accomplish because of the low incidence of MG. The fact that MG is often a life-threatening disease has also discouraged controlled studies. The lack of controlled studies is, of course, more troublesome when treatments such as thymectomy and cytotoxic drugs, with their slow

onset of effect, are being evaluated, than with rapidly acting treatments such as anti-cholinesterases and plasma exchange.

In the following the principles of the current treatment of MG will be outlined. Data from 213 MG patients, examined by the author during a 15-year period, will be used to illustrate the treatment results.

Patients

The diagnosis of MG was based on clinical criteria, neurophysiological investigations (response to repetitive nerve stimulation; single-fibre EMG recordings performed by E. Stålberg) and the presence of acetylcholine receptor antibodies in the serum (Lefvert et al., 1978).

Clinical data were obtained from standardized case reports. Clinical examination included standardized tests for muscle strength and physical performance (fatigue tests). The functions of the eye muscles, bulbar muscles and muscles of the neck, arms and legs were tested separately and graded on a scale from 0 to 4 (0: no fatigue; 4: complete paralysis). When these results are referred to, the sum of the individual muscle function scores (0–20) will be used.

MG was classified according to modified criteria proposed by Osserman (Perlo et al., 1966). Seventeen patients (8%) suffered from purely ocular MG (group I), 101 (47%) from mild generalized MG (group II A), 63 (30%) from mod-

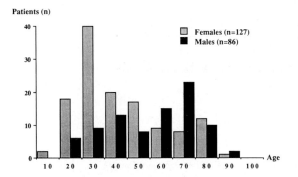

Patients (n)

Females (n=127)
Males (n=86)

Age

Fig. 1. Sex distribution and age at onset of myasthenia gravis in an essentially unselected population of 213 adult patients.

erately severe generalized MG (group II B) and 32 (15%) from early or late severe MG with crises (groups III and IV).

A total of 213 adult MG patients were treated by the author in 1974–1988 at the Department of Neurology of Akademiska sjukhuset, Uppsala. These patients represent an essentially unselected MG population. Probably all adult patients with this disease in the county of Uppsala (about 210,000 inhabitants ≥ 15 years) and most adult patients within the counties of Kopparberg, Väst-manland and Gävleborg (in total about 685,000 inhabitants ≥ 15 years) were examined. From these four counties 172 patients were referred for examination. Forty-two adult MG patients were resident in the county of Uppsala at the end of 1988, giving a prevalence figure of 20/100,000 adult inhabitants. Forty new cases were diagnosed in the county during the 15-year period, i.e. the annual incidence was about 1.3/100,000 adult inhabitants. These prevalence and incidence figures are about twice as high as those previously reported (Oosterhuis, 1984). In a recent Danish study, however, a similar incidence rate was found (Sørensen and Holm, 1989).

The mean length of time from the onset of the disease to the latest follow-up examination by the author was 10.1 years (SD: 9.3) and from the time of diagnosis 7.6 years. The length of time for which the author followed up the patients with regular examinations varied from 0 to 22 years.

Eighty-three patients (39%) were followed up for ≥ 5 years and 36 patients for ≥ 10 years.

The distribution by sex (60% women) and age at onset was similar to that found in previous large-sized study populations (Fig. 1) (Perlo et al., 1966; Oosterhuis, 1984).

For statistical comparison between groups the chi-square test and unpaired t test were used.

Symptomatic treatment

Myasthenia gravis was recognized as a separate entity about 100 years ago, but no effective treatment was available until 1934, when Mary Walker demonstrated the dramatic effect of physostigmine. Anticholinesterases still form the basic medical therapy in MG, but the patients seldom achieve normal strength. In the Uppsala material the initial effect of anticholinesterases could be evaluated in 200 patients. Only one patient became symptom-free; in 47% only moderate or slight improvement was achieved and in six patients there was no effect (Fig. 2). It is the general experience that the extraocular muscles react more poorly than other muscles, and four of the six patients who did not benefit from anticholinesterases had ocular MG. The mean score sum at the fatigue test in 119 patients was 5.7 (SD

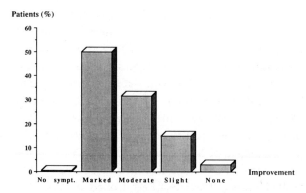

Patients (%)

No sympt. Marked Moderate Slight None

Improvement

Fig. 2. Improvement achieved after a few weeks of treatment with increasing doses of cholinesterase inhibitors in 200 MG patients.

3.0) before treatment and 4.0 (SD 2.2) after a few weeks of treatment with increasing doses of anticholinesterases, which further illustrates the limited effect of these drugs.

The clinical pharmacology of the two most commonly used drugs, neostigmine and pyridostigmine, has been thoroughly investigated (for references see Aquilonius and Hartvig, 1986). The oral bioavailability of these drugs is low. It is higher for pyridostigmine, 10–20%, than for neostigmine, about 2%. The plasma elimination half-lives are short, about 1.4 h and 0.9 h respectively. In spite of the short elimination half-life of pyridostigmine, the intraindividual variations in the plasma concentration are rather small during a dose interval during oral maintenance therapy. The smallness of the variations in steady-state concentration is probably the result of slow absorption from the gastrointestinal tract. In fasting subjects the time taken to reach the peak plasma concentration is similar for neostigmine and pyridostigmine, about 1.5 h. The time is almost doubled when pyridostigmine is taken with food, although the bioavailability is unchanged (Aquilonius et al., 1980). In clinical practice pyridostigmine is preferred to neostigmine and this preference thus finds support in pharmacokinetic data. Considering the limited variations in the steady-state concentration during oral maintenance treatment with pyridostigmine, there seems to be little advantage in using more long-acting anticholinesterases.

The interindividual differences in the steady-state plasma concentrations of neostigmine and pyridostigmine, even among patients receiving the same daily dose and having "optimal" therapy, are considerable. This variation has been found to be 4–7-fold (Aquilonius et al., 1983). In several studies no clear relationship has been found between dose and steady-state plasma concentration (Aquilonius et al., 1980; Chan et al., 1981; White et al., 1981). Although a positive correlation has been demonstrated between the plasma concentrations of these drugs and their effect, measured as decrement of muscle response to repetitive nerve stimulation, the relationship is less clear when a global evaluation of muscle function is used. As myasthenic weakness typically varies between different muscles a given dose of a cholinesterase inhibitor may improve the function of some muscles but not others. Davison et al. (1981) found that only two out of nine myasthenic patients showed a significant correlation between plasma levels of pyridostigmine and a global evaluation of muscle function, which was based on several standardized tests of muscle power and fatigue. At present, therefore, a generally useful "therapeutic interval" cannot be defined.

In practice the anticholinesterase dose is increased gradually, with adaptation of the dosage to the function of those muscle groups which are most important. Few patients gain any benefit from dosages of pyridostigmine higher than 120–180 mg 5 or 6 times a day. Cholinergic side-effects may limit the use of adequate doses. By gradually increasing the dosage over several weeks, by taking the drug with food and by treatment with anticholinergic drugs the muscarinic side-effects can be reduced. In the Uppsala study population 95 patients received anticholinergic drugs, but often for only a limited period of time.

It is a common experience that the clinical responsiveness to anticholinesterases slowly decreases in the first months of treatment, necessitating higher dosages to obtain the same effect. An intriguing question in this context is whether prolonged use of anticholinesterases causes damage to motor nerve terminals and/or motor end-plates. There is some evidence for this in animal experiments and in neurophysiological studies in patients (Hilton-Brown et al., 1982; Munsat, 1984), but at least some of the changes seem to be reversible by drug abstinence. At present the importance of these observations for therapeutic practice is unclear.

Ephedrine, aminophylline and potassium salts have been used as adjuvant therapies. Although they have been considered useful in selected cases, there is little documentation of their efficacy (Howard and Sanders, 1983; Oosterhuis, 1984).

Thymectomy

Despite great efforts to elucidate the role of the thymus in MG and the effect of thymectomy, our knowledge is still incomplete. The observation by Blalock, in 1939, of improvement of severe MG in a patient after thymomectomy, and his promising results of thymectomy in a subsequent small series of patients without demonstrable thymoma, stimulated interest in this treatment. In parallel with the advances in surgery and postoperative care in the last 30 years, thymectomy has gradually become adopted as a standard form of therapy. The complete lack of prospective controlled trials explains why controversies still exist concerning the efficacy of this treatment, its indications, the relation between the histological findings and the results, and the surgical approach (Howard and Sanders, 1983; Oosterhuis, 1984; Genkins et al., 1987; Grob et al., 1987).

The results of a computer-matched comparison of thymectomy and medical treatment (anticholinesterases only) clearly showed the beneficial effect of surgery (Buckingham et al., 1976). In the many uncontrolled investigations, significant improvement has been found after early thymectomy in 60–80% of the patients with generalized MG without a thymoma, and even higher figures have been reported from some recent studies (Olanow et al., 1987; Jaretzki et al., 1988). The improvement does not usually begin until after several months and is thought to go on for many years. It is therefore difficult in these uncontrolled studies to separate the effect of thymectomy from the natural course of the disease. Most clinical studies have indicated that the beneficial effect of thymectomy is greatest in patients between 10 and 40 years of age with a duration of illness shorter than 3 years (Oosterhuis, 1984). Reports on the effect of surgery in older patients are contradictory. The operation is usually not recommended for patients with purely ocular myasthenia. However, as the operation is relatively safe, the results are good (Schumm et al., 1985) and as generalization of MG occurs in about two-thirds of the

ocular cases thymectomy is increasingly used in such cases also. In my series six out of seven patients with ocular MG followed up for ≥ 1 year after thymectomy were symptom-free without medication at the latest follow-up examination.

It is not known why thymectomy is beneficial. Proposed mechanisms include the removal of an antigen source, as acetylcholine receptors are present in normal thymus cells, and the reduction of a reservoir of immunocompetent cells, or a source of antibodies or a thymic hormone.

Several reports indicate that with a transcervical approach to thymectomy the thymus is not completely removed and that the results of transcervical thymectomy are not as good as those obtained by sternal splitting (Matell et al., 1981b; Masaoka et al., 1982; Pirskanen et al., 1987). This matter is controversial, however (Papatestas et al., 1981; Genkins et al., 1987). In Uppsala the transcervical route was the standard procedure until 1980, when our Swedish multi-centre study indicated that sternal splitting gave better results (Matell et al., 1981b). In the author's series 79 patients were thymectomized via the transcervical approach and 69 by sternal splitting (plus 5 in whom both methods were used). The mean intervals between the onset of MG and operation were similar, 3.5 and 3.1 years respectively. The mean length of time from thymectomy to the latest follow-up examination was considerably shorter (4.0 years; SD 4.9) in the sternal split group than in the transcervical group (9.0 years; SD 5.6), which would probably favour the latter in a comparison of outcome. The age at onset and the severity of MG were similar in the two groups, but only six out of 25 thymoma patients were operated on by the transcervical method. For comparison between the groups, only patients followed up for ≥ 1 year after operation (58 in the sternal split group, 79 in the transcervical group) were included. At the latest follow-up examination significantly ($p < 0.05$) more patients operated on by the sternal split approach were free from symptoms (including patients subjectively healthy but with minor fatigue when tested) (Fig. 3). The

Patients (%)

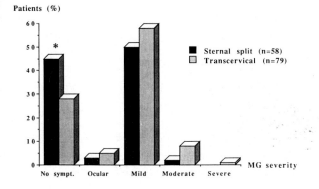

Fig. 3. Severity of MG at the latest follow-up examination in 137 patients followed up for ≥ 1 year after thymectomy via sternal splitting or the transcervical approach.

mean dose of anticholinesterases was significantly ($p < 0.05$) lower in the sternal split group at the latest follow-up examination. However, a higher proportion of the patients in the sternal split group (48 vs. 39%) had received steroids and/or cyto-toxic drugs and the mean preoperative anti-cholinesterase dose was higher in the transcervical group.

Thymomas have been found to be present in 9–16% of patients with MG (Oosterhuis, 1984). They occur most frequently at 40–60 years of age. In the present material 25 patients (11.7%) had a thymoma and in 12 of them it showed local inva-sion. Thymomas are associated with greater sever-ity of MG; 19 of the 25 patients had moderate or severe generalized MG and only six a mild form. The response to surgery is generally poorer in patients with thymoma than in those without. Fortunately, the response to steroids and/or cyto-toxic drugs is usually excellent. In the author's series 17 of the 25 patients were treated with steroids and 15 with cytotoxic drugs. In addition, patients with invasive thymoma received radiation therapy. Four patients have died; two had a malignant thymoma and one died at operation. At the latest follow-up examination 11 of the remain-ing 21 patients had no MG symptoms, nine had mild symptoms and one moderately severe MG.

Corticosteroids

The general adoption of corticosteroid treatment as part of the therapeutic arsenal against MG has greatly improved the prognosis in severe cases. Concerning this treatment again, conclusions have to be drawn from data gathered from uncontrolled retrospective studies in which varied dosage regi-mes and poorly standardized assessment methods have been used. The evidence in favour of its efficacy is mainly founded on observed rapid im-provements in patients with severe MG, and on exacerbations and remissions related to dose changes. Apart from plasma exchange, cortico-steroid treatment is the established therapy which most rapidly induces improvement in MG.

As far back as 40 years ago the effects of corticotrophin (ACTH) and cortisone were evaluated in several reports. Although improve-ment was observed in many patients, the fre-quently occurring initial life-threatening exacerba-tion was an obstacle for this therapy and occa-sional deaths occurred. Progress in the manage-ment of patients with respiratory insufficiency permitted new trials with corticotrophin in the 1960s (von Reis et al., 1965). Given as short intensive courses this treatment became a gener-ally accepted method to induce improvement in severe generalized MG. The duration of improve-ment following a course of corticotrophin varies considerably, but is usually not longer than a few months. Later studies indicated that short courses of corticotrophin and synthetic glucocorticoids (e.g. prednisone, methylprednisolone, dexametha-sone) produce approximately the same result in doses that are equivalent with respect to their glucocorticoid and anti-inflammatory effects (Brunner et al., 1976) and that improvement can be sustained by continuing with lower mainte-nance doses of steroids.

Since the 1970s corticosteroid treatment in the form of high-dose long-term oral prednisone ther-apy has been most commonly used (Mann et al., 1976; Howard and Sanders, 1983). The treatment is usually started with a high daily dose (equivalent to 60–150 mg prednisone) for rapid induction of improvement. When significant amelioration has been achieved, the dosage is changed to an alternate-day schedule. The dose is then gradually reduced in 5–10-mg steps, provided that improvement is maintained. In the early phase of treatment deterioration is common. This is unpredictable and may be severe. In a large series of patients reported by Johns (1987), severe exacerbation, usually requiring artificial ventilation, occurred in 9%. The patient should therefore be hospitalized during the initial phase of treatment. Severe exacerbation may also occur with lower steroid doses. Total remission, or marked amelioration, has been reported in 60–80% of the patients. In most cases improvement is noted within 2–3 weeks, but occasionally it does not begin until after 6–8 weeks. The best results are seen in patients with a late onset of MG.

A major drawback of high-dose oral treatment is the need for long-term administration to maintain improvement. Only a minority of the patients maintain maximum benefit when the treatment is discontinued, unless the drug is combined with cytotoxic therapy (Johns, 1987; Scherpbier and Oosterhuis, 1987). Adverse effects of the corticosteroid treatment are therefore common and occurred, for example, in 67% of the patients reported by Johns (1987).

To achieve more rapid improvement and to reduce the frequency of side-effects, repeated intensive courses of steroids may be advantageous. The experience with intravenous high-dose methylprednisolone pulse therapy seems promising in these respects (Matell et al., 1982; Arsura et al., 1985). In the author's series 37 patients were treated with methylprednisolone pulse therapy and the outcome of this treatment will be briefly reviewed and compared with that of high-dose oral prednisone treatment.

The dosage of intravenous methylprednisolone was 30 mg per kg body weight on two consecutive mornings. In 26 of the 37 patients repeated pulses were given (range 2–21), usually at intervals of 4–5 weeks. After the first pulse initial deteriora-

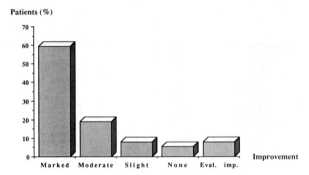

Fig. 4. Improvement achieved with the first intravenous methylprednisolone pulse in 37 patients with moderately severe or severe MG.

tion of myasthenic symptoms was common, reaching its maximum within 3–5 days. The exacerbation was marked in 24% and moderate or slight in about 50%. With repeated pulses, usually in patients receiving oral maintenance prednisone therapy, few patients experienced pronounced deterioration. Improvement after the first pulse commonly started within a week and reached its maximum within 2 weeks. Improvement after the first pulse was marked in 59% and moderate in 17% (Fig. 4). There was no significant correlation between age and effect, initial deterioration and effect or sex and effect, but slight or no effect was observed only in women ($n = 5$).

In 23 patients corticosteroid treatment was started with methylprednisolone pulse therapy, which was followed up with oral prednisone therapy, and in 17 cases with additional (range 2–14) pulses at intervals of 4–5 weeks. The mean initial oral prednisone dose corresponded to 60 mg a day (range 10–150 mg), although the therapy sometimes started with an alternate-day schedule. The effect of this treatment was compared with that of high-dose oral prednisone therapy, which was employed in 39 patients. In this group the mean initial prednisone dose corresponded to 87 mg a day (range 50–150 mg), although in a few patients the therapy started on an alternate-day schedule. After the first 1–2 months prednisone was regularly given as single-dose alternate-day treatment in both groups. The dose was gradually reduced,

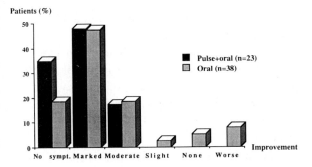

Patients (%)

Fig. 5. Improvement of MG in 23 patients after treatment for 3 months with methylprednisolone pulses plus oral prednisone maintenance therapy and in 38 patients treated with high-single-dose oral prednisone therapy.

the reduction in the first months being more rapid in the pulse therapy group. There was no difference between the groups concerning age at onset, sex distribution or severity of MG. There were eight thymoma patients in each group.

In patients started on oral high-dose prednisone therapy marked initial deterioration occurred in 22% and moderate or slight exacerbation in 44%. These figures are similar to those found after treatment with a methylprednisolone pulse. A higher proportion (35%) of the patients receiving pulse + oral therapy than of the oral prednisone group (18%) were symptom-free at 3 months (including those subjectively healthy, but with minor symptoms at a fatigue test), but the difference is not significant (Fig. 5). In the oral group three patients (all young women) were worse after treatment for 3 months and two patients showed no improvement. The difference between the groups in this respect was almost significant ($p = 0.07$). The mean change in the fatigue test score sum did not differ significantly between the groups.

Six patients who began with oral high-dose prednisone therapy later received pulse therapy. Twenty-six of the 33 patients who continued with oral therapy alone were treated with cytotoxic drugs, and in five additional patients azathioprine therapy was interrupted within the first months because of side-effects. In the pulse therapy group all but one patient received cytotoxic treatment; in one patient azathioprine treatment was inter-

rupted at an early stage because of side-effects. At the latest follow-up examination the mean duration of oral prednisone treatment was 1.8 years in the pulse + oral therapy group and 3.8 years in the oral group. In 11 patients in the former group and 19 in the latter, steroids had been discontinued. At the latest follow-up, 65% of the patients in the pulse + oral therapy group were symptom-free, compared with 42% of the patients in the oral group. The difference is not significant, however ($p = 0.09$). Significantly more patients in the oral group had moderate and severe symptoms at follow-up ($p = 0.02$). One possible explanation for this is that only two of the six patients with moderate and severe MG in the oral group had been treated with cytotoxic drugs.

The number of serious side-effects was considerably higher among the 33 patients in the oral high-dose prednisone group. Diabetes mellitus was provoked in three patients and was exacerbated in another four. Other adverse effects were: severe osteoporosis with compression fractures of the spine (2 patients), cataracts (4), psychological disturbances (2; one manic psychosis), pulmonary tuberculosis (1), septic infections (2) and perforation of the intestine (1). In the group receiving pulse + oral therapy one patient experienced a psychological disturbance with hypomania and one patient developed diabetes.

In conclusion, the results of the present study indicate that intravenous high-dose methylprednisolone pulse therapy, given as repeated pulses in combination with a lower oral maintenance dose of prednisone, is probably as effective as or more effective than high-single-dose oral prednisone therapy and is associated with fewer serious side-effects.

Cytotoxic drugs

Immunosuppression for long periods with azathioprine, 2–3 mg per kg body weight, is now a widely accepted form of treatment of severe generalized MG (Matell et al., 1981a; Mertens et al., 1981; Witte et al., 1984; Matell, 1987). As prospective controlled studies are lacking and most patients have received other forms of treatment, the efficacy of azathioprine is difficult to estimate. However, careful evaluation of the effect of withdrawal and reintroduction of treatment, using the patient as his own control, indicates that azathioprine is in fact effective. Exacerbation within 6 months of azathioprine withdrawal occurs in a majority of the patients, with delayed improvement after reinstatement of treatment (Matell et al., 1981a; Mertens et al., 1981; Hohlfeld et al., 1985). Addition of azathioprine treatment often makes it possible to considerably reduce the steroid dose in patients who repeatedly experience reactivation of MG when the steroid dose is tapered below a certain level. The improvement induced by long-term treatment with azathioprine is usually delayed for several months and may continue during the first 2–3 years. The best results are seen in late-onset rapidly progressive MG and in thymoma cases of all ages. In about 30% of the patients azathioprine does not give improvement, failures being most common in early-onset (< 35 years) MG. Cyclophosphamide and other cytotoxic drugs have been less extensively used than azathioprine, probably because they have more serious adverse effects.

In the Uppsala material 75 patients (35%) were treated with cytotoxic drugs. In 77% combined therapy with corticosteroids was used at some time. Azathioprine was administered to 72 patients. Twelve of these were also treated with cyclophosphamide, usually when azathioprine had to be withdrawn because of side-effects. In 11 patients, who improved while on azathioprine, treatment was discontinued after a median time of 4.5 years (range 1.5–10). In six of them exacerbation of MG occurred within 8 months. Although side-effects may be controlled with careful monitoring, they are frequent and sometimes serious (Kissel et al., 1986; Hohlfeld et al., 1988). In the present series adverse effects led to the withdrawal of azathioprine in 22% of the patients.

Ciclosporin, a new powerful immunosuppressive drug, was recently studied in a randomised, double-blind, placebo-controlled trial as the initial immunosuppressive treatment in MG of recent onset (Tindall et al., 1988). Ciclosporin gave significant improvement, which was usually evident within 2 weeks after the start of therapy, but the drug had to be withdrawn in four of the ten treated patients because of unacceptable side-effects. Ciclosporin also induced moderate to marked improvement in most patients with severe long-standing generalized MG in some recent open studies (Nyberg-Hansen and Gjerstad, 1988; Goulon et al., 1989). Immunosuppression of MG seems to be reversible and exacerbation on withdrawal or reduction of the ciclosporin dosage is common. The ultimate role of ciclosporin in the treatment of MG is still unclear and further controlled studies of its benefits and toxicity in comparison with established treatment are required.

High-dose intravenous immunoglobulin

Several investigators have reported rapid improvement of myasthenic weakness on treatment with high-dose intravenous gamma-globulin (Fateh-Moghadan et al., 1984; Gajdos et al., 1987; Arsura et al., 1988; Cook et al., 1988). The studies are uncontrolled and the numbers of patients small. The response rate is probably somewhat lower with this very expensive treatment than with corticosteroids (Arsura et al., 1988). High-dose intravenous immunoglobulin may possibly play a role as an adjunct in the management of severe MG, especially in patients with acute crises who do not respond satisfactorily to steroids or plasma exchange.

Plasma exchange

Beneficial effects of thoracic duct drainage in MG were reported in 1973 (Bergström et al.) and shortly thereafter the technically less complicated plasma exchange treatment was introduced (Pinching et al., 1976). By 1978 plasma exchange was a main theme at an international symposium on the immunobiology of MG (Dau, 1979) and since then numerous papers on the subject have been published (Seybold, 1987).

The efficacy of plasma exchange alone is difficult to evaluate because of the lack of controlled studies and the differences in techniques used at different centres. Significant improvement has been reported in about 75% of treated patients. Improvement has been noted during the first exchange, but most commonly starts after two or three exchanges. When this treatment is used alone, the duration of improvement is usually relatively short. Immunosuppression with steroids and/or cytotoxic drugs is therefore commonly added, although in one study no synergistic long-term effects were found between repeated plasma exchanges and immunosuppressive treatment (Newsom-Davis et al., 1979). Plasma exchange is expensive, technically complicated and not without risks and therefore should be reserved for selected patients. It is useful in the management of crises and for prevention of impending crises. The use of chronic intermittent plasma exchange treatment in patients with severe MG who respond poorly to other forms of treatment is rarely needed.

In the author's series 17 patients (8%) were treated with one to three plasma exchange courses. Each course lasted 1–2 weeks and consisted of three to seven individual exchanges of about one plasma volume. The treatment was combined with corticosteroids and/or azathioprine in all patients. Marked improvement within a week after the start of plasma exchange was noted in 60%.

Over-all treatment results

In the essentially unselected population of 213 MG patients treated by the author, anticholinesterases were used in 94%, thymectomy in 72%, some form of high-dose corticosteriod therapy in 34%, cytotoxic drugs in 35% and plasma exchange in 8%. At the latest follow-up examination 39 patients were symptom-free and 29 were subjectively healthy but showed minor fatigue when tested. Thus, 32% of the patients considered themselves to be symptom-free (Fig. 6) and 57% of

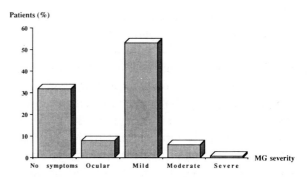

Patients (%)

Fig. 6. Severity of MG at the latest follow-up examination in 213 adult patients.

these were not using anticholinesterases. Only 7% had moderately severe or severe symptoms. A total of 148 patients were still using anticholinesterases, but the mean dose had been reduced from an amount corresponding to 12 tablets (SD 7.4) of 60 mg pyridostigmine a day, as the highest optimal dose, to 7 tablets (SD 4.4) daily at the latest follow-up examination.

Thirty-three of the 213 patients had died by January 1989; only nine of them died at the University Hospital, Uppsala. The hospital records and death certificates have been studied. The median age at the time of death was 76 years (range 30–89 years). In 27 patients death was not related to MG or its treatment. One of these patients died during an operation for a thymoma, another from a malignant thymoma. In one patient, who also suffered from severe multiple sclerosis, MG was the probable cause of death and in three patients MG may possibly have been a contributing factor. In two patients MG treatment was of importance. One of them suffered from a malignant thymoma with metastases. He died of an intestinal perforation in the postoperative period after a thoracotomy. At the time he was being treated with steroids for severe MG. A 72-year-old man died of pulmonary embolism, which emanated from a femoral vein thrombosis, a vein which had been catheterized during the plasma exchanges.

The therapeutic results achieved in the Uppsala study population confirm the low mortality figures now being reported from other special centres. Undoubtedly the introduction of immunosuppressive medication has also improved the quality of life for many myasthenic patients. However, these treatments are still non-specific and associated with serious adverse effects and, as immunosuppressive drugs often cannot be withdrawn without causing relapse, long-term administration is necessary to maintain improvement. It has even been questioned whether the saving of life achieved with anticholinesterases, thymectomy and improved intensive care facilities has in fact been further improved by immunosuppressive treatment, as patients now also die from conditions resulting from this treatment (Simpson and Thomaides, 1987). It is therefore important to optimize the use of what is considered to be established therapy today and to continue the search for more specific and less dangerous forms of treatment.

References

Aquilonius, S.-M. and Hartvig, P. (1986) Clinical pharmacokinetics of cholinesterase inhibitors. *Clin. Pharmacokin.,* 11: 236–249.

Aquilonius, S.-M., Eckernäs, S.-Å., Hartvig, P., Lindström, B. and Osterman, P.O. (1980) Pharmacokinetics and oral bioavailability of pyridostigmine in man. *Eur. J. Clin. Pharmacol.,* 18: 423–428.

Aquilonius, S.-M., Eckernäs, S.-Å., Hartvig, P., Lindström, B., Osterman, P.O. and Stålberg, E. (1983) Clinical pharmacology of pyridostigmine and neostigmine in patients with myasthenia gravis. *J. Neurol. Neurosurg. Psychiatr.,* 46: 929–935.

Arsura, E., Brunner, N.G., Namba, T. and Grob, D. (1985) High-dose intravenous methylprednisolone in myasthenia gravis. *Arch. Neurol.,* 42: 1149–1153.

Arsura, E.L., Bick, A., Brunner, N.G. and Grob, D. (1988) Effects of repeated doses of intravenous immunoglobulin in myasthenia gravis. *Am. J. Med. Sci.,* 295: 438–443.

Bergström, K., Franksson, C., Matell, G. and von Reis, G. (1973) The effect of thoracic duct lymph drainage in myasthenia gravis. *Eur. Neurol.,* 9: 157–167.

Brunner, N.G., Berger, C.L., Namba, T. and Grob, D. (1976) Corticotropin and corticosteroids in generalized myasthenia gravis: Comparative studies and role in management. *Ann. N.Y. Acad. Sci.,* 274: 577–595.

Buckingham, J.M., Howard, F.M., Bernatz, P.E., Payne, W.S., Harrison, E.G. Jr., O'Brien, P.C. and Weiland, L.H. (1976) The value of thymectomy in myasthenia gravis: A computer-assisted matched study. *Ann. Surg.,* 184: 453–458.

Chan, K., Davison, S.C., Dehghan, A. and Hyman, N. (1981) The effect of neostigmine on pyridostigmine bioavailability in myasthenic patients after oral administration. *Meth. Find. Exptl. Clin. Pharmacol.,* 3: 291–296.

Cook, L., Howard, J.F. Jr. and Folds J.D. (1988) Immediate effects of intravenous IgG administration on peripheral blood B and T cells and polymorphonuclear cells in patients with myasthenia gravis. *J. Clin. Immunol.,* 8: 23–31.

Dau, P.C. (Ed.) (1979) *Plasmapheresis and the Immunobiology of Myasthenia Gravis,* Houghton Mifflin Professional Publishers, Boston, 371 pp.

Davison, S.C., Hyman, N.M., Dehghan, A. and Chan, K. (1981) The relationship of plasma levels of pyridostigmine to clinical effect in patients with myasthenia gravis. *J. Neurol. Neurosurg. Psychiatr.,* 44: 1141–1145.

Fateh-Moghadam, A., Wick, M., Besinger, U. and Geursen, R.G. (1984) High-dose intravenous gammaglobulin for myasthenia gravis. *Lancet,* i: 848–849.

Gajdos, P., Outin, H.D., Morel, E., Raphael, J.C. and Goulon, M. (1987) High-dose intravenous gamma globulin for myasthenia gravis: An alternative to plasma exchange? *Ann. N.Y. Acad. Sci.,* 505: 842–844.

Genkins, G., Kornfeld, P., Papatestas, A.E., Bender, A.N. and Matta, R.J. (1987) Clinical experience in more than 2000 patients with myasthenia gravis. *Ann. N.Y. Acad. Sci.,* 505: 500–514.

Goulon, M., Elkharrat, D. and Gajdos. P. (1989) Traitement de la myasthénie grave par la ciclosporine. Etude ouverte de 12 mois. *La Presse Méd.,* 18: 341–346.

Grob, D., Arsura, E.L., Brunner, N.G. and Namba, T. (1987) The course of myasthenia gravis and therapies affecting outcome. *Ann. N.Y. Acad. Sci.,* 505: 472–499.

Hilton-Brown, P., Stålberg, E.V. and Osterman, P.O. (1982) Signs of reinnervation in myasthenia gravis. *Muscle Nerve,* 5: 215–221.

Hohlfeld, R., Toyka, K.V., Besinger, U.A., Gerhold, B. and Heininger, K. (1985) Myasthenia gravis: Reactivation of clinical disease and of autoimmune factors after discontinuation of long-term azathioprine. *Ann. Neurol.,* 17: 238–242.

Hohlfeld, R., Michels, M., Heininger, K., Besinger, U. and Toyka, K.V. (1988) Azathioprine toxicity during long-term immunosuppression of generalized myasthenia gravis. *Neurology,* 38: 258–261.

Howard, J.F. and Sanders, D.B. (1983) The management of patients with myasthenia gravis. In E.X. Albuquerque and A.T. Eldefrawi (Eds.), *Myasthenia Gravis,* Chapman and Hall, London, pp. 457–489.

Jaretzki, A., Penn, A.S., Younger, D.S., Wolff, M., Olarte, M.R., Lovelace, R.E. and Rowland, L.P. (1988) "Maximal" thymectomy for myasthenia gravis. *J. Thor. Cardiovasc. Surg.,* 95: 747–757.

Johns, T.R. (1987) Long-term corticosteroid treatment of myasthenia gravis. *Ann. N.Y. Acad. Sci.,* 505: 568–583.

Kissel, J.T., Levy, R.J., Mendell, J.R. and Griggs, R.C. (1986)

Azathioprine toxicity in neuromuscular disease. *Neurology,* 36: 35–39.

Lefvert, A.K., Bergström, K., Matell, G., Osterman, P.O. and Pirskanen, R. (1978) Determination of acetylcholine receptor antibody in myasthenia gravis: Clinical usefulness and pathogenetic implications. *J. Neurol. Neurosurg. Psychiatr.,* 41: 394–403.

Mann, J.D., Johns, T.R. and Campa, J.F. (1976) Long-term administration of corticosteroids in myasthenia gravis. *Neurology,* 26: 729–740.

Masaoka, A., Monden, Y., Seike, Y., Tanioka, T. and Kagotani, K. (1982) Reoperation after transcervical thymectomy for myasthenia gravis. *Neurology,* 32: 83–85.

Matell, G. (1987) Immunosuppressive drugs: Azathioprine in the treatment of myasthenia gravis. *Ann. N.Y. Acad. Sci.,* 505: 588–594.

Matell, G., Wedlund, J.-E., Osterman, P.O. and Pirskanen, R. (1981a) Effects of long-term azathioprine on the course of myasthenia gravis. In E. Satoyoshi (Ed.), *Myasthenia Gravis: Pathogenesis and Treatment,* University of Tokyo Press, Tokyo, pp. 373–382.

Matell, G., Lebram, G., Osterman, P.O. and Pirskanen, R. (1981b) Follow up comparison of suprasternal vs transsternal method for thymectomy in myasthenia gravis. *Ann. N.Y. Acad. Sci.,* 377: 844–845.

Matell, G., Baehrendtz, S., Hulting, J. and Malmlund, H.O. (1982) Effects on myasthenia of twin shock doses of methyl prednisolone (TSDMP). 5th International Congress on Neuromuscular Diseases, Marseille.

Mertens, H.G., Hertel, G., Reuther, P. and Ricker, K. (1981) Effect of immunosuppressive drugs (Azathioprine). *Ann. N.Y. Acad. Sci.,* 377: 691–699.

Munsat, T.L. (1984) Anticholinesterase abuse in myasthenia gravis. *J. Neurol. Sci.,* 64: 5–10.

Newsom-Davis, J., Wilson, S.G., Vincent, A. and Ward, C.D. (1979) Long-term effects of repeated plasma exchange in myasthenia gravis. *Lancet,,* i: 464–468.

Nyberg-Hansen, R. and Gjerstad, L. (1988) Myasthenia gravis treated with ciclosporin. *Acta Neurol. Scand.,* 77: 307–313.

Olanow, C.W., Wechsler, A.S., Sirotkin-Roses, M., Stajich, J. and Roses, A.D. (1987) Thymectomy as primary therapy in myasthenia gravis. *Ann. N.Y. Acad. Sci.,* 505: 595–606.

Oosterhuis, H.J.G.H. (1984) *Myasthenia Gravis,* Churchill Livingstone, London, 269 pp.

Papatestas, A.E., Genkins, G. and Kornfeld, P. (1981) Comparison of the results of transcervical and transsternal thymectomy in myasthenia gravis. *Ann. N.Y. Acad. Sci.,* 377: 766–778.

Perlo, V. P., Poskanzer, D.C., Schwab, R.S., Viets, H.R., Osserman, K.E. and Genkins, G. (1966) Myasthenia gravis: Evaluation of treatment in 1,355 patients. *Neurology,* 16: 431–439.

Pinching, A.J., Peters, D.K. and Newsom-Davis, J. (1976) Remission of myasthenia gravis following plasma-exchange. *Lancet, ii:* 1373–1376.

Pirskanen, R., Matell, G. and Henze, A. (1987) Results of transsternal thymectomy after failed transcervical "thymectomy". *Ann. N.Y. Acad. Sci.,* 505: 866–867.

Scherpbier, H.J. and Oosterhuis, H.J.G.H. (1987) Factors influencing the relapse risk at steroid dose reduction in myasthenia gravis. *Clin. Neurol. Neurosurg.,* 89: 145–150.

Schumm, F., Wiethölter, H., Fateh-Moghadam, A. and Dichgans, J. (1985) Thymectomy in myasthenia with pure ocular symptoms. *J. Neurol. Neurosurg. Psychiatr.,* 48: 332–337.

Seybold, M.E. (1987) Plasmapheresis in myasthenia gravis. *Ann. N.Y. Acad. Sci.,* 505: 584–587.

Simpson, J.A. and Thomaides, T. (1987) Treatment of myasthenia gravis: An audit. *Q. J. Med.,* 64: 693–704.

Sørensen, T.T. and Holm, E.-B. (1989) Myasthenia gravis in the county of Viborg, Denmark. *Eur. Neurol.,* 29: 177–179.

Tindall, R.S.A., Phillips, J.T., Rollins, J.A., Greenlee, R.G., Wells, L. and Belendiuk, G. (1988) Ciclosporin in the treatment of myasthenia gravis. *Monogr. Allergy,* 25: 135–147.

von Reis, G., Liljestrand, Å. and Matell, G. (1965) Results with ACTH and spironolactone in severe cases of myasthenia gravis. *Acta Neurol. Scand.,* 41 (Suppl. 13): 463–471.

White, M.C., De Silva, P. and Havard, C.W.H. (1981) Plasma pyridostigmine levels in myasthenia gravis. *Neurology,* 31: 145–150.

Witte, A.S., Cornblath, D.R., Parry, G.J., Lisak, R.P. and Schatz, N.J. (1984) Azathioprine in the treatment of myasthenia gravis. *Ann. Neurol.,* 15: 602–605.

S.-M. Aquilonius and P.-G. Gillberg (Eds.)
Progress in Brain Research, Vol. 84
© 1990 Elsevier Science Publishers B.V. (Biomedical Division)

CHAPTER 18

Current therapy of the Lambert-Eaton myasthenic syndrome

Håkan Lundh[1], Olle Nilsson[2] and Ingmar Rosén[3]

[1] *Department of Neurology, Halmstad Hospital, S-301 85 Halmstad, Sweden,* [2] *Department of Neurology and* [3] *Department of Clinical Neurophysiology, University Hospital, S-221 85 Lund, Sweden.*

Characteristics of LEMS

In the human disease now generally called the Lambert-Eaton myasthenic syndrome (LEMS) nearly all symptoms can be explained by peripheral blockade of somatic motor nerves and the parasympathetics, i.e. the cholinergic portions of the peripheral nervous system (Lambert and Rooke, 1965; O'Neill et al., 1988). In this respect it has great similarities to botulinum intoxication, and in both conditions neurally evoked quantal release of transmitter is reduced but with different mechanisms (Lambert and Elmqvist, 1971; Cull-Candy et al., 1976; Simpson, 1986; Wray et al., 1987).

LEMS seems to be caused by an autoimmune reaction against nerve terminal active zones mediated by plasma IgG. Electron microscopy using the technique of freeze-fracturing has shown reduction and disorganization of presynaptic active zone particles in LEMS (Fakunaga et al., 1982) and that type of lesion can be transferred to mice by LEMS IgG (Fukuoka et al., 1987a,b) like the electrophysiological features of LEMS (Lang et al., 1983). Since the active zone particles are thought to represent the calcium ionophore triggering transmitter release by permitting calcium into the nerve terminal (Pumplin et al., 1981), LEMS appears to be caused by an autoimmune attack on these calcium channels.

The clinical identification of LEMS often fails, and it is frequently mistaken for the more common disease myasthenia gravis although its clinical, pharmacological and electrophysiological characteristics are markedly different (Lambert and Rooke, 1965). In LEMS weakness and myasthenic fatiguability is located to proximal muscles in legs and arms and seldom to cranial nerve muscles as in myasthenia gravis. The cholinergic dysautonomia with dry mouth, absent sweating and bladder dysfunction present in LEMS is not found in myasthenia gravis. A most useful and consistent clinical sign to differentiate the two diseases is the absence or weakening of muscle stretch reflexes in LEMS, which is almost never found in myasthenia gravis, and the potentiation of these reflexes after 10 s maximal voluntary contraction never found in myasthenia gravis (Nilsson and Rosén, 1978). The enhancement of the stretch reflex after voluntary contraction is a pathognomonic diagnostic sign of LEMS and can be explained by the known pathophysiology of its presynaptic blockade (see below under electromyography and Fig. 1B). The edrophonium test cannot be used to differentiate LEMS and myasthenia gravis as it sometimes causes a long-lasting clinical improvement in LEMS (Henriksson et al., 1977). Cholinergic receptor antibodies are regularly not found in LEMS (O'Neill et al., 1988).

Two varieties of LEMS

LEMS was detected in the nineteen-fifties in patients with small cell bronchial carcinoma and rarely in other malignancies (Andersson et al., 1953; Henson, 1953; Lambert et al., 1956). It sometimes appears unassociated with carcinoma and clinical evidence indicates a possible autoimmune aetiology (Gutman et al., 1972; Lang et al., 1981). Both varieties of the disease, the paramalignant and the cryptogenetic forms, have similar symptoms and drug responses and can be differentiated only by the development of carcinoma. It is of great importance for the practical management of LEMS that carcinoma may be delayed up to 4 years after the diagnosis of LEMS (O'Neill et al., 1988).

The carcinomatous form often improves or remits after treatment of the lung cancer (Lambert and Rooke, 1965; O'Neill et al., 1988), but the cryptogenetic form is a chronic stable or slowly progressive disease (O'Neill et al., 1988).

Electromyography and treatment monitoring

The electromyography recordings of LEMS are different from myasthenia gravis and have characteristics in common with other presynaptic disorders such as magnesium intoxication and botulism. In LEMS the amplitude of the compound muscle action potential (CMAP) is reduced, decrement appears at low-frequency stimulation (< 10 Hz) and potentiation is typical at higher impulse frequencies (Fig. 1) (Lambert and Rooke, 1965). These electrophysiological findings are usually present in all muscles, i.e. also in muscles that are not clinically weak.

Two parameters are very reproducible in individual LEMS patients, namely the initial CMAP amplitude and its potentiation after 10 s maximal voluntary muscle contraction (Fig. 1B). These two parameters are now generally used as a clinical standard to monitor muscle status and drug response during drug introduction and the clinical follow-up of the individual LEMS patient.

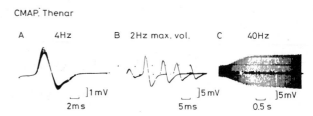

Fig. 1. Recordings of LEMS compound muscle action potential (CMAP) during repetitive nerve stimulation. Typical of LEMS is decreased amplitude of initial CMAP, decrement at low-frequency nerve stimulation (A) and increment at higher frequencies (C). In B CMAP is shown at 2 Hz stimulation before and 2, 5, 10 and 15 s after a 10-s period of maximal voluntary contraction (from Lundh et al., 1984).

Clinical muscle-power tests are less useful because they are often complicated by painful myalgia appearing on repetitive tests and may also be influenced by activation potentiation characteristic of LEMS.

Therapeutic principles

Since LEMS seems to be caused by cholinergic blockade of autoimmune aetiology therapeutic trials have included cholinergic drugs and immunosuppressive procedures.

Cholinergic drugs

The effects of cholinesterase inhibitors in LEMS are generally weak or unnoticeable (Figs. 4 and 5) (Lambert and Rooke, 1965), except in rare cases of mild LEMS where pyridostigmine alone may give acceptable relief (Lundh et al., 1984).

As the cholinergic dysfunction in LEMS seems to be caused by disturbance of the calcium mechanism of transmitter release, it is of interest to try drugs which modulate calcium ions at the nerve terminal. Such drugs are guanidine and the aminopyridines, which strongly enhance transmitter release (Kamenskaya et al., 1975; Lundh, 1978). Guanidine has been thought to act by increasing free intracellular calcium concentrations at critical nerve terminal sites through inhibition of mitochondrial respiration and divalent cation uptake to subcellular organelles (Lundh et al., 1977a). More recent experiments have suggested a mode of action for guanidine similar to that of the aminopyridines (Molgó and Mallart, 1988). These drugs increase transmitter release by their membrane potassium blocking effect (Yeh et al., 1976), which prolongs the nerve terminal action potential and thereby enhances calcium influx through voltage-dependent calcium channels (Lundh, 1978; Llinás et al., 1982). However, a direct facilitating action on nerve terminal calcium channels cannot be ruled out (Lundh and Thesleff, 1977). From a pharmacological standpoint such a mode of action would make guanidine and the aminopyridines ideal drugs in LEMS.

Guanidine

Guanidine has good therapeutic efficacy in LEMS and has long been the standard drug (Lambert, 1966; Oh and Kim, 1973). It markedly increases quantal transmitter release in LEMS intercostal muscles studied in vitro and also restores muscle twitches in paralysed LEMS muscles (Lambert and Elmqvist, 1971). Unfortunately, guanidine has been reported to cause serious side-effects on bone marrow and kidney (Cherington, 1976; Henriksson et al., 1977), and the drug has now been abandoned except in places where the aminopyridines are not yet available.

Aminopyridines

The administration intravenously of 4-amino-pyridine (4-AP) or 3,4-diaminopyridine (3,4-DAP) to a patient with LEMS often produces a "Lazarus effect", i.e., the paralysed immobile patient rises and walks around almost normally (Lundh et al., 1977b, 1984). These drugs are also active when given orally but with a slower time course (Figs. 4 and 5). Simultaneous recordings of the muscle action potential demonstrate normalization of initial amplitude and responses to repetitive nerve stimulation and maximal voluntary contraction (Fig. 2). Microelectrode recordings in vitro from LEMS intercostal muscle endplates have con-

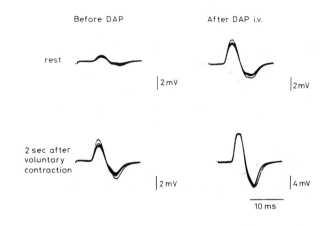

Fig. 2. Increase of CMAP of the thenar muscles after i.v. infusion of 9 mg 3,4-DAP. The CMAPs at rest and after maximal voluntary contraction are recorded. Note different amplification of the lower right record (from Lundh et al., 1983).

firmed the increase of quantal transmitter release by 4-AP (Sanders et al., 1980).

Anticholinesterases used as adjuvant drugs cause great potentiation of the 3,4-DAP effect (Fig. 3), although neostigmine and pyridostigmine usually have no significant effect when given alone (Figs. 4 and 5). Interestingly, such an effect is also achieved when anticholinesterases are added when the direct aminopyridine effect is vanishing (Fig. 4). The effect of 3,4-DAP after oral administration usually reaches its maximum within 2 h and disappears after 4 h. These observations form the basis

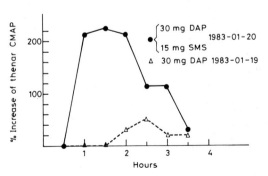

Fig. 3. Potentiation of 3,4-DAP by synstigmine (SMS) on CMAP after peroral administration. Note that recordings were made on consecutive days (from Lundh et al., 1984).

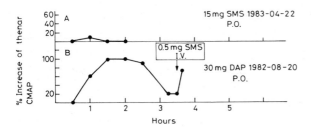

Fig. 4. Response and time course of single doses of synstigmine (SMS) (A) and 3,4-DAP (B) on CMAP. The marked potentiation of the SMS effect after 3,4-DAP remains when the direct 3,4-DAP effect is vanishing (from Lundh et al., 1984).

for the recommended treatment regimen, to give 3,4-DAP and pyridostigmine at 4-h intervals and extra pyridostigmine if needed between the 3,4-DAP doses. Such a regimen gives good and relatively stable symptomatic relief during the day clinically and electrophysiologically.

Side-effects of aminopyridines

4-AP and 3,4-DAP have both been used for continuous oral treatment of LEMS, but 4-AP has now been abandoned because of central nervous system stimulant side-effects, with epileptic seizures, mental confusion and ataxia at doses required to improve neuromuscular transmission (Murray and Newsom-Davis, 1981; Lundh, 1982).

3,4-DAP (Table I) has proved safer, and in Sweden 15 patients with LEMS have now been

TABLE I

Side effects of 3,4-DAP

Cough
Bronchial hypersecretion
Frequent micturation
Frequent defecation
Blurred vision
Palpitations
Ventricular extrasystoles?
Thoracic back pain
Paraesthesias
Coldness in extremities
Worsening of Raynaud
Dizziness
Insomnia
Chorea?
Epileptic fits

treated with 3,4-DAP continuously for up to 7 years. Incidents of epileptic fits have occurred with 3,4-DAP in clinical trials in the USA and Canada when high doses were used (> 60 mg/day). 3,4-DAP, however, has a more favourable therapeutic index than 4-AP, since it is 6–10-times more potent at the neuromuscular junction (Molgó et al., 1980) and 2-times less convulsant (Lemeignan et al., 1984).

Central nervous system stimulant side-effects of 3,4-DAP are infrequent and mild in doses below 40–60 mg/day. Rarely dose-dependent transient dizziness after dose intake appears and difficulty in sleeping may occur when the drug is taken after 5 p.m. One patient after 5 years of continuous treatment developed a mild form of chorea similar to that seen in chronic amphetamine users (Lundh and Tunving, 1981).

Usually, the cholinergic dysautonomia improves simultaneously with the muscle symptoms but sometimes autonomic side-effects appear, such as irritating cough and increased viscid secretion in the bronchi and frequency of micturation and defecation. Atropine or decrease of the pyridostigmine dose often ameliorates such symptoms. Blurred vision, itself a symptom of LEMS, often appears transiently after 3,4-DAP intake when autonomic and muscular symptoms improve in other parts of the body. This may indicate a local blocking effect in the eye of excess acetylcholine when cholinergic synapses at other places are not affected by depolarization block.

Repeated extensive blood tests in several patients for seven years at the longest have not shown any abnormality connected to 3,4-DAP.

Drug tolerance of 3,4-diaminopyridine

Besides the dose-dependent central nervous system side-effects the main treatment problem when using 3,4-DAP is its tendency to induce drug tolerance (Lundh et al., 1984). This may be observed after a few months of treatment with doses above 40–60 mg/day. It is signalled by the patient observing more pronounced weakness in the morning, and increasing doses of 3,4-DAP are needed to obtain a therapeutic effect. In such cases a "drug holiday" and decrease of dose are required and usually drug response is restored after a few weeks.

A related phenomenon is the reversion of the myasthenic day rhythm for the LEMS patient from normally being strongest in the morning to being weakest in the morning. This is generally observed during 3,4-DAP treatment and should not be mistaken for tolerance. It is dose-dependent and becomes more pronounced when the 3,4-DAP dose is increased or taken after 5 p.m., and it does not diminish during long-term medication.

Increasing the dose of 3,4-DAP in the individual LEMS patient may be like giving the patient what in Sweden would be called a " von Döbeln medicine', i.e., the better the drug makes the patient on one day the worse he will become the next day. This phenomenon, a type of rapidly developing tolerance, limits the usefulness of 3,4-DAP. It is probably not caused by depletion of available transmitter in the nerve terminals, since the synthesis and storage of acetylcholine in LEMS muscles are normal (Molenaar et al., 1982). It might be caused by calcium current failure in the LEMS nerve terminal membrane secondary to structural damage of ionic conductance channels.

Immunotherapy

The proposed autoimmune pathogenetic mechanism of LEMS has been strongly supported by empirical observations that immunosuppressive treatments have beneficial effects (Lang et al., 1981; Streib and Rothner, 1981; Dau and Denys, 1982; Newsom-Davis and Murray, 1984). Plasma exchange, corticosteroids and azathioprine are now successfully used in severe cases of LEMS not satisfactorily controlled by cholinergic drugs. Lung cancer has often appeared some time after starting immunosuppressive treatment (Newsom-Davis and Murray, 1984). Such therapy may in some way adversely influence *desired* immunity by disturbing the beneficial immunosuppressive control

of malignant cell change. Therefore immunosuppressive therapy is not recommended in non-cancer patients with a disease duration of less than 4 years, which is the longest delay observed for cancer development after LEMS diagnosis (O'Neill et al., 1988).

On the other hand, immunosuppressive therapy is usually superior to cholinergic drug treatment from the standpoint of symptom control, since its effects last far longer and act round the clock. Cholinergic drugs alone cause patients to be very drug-dependent and often compel them to plan daily activity in relation to the dose intakes of 3,4-DAP. Also morning weakness and the "von Döbeln medicine effect" of 3,4-DAP in LEMS (see above) are common problems.

Plasma exchange

In plasma exchange 3–4 litres of plasma are removed and replaced by some substitute. It is a popular but short-term method of producing immunosuppression. It is used to start immunotherapy when the effects of immunosuppressive agents are delayed as in LEMS. Five to ten exchanges during a 7–14-day period usually cause an obvious improvement, starting at the end of the treatment period, reaching its peak 2 weeks later and vanishing by 6 weeks (Newsom-Davis and Murray, 1984). The time course of improvement is much slower than for plasma exchange in myasthenia gravis, probably because of a slower time of turnover for the affected nerve terminal release structures compared to acetylcholine receptors.

Immunosuppressive agents

Corticosteroids in the form of prednisolone in doses similar to those used in myasthenia gravis (1–1.5 mg/kg/day) are effective but the combination with azathioprine (2–2.5 mg/kg/day) seems to produce an additive effect (Newsom-Davis and Murray, 1984). Azathioprine alone, however, is probably an inferior form of immunotherapy in LEMS. In cases intolerant or not responding to azathioprine, cyclosporine in combination with prednisolone may be effective (Lundh, unpublished observations).

Immunosuppressive drugs in LEMS take one to several months to act clinically and usually cannot be discontinued completely without the reappearance of symptoms. Because of the side-effects of immunosuppressive drugs and the difficulties with dosage of 3,4-DAP, treatment of LEMS is usually a complicated medical challenge. Often cholinergic drugs cannot be stopped totally during immunotherapy, but their doses may be decreased.

Recommended treatment regimen

Coexisting bronchial carcinoma should be investigated by performing lung roentgenogram every 3 months and broncoscopia every 6 months. When detected the lung cancer should be treated by suitable methods.

3,4-Diaminopyridine introduction

On a few consecutive days CMAP and its post-activation potentiation are followed every 30 min between 8 and 12 a.m. after oral administration of single drug doses (Fig. 5). Day one pyridostigmine is tested alone (60–120 mg), day two 3,4-DAP alone (usually 12 mg), day three another dose of

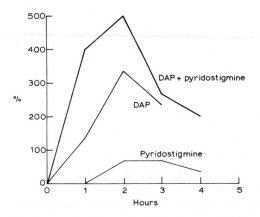

Fig. 5. Introduction of 3,4-DAP in an individual patient. Increase of CMAP response is followed in the mornings on consecutive days after oral doses of pyridostigmine (120 mg), 3,4-DAP (12 mg) and 3,4-DAP (12 mg)+ pyridostigmine (120 mg).

3,4-DAP (6, 18 or 24 mg) and day four 3,4-DAP + pyridostigmine (usually 12 mg 3,4-DAP + 120 mg pyridostigmine).

By this procedure a reasonable normalization of EMG response is achieved with the smallest possible 3,4-DAP dose and the individual drug response and duration of action can be determined. Also the potentiating capacity of pyridostigmine is measured. Treatment is then started with 3,4-DAP combined with pyridostigmine usually 3 (2–5) times a day and sometimes with 2 or 3 extra doses of pyridostigmine alone between 3,4-DAP doses if needed to maintain a stable drug response all day. Daily doses above 40–60 mg 3,4-DAP should not be used.

Immunotherapy

If the 3,4-DAP effect is insufficient prednisolone should be administered, but it is recommended only in cryptogenetic cases, i.e. after 4 years of observation without cancer development. In cancer cases not controlled by oncological treatment prednisolone can be used and often improves LEMS for some time. Azathioprine should only be used in cryptogenetic cases and is added after 1–2 months of inadequate response to prednisolone and 3,4-DAP. If effective the prednisolone dose is slowly reduced to maintenance therapy with an alternate-day regimen but it should not be discontinued. Prednisolone is given as a single dose after breakfast, but azathioprine is best given at bedtime or in divided doses at meals to minimize gastrointestinal side-effects. Spontaneous remissions of LEMS have not been reported and drug therapy cannot usually be stopped.

Acknowledgement

Miss Lena Klintefors is thanked for skilful typing.

References

Anderson, H.J., Churchill-Davidson, H.C. and Richardson, A.T (1953) Bronchial neoplasm with myasthenia: prolonged apnoea after administration of succinylcholine. *Lancet,* ii: 1291–1293.

Cherington, M. (1976) Guanidine and germine in Eaton-Lambert syndrome. *Neurology (Minneap.),* 26: 944–946.

Cull-Candy, S.G., Lundh, H. and Thesleff, S (1976) Effects of botulinum toxin on neuromuscular transmission in the rat. *J. Physiol. (Lond.),* 260: 177–203.

Dau, P.C. and Denys, E.H. (1981) Plasmapheresis and immunosuppressive drug therapy in Eaton-Lambert syndrome. *Ann. Neurol.,* 11: 570–575.

Fukunaga, H., Engel, A.G., Osame, M and Lambert, E.H. (1982) Paucity and disorganization of presynaptic membrane active zones in the Lambert-Eaton myasthenic syndrome. *Muscle Nerve,* 5: 686–697.

Fukuoka, T., Engel, A.G., Lang, B., Newsom-Davis, J., Prior, C. and Wray, D.W. (1987a) Lambert-Eaton myasthenic syndrome: I. Early morphological effects of IgG on the presynaptic membrane active zones. *Ann. Neurol.,* 22: 193–199.

Fukuoka, T., Engel, A.G., Lang, B., Newsom-Davis, J., Prior, C. and Wray, D.W. (1987b) Lambert-Eaton myasthenic syndrome. II. Immunoelectron microscopy localization of IgG at the mouse motor end-plate. *Ann. Neurol.,* 22: 200–211.

Henriksson, K.G., Nilsson, O., Rosén, J. and Schiller, H.H. (1977) Clinical, neurophysiological and morphological findings in Eaton-Lambert syndrome. *Acta Neurol. Scand.,* 56: 117–140.

Henson, R.A. (1953) Discussion of unusual manifestation of bronchial carcinoma. *Proc. R. Soc. Med.,* 46: 859–861.

Kamenskaya, M.A., Elmqvist, D. and Thesleff, S. (1975) Guanidine and neuromuscular transmission. *Arch. Neurol. (Chicago),* 32: 505–518.

Lambert, E.H. (1966) Defects of neuromuscular transmission in syndromes other than myasthenia gravis. *Ann. N.Y. Acad. Sci.,* 135: 367–384.

Lambert, E.H. and Elmqvist, D. (1971) Quantal components of end-plate potentials in the myasthenic syndrome. *Ann. N.Y. Acad. Sci.,* 183: 183–199.

Lambert, E.H. and Rooke, E.D. (1965) Myasthenic state and lung cancer. In W.R. Brain and F.H. Norris (Eds.) *The Remote Effects of Cancer on the Nervous System.* Grune and Stratton, New York and London, pp. 67–80.

Lambert, E.H., Eaton, L.M. and Rooke, E.D. (1956) Defect of neuromuscular conduction associated with malignant neoplasms. *Am. J. Physiol.,* 187: 612–613.

Lang, B., Newsom-Davis, J., Prior, C. and Wray, D. (1983) Antibodies to motor nerve terminals: an electrophysiological study of a human myasthenic syndrome transferred to mouse. *J. Physiol. (Lond.),* 344: 335–345.

Lang, B., Newsom-Davis, J., Wray, D., Vincent, A. and Murray, N. (1981) Autoimmune aetiology for myasthenic (Eaton-Lambert) syndrome. *Lancet,* ii: 224–226.

Lemeignan, M., Millart, H. Lamiable D., Molgo, J. and Lechat, P. (1984) Evaluation of 4-aminopyridine and 3,4-diaminopyridine penetrability into cerebrospinal fluid in anesthetized rats. *Brain Res.,* 304: 166–169.

Llinás, R., Walton, K., Sugimori, M. and Simon, S. (1982) 3- and 4-aminopyridine in synaptic transmission at the giant synapse. In P. Lechat, S. Thesleff and W.C. Bowman (Eds.) *Aminopyridines and Similar Acting Drugs. Advances in Biosciences, Vol. 35,* Pergamon Press, Oxford, pp. 69–79.

Lundh, H. (1978) Effects of 4-aminopyridine on neuromuscular transmission. *Brain Res.,* 153: 307–318.

Lundh, H. (1982) Therapeutic applications of aminopyridines in diseases of neuromuscular transmission. In P. Lechat, S. Thesleff and W.C. Bowman (Eds.) *Aminopyridines and Similar Acting Drugs. Advances in Biosciences. Vol. 35,* Pergamon Press, Oxford, pp. 287–296.

Lundh, H. and Thesleff, S. (1977) The mode of action of 4-aminopyridine and guanidine on transmitter release from motor nerve terminals. *Eur. J. Pharmacol.,* 42: 411–412.

Lundh, H. and Tunving, K. (1981) An extrapyramidal choreiform syndrome caused by amphetamine addiction. *J. Neurol. Neurosurg. Psychiatry,* 44: 728–730.

Lundh, H., Leander, S. and Thesleff, S. (1977a) Antagonism of the paralysis produced by botulinum toxin in the rat. *J. Neurol. Sci.,* 32: 29–43.

Lundh, H., Nilsson, O. and Rosén, I. (1977b) 4-Aminopyridine: a new drug tested in the treatment of Eaton-Lambert syndrome. *J. Neurol. Neurosurg. Psychiatry, 40:* 1109–1112.

Lundh, H., Nilsson, O. and Rosén, I. (1983) Novel drug of choice in Eaton-Lambert syndrome. *J. Neurol. Neurosurg. Psychiatry,* 46: 684–685.

Lundh, H., Nilsson, O. and Rosén, I. (1984) Treatment of Lambert-Eaton syndrome: 3,4-diaminopyridine and pyridostigmine. *Neurology (Cleveland),* 34: 1324–1330.

Molenaar, P.C., Newsom-Davis, J., Polak, R.L. and Vincent, A. (1982) Eaton-Lambert syndrome: acetylcholine and choline acetyltransferase in skeletal muscle. *Neurology (New York),* 32: 1061–1065.

Molgó, J. and Mallart, A. (1988) The mode of action of guanidine on mouse motor nerve terminals. *Neurosci. Lett.,* 89: 161–164.

Molgó, J., Lundh, H. and Thesleff, S. (1980) Potency of 3,4-diaminopyridine and 4-aminopyridine on mammalian neuromuscular transmission and the effect of pH changes. *Eur. J. Pharmacol.,* 61: 25–34.

Murray, N.M.F. and Newsom-Davis, J. (1981) Treatment with oral 4-aminopyridine in disorders of neuromuscular transmission. *Neurology (New York),* 31: 265–271.

Newsom-Davis, J. and Murray, N.M.F. (1984) Plasma exchange and immunosuppressive drug treatment in Lambert-Eaton myasthenic syndrome. *Neurology (Cleveland),* 34: 480–485.

Nilsson, O. and Rosén, I. (1978) The stretch reflex in the Eaton Lambert syndrome, myasthenia gravis and myotonic dystrophy. *Acta Neurol. Scand.,* 57: 350–357.

Oh, S.J. and Kim, K.W. (1973) Guanidine hydrochloride in Eaton-Lambert syndrome. *Neurology. (Minneap.),* 23: 1084–1090.

O'Neill, H., Murray N.M.F. and Newsom-Davis, J. (1988) The Lambert-Eaton myasthenic syndrome. A review of 50 cases. *Brain,* 111: 577–596.

Pumplin, D.W., Reese, T.S. and Llinas, R. (1981) Are the presynaptic membrane particles the calcium channels? *Proc. Natl. Acad. Sci. USA,* 78: 7210–7213.

Sanders, D.B., Kim, Y.I., Howard Jr, J.F. and Goetsch, C.A. (1980) Eaton-Lambert syndrome: a clinical and electrophysiological study of a patient treated with 4-aminopyridine. *J. Neurol. Neurosurg. Psychiatry,* 43: 978–985.

Simpson, L.L. (1986) Molecular pharmacology of botulinum toxin and tetanus toxin. *Annu. Rev. Pharmacol. Toxicol.,* 26: 427–453.

Streib, E.W. and Rothner, A.D. (1981) Eaton-Lambert myasthenic syndrome: Long-term treatment of three patients with prednisone. *Ann. Neurol.,* 10: 448–453.

Wray, D.W., Peers, C., Lang, B., Lande, S. and Newsom-Davis, J. (1987) Interference with calcium channels by Lambert Eaton myasthenic syndrome antibody. *Ann. N.Y. Acad. Sci.,* 505: 368–376.

Yeh, J.Z., Oxford, C.H., Wu, C.H. and Narahasi, T. (1976) Interactions of aminopyridines with potassium channels of squid axon membranes. *Biophys. J.,* 16: 77–81.

S.-M. Aquilonius and P.-G. Gillberg (Eds.)
Progress in Brain Research, Vol. 84
© 1990 Elsevier Science Publishers B.V. (Biomedical Division)

CHAPTER 19

Future prospects of cholinergic research on neuromuscular transmission

S. Thesleff (I) [1], E. Heilbronn (II) [2], P.C. Molenaar (III) [3] and A.G. Engel (IV) [4]

[1] *Department of Pharmacology, University of Lund, Sweden,* [2] *Department of Neurochemistry and Neurotoxicology, Stockholm University, Sweden,* [3] *Department of Pharmacology, University of Leiden, The Netherlands, and* [4] *Neuromuscular Research Laboratory, Mayo Clinic and Foundation, Rochester, MN, U.S.A.*

(I) S. Thesleff

It is difficult and perhaps always futile to speculate about the future but let me still try.

During the past decade tremendous progress has been made in our understanding of cholinergic neuromuscular transmission. Isolation of the nicotinic cholinergic receptor, in combination with molecular biology and new electrophysiological techniques, such as the patch-clamp, have given us a unique insight into the molecular structure and function of the receptor. This information is of importance not only for our understanding of cholinergic transmission but also for a more general appreciation of the mechanisms involved in chemically operated ion channels. Last but not least it has, as we have learned from several presentations, given us a much better understanding of a number of pathophysiological processes affecting the neuromuscular junction. These developments will no doubt continue with the characterization of other types of receptor.

It is also clear from the presentations that several steps in the physiology of neuromuscular transmission are still unknown or at least open to debate: for instance, the detailed mechanism for acetylcholine release from the motor nerve. Such aspects will, I am quite certain, be clarified during the nineties, since many laboratories are working on those issues. It is also clear that modulators of neuromuscular transmission are research fields which are rapidly gaining importance. Neuropeptides, ATP and other neuronal messengers which regulate synaptic formation and efficacy open new areas for research. Pre- and postsynaptic phosphorylation processes as well as the control of gene expressions in the muscle are areas for future research. The same applies to mechanisms which we so far have barely touched upon: I am thinking about chemical signals delivered by the muscle to the motor nerve. I am particularly referring to recent studies which suggest that the muscle secretes substances with nerve growth promoting and modulating activities. The identification of such factors will no doubt be of clinical importance.

(II) E. Heilbronn

Ever since the publication, in 1966, of Sir Bernard Katz's famous book "Nerve, Muscle and Synapse" the neuromuscular junction has been accepted as the main model of straightforward mammalian cholinergic neurotransmission. During the '70s, however, and as a consequence of the advent of receptorology and new analytical techniques, it became obvious that the neuromuscular junction is in fact a very specific synapse whose very high speed of transmission can be understood in terms of the structure and location in the muscle cell membrane of a glycoprotein–ion channel neurore-ceptor macromolecule. Molecular biological studies have revealed that a group of such nicotinic receptors, differing in subunit number or type, exists, but their relation to development and disease, i.e. to physiological and pathological function, remains to be found out. In the presynapse, pharmacological studies have implied the existence of both nicotinic and muscarinic cholinergic autoreceptors. Transmitter release at the neuromuscular junction, far from being completely understood, is obviously regulated by a number of different receptors, by the action of various other modulators and by enzyme actions, including those of kinases. Many of these have only just been recognized and their precise role in transmitter release needs to be explained and may provide, in fact, new pharmacological tools.

The occurrence of both low-molecular-weight substances and peptides in nerve and/or skeletal muscle cells or in the extracellular space around them, substances probably acting as cotransmitters or, perhaps more important, as modulators of transmission or postsynaptic efficacy, has very recently been recognized. One of them, ATP, released from both pre- and postsynapse upon depolarization, has been shown to control endogenous free Ca levels by increasing, via a P2-receptor–G-protein–phospholipase C cascade, the IP_3 content of myotubes in culture, which results in increases in their endogenous free Ca content. This Ca originates from both internal and external sources but neither these nor the mechanisms involving them have been completely identified. Levels of IP_3, as well as possibly those of other messenger-like substances, are clearly important to the muscle cell and seem to be under control of several modulator-receptor systems. The mechanisms by which they act (e.g. control of ion channels in external membrane and in intracellular Ca-store membranes, possibly as messengers in excitation-contraction coupling) have not yet been completely defined, nor is it clear exactly how they interact with the ACh-nicotinic receptor system or when they are of physiological importance.

They may turn out to be connected to developmental or ageing stages of skeletal muscle, i.e. to non-innervated muscle.

A role for membrane phospholipid turnover and its products, particularly in relation to the state of membrane depolarization, may exist but is not yet understood. Certain preliminary results point to a control function of ACh-receptor channel open state, perhaps receptor desensitization.

Peptides such as CGRP (VIP, somatostatin??) seem to be selectively localized in certain muscle fibers only. This observation so far has no explanation, but such may be found in the physiology of the relevant muscle fiber type or even in its liability to pathological states.

A review of important areas of future research around the neuromuscular junction should discuss many other questions more or less specific to this synapse and its components, including those of so far not described possible uptake/release functions of Ranviers nodes, neuron-myelin interactions, sprouting mechanisms and their control, the possible existence of "pioneer" neurons in innervation, trophic substances and their roles, control of receptor synthesis, migration and localization, identification and regulation of genes whose products are able to alter the further fate of early cells, etc. They are, one hopes, discussed by others. I would, however, like to conclude with an aspect close to my own interests, that of a possible involvment of cytokines in neuromuscular disease, especially in inflammatory and/or autoimmune disease.

(III) P.C. Molenaar

The neuromuscular junction has served as a model system for cholinergic transmission for about 40 years. As a model system it has been very successful, especially in the areas of electrophysiology and electron microscopy. (Skeletal muscle contains little acetylcholine, especially when compared to the nicotinic system of the electroplaque of the electric ray. Therefore, the neuromuscular junction is not particularly ideal for measuring release and content of ACh. Measurements of ACh have been of some importance, among other things for corroborating electrophysiological findings.)

Is the day of the neuromuscular junction now over? This, at least to some of us, embarrassing question is instigated by the astonishing progress made with the help of new methods in other systems such as patch-clamp analysis on oocytes and the molecular biology of transmitter receptors. It may be that the neuromuscular junction is gradually losing its role as an exemplary model. However, several colleagues in the audience put forward the idea that the neuromuscular junction, apart from meriting study for its specific properties, will be instrumental in solving questions bearing on matters of general importance. (i) Little is known, for instance, about the presynaptic membrane, how it functions and how the processes of exocytosis and endocytosis take place. (ii) It is clear that the nerve terminal and muscle membrane talk to each other, not only during formation and re-formation of synapses after injury but also in the normal situation. It will be fascinating to unravel the identity of the substances which form the words of this language. (iii) Finally, the neuromuscular junction is still the only synapse in which, with considerable detail, ACh release can be studied by both electrophysiological and chemical methods, while changes of structure can be assessed by electron microscopy, which has recently become even more powerful with the advent of monoclonal immuno-gold staining techniques.

(IV) A.G. Engel

My comments pertain to research on the neuromuscular junction (NMJ) and the diseases that affect the NMJ. Before considering future developments, I would like to reflect on some aspects of how our present knowledge of NMJ diseases was acquired. In this connection, I would like to dwell on three themes.

The first theme is that of a latent period be-tween a basic science observation and its clinical application. As knowledge of a given disease advances, the period between a relevant basic science discovery and its clinical application becomes shorter. Consider, for example, the basic science observations that led to our current knowledge of myasthenia gravis (MG). The light microscopic anatomy of the NMJ was clearly defined by Kühne's observations in 1870 and Dogiel's descriptions in 1890. Then hardly any observations were made on the NMJ until 1952, when Couteaux and Taxi localized acetylcholinesterase by enzyme cytochemistry at the NMJ. Two years later, Palade, and also Robertson, obtained the first glimpse of the NMJ in the electron microscope. Palade now recognized that the subneural apparatus observed by Kühne and Couteaux consisted of junctional folds, and that nerve terminals contained synaptic vesicles. These findings were directly relevant to the intracellular microelectrode studies of Fatt and Katz in 1952 and del Castillo and Katz in 1954, which established that the spontaneous or nerve impulse-induced release of ACh from the nerve terminals occurs in discrete quanta. On this basis, del Castillo and Katz could now postulate that the quantum resides in the synaptic vesicle. However, it was not until 1964 that Elmqvist and coworkers showed with intracellular microelectrode methods that there was a marked decrease of the miniature endplate potential amplitude in MG. In the early 1970s two other important basic science observations were made: the alpha-neurotoxins of elapid snakes were found to bind to AChR with high affinity, and the electric organs of fish proved to be an excellent source of AChR. Thus, the toxins could be used to purify AChR, and to quantitate it at the NMJ. The clinical applications now followed rapidly. In 1973, Fambrough and coworkers demonstrated AChR deficiency at the MG NMJ and, in the same year, Patrick and Lindstrom showed that rabbits immunized with AChR develop MG. By 1975, the autoimmune etiology of human MG and the effector mechanisms causing AChR loss from the NMJ were clearly established.

Acceleration in the application of basic science data to the study of a clinical disorder is also apparent in the history of the Lambert-Eaton syndrome. Without recounting the steps in detail, I will only mention the following. Impaired release of quanta from the nerve terminal by nerve impulse was noted in 1968 by Elmqvist and Lambert; that autoantibodies mediate the physiological defect was observed in 1981; and evidence that the disease is conditioned by a depletion of the presynaptic voltage-sensitive calcium channel was published in 1982. Further studies between 1982 and 1987 fully established that the autoantibodies in this disease are directed against the presynaptic voltage-sensitive calcium channel.

The second theme pertains to the manner in which basic science skills are transmitted from one investigator or laboratory to another. The transmission is by personal guidance of one investigator by another. For example, the application of in vitro microelectrode studies to the human intercostal muscles in Lund in the 1960s would not have come about without Stephen Thesleff's tutelage with Bernard Katz. The physiological defect in MG would not have been described by Elmqvist and coworkers without Thesleff's guidance. The introduction of microelectrode methods to the Mayo Clinic and the subsequent description of the physiological defect in the Lambert-Eaton syndrome by Elmqvist and Lambert in 1968 would not have come about without a visit by Dan Elmqvist to the Mayo Clinic that year. My own interest in the structure and function of the NMJ might not have been kindled had it not been for my association with Ed Lambert during that time.

The third theme relevant to future studies in NMJ disorders is the need for new investigators in basic and clinical research. New investigators require support, and this must come from several sources. An important source is a research grant from a private foundation or a government agency. Beyond that, there is the essential element of a sympathetic and enlightened academic environment which puts a premium on research. The growth of an investigator occurs over several years, and during this period the embryonic researcher must not be overburdened by clinical or teaching tasks. Further, investigators who show promise during their years of tutelage should be encouraged to continue with research rather than to provide a routine clinical or laboratory service.

As for the future, we can anticipate that new and exciting basic science observations pertaining to the NMJ will be made at an accelerated pace. One would hope that our knowledge of known NMJ disorders, e.g., autoimmune myasthenia gravis, the Lambert-Eaton syndrome, botulism, the slow-channel syndrome, etc., will become more precise and refined; and that heretofore unrecognized NMJ diseases will be discovered and characterized. In particular, one may anticipate (1) an increasing contribution from the molecular geneticist in explaining the basis of hereditary defects that affect the structure or function of the NMJ; (2) a better understanding of the manner in which calcium facilitates synaptic vesicle exocytosis and of the mechanisms that facilitate or interfere with the calcium-mediated process; (3) further knowledge of how molecular alterations in the acetylcholine receptor (AChR) can affect its affinity for acetylcholine (ACh), the kinetic properties of the AChR-associated ion channel, and the metabolic stability of AChR itself; and (4) a better understanding of the molecular architecture and physiological properties of the voltage-sensitive calcium channel of the motor nerve terminal.

SECTION II

Cholinergic Mechanisms in the Peripheral Nervous System

B: Autonomic Nervous System

S.-M. Aquilonius and P.-G. Gillberg (Eds.)
Progress in Brain Research, Vol. 84
© 1990 Elsevier Science Publishers B.V. (Biomedical Division)

CHAPTER 20

Structural and functional aspects of acetylcholine peptide coexistence in the autonomic nervous system

Björn Lindh[1,2] and Tomas Hökfelt [2]

Departments of [1] Anatomy and [2] Histology and Neurobiology, Box 60400, Karolinska Institutet, S-10401 Stockholm, Sweden

Introduction

The autonomic nervous system (ANS) consists of the sympathetic, parasympathetic and enteric nervous system. The efferent parts of the sympathetic and parasympathetic divisions of the ANS are structurally organized as a chain of two neurons from the central nervous system (CNS) to the peripheral effector organs. The sympathetic neurons in the CNS are located in the thoracic and upper lumbar spinal cord, whereas the parasympathetic neurons form a number of nuclei in the brain stem, and are also present in the sacral spinal cord. The autonomic ganglia constitute the relay organs of the ANS, where the central, preganglionic neurons make contacts with the peripheral, postganglionic neurons. On the basis of their anatomical localization autonomic ganglia are characterized as paravertebral, prevertebral and terminal ganglia. The paravertebral ganglia, which are located along the spinal cord, form the sympathetic chain whereas the prevertebral ganglia, which also are sympathetic, lie on the abdominal aorta. The terminal ganglia, which are mainly parasympathetic, are located near or within their target organs. The enteric nervous system, which consists of two ganglionated plexuses with nerves connected to them, extends throughout the whole gastrointestinal tract.

Acetylcholine (ACh) is the "classical" chemical mediator at the synapse between the preganglionic and postganglionic neurons, in both the sympathetic and parasympathetic nervous system. ACh is also the transmitter substance between the postganglionic neuron and the effector cell in the parasympathetic nervous system. In the sympathetic nervous system noradrenaline is the "classical" transmitter between the postganglionic neuron and the effector cell. The parasympathetic system is thus designated "cholinergic', whereas the sympathetic nervous system is said to be "noradrenergic". In the enteric nervous system ACh seems to be a major "classical" transmitter but 5-HT and non-5HT amine-handling neurons are also present in the enteric ganglia (see Furness and Costa, 1987).

From the last ten to fifteen years' research with isolation and characterization of the neuronal peptides, a new group of messenger molecules has emerged. Evidence has been obtained that neurons may use neuropeptides as messengers, and often they coexist with the "classical" neurotransmitters, such as ACh (Hökfelt et al., 1980, 1986; Cuello, 1982; Osborne, 1983; Chan-Palay and Palay, 1984). In the present paper, ACh and peptide coexistence in the ANS will be reviewed. The parasympathetic, sympathetic and enteric nervous system will be discussed separately, with emphasis on both structural and functional aspects. Some interesting experiments concerning neurotransmitter plasticity in autonomic neurons will be discussed in a separate section. Since the data in the present review are based on different histochemical techniques, these will be briefly mentioned in the Methodology section.

Methodology

Forty years ago, a histochemical technique for visualization of the ACh-metabolizing enzyme, acetylcholinesterase (AChE), was developed (Koelle and Friedenwald, 1949). This technique has been used to study presumably cholinergic neurons in the central as well as in the peripheral nervous system (see Silver, 1974; Butcher and Wolf, 1984). More recently, the ACh-synthesizing enzyme, choline acetyltransferase (ChAT), has been purified and by an indirect immuno-histochemical technique (see Coons 1958) ChAT antibodies have been used to analyse cholinergic systems (Kimura et al., 1981; Crawford et al., 1982; Eckenstein and Thoenen, 1982; Levey et al., 1983). Antibodies to AChE (Marsh et al., 1984) can in several cases also be used as markers for cholinergic neurons and the immunohistochemical technique is also useful for the study of peptide-containing neurons. In sympathetic ganglia, non-cholinergic neurons, i.e. the noradrenergic cell population, can be visualized with the formalin-induced histofluorescence technique (see Falck et al., 1962) or with antibodies raised to the catecholamine-synthesizing enzymes, tyrosine hydroxylase (TH) and dopamine β-hydroxylase (DβH) (Goldstein et al., 1973).

Many autonomic neurons contain multiple messenger molecules, and several methods for demonstration of multiple antigens in a neuron are available. First, with the adjacent-sections technique thin consecutive sections are incubated with different primary antisera (see Figs. 2A–C and 5A–C). The advantage with this approach is that cross-reactivity between the different antisera cannot occur, while the chief drawback is occasional difficulty in identifying the same cell with certainty in adjacent sections. Secondly, the elution-restaining technique (Tramu et al., 1978) may be used (see Fig. 2D–G). After photography, acid

potassium permanganate is used to elute the first antibody, and following control incubation the sections are incubated with the second primary antibody. The main disadvantage with this method is that the elution procedure may reduce the antigenicity of the second antigen, with false negative results as a possible consequence. Finally, direct double (Wessendorff and Elde, 1985) (see Figs. 1E–F, 3A–D and 4A–J) or triple staining (Staines et al., 1988) (see Figs. 1A–C) techniques can be used for simultaneous demonstration of two or three antigens in the same section. This approach requires the primary and secondary antisera to be raised in different species and the secondary antibodies to be labeled with different dyes.

The parasympathetic nervous system

The discussion of ACh and peptide coexistence in the parasympathetic nervous system will be focused on the innervation of the nasal mucosa and salivary glands, which, in this respect, are the most studied parts of the parasympathetic nervous system. Thus, the facial nerves convey preganglionic nerve fibers from the superior salivatory nucleus which continue in the major petrosal nerve and synapse in the sphenopalatine ganglion. The postganglionic parasympathetic neurons of this ganglion innervate the lacrimal gland and mucosal glands and blood vessels of the nose and the palate. Also in the superior salivatory nucleus preganglionic nerve fibers originate, which via the facial nerve and chorda tympani terminate in local ganglia, for instance, in the submandibular and sublingual ganglia, which supply the corresponding salivary glands with postganglionic fibers.

Several lines of evidence suggest that both the preganglionic terminals and most of the cell bodies of the cranial parasympathetic ganglia are cholinergic (see Koelle, 1955: Koelle and Koelle, 1959; Giacobini et al., 1979; Johnson and Pilar, 1980; Lundberg et al., 1982b; Leblanc et al., 1987). However, a number of neurons in the cranial parasympathetic ganglia of the chick (Teitelman et al., 1985), rat (Leblanc et al., 1987) and cat (Lindh et al., 1989) contain immunoreactivity to TH.

A large number of cholinergic neurons in the sphenopalatine ganglion are vasoactive intestinal polypeptide (VIP)-containing (Lundberg et al., 1980, 1981; Uddman et al., 1980), and VIP fibers are also abundant in the terminal areas of these neurons, for instance in the nasal mucosa where the VIP fibers are present around exocrine glands and blood vessels (Uddman et al., 1978, 1980; Lundberg et al., 1980, 1981). Stimulation of the preganglionic fibers to the sphenopalatine ganglion of the cat results in nasal secretion mediated via muscarinic receptors (Eccles and Wilson, 1973; Änggård, 1974) whereas the concomitant vasodilation is atropine-resistant (Malm, 1973; Änggård and Edvall, 1974). VIP, which is released upon parasympathetic nerve stimulation (Lundberg et al., 1981; Uddman et al., 1981), causes an atropine-resistant dilation of both resistance and capacitance vessels in the nasal mucosa and is thus a strong candidate for mediating the non-cholinergic vasodilation seen upon parasympathetic nerve stimulation. A peptide designated peptide histidine isoleucine (PHI), with a sequence homologous to VIP and sharing many of its biological actions, has subsequently been isolated (Tatemoto and Mutt, 1981). PHI is expressed on the same precursor gene as VIP (Itoh et al., 1983) and these peptides coexist in cholinergic autonomic neurons (Lundberg et al., 1984a). Thus, it is possible that PHI is also involved in mediating non-cholinergic vasodilation, for instance in the nasal mucosa of the cat.

Recently, it has been reported that neuropeptide Y (NPY)-containing cell bodies are also present in the sphenopalatine ganglion of the rat, pig and guinea pig but not in the cat or human (Leblanc et al., 1987; Lundberg et al., 1988; Lacroix et al., 1990). In the rat, analysis of consecutive sections revealed that virtually all NPY-positive cells in the sphenopalatine ganglion also contained immunoreactivity to VIP (Leblanc et al., 1987). Colocalization of NPY- and ChAT-LI could also be established in this ganglion, whereas

the few TH-positive cells appeared to be NPY-negative (Leblanc et al., 1987). The functional significance of a potent vasoconstrictor, NPY, coexisting with the two vasodilators, ACh and VIP, in postganglionic parasympathetic neurons remains to be established. The latter authors (Leblanc et al., 1987) suggest that NPY may have unknown physiological actions complementary rather than antagonistic to those of ACh and VIP.

VIP and PHI also coexist with ACh in postganglionic parasympathetic neurons innervating salivary glands (Lundberg et al., 1980, 1984a). The release of VIP, PHI and ACh in the submandibular salivary gland after parasympathetic nerve stimulation seems to be frequency-dependent. Thus, ACh is released upon low-frequency stimulation, whereas high-frequency activation also causes release of VIP and PHI (Lundberg et al., 1982b, 1984b). Interestingly, the release of these peptides increases after atropine administration, which points to the possibility that ACh, via muscarinic receptors, presynaptically inhibits VIP and PHI release. Infusion of ACh into the submandibular artery induces both vasodilation and salivary secretion, whereas infusion of VIP causes vasodilation, but no salivary secretion per se (Lundberg et al., 1982a). However, the salivatory volume response to ACh is potentiated by VIP, which may be an effect of the additional increase in blood flow, or a direct effect of VIP on secretory elements (Lundberg et al., 1982a).

Finally, as an example of peptide and ACh coexistence in preganglionic parasympathetic neurons, we present here some recent results obtained from studies in the guinea pig. Thus, preganglionic parasympathetic fibers originating in the dorsal motor nucleus (DMN X) travel in the vagus nerve and terminate, for instance, in enteric ganglia. In the gastrointestinal tract, especially in sphincter regions, VIP/PHI-immunoreactive nerve fibers are present in high numbers. Although most of these fibers are from the enteric neurons, some may have an extrinsic origin, for example in DMN X, where VIP/PHI-positive neurons are present (Triepel, 1982).

In order to find out whether or not vagal VIP/PHI-containing neurons project to the gastrointestinal tract a retrograde axonal tracing study was performed by injecting the subunit B of cholera toxin (CTB) into the guinea pig pylorus. After perfusion, sections of the brain stem were simultaneously incubated with antibodies to CTB, PHI and ChAT. A fair number of cells in the DMN X contained all three immunoreactivities (cf. Fig. 1A–C), demonstrating that VIP/PHI-containing cholinergic neurons in the medulla oblongata project to the guinea pig pylorus and contribute to the VIP/PHI-positive nerve fiber network present there. These VIP/PHI-containing cholinergic neurons may thus be involved in the control of the pyloric sphincter muscle in the guinea pig. In vivo experiments have shown that VIP can relax gastrointestinal sphincters (see Furness and Costa, 1987).

The sympathetic nervous system

Cholinergic preganglionic sympathetic neurons project to pre- and paravertebral ganglia, whereby ACh elicits both fast and slow excitatory postsynaptic potentials (see Skok, 1983; Kobayashi and Tosaka, 1983). The immunohistochemical evidence for the cholinergic nature of preganglionic sympathetic neurons is the presence of ChAT-positive neurons in the sympathetic lateral column (Houser et al., 1983; Kondo et al., 1985) and the demonstration of ChAT-immunoreactive nerve fibers in sympathetic ganglia (Fig. 1D) (Lindh et al., 1986b). Sympathetic ganglia also contain enkephalin (ENK)-positive nerve fibers (Schultzberg et al., 1979), most of which probably represent preganglionic fibers (Dalsgaard et al., 1982) and are possibly cholinergic. It has been shown in physiological experiments that ENK presynaptically inhibits cholinergic transmission in sympathetic ganglia (Konishi et al., 1979). In an early study in the cat it was demonstrated that neurotensin (NT) is also present in preganglionic sympathetic neurons (Lundberg et al., 1982c). More recently it has been shown that, in addition to

ENK and NT, substance P (SP) and somatostatin (SOM) are present in preganglionic sympathetic neurons of the cat (Krukoff, 1987). Furthermore, in the rat preganglionic sympathetic neurons seem to contain calcitonin gene-related peptide (CGRP) (Yamamoto et al., 1989).

Our knowledge of cholinergic postganglionic sympathetic neurons is mainly based on studies of the cat and rat. Early physiological studies of the cat suggested that a population of paravertebral sympathetic neurons innervating exocrine sweat glands in the foot pads (Langley, 1922; Dale and Feldberg, 1934) and blood vessels of the hind limbs (Folkow and Uvnäs, 1948) are cholinergic. Histochemical evidence for the cholinergic nature of these paravertebral sympathetic neurons was later obtained with the AChE-staining technique, demonstrating that 10–15% of the neurons in the stellate, lower lumbar and sacral sympathetic ganglia of the cat were strongly AChE-positive (Holmstedt and Sjöqvist, 1959; see also Sjöqvist, 1962). It was subsequently shown, using the Falck-Hillarp technique, that these AChE-containing cells seemed to lack catecholamines (Hamberger et al., 1965). Similar numbers of AChE-positive cells were found in a recent immunohistochemical study using antibodies to AChE (Fig. 2A, D) (Lindh et al., 1989a). With the double staining technique it can be shown that AChE- and TH-like immunoreactivities in these ganglia, in principle, have a complementary cellular distribution. However, occasional cells containing both immunoreactivities can be observed.

Cholinergic neurons in the paravertebral sympathetic ganglia of the cat contain immunoreactivity to VIP and PHI (Fig. 2C, F; cf. Fig. 3A with B) (Lundberg et al., 1979; Lindh et al., 1989a). Two types of cholinergic VIP/PHI-containing cell can be distinguished in these ganglia: one type with a strong VIP/PHI immunofluorescence clustered in groups, often found in the peripheral parts of the ganglia, and a second type with scattered cells of a weaker fluorescence (Figs. 2C, F and 3A) (Lundberg et al., 1979; Lindh et al., 1989a). More recently, it was shown that the

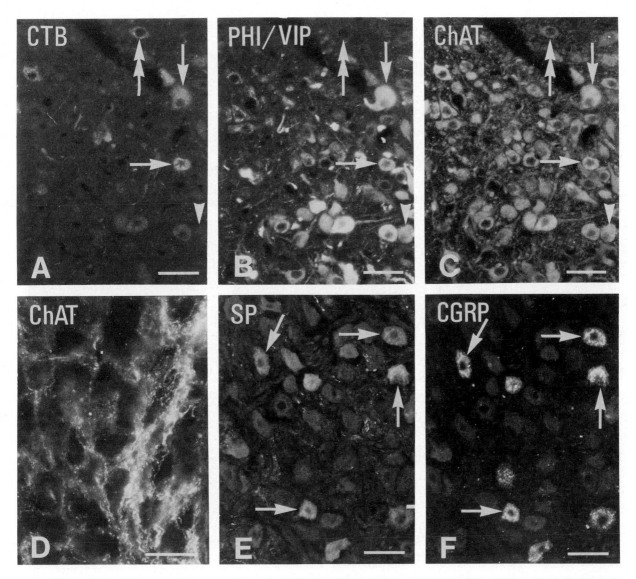

Fig. 1. Immunofluorescence micrographs of sections of the brain stem (A–C), the stellate ganglion of the guinea pig (D) and a cultured S1 sympathetic ganglion of the cat (E, F) after incubation with antisera to CTB (A), PHI (B), ChAT (C, D), SP (E) and CGRP (F). Micrographs A–C are taken from a triple staining experiment and show the same section. Micrographs E and F, which are from a double staining experiment, show the same section. Arrows in A point to CTB-positive cells which also contain immunoreactivity to PHI (B) and ChAT (C). Double arrows indicate a CTB-containing (A) cell which appears to lack PHI-LI (B) but contain ChAT-LI (C), while arrowheads point to a ChAT- (C) and PHI-positive (B) cell which is CTB-negative (A). The ChAT-positive fibers in the stellate ganglion have a fine varicose appearance (D). In E, arrows point to weakly stained SP-containing cells, which also display a strong CGRP-immunofluorescence (F). Bars indicate 50 μm.

scattered cells also contain immunoreactivity to CGRP (Fig. 2B, E, G; cf. Fig. 3C with D) (Lindh et al., 1987), and based on subsequent immunohistochemical analysis it has been suggested that the scattered cell population, in addition to ACh, VIP/PHI and CGRP, also contain SP (cf. Fig. 1E with F) (Kummer and Heym, 1988; Lindh et al., 1988a, 1989a). In a recent in situ hybridization

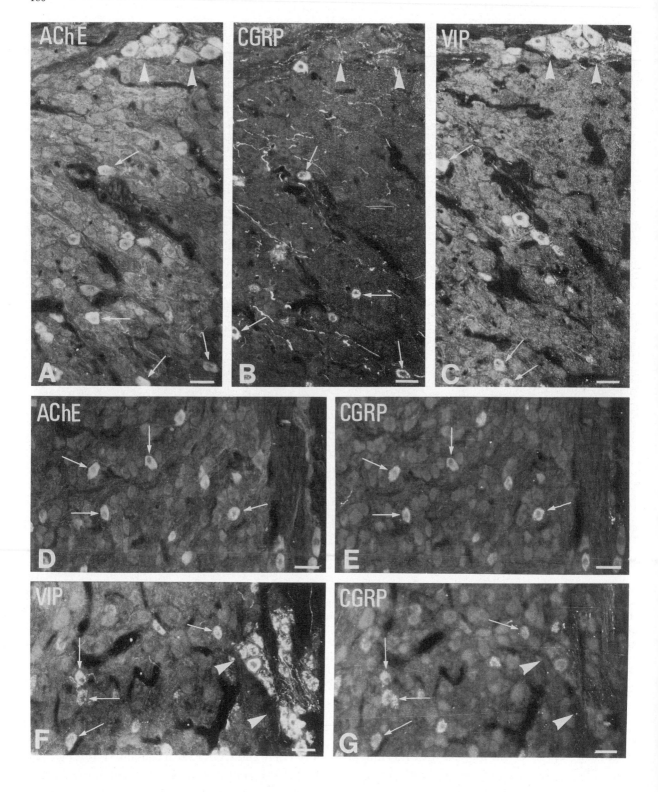

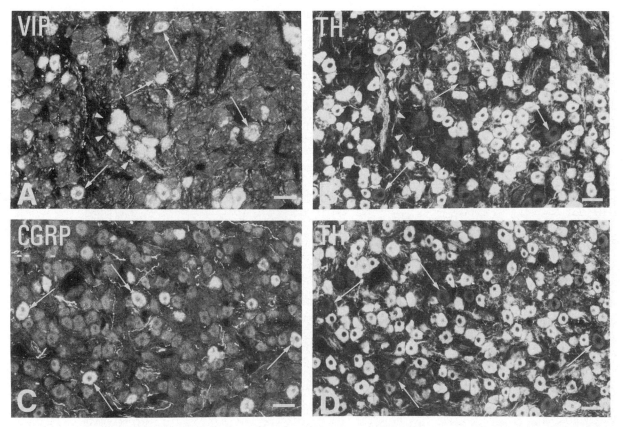

Fig. 3. Immunofluorescence micrographs of sections of stellate ganglion of the cat after incubation with antisera to VIP (A), TH (B and D) and CGRP (C). The micrographs are taken from a double staining experiment; A-B and C-D, respectively, show the same sections. In A arrows and arrowheads point to VIP-positive ganglion cells which are TH-negative (B). The VIP-containing cells are either scattered throughout the ganglia (arrows) or form small groups (arrowheads). The CGRP-positive neurons (arrows) (C) are all scattered and lack TH-LI (D). Bars indicate 50 μm.

study SP mRNA has been demonstrated in such cholinergic paravertebral sympathetic neurons of the scattered type (Lindh et al., 1989b).

It has been suggested that the two cholinergic cell populations project to different target areas (Lindh et al., 1989a). Thus, the scattered cell type, which in addition to ACh contain the four vasodi-

latory peptides VIP, PHI, CGRP and SP, would mainly innervate exocrine sweat glands in the foot pads whereas the clustered cell type "only" containing ACh, VIP and PHI would supply blood vessels in the skeletal muscle (cf. Fig. 4A–J). In the rat paravertebral sympathetic ganglia, VIP- (Hökfelt et al., 1977) and CGRP-immunoreactive

Fig. 2. Immunofluorescence micrographs of sections of the stellate ganglion (A–E) and an S1 paravertebral sympathetic ganglion (F–G) of the cat after incubation with antisera to AChE (A and D), CGRP (B, E and G) and VIP (C and F). The micrographs A–C show three consecutive sections, while D-E and F-G, respectively, show the same sections taken from an elution-restaining experiment. Arrowheads in A point to a group of clustered AChE-immunoreactive neurons which appear to be CGRP-negative (B) and VIP-positive (C), when the following two consecutive sections are analysed. Arrows point to AChE- (A), CGRP- (B) and VIP-containing (C) ganglion cells of the scattered type. In D are indicated AChE-positive cells which also contain CGRP-LI (E). Arrowheads in F outline a group of clustered VIP-positive cells apparently devoid of CGRP-LI (G). The scattered cells, however, contain both VIP- (F) and CGRP-immunoreactivity (G) (arrows). Bars indicate 50 μm.

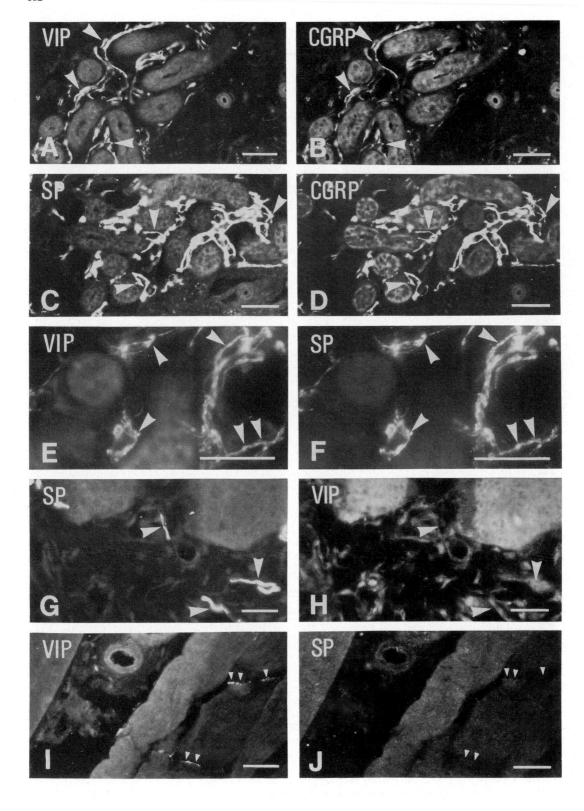

(Landis and Fredieu, 1986) neurons are present. These neurons appear to be cholinergic and innervate exocrine sweat glands in the paws (Landis and Fredieu, 1986; see also Landis, 1988).

The functional consequence of ACh coexisting with four vasodilatory peptides in postganglionic sympathetic neurons innervating exocrine sweat glands is at present unclear. However, a number of conclusions may be drawn from earlier physiological studies demonstrating that blockade of muscarinic receptors completely abolishes sweat secretion seen after sympathetic nerve stimulation, whereas the concomitant vasodilation is atropine-resistant. Thus, it is unlikely that any of the coexisting peptides induce sweat secretion per se, but may be responsible for the non-cholinergic vasodilation seen in the exocrine sweat glands. It may be suggested that sweat secretion is regulated similarly to secretion from the submandibular salivary gland (see above). The coexisting peptides would thus enhance ACh-induced sweat secretion by further increasing blood flow and/or by a direct effect on the secretory elements. It is, however, quite possible that one or more of the coexisting peptides are not directly involved in regulation of blood flow/sweat secretion, but have other functions. For instance, in the rat it has been demonstrated that CGRP may regulate SP levels by inhibiting an enzymatic breakdown of the peptide (Le Greves et al., 1985).

The enteric nervous system

Many gastrointestinal functions, for instance motility and secretion, and absorbtion of water and electrolytes are controlled or influenced by the neurons of the enteric nervous system. Thus, the enteric nervous system has a high capacity for reflex activity independently of the central nervous system, and in mammalian species there are, in fact, as many neurons in the enteric nervous system as in the spinal cord. The nerve cell bodies of the enteric nervous system, which are embedded in the wall of the digestive tube, are arranged in two ganglionated plexus extending virtually uninterrupted throughout the whole gastrointestinal tract. The myenteric plexus is located between the longitudinal and circular muscle layers, whereas the submucous plexus is present, as its name suggests, within the submucosa. Within the last ten years, above all thanks to the elegant studies of Costa, Furness and collaborators (see Furness and Costa, 1987), the circuitry and function of the enteric nervous system have begun to be unravelled. This group has, by combining different experimental techniques, i.e. lesions within the enteric plexus, immunohistochemical analysis of whole mount preparations, intracellular injection of tracer and electrophysiology, been able to characterize enteric neurons in the guinea pig small intestine on the basis of coexisting chemical messengers and to define their projections and functions. In the following a brief survey is given, mainly extracted from Furness and Costa (1987)

The nerve fibers innervating the circular muscle layer almost exclusively originate in the myenteric plexus. The circular muscles of the intestine are, in principle, supplied by three types of motor innervation, namely cholinergic excitatory, non-cholinergic excitatory and non-cholinergic, non-adrenergic inhibitory. Several lines of evidence suggest that SP is responsible for the non-

Fig. 4. Immunofluorescence micrographs of sections of the skin of the foot pads (A–H) and the soleus muscle (I, J) of the cat after incubation with antisera to VIP (A, E, H and I), CGRP (B, D) and SP (C, F, G and J). All sections are taken from double staining experiments, and A-B, C-D, E-F, G-H and I-J, respectively, show the same sections. In A, arrowheads point to VIP-positive fibers, distributed around sweat glands and also containing CGRP-LI (B). Arrowheads in C indicate SP-immunoreactive nerve fibers near some sweat glands in the skin of the foot pads; these fibers also contain CGRP-LI (D). In E arrowheads point to varicose, VIP-positive fibers which innervate a sweat gland and also contain SP-LI (F). Arrowheads in G point to SP-positive nerve fibers which lie beneath the epidermis; these nerves lack VIP-LI (H), probably being sensory. In I arrowheads point to some VIP-containing nerves in the soleus muscle which apparently are devoid of SP-LI (J). Bars indicate 50 μm.

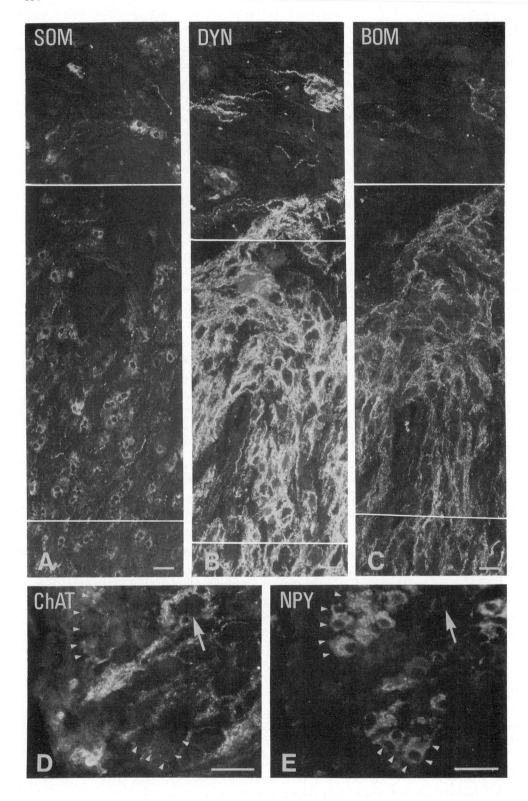

cholinergic excitatory motor transmission. The abundance of SP-immunoreactive nerve terminals in the circular muscle layer and the direct demonstration of SP and ChAT coexistence in myenteric neurons suggest that the cholinergic excitatory motor neurons and the SP-containing motor neurons are overlapping populations. It may be that these two compounds are differentially released from the same neurons upon nerve stimulation.

In the submucous plexus there are at least three different types of cholinergic neuron. One type, which receive a cholinergic excitatory input and project to the mucosa, are secretomotor. These cholinergic secretomotor neurons also contain CGRP, cholecystokinin (CCK), galanin (GAL), NPY and SOM. A second type of neuron, which in addition to ACh contain SP, are devoid of any significant excitatory synaptic input and are probably sensory. Finally, the third type of neuron appear to lack peptide immunoreactivity and terminate within the submucous plexus, probably acting as cholinergic interneurons.

In the myenteric plexus there also originate nerves which, via the mesenteric or colonic nerves, project to prevertebral sympathetic ganglia. Physiological experiments, where fast synaptic inputs from the intestine have been recorded in the prevertebral ganglia, suggest that these enteric nerves are cholinergic (see Szurszewski, 1981). Furthermore, a sparse network of ChAT-positive nerve fibers can be observed in the celiac–superior mesenteric ganglion (CSMG) of the guinea pig (Fig. 5D). In addition to ACh, these nerves contain immunoreactivity to ENK, CCK, VIP/PHI, dynorphin (DYN) (Fig. 5B), gastrin-releasing peptide (GRP)/bombesin (BOM) (Fig. 5C) and CGRP (Costa et al., 1986; Furness and Costa, 1987; Lindh et al., 1988b). The latter peptide-containing nerves terminate around two of the three main populations of noradrenergic neurons, i.e. noradrenergic neurons containing SOM (NA/SOM neurons) and noradrenergic neurons which have so far been found to lack peptide immunoreactivity (NA/– neurons) (cf. Fig. 5A–C) (Costa et al., 1986; Furness and Costa, 1987; Lindh et al., 1986a, 1988b; Macrae et al., 1986). Noradrenergic neurons containing NPY (NA/NPY neurons), which constitute the third noradrenergic cell population, seem to be devoid of this innervation (Costa et al., 1986; Furness and Costa, 1987; Lindh et al., 1986a, 1988b; Macrae et al., 1986) (cf. Fig. 5D with E). Denervation experiments have shown that the NA/SOM and the NA/– neurons, respectively, project to the submucous and myenteric plexus (Costa and Furness, 1984), whereas the NA/NPY neurons innervate intestinal blood vessels (Furness et al., 1983). Taken together, these findings suggest that a peripheral reflex arc, of importance for controlling intestinal motility and mucosal functions but not for regulation of intestinal blood flow, originates in the enteric ganglia and is relayed in the guinea pig CSMG (Costa et al., 1986; Furness and Costa, 1987; Lindh et al., 1988b).

Neurotransmitter plasticity

In vivo and in vitro studies have shown that postmitotic sympathetic neurons have the capacity to alter their expression of neurotransmitters (Potter et al., 1986; Landis, 1988). This may be seen as an increased or decreased synthesis of

Fig. 5. Immunofluorescence micrographs (A–C are montages) of sections of the guinea pig CSMG of an operated animal with only the mesenteric nerve supply intact (A–C) and from an unoperated animal (D, E) after incubation with antisera to SOM (A), DYN (B), BOM (C), ChAT (D) and NPY (E). Sections in A–C are semi-consecutive, whereas D and E show the same section. The latter section (D, E) was first stained with a ChAT antiserum and subsequently, after photography, NPY antiserum was applied. The SOM-positive cell bodies are mainly found in the superior mesenteric pole (SMP) of the ganglion (A). The DYN- (B) and BOM-immunoreactive (C) nerve fiber networks seem to be confined to SMP of the CSMG. In D the arrow points to a cell which is surrounded by a dense ChAT-positive nerve fiber network; this cell appears to be NPY-negative (E). Two groups of NPY-containing cells are outlined (E) which seem to be almost devoid of ChAT innervation (D). Bars indicate 50 μm.

messenger molecules, or even as complete "switch', where the neurons change the "classical" transmitter they use and become, for instance, cholinergic instead of noradrenergic. Several lines of evidence suggest that environmental factors may play an important role in the choice of neurotransmitters.

Cultures of neurons dissociated from superior cervical ganglia (SCG) of newborn rats were, originally, used for in vitro studies of the neurotransmitter choice of sympathetic neurons. Neurons from young cultures only synthesize catecholamines (Mains and Patterson, 1973), in accordance with the adrenergic signal sympathetic neurons receive early in development. If the dissociated sympathetic neurons are grown in cultures without any non-neuronal elements they continue, in principle, to differentiate into a noradrenergic phenotype (Mains and Patterson, 1973; Rees and Bunge, 1974; Burton and Bunge, 1975; Patterson and Chun, 1977). However, if these cultures also contain non-neuronal cells, for instance heart myocytes, both noradrenergic and cholinergic properties will develop (O'Lague et al., 1974; Patterson and Chun, 1974, 1977; Johnson et al., 1976). The cholinergic properties may also be induced by a conditioned medium, i.e. a culture medium taken from another cell culture containing a diffusible factor secreted from these latter cells (Patterson and Chun, 1977). The cholinergic factor, which has recently been purified from conditioned medium (Fukada, 1985; Weber et al., 1985) appears not only to increase ChAT activity but also to decrease catecholamine synthesis (Patterson and Chun, 1977; Reichardt and Patterson, 1977).

Experimental evidence is now available suggesting that changes from a noradrenergic to a cholinergic phenotype may also occur in sympathetic neurons in vivo (Landis and Keefe, 1983; Leblanc and Landis, 1986; see also Landis, 1988). Thus, sympathetic nerves, which at day 4 become associated with sweat glands in the foot pads of postnatal rats, express noradrenergic traits. However, the catecholamine histofluorescence will sub-

sequently disappear and TH- and DβH-LI will diminish. Around day 10, AChE staining and VIP-LI will be present around the sweat glands, and ChAT activity will be detectable. Ultrastructural analysis (Landis and Keefe, 1983), catecholamine-uptake studies (Landis and Keefe, 1983) and neurotoxic lesions (Yodlowski et al., 1984) all suggest that a change from noradrenergic to cholinergic properties takes place in a single population of sympathetic fibers, rather than that later-arriving cholinergic fibers replace noradrenergic fibers, which would subsequently disappear. An interesting cross-innervation experiment (Schotzinger and Landis, 1988) illustrates that the switch from a noradrenergic to a cholinergic phenotype is probably regulated by environmental factors from the target area. In this experiment, sweat glands containing glabrous skin from the foot pads of the rat were transplanted to the hairy skin of the thorax, which is devoid of cholinergic innervation. Sympathetic neurons normally innervating noradrenergic targets in the hairy skin would thus innervate sweat glands of the transplanted glabrous skin. Similar to the normal situation, the sympathetic innervation of the transplanted glands first expressed noradrenergic traits, with a subsequent development of cholinergic properties.

The regulation of expression of neuropeptides in sympathetic neurons has also been extensively studied, both in vivo and in vitro. In a series of experiments Kessler, Black and collaborators have studied the expression of SP and SOM in the rat SCG. In adult animals, decentralization and treatment with ganglionic blocking agents increase SP levels in the ganglion (Kessler and Black, 1982). When sympathetic ganglia from newborn rats were explanted into cell culture, a more than 20-fold increase in SP immunoreactivity was observed after 24 h (Kessler et al., 1981, 1983). Also SOM levels increased markedly after 24 h in culture (Kessler et al., 1983). The increase in SP and SOM in vitro could be blocked by veratridine, a depolarizing agent (Kessler et al., 1981, 1983). In situ hybridization studies (Roach et al., 1987; Spiegel et al., 1989) have shown that the increased SP and SOM levels are due to an increased net synthesis of SP and SOM precursors, and not merely to an inhibited release of the peptides with a subsequent accumulation. Taken together these experimental data suggest that decentralization and a lack of presynaptic impulse activity, a consequence of the explantation, are responsible for the increased synthesis of SP and SOM. Thus, cholinergic stimulation of postsynaptic nicotinic receptors would normally suppress the synthesis of SP, SOM and their precursors in vivo. This inhibitory action of presynaptic impulse activity contrasts with the effects on the catecholamine-synthesizing enzymes, which are induced by membrane depolarization (see Kessler, 1985).

Interestingly, changes in cell culture environments which cause increased ChAT activity, for instance co-culture with non-neuronal cells and conditioned medium, increase SP levels but decrease SOM levels. Thus, cell culture conditions which increase ChAT activity and SP levels result in decreased TH activity and SOM content (Kessler, 1985).

Summary

The present article is an attempt to briefly review acetylcholine and peptide coexistence in the ANS. For more detailed information the reader is referred to the book by Furness and Costa (1987) and books edited by Elfvin (1983) and Björklund et al. (1988). Acetylcholine is the "classical" transmitter substance between preganglionic and postganglionic neurons in both the sympathetic and parasympathetic nervous system but also between postganglionic parasympathetic neurons and effector cells. ENK and NT were early on shown to be present in preganglionic sympathetic neurons whereas SP and SOM have more recently been associated with these cells. Physiological experiments have shown that ENK may presynaptically inhibit cholinergic transmission in sympathetic ganglia. The cholinergic postganglionic parasympathetic neurons contain VIP/PHI. These peptides may be responsible for the atropine-resistant vasodilation seen after stimulation of parasympathetic nerves. In salivary glands VIP has been shown to potentiate the salivatory volume response to ACh. A number of postganglionic sympathetic neurons innervating exocrine sweat glands in the skin are also cholinergic. In addition to VIP/PHI, these neurons contain CGRP and probably also SP. The functional significance of acetylcholine coexisting with four vasodilatory peptides in this cell population is at present unclear.

In the enteric ganglia the coexistence situation is very complex. Thus, in the myenteric plexus cholinergic SP-containing excitatory motor neurons seem to be present. In the myenteric plexus other cholinergic neurons may contain at least six different neuronal peptides. These latter neurons seem to be part of the peripheral intestino-intestinal reflex arc which is involved in regulation of gastrointestinal motility and mucosal functions. In the submucous plexus three populations of cholinergic neurons are present, one of which has secretomotor properties and contains CGRP, CCK, GAL, NPY and SOM.

In vivo and in vitro studies have shown that developing sympathetic neurons can "change" the "classical" transmitter they use and alter their neuropeptide expression. If dissociated sympathetic neurons are grown in cultures without any non-neuronal elements they differentiate into a noradrenergic phenotype. However, if the cultures also contain non-neuronal cells, both noradrenergic and cholinergic properties will develop. These changes may also by induced by a conditioned medium, containing a diffusible factor secreted from the non-neuronal cells.

In conclusion, the present article underlines the complexity of the chemical neuroanatomy of the ANS and emphasizes the abundance of the peptides in both noradrenergic and cholinergic neurons. Although these peptides can be shown to exert a number of interesting effects in various experimental paradigms, much work is needed to define their exact role in nervous system function.

188

Acknowledgements

The skilful technical assistance of Ms. A.-S. Höijer is gratefully acknowledged. We thank Professor L.-G. Elfvin for support and valuable discussion. The present study was supported by grants from the Karolinska Institutet, the Swedish Medical Research Council (12x-5189; 04x-2887) and Ruth and Richard Julins Stiftelse. The immunohistochemical studies illustrated in the present paper were made possible by the generous gift of antisera from Drs. A. C. Cuello, Department of Pharmacology and Therapeutics, McGill University, Montreal, Canada (TH, SP), G. Dockray, Department of Physiology, University of Liverpool, Liverpool, UK (BOM), J. Fahrenkrug, Bispebjerg Hospital, Copenhagen, Denmark (VIP and PHI), J. Fischer, Department of Orthopedic Surgery and Medicine, University of Zürich, Switzerland (CGRP), L. Hersh, Department of Biochemistry, Southwestern Medical School, University of Texas, Dallas, Texas, USA (ChAT), J. Massoulié, Laboratoire de Neurobiologie, Ecole Normale Supérieure, Paris, France (AChE), P.M. Salvaterra, Division of Neuroscience, Beckman Research Institute of the City of Hope, Duarte, CA, USA (ChAT) and L. Terenius, Department of Pharmacology, Uppsala University, Uppsala, Sweden (DYN, NPY, CGRP).

References

Änggård, A. (1974) The effects of parasympathetic nerve stimulation on the microcirculation and secretion in the nasal mucosa of the cat. *Acta Otolaryngol.*, 78: 98–105.

Änggård, A. and Edvall, L. (1974) The effects of sympathetic nerve stimulation on the tracer disappearance rate and local blood flow content in the nasal mucosa of the cat. *Acta Otolaryngol.*, 77: 131–139.

Björklund, A., Hökfelt, T. and Owman, C. (Eds.) (1988) *Handbook of Chemical Neuroanatomy, Vol. 6, The Peripheral Nervous System,* Elsevier, Amsterdam.

Burton, H. and Bunge, R.P. (1975) A comparison of the uptake and release of [^{3}H] norepinephrine in rat autonomic and sensory ganglia in tissue culture. *Brain Res.,* 97: 157–162.

Butcher, L.L. and Wolf, N.J. (1984) Histochemical distribution of acetylcholinesterase in the central nervous system: Clues to the localization of cholinergic neurons. In A. Björklund,

T. Hökfelt and N.J. Kuhar (Eds.), *Handbook of Chemical Neuroanatomy, Vol. 3,* Elsevier, Amsterdam, pp. 1–45.

Chan-Palay, V, and Palay, S.L. (1984) *Coexistence of Neuroactive Substances in Neurons,* John Wiley & Sons, New York.

Coons, A.H. (1958) Fluorescent antibody methods. In J.F. Danielli (Ed.), *General Cytochemical Methods,* Academic Press, New York, pp. 399–422.

Costa, M. and Furness, J.B. (1984) Somatostatin is present in a subpopulation of noradrenergic nerve fibers supplying the intestine. *Neuroscience,* 13: 911–919.

Costa, M., Furness, J.B. and Gibbins, I.L. (1986) Chemical coding of enteric neurons. In T. Hökfelt, K. Fuxe and B. Pernow (Eds.), *Coexistence of Neuronal Messengers: A New Principle in Chemical Transmission, Progress in Brain Research, Vol. 68,* Elsevier, Amsterdam, pp. 217–239.

Crawford, G.D., Correa, L. and Salvaterra, P.M. (1982) Interaction of monoclonal antibodies with mammalian choline acetyltransferase. *Proc. Natl. Acad. Sci. USA,* 79: 7031–7035.

Cuello, A.C. (Ed.) (1982) *Co-transmission,* MacMillan, London and Basinstoke.

Dale, H.H. and Feldberg, W. (1934) The chemical transmission of secretory impulses to the sweat glands of the cat. *J. Physiol. (Lond.),* 82: 121–128.

Dalsgaard, C.-J., Hökfelt, T., Elfvin, L.-G. and Terenius, L. (1982) Enkephalin-containing sympathetic preganglionic neurons projecting to the inferior mesenteric ganglion: Evidence from retrograde tracing and immunohistochemistry. *Neuroscience,* 7: 2039–2050.

Eccles, R. and Wilson, H. (1973) The parasympathetic secretory nerves of the nose of the cat. *J. Physiol. (Lond.),* 230: 213–223.

Eckenstein, F. and Thoenen, H. (1982) Production of specific antisera and monoclonal antibodies to choline acetyltransferase: characterization and use for identification of cholinergic neurons. *EMBO J.,* 1: 363–368.

Elfvin, L.-G. (Ed.), (1983) *Autonomic Ganglia,* John Wiley & Sons, Chichester.

Falck, B., Hillarp, N.-Å., Thieme, G. and Torp, A. (1962) Fluorescence of catecholamines and related compounds condensed with formaldehyde. *J. Histochem. Cytochem.,* 10: 348–354.

Folkow, B. and Uvnäs, B. (1948) The distribution and functional significance of sympathetic vasodilators to hind limbs of the cat. *Acta Physiol. Scand.,* 15: 389–400.

Fukada, K. (1985) Purification and partial characterization of a cholinergic differentiation factor. *Proc. Natl. Acad. Sci. USA,* 82: 8795–8799.

Furness, J.B. and Costa, M. (1987) *The Enteric Nervous System,* Churchill Livingstone, Edinburgh.

Furness, J.B., Costa, M., Emson, P.C., Håkanson, R., Moghimzadeh, E., Sundler, F., Taylor, I.L. and Chance, R.E. (1983) Distribution, pathways and reactions to drug treatment of nerves with neuropeptide Y- and pancreatic polypeptide-like immunoreactivity in the guinea pig digestive tract. *Cell Tissue Res.,* 234: 71–92.

Giacobini, E., Pilar, G., Suszkiv, J. and Uchimura, H. (1979) Normal distribution and denervation changes of neurotransmitter related enzymes in cholinergic neurons. *J. Physiol. (Lond.)*, 286: 233–253.

Goldstein, M., Anagnoste, B., Freedman, L.S., Roffman, M., Ebstein, R.B., Park, D.H., Fuxe, K. and Hökfelt, T. (1973) Characterization, localization and regulation of the catecholamine synthesizing enzymes. In E. Usdin and S. Snyder (Eds.), *Frontiers of Catecholamine Research,* Pergamon Press, New York, pp. 69–78.

Hamberger, B., Norberg, K.-A. and Sjöqvist, F. (1965) Correlated studies on monoamines and acetylcholinesterase in sympathetic ganglia, illustrating the distribution of adrenergic and cholinergic neurons. In G.B. Koelle, W.W. Douglas and A. Carlsson (Eds), *Pharmacology of Cholinergic and Adrenergic Transmission,* Pergamon Press, Oxford, pp. 41–54.

Holmstedt, B. and Sjöqvist, F. (1959) Distribution of acetocholinesterase in various sympathetic ganglia. *Acta Physiol. Scand.,* 47: 284–296.

Houser, C.R., Crawford, G.D., Barber, R.P., Salvaterra, P.M. and Vaughn, J.E. (1983) Organization and morphological characteristics of cholinergic neurons: an immunocytochemical study with a monoclonal antibody to choline acetyltransferase. *Brain Res.,* 266: 97–119.

Hökfelt, T., Elfvin, L.-G., Schultzberg, M., Fuxe, K., Said, S.I. and Goldstein, M. (1977) Immunohistochemical evidence of vasoactive intestinal polypeptide-containing neurons and nerve fibers in sympathetic ganglia. *Neuroscience,* 2: 885–896.

Hökfelt, T., Johansson, O., Ljungdahl, Å., Lundberg, J.M., and Schultzberg, M. (1980) Peptidergic neurons. *Nature,* 284: 515–521.

Hökfelt, T., Fuxe, K. and Pernow, B. (Eds.) (1986) *Coexistence of Neuronal Messengers: A New Principle in Chemical Transmission. Progress in Brain Research, Vol. 68,* Elsevier, Amsterdam.

Itoh, N., Obata, K., Yanaihara, N. and Okamoto, H. (1983) Human preprovasoactive intestinal polypeptide contains a novel PHI-27-like peptide, PHM-27. *Nature,* 304: 547–549.

Johnson, D.A. and Pilar, G. (1980) The release of acetylcholine from postganglionic cell bodies in response to depolarization. *J. Physiol. (Lond.),* 299: 605–619.

Johnson, M., Ross, D., Meyers, M., Rees, R., Bunge, R., Wakshull, E. and Burton, H. (1976) Synaptic vesicle cytochemistry changes when cultured sympathetic neurones develop cholinergic interactions. *Nature,* 262: 308–310.

Kessler, J.A. (1985) Differential regulation of peptide and catecholamine characters in cultured sympathetic neurons. *Neuroscience,* 15: 827–839.

Kessler, J.A. and Black, I.B. (1982) Regulation of substance P in adult rat sympathetic ganglia. *Brain Res.,* 234: 182–187.

Kessler, J.A., Adler, J., Bohn, M. and Black, I.B (1981) Substance P in sympathetic neurons: regulation by impulse activity. *Science,* 214: 335–336.

Kessler, J.A., Adler, J.E., Bell, W.O. and Black, I.B. (1983) Substance P and somatostatin metabolism in sympathetic and special sensory ganglia in vitro. *Neuroscience,* 9: 309–318.

Kimura, H., McGeer, P.L., Peng, J.H. and McGeer, E.D.

(1981) The central cholinergic system studied by choline acetyltransferase immunohistochemistry in the cat. *J. Comp. Neurol.,* 200: 151–200.

Kobayashi, H. and Tosaka, T. (1983) Slow synaptic actions in mammalian sympathetic ganglia, with special reference to the possible roles played by cyclic nucleotides. In L.-G. Elfvin (Ed.), *Autonomic Ganglia,* John Wiley & Sons, Chichester, pp. 281–307.

Koelle, G.B. (1955) The histochemical identification of acetylcholinesterase in cholinergic, adrenergic and sensory neurons. *J. Pharmacol. Exp. Ther.,* 114: 167–184.

Koelle, G.B. and Friedenwald, J.S. (1949) A histochemical method for localizing cholinesterase activity. *Proc. Soc. Exp. Biol. Med.,* 70: 617–622.

Koelle, W.A. and Koelle, G.B. (1959) The localization of external or functional acetylcholinesterase at the synapse of autonomic ganglia. *J. Pharmacol. Exp. Ther.,* 126: 1–8.

Kondo, H., Kuramoto, H., Wainer, B.H. and Yanaihara, N. (1985) Evidence for the coexistence of acetylcholine and enkephalin in the sympathetic preganglionic neurons of rats. *Brain Res.,* 335: 309–314.

Konishi, S., Tsunoo, A. and Otsuka, M. (1979) Enkephalin presynaptically inhibits cholinergic transmission in sympathetic ganglia. *Nature,* 282: 515–516.

Krukoff, T.L. (1987) Coexistence of neuropeptides in sympathetic preganglionic neurons of the cat. *Peptides,* 8: 109–112.

Kummer, W. and Heym, C. (1988) Neuropeptide distribution in the cervicothoracic paravertebral ganglia of the cat with particular reference to calcitonin gene-related peptide immunoreactivity. *Cell Tissue Res.,* 252: 463–471.

Lacroix, J.S., Änggård, A., Hökfelt, T. and Lundberg, J.M. (1990) Neuropeptide Y: presence in sympathetic and parasympathetic innervation of the nasal mucosa. *Cell Tissue Res.,* 259: 119–128.

Landis, S.C. (1988) Neurotransmitter plasticity in sympathetic neurons. In A. Björklund, T. Hökfelt and C. Owman (Eds.), *Handbook of Chemical Neuroanatomy, Vol. 6, The Peripheral Nervous System,* Elsevier, Amsterdam, pp. 65–115.

Landis, S.C. and Fredieu, J.R. (1986) Coexistence of calcitonin gene-related peptide and vasoactive intestinal peptide in cholinergic sympathetic innervation of rat sweat glands. *Brain Res.,* 377: 177–181.

Landis, S.C. and Keefe, D. (1983) Evidence for neurotransmitter plasticity in vivo: developmental properties of cholinergic sympathetic neurons. *Dev Biol.,* 98: 349–372.

Langley, J.N. (1922) The secretion of sweat. Part I. Supposed inhibitory nerve fibers on the posterior nerve roots. Secretion after denervation. *J. Physiol. (Lond.),* 56: 110–119.

Le Greves, P., Nyberg, F., Terenius, L. and Hökfelt, T. (1985) Calcitonin gene-related peptide is a potent inhibitor of substance P degradation. *Eur. J. Pharmacol.,* 115: 309–311.

Leblanc, G.G. and Landis, S.C. (1986) Development of choline acetyltransferase activity in the cholinergic sympathetic innervation of sweat glands. *J. Neurosci.,* 6: 260–265.

Leblanc, G.G., Trimmer, B.A. and Landis, S.C. (1987) Neuropeptide Y-like immunoreactivity in rat cranial parasympathetic neurons: Coexistence with vasoactive intestinal peptide and choline acetyltransferase. *Proc. Natl. Acad. Sci. USA*, 84: 3511–3515.

Levey, A.I., Armstrong, D.M, Atwich, S.F., Terry, R.D. and Wainer, B.H. (1983) Monoclonal antibodies to choline acetyltransferase: production, specificity, and immunohistochemistry. *J. Neurosci.*, 3: 1–9.

Lindh, B., Hökfelt, T., Elfvin, L.-G., Terenius, L., Fahrenkrug, J., Elde, R. and Goldstein, M. (1986a) Topography of NPY-, somatostatin-, and VIP-immunoreactive neuronal subpopulations in the guinea pig celiac-superior mesenteric ganglion and their projections to the pylorus. *J. Neurosci.*, 6: 2371–2383.

Lindh, B., Staines, W., Hökfelt, T., Terenius, L. and Salvaterra, P.M. (1986b) Immunohistochemical demonstration of choline acetyltransferase-immunoreactive preganglionic nerve fibers in guinea pig autonomic ganglia. *Proc. Natl. Acad. Sci. USA*, 83: 5316–5320.

Lindh, B., Lundberg, J.M., Hökfelt, T., Elfvin, L.-G., Fahrenkrug, J. and Fischer, J. (1987) Coexistence of CGRP- and VIP-like immunoreactivities in a population of neurons in the cat stellate ganglia. *Acta physiol. Scand.*, 131: 475–476.

Lindh, B., Hægerstrand, A., Lundberg, J.M., Hökfelt, T., Fahrenkrug, J., Cuello, A.C., Grassi, J. and Massoulié, J. (1988a) Substance P-, VIP-, and CGRP-like immunoreactivities coexist in a population of cholinergic postganglionic sympathetic nerves innervating sweat glands in the cat. *Acta Physiol. Scand.*, 134: 569–570.

Lindh, B., Hökfelt, T. and Elfvin, L.-G. (1988b) Distribution and origin of peptide-containing fibers in the celiac superior mesenteric ganglion of the guinea-pig. *Neuroscience*, 26: 1037–1071.

Lindh, B., Lundberg, J.M. and Hökfelt, T. (1989a) NPY-, galanin-, VIP/PHI-, CGRP- and substance P-immunoreactive neuronal subpopulations in cat autonomic and sensory ganglia and their projections. *Cell Tissue Res.*, 256: 259–273.

Lindh, B., Pelto-Huikko, M., Schalling, M., Lundberg, J.M. and Hökfelt, T. (1989b) Substance P is present in CGRP-containing cholinergic paravertebral sympathetic neurons in the cat. Evidence from combined in situ hybridization and immunohistochemistry. *Neurosci. Lett.*, 107: 1–5.

Lundberg, J.M., Hökfelt, T., Schultzberg, M., Uvnäs-Wallensten, K., Köhler, C., and Said, S.I. (1979) Occurrence of vasoactive intestinal polypeptide (VIP)-like immunoreactivity in certain cholinergic neurons of the cat. Evidence from combined immunohistochemistry and acetylcholinesterase staining. *Neuroscience*, 4: 1539–1559.

Lundberg, J.M., Änggård, A., Fahrenkrug, J., Hökfelt, T. and Mutt, V. (1980) Vasoactive intestinal polypeptide in cholinergic neurons of exocrine glands: functional significance of coexisting transmitters for vasodilation and secretion. *Proc. Natl. Acad. Sci. USA*, 77: 1651–1655.

Lundberg, J.M., Änggård, A., Emson, P., Fahrenkrug, J. and Hökfelt, T. (1981) Vasoactive intestinal polypeptide and cholinergic mechanisms in the nasal mucosa. Studies on choline acetyl-transferase and release of vasoactive intestinal polypeptide. *Proc. Natl. Acad. Sci. USA*, 78: 5255–5259.

Lundberg, J.M., Änggård, A. and Fahrenkrug, J. (1982a) Com-

plementary role of vasoactive intestinal polypeptide (VIP) and acetylcholine for cat submandibular gland blood flow and secretion. III. Effects of local infusions. *Acta Physiol. Scand.*, 114: 329–338.

Lundberg, J.M., Änggård, A., Fahrenkrug, J., Lundgren, C. and Holmstedt, B. (1982b) Co-release of VIP and acetylcholine in relation to blood flow and salivary secretion in cat submandibular salivary gland. *Acta Physiol. Scand.*, 115: 525–528.

Lundberg, J.M., Rökaeus, Å., Hökfelt, T., Rosell, S., Brown, M. and Goldstein, M. (1982c) Neurotensin-like immunoreactivity in the preganglionic sympathetic nerves and in the adrenal medulla of the cat. *Acta Physiol. Scand.*, 114: 153–155.

Lundberg, J.M., Fahrenkrug, J., Hökfelt, T., Martling, C.-R., Larsson, O., Tatemoto, K. and Änggård, A. (1984a) Coexistence of peptide HI (PHI) and VIP in nerves regulating blood flow and bronchial smooth muscle tone in various mammals including man. *Peptides*, 5: 593–606.

Lundberg, J.M., Fahrenkrug, J., Larsson, O. and Änggård, A. (1984b) Corelease of vasoactive intestinal polypeptide and peptide histidine isoleucine in relation to atropine-resistant vasodilation in cat submandibular salivary gland. *Neurosci. Lett.*, 52: 37–42.

Lundberg, J.M., Martling, C.-R., and Hökfelt, T. (1988) Airways, oral cavity and salivary glands: classical transmitters and peptides in sensory and autonomic motor neurons. In A. Björklund, T. Hökfelt and C. Owman (Eds.), *Handbook of Chemical Neuroanatomy, Vol. 6, The peripheral nervous system*, Elsevier, Amsterdam, pp. 391–444.

Macrae, I.M., Furness, J.B. and Costa, M. (1986) Distribution of subgroups of noradrenaline neurons in the coeliac ganglion of the guinea pig. *Cell Tissue Res.*, 244: 173–180.

Mains, R.E. and Patterson, P.H. (1973) Primary cultures of dissociated sympathetic neurons. I. Establishment of long-term growth in culture and studies of differentiated properties. *J. Cell Biol.*, 59: 329–345.

Malm, L. (1973) Vasodilatation in the nasal mucosa of the cat and the effects of parasympathetic and beta-adrenergic blocking agents. *Acta Otolaryngol.*, 76: 277–282.

Marsh, D., Grassi, J., Vigny, M. and Massoulié, J. (1984) An immunological study of rat acetylcholinesterase: comparison with acetylcholinesterases from other vertebrates. *J. Neurochem.*, 43: 204–213.

Osborne, N.N. (Ed.) (1983) *Dale's Principle and Communication Between Neurones*, Pergamon Press, Oxford and New York.

O'Lague, P.H., Obata, K., Claude, P., Furshpan, E.J. and Potter, D.D. (1974) Evidence for cholinergic synapse between dissociated rat sympathetic neurons in cell culture. *Proc. Natl. Acad. Sci. USA*, 71: 3602–3606.

Patterson, P.H. and Chun, L.L.Y. (1974) The influence of non-neuronal cells on catecholamines and acetylcholine synthesis and accumulation in cultures of dissociated sympathetic neurons. *Proc. Natl. Acad. Sci. USA*, 71: 3607–3610.

Patterson, P.H. and Chun, L.L.Y. (1977) Induction of acetylcholine synthesis in primary cultures of dissociated rat sympathetic neurons. I. Effects of conditioned medium. *Dev. Biol.,* 56: 263–280.

Potter, D.D., Matsumoto, S.G., Landis, S.C., Sah, D.W.Y and Furshpan, E.J. (1986) Transmitter status in cultured sympathetic principal neurons: plasticity, graded expression and diversity. In T. Hökfelt, K. Fuxe, B. Pernow (Eds.), *Coexistence of Neuronal Messengers: A New Principle in Chemical Transmission, Progress in Brain Research, Vol. 6,* Elsevier, Amsterdam, pp. 103–120.

Rees, R. and Bunge. R.P. (1974) Morphological and cytochemical studies of synapses formed in culture between isolated rat superior cervical ganglion neurons. *J. Comp. Neurol.,* 157: 1–12.

Reichardt, L.F. and Patterson, P.H. (1977) Neurotransmitter synthesis and uptake by isolated sympathetic neurons in microcultures. *Nature,* 270: 147–151.

Roach, A., Adler, J.E. and Black, I.B. (1987) Depolarizing influences regulate preprotachykinin mRNA in sympathetic neurons. *Proc. Natl. Acad. Sci. USA,* 84: 5078–5081.

Schotzinger, R.J. and Landis, S.C. (1988) Cholinergic phenotype developed by noradrenergic sympathetic neurons after innervation of a novel cholinergic target in vivo. *Nature,* 355: 637–639.

Schultzberg, M., Hökfelt, T., Terenius, L., Elfvin, L.-G., Lundberg, J.M. Brandt, J., Elde, R.P. and Goldstein, M. (1979) Enkephalin immunoreactive nerve fibers and cell bodies in sympathetic ganglia of the guinea-pig and rat. *Neuroscience,* 4: 249–270.

Silver, A. (1974) *The Biology of Cholinesterases,* North-Holland Publ. Co., Amsterdam.

Sjöqvist, F. (1962) Cholinergic sympathetic ganglion cells. M.D. Thesis, Stockholm

Skok, V.I. (1983) Fast synaptic transmission in autonomic ganglia. In L.-G. Elfvin (Ed.), *Autonomic Ganglia,* John Wiley & Sons, Chichester, pp. 265–279.

Spiegel, K., Kremer, N.E. and Kessler, J.E. (1989) Differences in the effects of membrane depolarization on levels of preprosomatostatin mRNA and tyrosine hydroxylase mRNA in rat sympathetic neurons in vivo and in culture. *Mol. Brain Res.,* 5: 23–29.

Staines, W. A., Meister, B., Melander, T., Nagy, J.I. and Hökfelt, T. (1988) Three-color immunofluorescence histochemistry allowing triple labeling within a single section. *J. Histochem. Cytochem.,* 36: 145–151.

Szurszewski, J.H. (1981) Physiology of mammalian prevertebral ganglia. *Annu. Rev. Physiol.,* 43: 53–68.

Tatemoto, K. and Mutt, V. (1981) Isolation and characterization of the intestinal peptide porcine PHI (PHI-27), a new member of the glucagon-secretin family. *Proc. Natl. Acad. Sci. USA,* 78: 6603–6607.

Teitelman, G., Joh, T.H., Frayson, L., Park, D.H., Reis, D.J. and Iacovitti, L. (1985) Cholinergic neurons of the chick ciliary ganglia express adrenergic traits in vivo and in vitro. *J. Neurosci.,* 5: 29–39.

Tramu, G., Pillez, A. and Leonardelli, J. (1978) An efficient method of antibody elution for the successive or simultaneous localization of two antigens by immunocytochemistry. *J. Histochem. Cytochem.,* 26: 322–324.

Triepel, J. (1982) Vasoactive intestinal polypeptide (VIP) in the medulla oblongata of the guinea pig. *Neurosci. Lett.,* 29: 73–78.

Uddman, R., Alumets, J., Densert, O., Håkanson, R. and Sundler, F. (1978) Occurrence and distribution of VIP nerves in the nasal mucosa and tracheobronchial wall. *Acta Otolaryngol.,* 85: 443–448.

Uddman, R., Malm, L., Fahrenkrug, J. and Sundler, F. (1981) VIP increases in nasal blood during stimulation of the vidian nerve. *Acta Otolaryngol.,* 91: 135–138.

Uddman, R., Malm, L. and Sundler, F. (1980) The origin of vasoactive intestinal polypeptide (VIP) nerves in the feline nasal mucosa. *Acta Otolaryngol.,* 89: 152–156.

Weber, M., Raynaud, B. and Delteil, C. (1985) Molecular properties of a cholinergic differentiation factor from muscle-conditioned medium. *J. Neurochem.,* 45: 1541–1547.

Wessendorff, M.W. and Elde, R.P. (1985) Characterization of immunofluorescence technique for the demonstration of coexisting neurotransmitters within nerve fibers and terminals. *J. Histochem. Cytochem.,* 33: 984–994.

Yamamoto, K., Senba, E., Matsunaga, T. and Tohyama, M. (1989) Calcitonin gene-related peptide containing sympathetic preganglionic and sensory neurons projecting to the superior cervical ganglion of the rat. *Brain Res.,* 487: 158–164.

Yodlowski, M., Fredieu, J.R. and Landis, S.C. (1984) Neonatal 6-hydroxydopamine treatment eliminates cholinergic sympathetic innervation and induces sensory sprouting in rat sweat glands. *J. Neurosci.,* 4: 1535–1548.

S.-M. Aquilonius and P.-G. Gillberg (Eds.)
Progress in Brain Research, Vol. 84
© 1990 Elsevier Science Publishers B.V. (Biomedical Division)

CHAPTER 21

Pharmacological muscarinic receptor subtypes

Herbert Ladinsky, Giovanni B. Schiavi, Eugenia Monferini and Ettore Giraldo

Department of Biochemistry, Istituto De Angeli, Boehringer-Ingelheim Italia, Milan, Italy

Pirenzepine and M_1/M_2 muscarinic receptor subtypes

A number of drugs have been identified in recent years which can discriminate between muscarinic receptor types, most notably the antagonist pirenzepine (PZ). The discovery that PZ distinguished between muscarinic receptors in membranes of different peripheral tissues and regions of the brain significantly strengthened the earlier concept that more than one muscarinic receptor existed and has formed the basis for the classification of the receptors as M_1 and M_2 *. In Fig. 1 (taken from Hammer, 1979), the inhibition curves generated by atropine and PZ in displacing [^{3}H]QNB from specific muscarinic receptor sites in the cerebral cortex are compared. In contrast with atropine binding, PZ binding did not conform to the simple case of interaction with a uniform population of sites. The displacement curve was flattened, the data suggesting that there are subclasses of binding sites within the tissue which differ in their affinities.

In a more detailed study, Hammer and colleagues (1980) demonstrated that PZ, in contrast with the classical antagonist *N*-methylscopolamine (NMS), showed large affinity variations also between tissues. PZ bound strongly to muscarinic

receptors in nervous tissues and weakly to receptors in heart, salivary glands and intestinal smooth muscle. The tissue selectivity profile correlated well with the pharmacological activity of the drug determined in vivo, and in vitro on isolated organ preparations (Hammer and Giachetti, 1982). With the discovery of the heterogeneous binding profile of PZ, it might be said that the molecular pharmacology of muscarinic receptors began.

Affinity constants for equilibrium binding of PZ to muscarinic receptors in membranes from brain and peripheral tissues are shown in Table I. It can be seen that PZ showed high affinity for

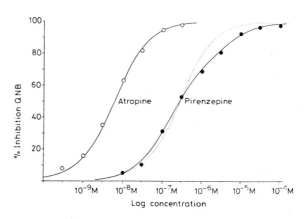

Fig. 1. Binding of atropine and pirenzepine to muscarinic receptors in membranes from rat cerebral cortex determined by competition with [^{3}H]QNB (tritiated quinuclidinyl benzilate). The inhibition curve generated by PZ, differently from that of atropine, deviates significantly from a simple Langmuir isotherm (indicated by a dotted line). The data are compatible with binding to a heterogeneous population of sites which differ in their affinities. (Reproduced from Hammer, 1979, with permission.)

---

* The nomenclature used here for pharmacological and molecular subtypes is that recommended by the Symposium Committee, Subtypes of Muscarinic Receptors IV (Levine and Birdsall, 1989).

TABLE I

Binding affinity values of pirenzepine for brain and peripheral tissue muscarinic receptor subtypes

Tissue	Sub-type	n_H	K_D (nM)
Cerebral cortex	M_1	0.98	14 ± 2
Heart	M_2	0.87	683 ± 42
Subm. glands	M_3	0.88	323 ± 33
Striatum		0.77 [a]	$36 \pm 4 \ (30 \pm 3\%)$
			$393 \pm 37 \ (70 \pm 3\%)$
Ileum long. sm. muscle		0.94	500 ± 16 [b]

Tissues from rats and guinea pigs (ileum) were prepared, and binding curves were derived, as already described (Giraldo et al., 1987a,b); 0.5 nM [^{3}H]PZ was used to label the M_1 receptor in cerebral cortex and 0.3 nM [^{3}H]NMS was used to label receptors in the other tissues. Free radioligand was separated from bound by filtration or centrifugation techniques. Data were evaluated by non-linear least-squares regression analysis of competition curves on the basis of a one- or two-binding-site model using standard computer programs. K_D values were calculated after correcting for the radioligand occupancy shift. n_H was calculated by linear regression analysis and assessed for statistically significant deviation from unity. The data are the means and S.E.M. of three or four experiments run in quadruplicate. Numbers in brackets represent the percentage of total receptors. [a] Significantly less than unity ($p < 0.01$); [b] expressed as K_i (heterogeneous population of receptors, see text).

receptors in the cerebral cortex (K_D 14 nM) (M_1 site) and distinguished these sites from those of the heart (K_D 683 nM) and submandibular glands (K_D 323 nM) (M_2 sites) with a selectivity of 25–50-fold. Since the difference in affinity of PZ for the sites in heart and glands is small (around 2-fold), this compound cannot be considered to discriminate between the two.

AF-DX 116, methoctramine, hexahydrosiladifenidol and $M_2/M_3/M_4$ muscarinic receptor subtypes

The introduction of the novel antimuscarinic PZ analogue, AF-DX 116, has provided deeper insight into the classification of the muscarinic subtypes. The M_2 subtype in heart and glands, as defined by PZ, could be further divided into two different subclasses (Table II); the receptors in the

TABLE II

Binding affinity values of AF-DX 116 for brain and peripheral tissue muscarinic receptor subtypes

Tissue	Sub-type	n_H	K_D (nM)
Cerebral cortex	M_1	0.93	764 ± 81
Heart	M_2	0.96	113 ± 15
Subm. glands	M_3	0.96	2923 ± 238
Striatum		0.94	1598 ± 208 [b]
Ileum long. sm. muscle		0.87 [a]	$110 \pm 4 \ (82 \pm 3\%)$
			$2541 \pm 356 \ (18 \pm 3\%)$

See legend to Table I for details.

heart displayed high affinity for the compound (K_D 113 nM), those in the glands showed low affinity (K_D 2.92 μM), thus indicating that the two receptors are different (Hammer et al., 1986). The binding profile of AF-DX 116 correlated well with its pharmacological profile determined in vitro and in vivo (Giachetti et al., 1986; Micheletti et al., 1987).

In general, muscarinic receptors are classified as neuronal M_1 (high affinity for PZ), cardiac M_2 (low affinity for PZ/high affinity for AF-DX 116) and glandular M_3 (low affinity for both PZ and AF-DX 116). This well-established system for classifying the muscarinic receptors into subtypes is thus essentially based on data obtained with these two selective antagonists, but supporting results with other antagonists, including the allosteric, cardioselective compound methoctramine (METH) (Melchiorre et al., 1987; Giraldo et al.,

TABLE III

Binding affinity values of methoctramine for brain and peripheral tissue muscarinic receptor subtypes

Tissue	Subtype	n_H	K_D (nM)
Cerebral cortex	M_1	0.96	254 ± 19
Heart	M_2	0.98	35 ± 5
Subm. glands	M_3	0.86 [a]	4427 ± 508 [c]
Striatum		0.97	184 ± 9 [b]

See legend to Table I for details. [c] Expressed as corrected IC_{50} (allosteric action).

TABLE IV

Binding affinity values of hexahydrosiladiphenidol for brain and peripheral tissue muscarinic receptor subtypes

Tissue	Sub-type	n_H	K_D (nM)
Cerebral cortex	M_1	0.96	18 ± 2
Heart	M_2	0.98	182 ± 14
Subm. glands	M_3	0.86	15 ± 1
Striatum		0.90	$36 (n = 2)$ [b]
Ileum long. sm. muscle		0.86 [a]	$24 \pm 4 (25 \pm 5\%)$
			$355 \pm 18 (76 \pm 4\%)$

See legend to Table I for details.

1988a) and the smooth muscle selective one hexahydrosiladifenidol (HHSiD) (Mutchler and Lambrecht, 1984), have contributed invaluably to the classification. METH, a tetraamine derivative, is one of the few muscarinic antagonists to show more than 100-fold discrimination between one receptor (M_2) (K_D 35 nM) and another (M_3) (K_D 4.43 μM) in binding studies (Table III) and between the heart and smooth muscle in functional studies. It will be shown below that the high selectivity of this compound has been useful in providing evidence for an M_4 subtype in striatum. HHSiD exhibits 30-fold selectivity for smooth muscle vs. atrium in isolated organ preparations and shows reverse selectivity for the M_3/M_2 subtypes with respect to AF-DX 116 in receptor binding experiments (Table IV). Indeed, this silicon-containing compound shows high affinity for the M_3 subtype (K_D 15 nM), and low affinity for the cardiac M_2 subtype (K_D 182 nM).

Pharmacological M_1–M_4 and molecular m1–m4 receptor subtypes

The question of whether the pharmacologically described receptor subclasses constituted structural or conformational subtypes was resolved with the cloning of a complementary DNA (cDNA) for the M_1 muscarinic receptor from pig brain (Kubo et al., 1986a) and of a cDNA for the M_2 receptor

from pig heart (Kubo et al., 1986b), establishing that the muscarinic receptor subtypes are indeed distinct gene products. Subsequently, a family of five mammalian receptor genes (m1, m2, m3, m4, m5) (Bonner et al., 1987, 1988; Peralta et al., 1987) was isolated from rat and human cDNA or genomic libraries, while as many as four or five more molecular forms have been proposed to exist on the basis of genomic blot hybridization analysis (Bonner et al., 1987). The m1 and m2 genes encode, respectively, the pharmacologically defined M_1 and M_2 muscarinic receptors. The types of muscarinic receptor encoded by the other three genes are not clear. The m1–m5 receptors have been expressed in several cell lines and their binding properties assessed (Buckley et al., 1989). Their coupling to guanine nucleotide binding proteins to activate several different second-messenger systems and ion channels has also often been reported. m1, m3 and m5 receptors in transformed cells are generally associated with metabolism of phosphatidyl inositol, similarly to M_1 receptors in brain; m2 and m4 cloned receptors are generally associated with inhibition of adenylate cyclase, similarly to M_2 receptors in mammalian heart and M_4 receptors in striatum (see Levine and Birdsall, 1989).

From hybridization experiments, the m1–m3 mAChR subtypes are found to be widely and non-homogeneously distributed in the mammalian CNS and peripheral tissues (Maeda et al., 1988; their data are illustrated in Table I of Chapter 25 of this volume) and support pharmacological data for the similarly wide distribution of the M_1–M_3 subtypes (Hammer et al., 1986; Giraldo et al., 1987a,b). mRNAs encoding m4 and m5 receptors have so far been found only in brain (Maeda et al., 1988; Weiner and Brann, 1989). In addition, many tissues contain the same receptor subtype, and different receptor mRNAs are frequently co-expressed in the same tissue. It is conceivable that some of the pharmacologically defined receptor subtypes in a tissue probably comprise more than one receptor species, not readily distinguished by the currently available selective agents. The impact of the identification of subtypes of muscarinic receptors is easily understood in the light of such ubiquity of the receptor subtypes. It provides an explanation of the composite pharmacological actions and the side-effects produced by classical non-selective antimuscarinic agents, and a rationale for understanding the heterogeneous binding curves that are frequently observed when antagonists are used to label receptors in the tissues. The ability to distinguish between the types of receptor in tissues has important clinical implications. An understanding of the differences between the different subtypes in location and in function makes it possible to direct drug therapy toward the appropriate type (Goyal, 1989).

In current studies we are attempting to delineate the different receptor subtype populations present in brain and peripheral tissues by an approach first described by Giraldo et al. (1987a). Since AF-DX 116 and METH have binding profiles different from those of PZ and HHSiD, which in turn differ from each other, we used these agents in binding studies in guinea pig ileal smooth muscle and rat striatum in comparison with each other.

Pharmacological muscarinic receptor subtypes in guinea pig ileal longitudinal smooth muscle

The property of AF-DX 116 to discriminate highly between M_2 and M_3 receptors has led to the detection of heterogeneity in the longitudinal smooth muscle of the guinea pig ileum (Fig. 2) and in the characterization of the muscarinic receptor subtypes present therein. In this tissue, the AF-DX 116/[3H]NMS inhibition curve was shallow, with a Hill coefficient (n_H) significantly less than one. The data points fitted best to a two-binding-site model. AF-DX 116 recognized 82% of total receptors with high affinity (K_D 110 nM) and 18% of receptors with much lower affinity (K_D 2.54 μM) (Table II).

The affinity constants of AF-DX 116 for the receptors in the smooth muscle and the respective values for the heart and glands, seen in Table II,

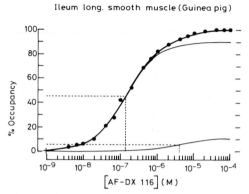

Fig. 2. Binding profile of AF-DX 116 in guinea pig ileal longitudinal smooth muscle determined by competition with [3H]NMS. The curve indicates the computer fit of the experimental data points of a representative experiment after correction for the radioligand occupancy shift, according to a two-binding-site model with visualization of the individual components of the curve and their dissociation constants.

are similar enough to suggest that the smooth muscle contains a substantial population of the cardiac M_2 receptors and a smaller population of the glandular M_3 type.

Evidence for the presence of the two different receptor populations in smooth muscle was supported by data obtained with HHSiD. In HHSiD/[3H]NMS competition experiments, a shallow curve was also generated with an n_H significantly less than unity. According to a two-binding-site model, HHSiD distinguished 25% of total receptors with high affinity (K_D 24 nM) and 76% of receptors with low affinity (K_D 355 nM). In Table IV, the HHSiD affinity values for the smooth muscle are compared with those for the heart and glands; the binding constants of the smooth muscle receptors showing high and low affinity for HHSiD were similar to the respective values for the glands and heart.

In a similar type of inhibition experiment, METH was reported to recognize the two receptor populations in rat and guinea pig ileal longitudinal and circular smooth muscles (Michel and Whiting, 1988a,b) and AF-DX 116 revealed the two receptor populations in rat bladder (Monferini et al., 1988) and bovine tracheal smooth muscle (Roffel et al., 1987). Both cardioselective agents recognized, as well, the M_2 and M_3 receptor populations in the porcine ileal muscles and coronary artery (van Charldorp et al., 1990). In all cases, the percentages of total receptors amounted to around 70% cardiac type and 30% glandular type. No other selective antagonists have been reported to be capable of discriminating between subtypes in smooth muscle in equilibrium binding experiments.

m2 and m3 mRNA species have recently been detected in the large and small intestine, trachea and bladder of the pig and rat by Northern blot hybridization analysis (Maeda et al., 1988), confirming in this elegant manner that m2 and m3 receptors are expressed in the smooth muscles.

A significant consequence of these findings has been to verify that smooth muscle contraction appears to be due mainly to agonist stimulation of the M_3 receptors, located postjunctionally on smooth muscle cells. This was ascertained from direct correlations of the affinity constants of several selective drugs, i.e. AF-DX 116 (Giachetti et al., 1986; Micheletti et al., 1987; others), METH (Giraldo et al., 1988a), HHSiD (Mutchler and Lambrecht, 1984) and 4-DAMP (Barlow et al., 1976; Monferini et al., 1988) obtained from binding and functional data in isolated organ preparations. Indeed, both AF-DX 116 and METH showed low potency in blocking agonist-induced ileal, tracheal and urinary bladder contraction whereas HHSiD and 4-DAMP demonstrated high potency in this regard. The role of the large M_2 subtype population in the smooth muscle is unclear.

Pharmacological muscarinic receptor subtypes in rat striatum

The property of PZ to discriminate highly between the M_1 and M_2 receptors has led to the detection of heterogeneity of receptors in the rat striatum (Fig. 3) and to the characterization of the receptor subtypes with other selective compounds. In this tissue, the PZ/[³H]NMS displacement curve was shallow, with an n_H significantly less than one,

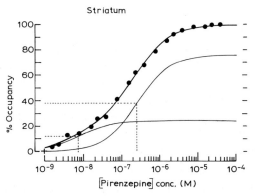

Fig. 3. Binding profile of pirenzepine in rat striatum determined by competition with [³H]NMS. The curve indicates the computer fit of the experimental data points of a representative experiment after correction for the radioligand occupancy shift, according to a two-binding-site model with visualization of the individual components of the curve and their dissociation constants.

and the data points fitted best to a two-binding-site model, indicating the presence of two large populations of receptors. One receptor population, amounting to 30% of total receptors, bound PZ with high affinity (K_D 36 nM) (Table I), suggesting it to be the M_1 subtype. The second and larger (70%) population of sites bound PZ with low affinity (K_D 393 nM). The presence of the M_1 receptor in striatum was confirmed by determining that [³H]PZ bound to the striatal membranes with high affinity (Watson et al., 1984) and by the demonstration that m1 mRNA was uniformly distributed in rat striatum by blot and in situ hybridization analysis employing a radiolabeled oligonucleotide probe uniquely specific for m1 mRNA (Buckley et al., 1988).

From the binding experiments with PZ alone, the nature of the second receptor population cannot be more closely defined, since PZ does not discriminate between the M_2 and M_3 low-affinity binding sites. AF-DX 116/[³H]NMS competition experiments in the striatal membrane preparation generated a steep curve, with n_H not significantly different from unity, suggesting that AF-DX 116 bound to a uniform population of sites. The affinity constant, 1.6 μM, fell within a range similar to the K_D value, 2.9 μM, shown for the glandular

M_3 subtype (Table II), indicating intermediate–low affinity for the antagonist. Based on these findings, we had proposed earlier (Giraldo et al., 1987a) that, firstly, the striatum was devoid of the M_2 type. Our finding was subsequently supported by blot and in situ hybridization analysis where a signal for m2 mRNA in this region was not detected (Buckley et al., 1988). The rather weak signal for the m3 mRNA in the latter study did not support another of our conclusions, however; i.e. that, secondly, the M_3 subtype was the major receptor present in striatum. On the other hand, the rather strong signal generated for the m4 mRNA as observed by Buckley and colleagues prompted us to reinvestigate whether an M_4 (non-M_1, non-M_2 and non-M_3) subtype might be detected in the tissue.

The inhibition curves generated by METH/[³H]NMS displacement experiments were steep and fitted best to a one-binding-site model. The affinity constant of METH (K_D 184 nM), was consistent with its affinity (K_D 254 nM) for the M_1 receptor, but inconsistent with its affinities for the M_2 (K_D 35 nM) or M_3 (K_D 4.43 μM) receptors (Table III). This result suggests that METH bound to both the M_1 site and to a novel, non-M_2, non-M_3 binding site of similar affinity to M_1. Otherwise, it is likely that the presence of a significant amount of low-affinity M_3 receptor sites would have generated a shallow curve. It is suggested that this novel site, showing low affinity for PZ, intermediate affinity for METH, and intermediate—low affinity for AF-DX 116, is presumably the m4 mAChR revealed in striatum by blot and in situ hybridization studies (Buckley et al., 1988). Furthermore, the tissue binding profiles of these compounds were not dissimilar to those described in CHO-K1 cells transfected with the cloned m1–m4 subtypes (Buckley et al., 1989). Further experiments are needed in any event to clarify this point, and perhaps must await the discovery of novel selective agents.

The HHSiD/[³H]NMS competition curve fitted best to a one-binding-site model, its affinity constant of 36 nM (Table IV) being more consistent with its affinity for M_1 (K_D 18 nM) and M_3 (K_D 15 nM) than with its affinity for M_2 (K_D 182 nM). This compound does not help to delineate the fourth subtype except to indicate that it may have high affinity for HHSiD.

It is premature to suggest the functional consequences of these results. A low-affinity site for both PZ (Consolo et al., 1987) and AF-DX 116 (Consolo et al., 1988) appears to regulate cholinergic neurotransmission in rat striatum post-synaptically, whereas the high-affinity M_1 site for PZ appears to be responsible for the regulation of dopamine release from synaptosomes of this region via a presynaptic mechanism (Raiteri et al., 1984). Clarification of the receptor subtype involved in cholinergic neurotransmission must await the introduction of m4-selective compounds. In humans, antimuscarinic agents improve the psychomotor performance of Parkinson's patients. It is tempting to speculate that if drugs can be developed which are selective for this particular muscarinic receptor subtype, they will be useful in treating this disease. The restricted localization of the m4 subtype to the CNS holds promise, too, for finding a drug with minimal peripheral side-effects.

Conclusions

The introduction of several selective muscarinic receptor antagonists over the last decade has permitted the classification of muscarinic receptors into three pharmacological receptor subtypes, M_1, M_2 and M_3, with indications for a fourth type, and has certainly played a role in prompting the discovery of the molecular forms of the receptor, now known to number five. The distribution of muscarinic receptor subtypes in body tissues has been described by hybridization techniques and has provided insight in elucidating the pharmacologically defined receptors present in smooth muscle (M_2 and M_3) and striatum (M_1 and M_4) using PZ, AF-DX 116, HHSiD and METH. It is still to be expected that other, as yet undetected pharmacological receptor subtypes are present in these tissues. The alliance of molecular genetics with molecular pharmacology has paved the way for the search for selective muscarinic receptor agonists and antagonists. One might expect that when new selective agents are developed, they will have a variety of therapeutic uses in disorders of the central and peripheral nervous systems.

References

Barlow, R.B., Berry, K.J., Glenton, P.A.M., Nikolaou, N.M. and Soh, K.S. (1976) A comparison of affinity constants for muscarine-sensitive acetylcholine receptors in guinea pig atrial pacemaker cells at 29°C and 37°C. *Br. J. Pharmacol.,* 58: 613–620.

Bonner, T.I., Buckley, N.J., Young, A.C. and Brann, M.R. (1987) Identification of a family of muscarinic acetylcholine receptor genes. *Science,* 237: 527–532.

Bonner, T.I., Young, A.C., Brann, M.R. and Buckley, N.J. (1988) Cloning and expression of the human and rat m5 muscarinic acetylcholine receptor genes. *Neuron,* 1: 403–410.

Buckley, N.J., Bonner, T.I. and Brann, M.R. (1988) Localization of a family of muscarinic receptor mRNAs in rat brain. *J. Neurosci.,* 8: 4646–4652.

Buckley, N.J., Bonner, T.I., Buckley, C.M. and Brann, M.R. (1989) Antagonist binding properties of five cloned muscarinic receptors expressed in CHO-K1 cells. *Mol. Pharmacol.,* 35: 469–476.

Consolo, S., Ladinsky, H., Vinci, R., Palazzi, E. and Wang, J.-X. (1987) An in vivo pharmacological study on muscarinic receptor subtypes regulating cholinergic neurotransmission in rat striatum. *Biochem. Pharmacol.,* 36: 3075–3077.

Consolo, S., Palazzi, E., Carelli, M. and Ladinsky, H. (1988) Glandular M2 muscarinic receptor subtype modulates cholinergic neurotransmission in rat brain: an in vivo study with AF-DX 116. *Trends Pharmacol. Sci.,* 9 (Suppl): 92.

Giachetti, A., Micheletti, R. and Montagna, E. (1986) Cardioselective profile of AF-DX 116, a muscarinic M2 receptor antagonist. *Life Sci.,* 38: 1663–1672.

Giraldo, E., Hammer, R. and Ladinsky, H. (1987a) Distribution of muscarinic receptor subtypes in rat brain as determined in binding studies with AF-DX 116 and pirenzepine. *Life Sci.,* 40: 833–840.

Giraldo, E., Monferini, E., Ladinsky, H. and Hammer, R. (1987b) Muscarinic receptor heterogeneity in guinea pig intestinal smooth muscle: binding studies with AF-DX 116. *Eur. J. Pharmacol.,* 141: 475–477.

Giraldo, E., Micheletti, R., Montagna, E., Giachetti, A., Viganò, A.M., Ladinsky, H. and Melchiorre, C. (1988a) Binding and functional characterization of the cardioselective muscarinic antagonist methoctramine. *J. Pharmacol. Exp. Ther.,* 244: 1016–1020.

Giraldo, E., Viganò, M.A., Hammer, R. and Ladinsky, H. (1988b) Characterization of muscarinic receptors in guinea

pig ileum longitudinal smooth muscle. *Mol. Pharmacol.,* 33: 617–625.

Goyal, R.K. (1989) Muscarinic receptor subtypes: physiology and clinical implications. *N. Engl. J. Med.,* 321: 1022–1029.

Hammer, R. (1979) Bindungsstudien mit Pirenzepin am muskarinischen Rezeptor. In A.L. Blum and R. Hammer (Eds.), *Die Behandlung des Ulcus pepticum mit Pirenzepin,* Demeter Verlag, Graefelfing, F.R.G., pp. 49–52.

Hammer, R. and Giachetti, A. (1982) Muscarinic receptor subtypes: M1 and M2 biochemical and functional characterization. *Life Sci.,* 31: 2991–2998.

Hammer, R., Berrie, C.P., Birdsall, N.J.M., Burgen, A.S.V. and Hulme, E.C. (1980) Pirenzepine distinguishes between different subclasses of muscarinic receptors. *Nature (Lond.),* 283: 90–92.

Hammer, R., Giraldo, E., Schiavi, G.B., Monferini, E. and Ladinsky, H. (1986) Binding profile of a novel cardioselective muscarine receptor antagonist, AF-DX 116, to membranes of peripheral tissues and brain of the rat. *Life Sci.,* 38: 1653–1662.

Kubo, T., Fukuda, K., Mikami, A., Maeda, A., Takahashi, H., Mishina, M., Haga, T., Haga, K., Ichyama, A., Kangawa, K., Kojima, M., Matsuo, H., Hirose, T., and Numa, S. (1986a) Cloning, sequencing and expression of complementary DNA encoding the muscarinic acetylcholine receptor. *Nature (Lond.),* 323: 411–416.

Kubo T., Maeda, A., Sugimoto, K., Akiba, I., Mikami, A., Takahashi, H., Haga, T., Haga, K., Ichyama, A., Kangawa, K., Matsuo, H., Hirose, T., and Numa, S. (1986b) Primary structure of porcine cardiac muscarinic acetylcholine receptor deduced from the cDNA sequence. *FEBS Lett.,* 209: 367–372.

Levine, R. R. and Birdsall, N.J.M. (Eds.) (1989) Subtypes of Muscarinic receptors IV. *Trends Pharmacol. Sci.,* 10 (Suppl.).

Maeda, A., Kubo, T., Mishina, M. and Numa, S. (1988) Tissue distribution of mRNAs encoding muscarinic acetylcholine receptor subtypes. *FEBS Lett.,* 239: 339–342.

Melchiorre, C.A., Cassinelli, A. and Quaglia, W. (1987) Differential blockade of muscarinic receptor subtypes by polymethylene tetraamines: novel class of selective antagonists of cardiac M2 muscarinic receptors. *J. Med. Chem.,* 30: 201–204.

Michel, A.D. and Whiting, R.L. (1987) Direct binding studies on ileal and cardiac muscarinic receptors. *Br. J. Pharmacol.,* 92: 755–767.

Michel, A.D. and Whiting, R.L. (1988a) Methoctramine, a polymethylene tetraamine, differentiates three subtypes of muscarinic receptor in direct binding studies. *Eur. J. Pharmacol.,* 145: 61–66.

Michel, A.D. and Whiting, R.L. (1988b) Methoctramine reveals heterogeneity of M_2 muscarinic receptors in longitudinal ileal smooth muscle membranes. *Eur. J. Pharmacol.,* 145: 305–311.

Micheletti, R., Montagna, E. and Giachetti, A. (1987) AF-DX 116, a cardioselective muscarinic antagonist. *J. Pharmacol. Exp. Ther.,* 241: 628–634.

Monferini, E., Giraldo, E. and Ladinsky, H. (1988) Characterization of the muscarinic receptor subtypes in the rat urinary bladder. *Eur. J. Pharmacol.*, 147: 453–458.

Mutchler, E. and Lambrecht, G. (1984) Selective muscarinic agonists and antagonists in functional tests. *Trends Pharmacol. Sci.*, 5 (Suppl.): 39–44.

Peralta, E.G., Ashkenazi, A., Winslow, J.W., Smith, D.H., Ramachandran, J. and Capon, D.J. (1987) Distinct primary structures, ligand binding properties and tissue specific expression of four human muscarinic acetylcholine receptors. *EMBO J.*, 6: 3923–3929.

Raiteri, M., Leardi, R. and Marchi, M. (1984) Heterogeneity of presynaptic muscarinic receptors regulating neurotransmitter release in the rat brain. *J. Pharmacol. Exp. Ther.*, 228: 209–214.

Roffel, A.F., in't Hout, W.G., De Zeeuw, R.A. and Zaagsma, J.

(1987) The M2 selective antagonist AF-DX 116 shows high affinity for muscarinic receptors in bovine tracheal membranes. *Naunyn-Schmiedeberg's Arch. Pharmacol.*, 335: 593–595.

van Charldorp, K.J., Mol, F., Batink, H.D., de Jonge, A. and van Zwieten, P.A. (1990) Similarity between muscarinic receptors/binding sites in porcine coronary artery and ileum. *Eur. J. Pharmacol.*, in press.

Watson, M., Vickroy, T.W., Roeske, W.R. and Yamamura, H.I. (1984) Subclassification of muscarinic receptors based upon the selective antagonist pirenzepine. *Trends Pharmacol. Sci.*, 5 (Suppl.): 9–11.

Weiner, D.M. and Brann, M.R. (1989) Distribution of m1–m5 muscarinic receptor mRNAs in rat brain. *Trends Pharmacol. Sci.*, 10 (Suppl.): 115.

S.-M. Aquilonius and P.-G. Gillberg (Eds.)
Progress in Brain Research, Vol. 84
© 1990 Elsevier Science Publishers B.V. (Biomedical Division)

CHAPTER 22

Basic and clinical aspects of cholinergic agents in bladder dysfunction

K.-E. Andersson and H. Hedlund

Departments of Clinical Pharmacology and Urology, University Hospital, Lund, Sweden

Introduction

Through the pelvic nerves, the urinary bladder of both animals and man receives a rich cholinergic innervation (Mobley, et al., 1966; Ek et al., 1977; Elbadawi, 1982). It is therefore not surprising that muscarinic receptors play an important role in bladder function. There are, however, marked differences between species. This review will focus mainly on the human bladder as a target organ for agents stimulating or blocking muscarinic receptors, normally and in different types of bladder dysfunction.

Muscarinic receptors and bladder contraction

Normal bladder

In contrast to most animal species, where bladder contraction is mediated by both cholinergic and non-cholinergic, non-adrenergic mechanisms (Ambache and Zar, 1970; Taira, 1972) contraction of the normal human detrusor seems to be mediated mainly, if not exclusively, through muscarinic receptor stimulation (Sjögren et al., 1982; Sibley, 1984; Kinder and Mundy, 1985; Craggs et al., 1986). Thus, atropine caused more than 95% inhibition of electrically evoked contrac-

tions in morphologically normal bladder samples from patients undergoing bladder surgery for different reasons (Sjögren et al., 1982). Comparing the effects of atropine on contractions induced by electrical-field stimulation in isolated bladder preparations from rabbit, pig and man, Sibley (1984) concluded that nerve-mediated activity in human bladder is exclusively cholinergic. The results obtained by Craggs et al. (1986) comparing the effects of atropine on bladder contractions evoked by sacral ventral root stimulation in cats, monkeys and paraplegic man supported this conclusion.

Not all investigators have been able to show a complete atropine sensitivity in the human bladder. Hindmarsh et al. (1977) found that electrically induced contractions were partially resistant to atropine, and Cowan and Daniel (1983) found that acetylcholine was responsible for approximately 50% of the electrically induced contraction in strips of the normal human bladder. These findings supported the view that in the human bladder, as in the bladder of most animals, acetylcholine was the main, but not the sole, motor transmitter. Varying experimental approaches and differences in the tissue materials investigated may partly explain these apparently conflicting data. Taken together, however, the available results strongly favour the view that in normal human bladder muscle non-cholinergic, non-adrenergic mechanisms have no significant role in bladder contraction.

Correspondence to: K.-E. Andersson, Department of Clinical Pharmacology, University Hospital, S-221 85 Lund, Sweden.

Bladder dysfunction

Resistance to atropine has been reported in morphologically and/or functionally changed bladders. In bladder strips from male patients with a diagnosis of unstable bladder, and in particular from patients with bladder hypertrophy, up to 50% of the electrically induced contraction was resistant to atropine (Sjögren et al., 1982). A varying degree of atropine resistance (0–65%) was found in isolated detrusor preparations from male patients, most of them having prostatic hypertrophy (Nergårdh and Kinn, 1983). However, Sibley (1984) showed that the atropine-resistant response in hypertrophic bladder muscle was also resistant to tetrodotoxin (TTX), suggesting that this response was not nerve-mediated, but dependent on direct muscle stimulation.

Comparison between isolated detrusor muscle from normal bladders and bladders with different types of hyperactivity (idiopathic instability and hyperreflexia) revealed no significant differences in the degree of inhibition of electrically induced contractions by TTX and atropine (Kinder et al., 1985). The concentration-response curves for acetylcholine were similar. These data suggest that in both normal and hyperactive detrusor muscle acetylcholine may be the only contractile transmitter. Restorick and Mundy (1989) showed that in bladder tissue from patients with bladder hyperactivity, but without overt neurological disease, there was a significant reduction in the density of muscarinic receptors. In contrast, the density of alpha-adrenoceptors was significantly increased. Whether these changes in receptor densities are causally related to the bladder hyperactivity, or a consequence of it, remains to be established.

Parasympathetic denervation or decentralization leads to an impaired ability of the bladder to empty. An increased responsiveness to muscarinic receptor stimulation can often be demonstrated, and this has been the basis for the use of bethanechol or carbachol as a test to diagnose neurogenic bladder disorders (Lapides et al., 1962; Glahn, 1970). It has been assumed that the increased response to cholinergic agents is due primarily to changes in muscarinic receptor functions secondary to the denervation/decentralization. An increased density of muscarinic receptors might thus be conceivable. However, Nilvebrant et al. (1986) found no changes in the muscarinic receptor density in the denervated rat bladder that could explain supersensitivity and suggested that the regulation of the receptor levels is influenced by the functional state of the bladder. In support of this, Mattiasson et al. (1984) were unable to demonstrate any supersensitivity to muscarinic receptor stimulation in decentralized cats provided that the urine was diverted and the bladder did not hypertrophy.

Prejunctional muscarinic receptors

As in other tissues, the release of noradrenaline and acetylcholine in the human bladder and urethra can be influenced by prejunctional muscarinic receptors (Mattiasson et al., 1987, 1988). The release from adrenergic nerve terminals could be concentration-dependently decreased and increased by carbachol and scopolamine, respectively; in both bladder and urethral tissue. Muscarinic receptors inhibiting acetylcholine release were demonstrated on the cholinergic axon terminals in human urethral smooth muscle (Mattiasson et al., 1988) and in the rat urinary bladder (D'Agostino et al., 1986).

The importance of prejunctional muscarinic receptors for bladder function can only be speculated upon. Immediately before bladder contraction starts during voiding, the intraurethral pressure falls (Tanagho and Miller, 1970; Ulmsten et al., 1977; Rud et al., 1978). The possibility cannot be excluded that this fall in intraurethral pressure is caused by stimulation of prejunctional muscarinic receptors on noradrenergic nerves diminishing noradrenaline release and thereby tone in the proximal urethra (Mattiasson et al., 1987). Such an effect would facilitate micturition. There may be a mutual influence of adrenergic and cholinergic nerves at different levels. Thus, de Groat and Saum (1972) demonstrated inhibition of the cholinergic influence on the bladder by adrenergic nerves at the ganglionic level. Such an inhibition was suggested also to exist at the axon terminal level (Mattiasson et al., 1987).

Muscarinic receptor characteristics

Using ^{3}H-QNB binding Levin et al. (1982) found a density of muscarinic receptors in homogenates of the human urinary bladder of 63 ± 10 fmol/mg protein and a K_d value of 5×10^{-9} M. Similar values were found by Anderson et al. (1985) using both post-surgical and post-mortem bladder material. Nilvebrant et al. (1985) found receptor densities in human detrusor muscle varying between 77 and 231 fmol/mg protein. The binding of ^{3}H-QNB was of high affinity ($K_d = 1.2 \times 10^{-11}$ M). Batra et al. (1987), comparing the muscarinic receptors in human urinary bladder and parotid gland, found a receptor density of 234 fmol/mg protein and a K_d value of 2×10^{-11} M in the urinary bladder. It was found that muscarinic receptor agonists recognized more than one population of receptor sites, whereas muscarinic receptor antagonists were bound to a virtually uniform population of sites (Nilvebrant et al., 1985). This suggested that a selective effect on the muscarinic receptors of human bladder cannot be obtained with currently available antimuscarinic agents.

The effects of pirenzepine on contractions induced by acetylcholine or bethanechol and by electrical stimulation were investigated in isolated strips of human urinary bladder (Zappia et al., 1986). Pirenzepine was found to behave like atropine, but its potency was 100–300 times lower. It was concluded that according to the M_1/M_2 classification the muscarinic receptors of the human bladder were of M_2 type. This conclusion was supported by receptor binding experiments (Batra et al., 1987; Ruggieri et al., 1987; Levin et al., 1988). These findings are in line with the results of other investigators studying muscarinic receptor subtypes in rat bladder (Adami et al., 1985; van Charldorp et al., 1985).

van Charldorp et al. (1985) found evidence that the M_2 receptors in the bladder of pithed rats were heterogeneous. Monferini et al. (1988) classified by means of AF-DX 116 the muscarinic receptors of the rat urinary bladder (M_2) into cardiac and glandular subtypes. They identified a small proportion of glandular muscarinic receptors which could represent the functional receptor responsible for muscarinic agonist-induced contraction, and proposed to call this receptor subtype M_3.

Muscarinic receptor coupling

In the bladder, little is known about the coupling between the muscarinic receptors and intracellular messenger systems. In isolated human bladder, Fovaeus et al. (1987) demonstrated differences in the dependence on extracellular calcium between activation through acetylcholine released by electrical stimulation and activation via exogenous carbachol. In calcium-free medium containing 10^{-4} M EGTA, electrically induced contractions disappeared within 15–20 min, whereas pretreatment in calcium-free medium for 30 min reduced the carbachol (10^{-4} M) induced contraction by approximately 70%. Both types of activation could be blocked by atropine. These results suggested heterogeneity between muscarinic bladder receptors, and the possibility that more than one messenger system may be involved.

Ruggieri et al. (1987) found that carbachol inhibited adenylate cyclase in both rabbit and human urinary bladder. They reported no effect of acetylcholine or carbachol on the turnover of phosphoinositides. Andersson et al. (1989) compared the contractile effects of carbachol and acetylcholine, and their abilities to stimulate production of inositol phosphates in human detrusor muscle. Carbachol and acetylcholine (combined with physostigmine) produced almost identical concentration-contraction curves. Carbachol caused a concentration-dependent increase in the accumulation of inositol phosphates, amounting to more than 300% at a concentration of 10^{-5} M.

However, acetylcholine (combined with physostigmine) was significantly less effective than carbachol (in terms of both potency and efficacy), suggesting that the importance of inositol phosphates in contractile activation differed between the two agonists. This supports the view that the muscarinic receptors of the human bladder are heterogeneous.

Clinical effects of cholinergic agents on the bladder

The central role of muscarinic receptors in bladder function makes it logical to use drugs stimulating or blocking muscarinic receptors to treat bladder function disorders. These drugs have been used to treat both disturbances of the emptying function of the bladder and disturbances of the storage function (Andersson, 1988).

Stimulation of bladder emptying

Bladder emptying requires a coordinated contraction of adequate magnitude of the detrusor muscle, a concomitant lowering of the outflow resistance at the level of the smooth and striated sphincter, and absence of anatomic obstruction (Wein, 1987). If these requirements are not fulfilled, urinary retention or residual urine will result. When the primary cause of emptying failure may be insufficient strength of the detrusor, drugs stimulating bladder contraction may be indicated.

Carbachol and bethanechol are the two main agents used clinically and both are considered to have some selectivity for the urinary bladder (Finkbeiner, 1985; Taylor, 1985). Despite doubts about its clinical effectiveness in promoting bladder emptying (Blaivas, 1984; Downie, 1984; Finkbeiner, 1985), bethanechol is widely used both injected subcutaneously and given orally. When bethanechol is given subcutaneously to neurologically normal individuals, the effect on the bladder is characterized by an increased stiffness of the bladder wall at rest. This is reflected in high pressures in the cystometrogram, decreased capacity, and an increased awareness of the distended bladder, effects which may not result in an in-

crease in urine flow rate during voiding (Downie, 1984). It might be that bethanechol-induced bladder contraction and voiding requires intact bladder reflex pathways, as was demonstrated in cats (Twiddy et al., 1980).

Bethanechol and other muscarinic receptor agonists may have effects on the decompensated (myogenic, "atonic") bladder which are different from those on the normal bladder. Outflow obstruction, which may cause bladder decompensation, has been shown to be associated with a reduction in the autonomic innervation of the bladder sometimes leading to "denervation supersensitivity" (Gosling et al., 1986). In such patients, a change of the response to muscarinic receptor stimulation can be expected. However, neither bethanechol nor carbachol has been shown convincingly to have a beneficial effect on bladder emptying, not even in bladders with morphological and/or functional disturbances, including the decompensated bladder. Patients with benign prostatic hyperplasia, who received prazosin to relieve their outflow obstruction, were treated with oral carbachol in a dose that caused side-effects (perspiration, gastrointestinal discomfort) in all of them. However, none had any effect on urodynamic variables, or improved bladder emptying (Hedlund and Andersson, 1988).

Inhibition of bladder contraction

Motor urge incontinence is characterized by a strong desire to void and is associated with an increased contractile activity in the detrusor muscle during the filling phase of the bladder, in the form of either unstable (involuntary) bladder contractions and/or decreased compliance. Uncontrolled bladder contractions may occur in connection with neurological diseases or lesions, but can also be associated with outflow obstruction, inflammation and irritative processes in the bladder, or they may by idiopathic.

It is well known that atropine (Cullumbine et al., 1955) and other anticholinergic drugs produce an almost complete paralysis of the normal bladder when injected intravenously. Despite several reports on insufficient efficacy of anticholinergic drugs given orally to patients with unstable detrusor contractions (Ritch et al., 1977; Walter et al., 1982; Bonnesen et al., 1984; Zorzitto et al., 1986), there are several studies suggesting that muscarinic receptors mediate not only normal bladder contraction, but also the main part of the contraction in hyperactive bladders (Low, 1977; Cardozo and Stanton, 1979; Naglo et al., 1981). Lack of effect can be attributed to low bioavailability of available anticholinergics (Sundwall et al., 1973; Vose et al., 1979) making it difficult to achieve sufficient concentrations in the effector organ, or to side-effects, limiting the dose that can be given. Theoretically, it may be due to the occurrence of a non-adrenergic, non-cholinergic transmitter substance producing an atropine-resistant contraction. The fact that intramuscular emepronium bromide was ineffective in patients suffering from urinary incontinence due to small capacity, hyperreflexic bladders (Perera et al., 1982) seemed to support the occurrence of "true" atropine resistance.

Propantheline bromide and emepronium bromide are probably the most widely used drugs in the treatment of bladder hyperactivity. Both drugs have pronounced effects on both normal bladder emptying and unstable bladder contractions when given parenterally (Boman and Von Garrelts, 1973; Syversen et al., 1976; Low, 1977; Ulmsten et al., 1977; Cardozo and Stanton, 1979; Blaivas et al., 1980).

The incomplete and individually varying biological availability of both propantheline bromide (Vose et al., 1979) and emepronium bromide (Sundwall et al., 1973) makes individual titration of the optimal dose necessary. The dose is increased until incontinence is abolished or until untoward side-effects preclude further increase. With this approach, good clinical responses were obtained in a majority of patients with uninhibited detrusor contractions (propantheline bromide: Blaivas et al., 1980; emepronium carragenate: Massey and Abrams, 1986). An important factor limiting the clinical use of available

anticholinergic agents is their lack of selectivity for the muscarinic receptors of the bladder. This will lead to systemic side-effects independent of what drug is tried. Atropine and related tertiary amines are well absorbed from the gastrointestinal tract, and have good penetration to the central nervous system (CNS). Side-effects from the CNS will therefore often limit their use. Quarternary ammonium compounds have a lower incidence of side actions from the CNS, but produce well-known peripheral anticholinergic side-effects such as accommodation paralysis, tachycardia and dryness of mouth.

Despite the limitations of available anticholinergics, agents with other modes of action have not been demonstrated to be clinically more effective in the treatment of bladder storage dysfunction (Andersson, 1988).

Conclusion

Current treatment of bladder emptying and storage failure with cholinergic agents is far from optimal. Improvement can be expected with increased knowledge of the muscarinic receptor functions in the human bladder.

References

Adami, M., Bertaccini, G., Coruzzi, G. and Poli, E. (1985) Characterization of cholinoreceptors in the rat urinary bladder by the use of agonists and antagonists of the cholinergic system. *J. Auton. Pharmacol.*, 5: 197–205.

Ambache, H. and Zar, M.A. (1970) Non-cholinergic transmission by postganglionic motor neurones in the mammalian bladder. *J. Physiol. (Lond.)*, 210: 761–783.

Anderson, G.F., Skender, J.G. and Nauarro, S.P. (1985) Quantitation and stability of cholinergic receptors in human bladder tissue from post surgical and postmortem sources. *J. Urol.*, 133: 897–899.

Andersson, K.-E. (1988) Current concepts in the treatment of disorders of micturition. *Drugs*, 35: 477–494.

Andersson, K.-E., Fovaeus, M., Hedlund, H., Holmquist, F. and Sundler, F. (1989) Muscarinic receptor stimulation of phosphoinositide hydrolysis in the human urinary bladder. *J. Urol.*, 141: 324A (abstract 619).

Bartra, S., Björklund, A., Hedlund, H. and Andersson, K.-E. (1987) Identification and characterization of muscarinic cholinergic receptors in the human urinary bladder and parotid gland. *J. Auton. Nerv. Syst.,* 20: 129–135.

Blaivas, J.G. (1984) If you currently prescribe bethanechol chloride for urinary retention, please raise your hand. *Neurourol. Urodyn.,* 3: 209–210.

Blaivas, J.G., Labib, K.B., Michalik, S.J. and Zayed, A.A.H. (1980) Cystometric response to propantheline in detrusor hyperreflexia: therapeutic implications. *J. Urol.,* 124: 259–262.

Boman, J. and von Garrelts, B. (1973) Emepronium bromide (Cetiprin). Its effect on bladder pressure and urinary flow in healthy subjects. *Scand. J. Urol. Nephrol.,* 7: 153–157.

Bonnesen, T., Tikjøb, G., Kamper, A.L., Bay Nielsen, A.M., Thorup Andersen, J. and Juul Jørgensen, S. (1984) Effect of emepronium bromide (Cetiprin) on symptoms and urinary bladder function after transurethral resection of the prostate. *Urol. Int.,* 39: 318–320.

Cardozo, L.D. and Stanton, S.L. (1979) An objective comparison of the effects of parenterally administered drugs in patients suffering from detrusor instability. *J. Urol.,* 122: 58–59.

Cowan, W.D. and Daniel, E.E. (1983) Human female bladder and its noncholinergic contractile function. *Can. J. Physiol. Pharmacol.,* 61: 1236–1246.

Craggs, M.D., Rushton, D.N. and Stephenson, J.D. (1986) A putative non-cholinergic mechanism in urinary bladders of new but not old world primates. *J. Urol.,* 136: 1348–1350.

Cullumbine, H., McKee, W. and Creasey, N.H. (1955) The effects of atropine sulphate upon healthy male subjects. *Q. J. Exp. Physiol.,* 30: 309–319.

D'Agostino, G., Kilbinger, H., Chiari, M.C. and Grana, E. (1986) Presynaptic inhibitory muscarinic receptors modulating ^{3}H-acetylcholine release in the rat urinary bladder. *J. Pharmacol. Exp. Ther.,* 239: 522–528.

de Groat, W.C. and Saum W.R. (1972) Sympathetic inhibition of the urinary bladder and of pelvic ganglionic transmission in the cat. *J. Physiol. (Lond.),* 220: 297–314.

Downie, J.W. (1984) Bethanechol in urology–a discussion of issues. *Neurourol. Urodyn.,* 3: 211–222.

Ek, A., Alm, P., Andersson, K.-E. and Persson, C.G. (1977) Adrenergic and cholinergic nerves of the human urethra and urinary bladder. A histochemical study. *Acta Physiol. Scand.,* 99: 345–352.

Elbadawi, A. (1982) Neuromorphological basis of vesicourethral function. I. Histochemistry, ultrastructure, and function of intrinsic nerves of the bladder and uretra. *Neurourol. Urodyn.,* 1: 3–50,

Finkbeiner, A.E. (1985) Is bethanechol chloride clinically effective in promoting bladder emptying? A literature review. *J. Urol.,* 134: 443–449.

Fovaeus, M., Andersson, K.-E., Batra, S., Morgan, E. and Sjögren, C. (1987) Effects of calcium, calcium channel blockers and Bay K 8644 on contractions induced by muscarinic receptor stimulation of isolated bladder muscle from rabbit and man. *J. Urol.,* 137: 798–803.

Glahn, B.E. (1970) Neurogenic bladder diagnosed pharmacologically on the basis of denervation supersensitivity. *Scand. J. Urol. Nephrol.,* 4: 13–24.

Gosling, J.A., Gilpin, S.A., Dixon, J.S. and Gilpin, C.J. (1986) Decrease in the autonomic innervation of human detrusor muscle in outflow obstruction. *J. Urol.,* 136: 501–504.

Hedlund, H. and Andersson, K.-E. (1988) Effects of prazosin and carbachol in patients with benign prostatic obstruction. *Scand. J. Urol. Nephrol.,* 22: 19–22.

Hindmarsh, J.R., Idowu, O.A., Yeates, W.K. and Zar, M.A. (1977) Pharmacology of electrically evoked contractions of human bladder. *Br. J. Pharmacol.,* 61: 115P.

Kinder, R.B. and Mundy, A.R. (1985) Atropine blockade of nerve-mediated stimulation of the human detrusor. *Br. J. Urol.,* 57: 418–421.

Kinder, R.B., Restorick, J.M. and Mundy, A.R. (1985) A comparative study of detrusor muscle from normal, idiopathic unstable and hyperreflexic bladder. In *Proceedings of the 15th Annual Meeting of the International Continence Society.* London, pp. 170–171.

Lapides, J., Friend, C.R., Ajemian, E.P. and Reus, W.F. (1962) A new method for diagnosing the neurogenic bladder. *Univ. Mich. Med. Bull.,* 28: 166–180.

Levin, R.M., Staskin, D.R. and Wein, A.J. (1982) The muscarinic cholinergic binding kinetics of the human urinary bladder. *Neurourol. Urodyn.,* 1: 221–225.

Levin, R.M., Ruggieri, M.R. and Wein, A.J. (1988) Identification of receptor subtypes in the rabbit and human urinary bladder by selective radio-ligand binding. *J. Urol.,* 139: 844–848.

Low, J.A. (1977) Urethral behaviour during the involuntary detrusor contraction. *Am. J. Obstet. Gynecol.,* 128: 32–39.

Massey, J.A. and Abrams, P. (1986) Dose titration in clinical trials. An example using emepronium carrageenate in detrusor instability. *Br. J. Urol.,* 58: 125–128.

Mattiasson, A., Andersson, K.-E., Sjögren, C., Sundin, T. and Uvelius, B. (1984) Supersensitivity to carbachol in the parasympathetically decentralized feline urinary bladder. *J. Urol.,* 131: 562–565.

Mattiasson, A., Andersson, K.-E., Elbadawi, A., Morgan, E. and Sjögren, C. (1987) Interactions between adrenergic and cholinergic nerve terminals in the urinary bladder of rabbit, cat and man. *J. Urol.,* 137: 1017–1019.

Mattiasson, A., Andersson, K.-E. and Sjögren, C. (1988) Inhibitory muscarinic receptors and α-adrenoceptors on cholinergic axon terminals in the urethra of rabbit and man. *Neurourol. Urodyn.,* 6: 449–456.

Mobley, T.L., El-Badawi, A., McDonald, D. and Schenk, E. (1966) Innervation of the human urinary bladder. *Surg. Forum,* 17: 505–506.

Monferini, E., Giraldo, E. and Ladinsky, H. (1988) Characterization of the muscarinic receptor subtypes in the rat urinary bladder. *Eur. J. Pharmacol.,* 147: 453–458.

Naglo, A.S., Nergårdh, A. and Boreus, L.O. (1981) Influence of atropine and isoprenaline on detrusor hyperactivity in children with neurogenic bladder. *Scand. J. Urol. Nephrol.,* 15: 97–102,

Nergårdh, A. and Kinn, A.-C. (1983) Neurotransmission in activation of the contractile response in the human urinary bladder. *Scand. J. Urol. Nephrol.* 17: 153–157.

Nilvebrant, L., Andersson, K.-E. and Mattiasson, A. (1985)

Characterization of the muscarinic cholinoreceptors in the human detrusor. *J. Urol.,* 134: 418–423.

Nilvebrant, L., Ekström, J. and Malmberg, L. (1986) Muscarinic receptor density in the rat urinary bladder after denervation, hypertrophy and urinary diversion. *Acta Pharmacol. Toxicol.,* 59: 306–314.

Perera, G.L.S., Ritch, A.E.S. and Hall, M.R.P. (1982) The lack of effect of intramuscular emepronium bromide for urinary incontinence. *Br. J. Urol.,* 54: 259–260.

Restorick, J.M. and Mundy, A.R. (1989) The density of cholinergic and alpha and beta adrenergic receptors in the normal and hyper-reflexic human detrusor. *Br. J. Urol.,* 63: 32–35.

Ritch, A.E.S., Castleden, C.M., George, C.F. and Hall, M.R.P. (1977) A second look at emepronium bromide in urinary incontinence. *Lancet,* 1: 504–506.

Rud, T., Ulmsten, U. and Andersson, K.-E. (1978) Initiation of voiding in healthy women and those with stress incontinence. *Acta Obstet. Gynecol. Scand.,* 57: 457–462.

Ruggieri, M.R., Bode, D.C., Levin, R.M. and Wein, A.J. (1987) Muscarinic receptor subtypes in human and rabbit bladder. *Neurourol. Urodyn.,* 6: 119–128.

Sibley, G.N.A. (1984) A comparison of spontaneous and nerve-mediated activity in bladder muscle from man, pig and rabbit. *J. Physiol. (Lond.),* 354: 431–443.

Sjögren, C., Andersson, K.-E., Husted, S., Mattiasson, A. and Møller-Madsen, B. (1982) Atropine resistance of transmurally stimulated human bladder muscle. *J. Urol.,* 128: 1368–1371.

Sundwall, A., Vessman, J. and Strindberg, B. (1973) Fate of emepronium in man in relation to its pharmacological effects. *Eur. J. Clin. Pharmacol.,* 6: 191–195.

Syversen, J.H.N., Møllestad, E. and Semb, L.S. (1976) Emepronium bromide (Cetiprin) as spasmolytic agent in transvesical prostatectomy. *Scand. J. Urol. Nephrol.,* 10: 201–203.

Taira, N. (1972) The autonomic pharmacology of the bladder. *Annu. Rev. Pharmacol. Toxicol.,* 12: 197–208.

Tanagho, E.A. and Miller, E.R. (1970) Initiation of voiding. *Br. J. Urol.,* 42: 175–183.

Taylor, P. (1985) Cholinergic agonists. In A. Goodman Gilman, L.S. Goodman, T.W. Rall and F, Murad (Eds.), *The Pharmacological Basis of Therapeutics,* 7th edn., MacMillan Publishing Co, New York, pp. 100–109.

Twiddy, D.A.S., Downie, J.W. and Awad, S.A. (1980) Response of the bladder to bethanechol after acute spinal cord transection in cats. *J. Pharmacol. Exp. Ther.,* 215: 500–506.

Ulmsten, U, Andersson, K.-E. and Persson, C.G.A. (1977) Diagnostic and therapeutic aspects of urge urinary incontinence. *Urol. Int.,* 32: 88–96.

van Charldorp, K.J., de Jonge, A., Thoolen, M.J. and van Zwieten, P.A. (1985) Subclassification of muscarinic receptors in the heart, urinary bladder and sympathetic ganglia in the pithed rat. Selectivity of some classical agonists. *Naunyn Schmiedebergs Arch. Pharmacol.,* 331: 301–306.

Vose, C.W., Ford, G.C., Grigson, S.J.W., Haskins, N.J., Prout, M., Stevens, P.M., Rose, D.A. and Palmer, R.F. (1979) Pharmacokinetics of propantheline bromide in normal man. *Br. J. Clin. Pharmacol.,* 7: 89–93.

Walter, S., Hansen, J., Hansen, L., Maegaard, E., Meyhoff, H.H. and Nordling, J. (1982) Urinary incontinence in old age. A controlled clinical trial of emepronium bromide. *Br. J. Urol.,* 54: 249–251.

Wein, A.J. (1987) Lower urinary tract function and pharmacological management of lower urinary tract dysfunction. *Urol. Clin. North Am.,* 14: 273–296.

Zappia, L., Cartella, A., Potenzoni, D. and Bertaccini, G. (1986) Action of pirenzepine on the human urinary bladder in vitro. *J. Urol.,* 136: 739–742.

Zorzitto, M.L., Jewett, M.A.S., Fernie, G.R., Holliday, P.J. and Bartlett, S. (1986) Effectiveness of propantheline bromide in the treatment of geriatric patients with detrusor instability. *Neurourol. Urodyn.,* 5: 133–140.

S.-M. Aquilonius and P.-G. Gillberg (Eds.)
Progress in Brain Research, Vol. 84
© 1990 Elsevier Science Publishers B.V. (Biomedical Division)

CHAPTER 23

Cholinergic regulation of the endocrine pancreas

Bo Ahrén [1,2], Sven Karlsson [1] and Stefan Lindskog [1]

Departments of [1] Pharmacology and [2] Surgery, Lund University, Lund, Sweden

Cholinergic activation of the endocrine pancreas

It has been known since 1869 that the pancreatic islets are innervated (Langerhans, 1869). Today it is known that these nerves are cholinergic, adrenergic and neuropeptidergic (Ahrén et al., 1986a). The cholinergic, preganglionic, nerve fibers traverse within the vagus and enter the pancreas together with the arteries. They terminate in intrapancreatic ganglia, which is the origin of postganglionic fibers which reach the islets (Coupland, 1958; Miller, 1981). The existence of a dense cholinergic islet innervation has been demonstrated not only in experimental animals but also in human islets, where a periinsular cholinergic plexus has been visualized (Amenta et al., 1983). Individual fibers from this plexus penetrate islets and terminate close to the endocrine cells. Within the islets, synaptic-like structures and even gap junctions between nerve terminals and endocrine cells have been seen (Orci et al., 1973; Smith and Porte, 1976). Hence, an intimate neural-islet relationship exists. It has also been demonstrated that islets have a 10-fold higher concentration of choline acetyltransferase than the surrounding exocrine tissue (Godfrey and Matschinsky, 1975). Most likely, therefore, acetylcholine is an intraislet neurotransmitter. However, it should be noted that the neuropeptides vasoactive intestinal polypeptide (VIP) and gastrin-releasing polypeptide (GRP) might also be of some importance as intraislet neurotransmitters, since they occur in intrapancreatic nerves (Bishop et al., 1980; Knuhtsen et al., 1987) and are liberated from the pancreas upon vagal nerve activation (Holst et al., 1984; Knuhtsen et al., 1985). Thus, the islet cholinergic nerves might use acetylcholine as well as VIP and/or GRP as mediator.

Vagal nerve activation, cholinergic agonism and islet hormone secretion

It was demonstrated in the 1920s that electrical vagal activation in adrenalectomized cats caused hypoglycemia, a finding that was interpreted as a consequence of stimulated insulin secretion (Britton, 1925). Later studies also revealed an increase in the number of insulin cells within the islets after long-term vagal nerve activation in cats (Sergeyeva, 1940). Finally, after the development of insulin radioimmunoassays it could be clearly established that electrical vagal activation stimulates insulin secretion. This was demonstrated in a number of species, for example the dog (Kaneto et al., 1967; Ahrén and Taborsky, 1986), the calf (Bloom and Edwards, 1981), the pig (Holst et al., 1981a), the cat (Uvnäs-Wallensten and Nilsson, 1978) and the rat (Sakaguchi and Tamaguchi, 1980). In the dog and the calf, this effect seems to be muscarinic, since it was antagonized by atro-

---

Correspondence to: Dr. Bo Ahrén, Department of Pharmacology, Lund University, Sölvegatan 10, S-223 62 Lund, Sweden.

pine (Bloom and Edwards, 1981: Ahrén and Taborsky, 1986). However, in the pig and the cat, atropine was unable to inhibit vagally induced insulin secretion (Uvnäs-Wallensten and Nilsson, 1978; Holst et al., 1981a). This indicates a contribution of non-cholinergic, presumably peptidergic, mechanisms, at least in these species. However, a clear stimulation of insulin secretion after vagal nerve activation is evident in all species.

Studies on the receptor type involved in the cholinergic activation of insulin secretion have revealed that intrapancreatic ganglia possess nicotinic receptors regulating the islets by complex postganglionic mechanisms involving both stimulatory and inhibitory components (Stagner and Samols, 1986). Furthermore, acetylcholine or carbachol has repeatedly been shown to stimulate insulin secretion by a mechanism which is inhibited by atropine both in vivo and in vitro in several species (Iversen, 1973; Miller, 1981; Holst et al., 1981b; Ahrén and Lundquist, 1981; Ahrén et al., 1986a). This suggests that besides nicotinic, ganglionic receptors, the cholinergic nerves regulate islet hormone secretion by muscarinic receptors, which are presumably located within the islets. It is worth emphasizing the dependence of this muscarinic stimulation of insulin secretion on the ambient glucose level: the direct stimulation of insulin secretion by acetylcholine is glucose-dependent (Holst et al., 1981b; Garcia et al., 1988) and the affinity for agonist of islet muscarinic receptors is enhanced by a long-term glucose environment (Grill and Östenson 1983; Östenson and Grill, 1987).

It is known that the muscarinic receptors may be divided into four different subtypes, designated M_1, M_2, M_3 and M_4, respectively (Kerlavage et al., 1987). Studies have therefore been undertaken to identify the subtype involved in the stimulation of insulin secretion. It has, however, been shown that the specific antagonists pirenzepine (M_1-receptor antagonist) and AF-DX 116 (M_2-receptor antagonist) have no or only a weak inhibitory action on cholinergically stimulated insulin secretion (Henquin and Nenquin, 1988). This indicates

that the insulin cell muscarinic receptor subtype probably does not belong to either of these subtype categories.

Glucagon secretion has also been demonstrated to be increased by vagal nerve activation in the dog (Ahrén and Taborsky, 1986), the calf (Bloom and Edwards, 1981) and the pig (Holst et al., 1981a). However, in both the dog and the pig, atropine does not inhibit this effect, making it likely that it is non-cholinergic. This is also supported by the failure of the cholinergic agonist bethanechol to stimulate glucagon secretion in man (Palmer et al., 1979). However, in several other species, like the dog, the rat and the mouse, exogenous administration of cholinergic agonists has been demonstrated to stimulate glucagon secretion (Iversen, 1973; Kimura et al., 1982; Ahrén and Lundquist, 1986). This suggests that species differences exist with regard to involvement of muscarinic mechanisms in the regulation of glucagon secretion. However, the demonstration of a direct glucagonotropic action of acetylcholine does not necessarily imply that acetylcholine mediates the stimulated glucagon secretion during vagal nerve activation. For example, in the dog, acetylcholine stimulated glucagon secretion (Iversen, 1973), but, nevertheless, also in the dog, vagally induced glucagon secretion was not inhibited by atropine (Ahrén and Taborsky 1986). Hence, the exact nature of the effect of vagal nerve activation on glucagon secretion remains to be established; suffice it to say that in most species, vagal nerve activation stimulates glucagon secretion.

Electrical vagal nerve activation also increases somatostatin secretion from the pancreas in dogs (Ahrén et al., 1986b) and the secretion of pancreatic polypeptide (PP) in dogs, calves and pigs (Schwartz et al., 1978; Bloom and Edwards, 1981; Ahrén et al., 1986b). In the dog, these responses are partially but not totally reversible by atropine (Ahrén et al., 1986b). In contrast, studies on the direct action of cholinergic agonists on the secretion of somatostatin have resulted in conflicting reports. Thus, reports demonstrating inhibition, no effect, and stimulation exist (Hermansen, 1980; Kimura et al., 1982; Holst et al., 1983). However, the secretion of PP has consistently been shown to be markedly stimulated by acetylcholine in the dog (Hermansen, 1980). Hence, vagal activation stimulates the secretion of all four islet endocrine peptides, insulin, glucagon, somatostatin and PP. Some of these actions, like the stimulation of insulin secretion in the dog, seem cholinergically mediated, whereas others, like the stimulation of glucagon secretion in the dog, seem to be non-cholinergic effects (Ahrén et al., 1986a).

Physiology and pathophysiology of cholinergic actions on islet hormone secretion

It has been demonstrated in rats and humans that immediately postprandially, even prior to any alterations in the glycemia, a rapid insulin secretion occurs (Sjöström et al., 1980; Berthoud and Jeanrenaud, 1982; Steffens and Strubbe, 1983; Simon et al., 1986). This effect is most likely mainly cholinergic, muscarinic, in nature, since it is inhibited to a large degree by atropine (Sjöström et al., 1980; Berthoud and Jeanrenaud, 1982). In fact, almost 50% of the insulin secretion in the immediate (first 6 min) postprandial period in rats has been shown to be cholinergically dependent (Berthoud, 1984). Whether the cholinergic system is involved in the regulation of insulin secretion also after this immediate postprandial period is more difficult to study due to its multifactorial regulation by gastrointestinal hormones, intestinal motility and absorbed nutrients. A contribution by atropine-sensitive mechanisms to the intestinal phase of postprandial insulin secretion has, however, been demonstrated in rats (Schusdziarra et al., 1983; Berthoud, 1984). It remains to be established, though, whether these mechanisms are related to islet or intestinal functions. Therefore, the most convincingly demonstrated cholinergic contribution to the regulation of islet function in relation to meal intake is, so far, the cephalic phase. It has even been hypothesized that this particular phase is of importance for prevention of

glucose intolerance after meal intake (Steffens and Strubbe, 1983).

Evidence has also been put forward that cholinergic mechanisms are involved in the hypoglycemia-induced glucagon secretion, as shown by inhibition of this response by atropine in calves (Bloom et al., 1974) and rats (Patel, 1984) and by vagotomy in humans (Russell et al., 1974). A similar response is the acute glucagon secretion that occurs during neuroglycopenia induced by 2-deoxyglucose, and this response in man (Hedo et al., 1978) and mice (Karlsson and Ahrén, 1987), is also inhibited by atropine. Also, neuroglycopenia-induced insulin secretion in mice is inhibited by atropine (Karlsson et al., 1987). Thus, it seems that the islet responses to hypoglycemia and neuroglycopenia are to a large degree governed by cholinergic mechanisms.

The cholinergic system has also been suggested to be implicated in certain pathophysiological processes related to obesity (Steffens and Strubbe, 1983). Thus, cholinergic overactivity seems to a large extent responsible for the hyperinsulinemia in the obese mouse (Ahrén and Lundquist, 1982) and for the insulin and glucagon hypersecretion in the obese Zucker rat (Rohner-Jeanrenaud and Jeanrenaud, 1985; Fletcher and McKenzie, 1988). Hence, it may be safe to conservatively conclude that, physiologically, the cholinergic system is involved both in the cephalic phase of postprandial insulin secretion and in the islet defense response to hypoglycemia or neuroglycopenia. Furthermore, pathophysiologically, the cholinergic system might be of importance for the development of obesity. However, the exact role of cholinergic neurotransmission under these conditions, as well as whether it also participates in other physiological or pathophysiological events, is not yet established and needs to be studied in more detail.

Mechanism of islet muscarinic action

When studies on the mechanism of action of cholinergic activation of islets have been designed, most authors have started to compare the mechanistic effects of cholinergic agonists with those of glucose. Glucose is known to stimulate insulin secretion by increasing the cytoplasmic concentration of Ca^{2+}. This is obtained by at least two different processes: an inward Ca^{2+} current caused by opening of voltage-sensitive Ca^{2+} channels and a liberation of intracellularly stored Ca^{2+} (Prentki and Matschinsky, 1987).

The opening of the voltage-sensitive Ca^{2+} channels by glucose is mediated by depolarization, which in turn is induced by closure of the ATP-sensitive K^+ channels (Petersen, 1988). Hence, glucose increases the formation of ATP through its metabolism, and ATP closes, or at least decreases the mean opening time of, the ATP-sensitive K^+ channels. This in turn leads to depolarization and opening of the voltage-sensitive Ca^{2+} channels. To study whether mechanisms similar to these might explain the stimulated insulin secretion observed after cholinergic activation, we used isolated rat islets prelabelled with various isotopes and then perifused. Thereafter, they were stimulated with the cholinergic agonist carbachol. Initially, we established the dose of carbachol to be used by performing static batch incubations of single islets and determining the insulin secretion. We then found a dose level of 10^{-4} M of carbachol to be suitable for the subsequent perifusion experiments (Fig. 1). When the islets were then prelabelled with $^{45}Ca^{2+}$ and perifused in a KRB medium supplemented with 8.3 mM glucose, it was found, as is seen in Fig. 2, that addition of the cholinergic agonist carbachol (10^{-4} M) rapidly stimulated a marked but short-lived $^{45}Ca^{2+}$ efflux. This has also previously been shown in islets from both rats (Mathias et al., 1985) and mice (Hermans et al., 1987; Garcia et al., 1988). This stimulation of $^{45}Ca^{2+}$ efflux is similar to that obtained after glucose stimulation (Prentki and Matschinsky, 1987; Skoglund et al., 1988) and reflects the increase in the cytoplasmic concentration of Ca^{2+}. It might be caused either by increased $^{45}Ca^{2+}$–$^{40}Ca^{2+}$ exchange over the plasma membrane due to opening of membraneous Ca^{2+} channels and/or to liberation of Ca^{2+} from intracellular

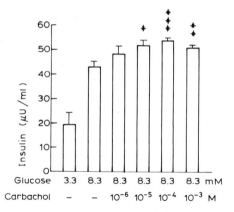

Fig. 1. Effects of the cholinergic agonist carbachol at different dose levels on insulin secretion from single isolated, overnight cultured, rat islets incubated in a KRB medium with 8.3 mM glucose and 1.28 mM Ca^{2+}. The islets were isolated with the collagenase isolation technique (Lacy and Kostianovsky, 1967) and cultured overnight in RPMI medium. After 45 min preincubation of single islets in 0.1 ml of the KRB medium, carbachol was introduced and a 60 min incubation was performed, whereafter medium was analysed for its concentration of insulin by a radioimmunoassay (Heding, 1966). Means ± SEM for 16 islet incubations are shown for each column. Asterisks indicate the probability level of random difference versus 8.3 mM glucose alone. * $p < 0.05$; ** $p < 0.01$; *** $p < 0.001$.

stores leading to enhanced cytoplasmic Ca^{2+} concentration and extrusion of Ca^{2+}. However, it has previously been demonstrated that a large degree of the stimulation of $^{45}Ca^{2+}$ efflux by cholinergic agonists is also seen in Ca^{2+}-deprived medium (Morgan et al., 1985; Mathias et al., 1985; Hellman and Gylfe, 1986; Hermans et al., 1987; Garcia et al., 1988; Henquin et al., 1988). Under such conditions exchange of Ca^{2+} over the plasma membrane is not possible. This suggests that the underlying mechanism of carbachol-stimulated $^{45}Ca^{2+}$ efflux depends to a large degree on mobilization of Ca^{2+} from intracellular stores. However, the contribution of calcium exchange over the plasma membrane, in the presence of extracellular calcium, is also likely to be important, and, therefore, cholinergic agonists seem to exert two actions on the cellular calcium homeostasis.

The process of liberating Ca^{2+} from intracellular stores might be mediated by inositol 1,4,5-trisphosphate (IP_3). IP_3 is formed by hydrolysis of

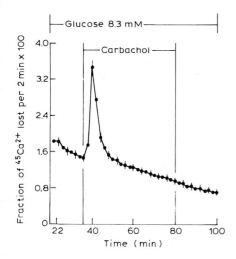

Fig. 2. Effects of the cholinergic agonist carbachol (10^{-4} M) on $^{45}Ca^{2+}$ efflux from $^{45}Ca^{2+}$-loaded isolated rat islets perifused in a medium with 8.3 mM glucose and 1.28 mM Ca^{2+}. The islets were isolated with the collagenase isolation technique (Lacy and Kostianovsky, 1967) and cultured overnight in RPMI medium. After loading for 120 min in KRB medium with $^{45}CaCl_2$ at 1.28 mM Ca^{2+} and 16.7 mM glucose, the islets were pre-perifused at 8.3 mM glucose for 20 min prior to introduction of carbachol. Perifusion was performed in columns with 35–40 islets in each at a flow rate of 0.1 ml/min as previously described (Skoglund et al., 1988). The results are demonstrated as the fraction (%) of $^{45}Ca^{2+}$ in each 2 min sample of the total islet content of $^{45}Ca^{2+}$. Means ± SEM of four experiments are shown.

phosphatidylinositol 4,5-biphosphate (PIP_2) after activation of the membrane-bound phospholipase C (PLC; Prentki and Matschinsky, 1987). We studied whether carbachol affects this process by the use of perifusion of isolated islets prelabelled with *myo*-[2-^{3}H]inositol. We found, as is seen in Fig. 3, that when isolated rat islets prelabelled with *myo*-[2-^{3}H]inositol were perifused in a KRB medium supplemented with 8.3 mM glucose, carbachol (10^{-4} M) stimulated a large and sustained release of [^{3}H]inositol. Such an action has previously been demonstrated by other groups (Best and Malaisse, 1984; Best et al., 1984; Morgan et al., 1985; Garcia et al., 1988). This release of [^{3}H]inositol is interpreted as being secondary to hydrolysis of PIP_2 by PLC (Zawalich and Zawalich, 1988). It could therefore indeed be postulated that cholinergic agonists stimulate the hydrolysis

of PIP_2 in normal islets. The IP_3 which is formed then diffuses into the cytoplasm and stimulates the liberation of Ca^{2+} from intracellular stores. This process is in turn reflected as the stimulation of $^{45}Ca^{2+}$ efflux from prelabelled islets in the Ca^{2+}-deprived medium. However, this is probably not the only mechanism behind the release of intracellular Ca^{2+} from stores. For example, acetylcholine-induced stimulation of $^{45}Ca^{2+}$ efflux in Ca^{2+}-deficient medium has been demonstrated to be inhibited by exclusion of Na^+ (Hellman and Gylfe, 1986; Henquin et al., 1988). This suggests that besides the release of intracellular Ca^{2+} mediated by IP_3, acetylcholine also liberates Ca^{2+} from intracellular stores by an Na^+-dependent mechanism. In fact, it has been hypothesized that IP_3 and Na^+ generate the liberation of intracellular Ca^{2+} from two different storage sites: IP_3 from

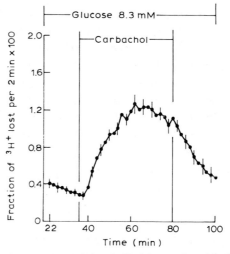

Fig. 3. Effects of the cholinergic agonist carbachol (10^{-4} M) on [^{3}H]-inositol-efflux from *myo*-[2-^{3}H]inositol-loaded isolated rat islets perifused in a medium with 8.3 mM glucose and 1.28 mM Ca^{2+}. The islets were isolated with the collagenase isolation technique (Lacy and Kostianovsky, 1967) and cultured overnight in RPMI medium. After loading for 120 min in KRB medium with *myo*-[2-^{3}H]inositol at 1.28 mM Ca^{2+} and 3.3 mM glucose, the islets were pre-perifused at 8.3 mM glucose for 20 min prior to introduction of carbachol. Perifusion was performed in columns with 35–40 islets in each at a flow rate of 0.1 ml/min as previously described (Skoglund et al., 1988). The results are demonstrated as the fraction (%) of ^{3}H in each 2 min sample of the total islet content of ^{3}H. Means ± SEM of four experiments are shown.

the endoplasmic reticulum and Na^+ from the mitochondria (Hellman and Gylfe, 1986; Henquin et al., 1988). In any case, cholinergic agonists seem able to markedly stimulate the hydrolysis of PIP_2 and to induce liberation of Ca^{2+} from intracellular stores.

It is known that PLC-induced hydrolysis of PIP_2 also generates 1,2-diacylglycerol (DAG), and carbachol has been shown to stimulate DAG formation in rat islets (Peter-Riesch et al., 1988). The DAG thus formed remains in the plasma membrane and activates protein kinase C (PKC). It is possible that activated PKC sensitizes the exocytotic process for Ca^{2+} and, hence, augments stimulated insulin secretion (Prentki and Matschinsky, 1987). However, strong experimental evidence for this hypothesis is still lacking (Metz, 1988). There exists the possibility, though, that cholinergic agonists potentiate insulin secretion by the two processes of increasing the cytoplasmic Ca^{2+} concentrations and by increasing the sensitivity for Ca^{2+} in the exocytotic process by PKC. In this context, it must be remembered that for acetylcholine-stimulated insulin secretion to occur, enhancement of the ambient concentrations of glucose is necessary. For example, despite stimulation by acetylcholine of $^{45}Ca^{2+}$ efflux at low glucose levels, no insulin secretion was observed (Garcia et al., 1988). This might suggest that a certain threshold for the cytoplasmic Ca^{2+} concentration must be reached before insulin secretion is potentiated by acetylcholine.

It should be emphasized that the model outlined above is simplified. For example, although the $^{45}Ca^{2+}$ efflux stimulated by acetylcholine remains in a Ca^{2+}-deficient medium, it is clearly diminished (Garcia et al., 1988). This indicates that it is governed not only by increased liberation of Ca^{2+} from intracellular storage sites, but also by increased $^{45}Ca^{2+} - {}^{40}Ca^{2+}$-exchange mechanisms over the plasma membrane (Sánchez-Andrés et al., 1988). When studying possible mechanisms underlying such an effect, it is of interest to remember that glucose stimulates the uptake of extracellular Ca^{2+} by gating the voltage-sensitive

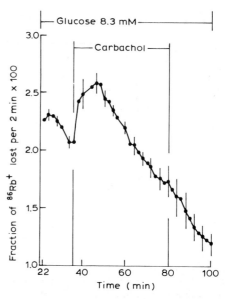

Fig. 4. Effects of the cholinergic agonist carbachol (10^{-4} M) on $^{86}Rb^+$ efflux from $^{86}Rb^+$-loaded isolated rat islets perifused in a medium with 8.3 mM glucose and 1.28 mM Ca^{2+}. The islets were isolated with the collagenase isolation technique (Lacy and Kostianovsky, 1967) and cultured overnight in RPMI medium. After loading for 90 min in KRB medium with $^{86}RbCl$ at 1.28 mM Ca^{2+} and 3.3 mM glucose, the islets were pre-perifused at 8.3 mM glucose for 20 min prior to introduction of carbachol. Perifusion was performed in columns with 35–40 islets in each at a flow rate of 0.1 ml/min as previously described (Skoglund et al., 1988). The results are demonstrated as the fraction (%) of $^{86}Rb^+$ in each 2 min sample of the total islet content of $^{86}Rb^+$. Means ± SEM of four experiments are shown.

Ca^{2+} channels, a process mediated by closure of the ATP-dependent K^+ channels (Prentki and Matschinsky, 1987; Petersen, 1988). That cholinergic agonists exert a similar action is thus possible. This was studied by perifusing islets pre-labelled with $^{86}Rb^+$. Since glucose closes the ATP-dependent K^+ channels, or reduces their mean opening time, the hexose reduces $^{86}Rb^+$ efflux from such islets (Sehlin and Täljedal, 1975). We found, in contrast, that carbachol (10^{-4} M) increased the $^{86}Rb^+$ efflux (Fig. 4), which confirms previous studies (Hermans et al., 1987; Henquin et al., 1988; Garcia et al., 1988). Hence, the action of cholinergic agonists clearly differs from that of glucose. The stimulation of $^{86}Rb^+$ efflux induced by cholinergic agonists might have at least two explanations: (1) opening of Ca^{2+}-sensitive K^+ channels mediated by the increased cytoplasmic concentration of Ca^{2+} and/or (2) opening of voltage-sensitive K^+ channels mediated by depolarization primarily induced by the cholinergic agonist (Henquin et al., 1987). It was recently proposed that acetylcholine depolarizes the cell by increasing the membrane permeability for Na^+, since omission of Na^+ from the medium abolished the stimulated $^{86}Rb^+$ efflux, as it reduced the stimulated $^{45}Ca^{2+}$ efflux (Henquin et al., 1988). Acetylcholine has also been shown to increase the $^{22}Na^+$ uptake by isolated islets (Gagerman et al., 1980; Henquin et al., 1988). It is thus possible that carbachol increases the $^{86}Rb^+$ efflux by opening voltage-sensitive K^+ channels through depolarization induced by increased membrane permeability of Na^+. The exact mechanism underlying the increased $^{86}Rb^+$ efflux after cholinergic activation remains, however, to be established. In any case, it is clear that cholinergic agonists do not stimulate insulin secretion by the same cellular physiological mechanisms as does glucose.

The activation of adenylate cyclase with the subsequent formation of cyclic AMP has been suggested to be a potentiating mechanism in glucose-stimulated insulin secretion (Prentki and Matschinsky, 1987). We examined the possibility that carbachol, similarly to glucose, stimulates the formation of cyclic AMP by the use of isolated rat islets. The islets were incubated for 30 min in the presence of glucose (3.3, 8.3 or 16.7 mM) and/or carbachol (10^{-4} M). It was found that whereas glucose increased the concentration of cyclic AMP in islet homogenate, carbachol had no effect (Table I). Therefore, it is unlikely that changes in the cellular content of cyclic AMP participate in the mechanism whereby carbachol stimulates insulin secretion. Similar findings have been presented by several other groups (Gagerman et al., 1978; Wollheim et al., 1980; Mathias et al., 1985).

A possible mechanism for the stimulation of insulin secretion by carbachol/acetylcholine is illustrated in Fig. 5. It suggests that muscarinic

TABLE I

Effects of glucose and carbachol on the concentration of cyclic AMP in isolated rat islets

Glucose (mM)	Carbachol (M)	Cyclic AMP (fmol/islet)	n
3.3	–	62± 8	7
8.3	–	73±15	8
8.3	10^{-4}	88±19 [a]	6
16.7	–	124±20 [b]	2

Twenty overnight incubated rat islets were incubated for 30 min in 0.2 ml KRB medium supplemented with isobutyl methylxanthine (10^{-3} M) at various glucose concentrations without or with carbachol (10^{-4} M). After incubation, the islets were sonicated, deproteinized, and, after lyophilization, assayed for their content of cyclic AMP with a commercially available radioimmunoassay (Amersham Int., Amersham, UK) using a rabbit anti-succinyl-cyclic AMP antiserum and as tracer ^{125}I-2-O-succinyl-cyclic AMP-tyrosine methyl esther. Mean±SEM for 2–8 different incubations are shown. [a] indicates not significantly different from the value at 8.3 mM glucose, and [b] indicates a probability level of random difference from the value at 3.3 mM glucose of $p < 0.05$.

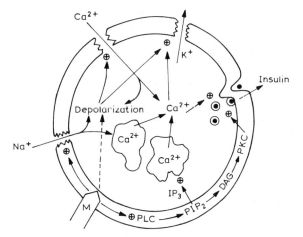

Fig. 5. Scheme for possible mechanisms of cholinergic agonists underlying their stimulatory action on insulin secretion. For detailed explanation see text. M = muscarinic receptor, PLC = phospholipase C, PIP_2 = phosphatidylinositol 4,5-biphosphate, DAG = 1,2-diacylglycerol, PKC = protein kinase C, IP_3 = inositol 1,4,5-trisphosphate. Ion channels, intracellular Ca^{2+} storage sites (presumably endoplasmic reticula and mitochondria), secretory granules undergoing exocytosis and plasma membrane are all shown schematically. Arrows indicate causative processes, and + indicates stimulation.

receptor activation of the insulin cells induces depolarization by increasing the membrane permeability for Na^+; this depolarization gates both voltage-sensitive Ca^{2+} channels and K^+ channels. The cholinergic agonists also initiate cleavage of PIP_2 to IP_3 and DAG through activation of PLC. IP_3 in turn causes liberation of intracellular Ca^{2+} and DAG activates PKC, which might increase the sensitivity in the exocytotic machinery for Ca^{2+}. Both the increased uptake of Ca^{2+} from the extracellular space through gated Ca^{2+} channels and the liberation of Ca^{2+} from intracellular stores elevate the cytoplasmic concentration of Ca^{2+}. This then forms, perhaps together with the activated PKC, the basis for potentiation of insulin secretion. The increased cytoplasmic Ca^{2+} concentration might also induce gating of K^+ channels, which might be regarded as rectifying impulses, of importance for the subsequent repolarization.

Concluding remarks

Pancreatic islets are abundantly innervated by cholinergic nerves, the activation of which stimulates the secretion of insulin, glucagon, somatostatin and PP. Physiologically, this action might be of importance in the immediate postprandial situation and as a safeguard against hypoglycemia and neuroglycopenia. Pathophysiologically, the action might be of importance during the development of obesity. Mechanistically, cholinergic agonists stimulate insulin secretion by activating cellular events related to liberation of intracellular Ca^{2+} and cleavage of membrane-bound phosphoinositides. Most important for future research is to establish the contribution of non-cholinergic (peptidergic) mechanisms to the function of islet vagal activation, and to define in more detail the mechanism of action of cholinergic agonists in the islets. Furthermore, the islet muscarinic receptor subtype awaits to be defined, as does the exact involvement of the cholinergic system in physiological conditions and pathophysiologically in relation to obesity and diabetes.

Acknowledgements

The studies performed by the authors have been supported by the Swedish Medical Research Council (grant No. 14X-6834), Nordisk Insulinfond, Swedish Diabetes Association, Albert Påhlssons and Magnus Bergvalls Foundations, Swedish Hoechst Diabetes Fund, Diabetesföreningen i Malmö, Crafoordska Stiftelsen, and the Faculty of Medicine, Lund University. For technical assistance, the authors are grateful to Lena Kvist.

References

Ahrén, B. and Lundquist, I. (1981) Effects of autonomic blockade by methylatropine and optical isomers of propranolol on plasma insulin levels in the basal state and after stimulation. *Acta Physiol. Scand.*, 112: 57–63.

Ahrén, B. and Lundquist, I. (1982) Modulation of basal insulin secretion in the obese, hyperglycemic mouse. *Metabolism*, 31: 172–179.

Ahrén, B. and Lundquist, I. (1986) Secretin potentiates cholinergically induced glucagon secretion in the mouse. *Acta Physiol. Scand.*, 128: 575–578.

Ahrén, B. and Taborsky Jr, G.J. (1986) The mechanism of vagal nerve stimulation of glucagon and insulin secretion in the dog. *Endocrinology*, 118: 1551–1557.

Ahrén, B., Taborsky Jr, G.J. and Porte Jr, D. (1986a) Neuropeptidergic versus cholinergic and adrenergic regulation of islet hormone secretion. *Diabetologia*, 29: 827–836.

Ahrén, B., Paquette, T.L. and Taborsky Jr, G.J. (1986b) Effect and mechanism of vagal nerve stimulation on somatostatin secretion in dogs. *Am. J. Physiol.*, 250: E212–E217.

Amenta, F., Cavallotti, C., de Rossi, M., Tonelli F. and Vatrella, F. (1983) The cholinergic innervation of human pancreatic islets. *Acta Histochem.*, 73: 273–278.

Berthoud, H.R. (1984) The relative contribution of the nervous system, hormones, and metabolites to the total insulin response during a meal in the rat. *Metabolism*, 33: 18–25.

Berthoud, H.R. and Jeanrenaud, B. (1982) Sham feeding-induced cephalic phase insulin release in the rat. *Am. J. Physiol.*, 242: E280–E285.

Best, L. and Malaisse, W.J. (1984) Nutrient and hormone-neurotransmitter stimuli induce hydrolysis of phosphoinositides in rat pancreatic islets. *Endocrinology*, 115: 1814–1820.

Best, L., Dunlop, M. and Malaisse, W.J. (1984) Phospholipid metabolism in pancreatic islets. *Experientia*, 40: 1085–1091.

Bishop, A.E., Polak, J.M., Green, I.C., Bryant, M.G. and Bloom, S.R. (1980) The location of VIP in the pancreas of man and rat. *Diabetologia*, 18: 73–78.

Bloom, S.R. and Edwards, A.V. (1981) Pancreatic endocrine responses to stimulation of the peripheral ends of the vagus nerve in conscious calves. *J. Physiol.*, 315: 31–41.

Bloom, S.R., Edwards, A.V. and Vaughan, N.J.A. (1974) The role of the autonomic innervation in the control of glucagon release during hypoglycemia in the calf. *J. Physiol.,* 236: 611–623.

Britton, S.W. (1925) Studies on the conditions of activity in endocrine glands. XVII. The nervous control of insulin secretion. *Am. J. Physiol.,* 24: 291–308.

Coupland, R.E. (1958) The innervation of the pancreas of the rat, cat and rabbit as revealed by the cholinesterase technique. *J. Anat.,* 92: 143–149.

Fletcher, J.M. and McKenzie, N.M. (1988) The parasympathetic nervous system and glucocorticoid-mediated hyperinsulinaemia in the genetically obese (fa/fa) Zucker rat. *J. Endocr.,* 118: 87–92.

Gagerman, E., Idahl, L.-Å., Meissner, H.P. and Täljedal, I.B. (1978) Insulin release, cGMP, cAMP, and membrane potential in acetylcholine-stimulated islets. *Am. J. Physiol.,* 235: E493–E500.

Gagerman, E., Sehlin, J.O. and Täljedal, I.B. (1980) Effects of acetylcholine on ion fluxes and chlorotetracycline fluorescence in pancreatic islets. *J. Physiol.,* 300: 505–513.

Garcia, M.C., Hermans, M.P. and Henquin, J.C. (1988) Glucose-, calcium- and concentration-dependence of acetylcholine stimulation of insulin release and ionic fluxes in mouse islets. *Biochem. J.,* 254: 211–218.

Godfrey, D.A. and Matschinsky, F.M. (1975) Enzymes of the cholinergic system in islets of Langerhans. *J. Histochem. Cytochem.,* 23: 645–651.

Grill, V. and Östenson, C.G. (1983) Muscarinic receptors in pancreatic islets of the rat. Demonstration and dependence on long-term glucose environment. *Biochim. Biophys. Acta,* 756: 159–162.

Heding, L. (1966) A simplified insulin radioimmunoassay method. In L. Donato, G. Milhaud and J. Sirchis (Eds.), *Labelled Proteins in Tracer Studies,* Euratom, Brussels, pp. 345–350.

Hedo, J.A., Villanueva, M.L. and Marco, J. (1978) Stimulation of pancreatic polypeptide and glucagon secretion by 2-deoxy-D-glucose in man: evidence for cholinergic mediation. *J. Clin. Endocrinol. Metab.,* 47: 366–371.

Hellman, B. and Gylfe, E. (1986) Mobilization of different intracellular calcium pools after activation of muscarinic receptors in pancreatic beta cells. *Pharmacology,* 32: 257–267.

Henquin, J.C. and Nenquin, M. (1988) The muscarinic receptor subtype in mouse pancreatic B-cells. *FEBS Lett.,* 236: 89–92.

Henquin, J.C., Garcia, M.C., Bozem, M., Hermans, M.P. and Nenquin, M. (1988) Muscarinic control of pancreatic B cell function involves sodium-dependent depolarization and calcium influx. *Endocrinology,* 122: 2134–2142.

Hermans, M.P., Schmeer, W. and Henquin, J.C. (1987) Modulation of the effect of acetylcholine on insulin release by the membrane potential of B cells. *Endocrinology,* 120: 1765–1773.

Hermansen, K. (1980) Secretion of somatostatin from the normal and diabetic pancreas. Studies in vitro. *Diabetologia,* 19: 492–504.

Holst, J.J., Gronholt, R., Schaffalitzky de Muckadell, O.B. and Fahrenkrug, J. (1981a) Nervous control of pancreatic endocrine secretion in pigs. 2. The effect of pharmacological blocking agents on the response to vagal stimulation. *Acta Physiol. Scand.,* 111: 9–14.

Holst, J.J., Schaffalitzky de Muckadell, O.B., Fahrenkrug, J., Lindkaer, S., Nielsen, O.V. and Schwartz, T.W. (1981b) Nervous control of pancreatic endocrine secretion in pigs. III. The effect of acetylcholine on the pancreatic secretion of insulin and glucagon. *Acta Physiol. Scand.,* 111: 15–22.

Holst, J.J., Jensen, S.L., Knuhtsen, S. and Nielsen, O.V. (1983) Autonomic nervous control of pancreatic somatostatin secretion. *Am. J. Physiol.,* 245: E542–548.

Holst, J.J., Fahrenkrug, J., Knuthsen, S., Jensen, S.L., Poulsen, S.S. and Nielsen, O.V. (1984) Vasoactive intestinal polypeptide (VIP) in the pig pancreas: role of VIPergic fibers in control of fluid and bicarbonate secretion. *Regul. Pept.,* 8: 245–249.

Iversen, J. (1973) Effect of acetylcholine on the secretion of glucagon and insulin from the isolated, perfused canine pancreas. *Diabetes,* 22: 381–387.

Kaneto, A., Kosaka, K. and Nakao, K. (1967) Effects of stimulation of the vagus nerve on insulin secretion. *Endocrinology,* 80: 530–536.

Karlsson, S. and Ahrén, B. (1987) Inhibition of 2-deoxy-glucose-induced glucagon secretion by muscarinic and α-adrenoceptor blockade in the mouse. *Diab. Res. Clin. Pract.,* 3: 239–242.

Karlsson, S., Bood, M. and Ahrén, B. (1987) The mechanism of 2-deoxyglucose-induced insulin secretion in the mouse. *J. Auton. Pharmacol.,* 7: 135–144.

Kerlavage, A.R., Fraser, C.M. and Venter, J.C. (1987) Muscarinic cholinergic receptor structure; molecular biological support for subtypes. *Trends. Pharmacol. Sci.,* 8: 426–431.

Kimura, H., Katagiri, K., Ohno, T., Harada, N., Imanishi, H., Iwasaki, M., Ito, M. and Takeuchi, T. (1982) Effect of acetylcholine and new cholinergic derivative on amylase output, insulin, glucagon, and somatostatin secretions from perfused isolated rat pancreas. *Horm. Metab. Res.,* 14: 356–360.

Knuhtsen, S., Holst, J.J., Jensen, S.L. and Nielsen, O.V. (1985) Gastrin releasing peptide: effect on exocrine secretion, and release from isolated perfused pig pancreas. *Am. J. Physiol.,* 248: G281–G287.

Knuhtsen, S., Holst, J.J., Baldissera, F.G., Skak-Nielsen, T., Poulsen, S.S., Jensen, S.L. and Nielsen, O.V. (1987) Gastrin releasing peptide in the porcine pancreas. *Gastroenterology,* 92: 1153–1158.

Lacy, P.E. and Kostianovsky, M. (1967) Method for the isolation of intact islets of Langerhans from the rat pancreas. *Diabetes,* 16: 35–39.

Langerhans, P. (1869) Beiträge zur mikroskopischen Anatomie der Bauchspeicheldrüse. Inaugural-Dissertation. Friedrich-Wilhelms-Universität, Berlin, pp 1–32.

Mathias, P.C.F., Carpinelli, A.R., Billaudel, B., Garcia-Morales, P., Valverde, I. and Malaisse, W.J. (1985) Cholinergic

218

stimulation of ion fluxes in pancreatic islets. *Biochem. Pharmacol.*, 34: 3451–3457.

Metz, S.A. (1988) Is protein kinase C required for physiologic insulin release? *Diabetes*, 37: 3–7.

Miller, R.E. (1981) Pancreatic neuroendocrinology: peripheral neural mechanisms in the regulation of the islets of Langerhans. *Endocr. Rev.*, 4: 471–494.

Morgan, N.G., Rumford, G.M. and Montague, W. (1985) Studies on the role of inositol triphosphate in the regulation of insulin secretion from isolated rat islets of Langerhans. *Biochem. J.*, 228: 713–718.

Orci, L., Perrelet, A., Ravazzola, M., Malaisse-Lagae, F. and Renold, A.E. (1973) A specialized membrane junction between nerve endings and B-cells in islets of Langerhans. *Eur. J. Clin. Invest.*, 3: 443–445.

Östenson, C.G. and Grill, V. (1987) Evidence that hyperglycemia increases muscarinic binding in pancreatic islets of the rat. *Endocrinology*, 121: 1705–1710.

Palmer, J.P., Werner, P.L., Hollander, B. and Ensinck, J.W. (1979) Evaluation of the control of glucagon secretion by the parasympathetic nervous system in man. *Metabolism*, 28: 549–552.

Patel, D.G. (1984) Role of parasympathetic nervous system in glucagon response to insulin-induced hypoglycemia in normal and diabetic rats. *Metabolism*, 33: 1123–1127.

Peter-Riesch, B., Fathi, M., Schlegel, W. and Wollheim, C.B. (1988) Glucose and carbachol generate 1,2-diacylglycerols by different mechanisms in pancreatic islets. *J. Clin. Invest.*, 81: 1154–1161.

Petersen, O.H. (1988) Control of potassium channels in insulin-secreting cells. *ISI. Atlas Sci. Biochem.*, 1: 144–149.

Prentki, M. and Matschinsky, F.M. (1987) Ca^{2+}, cAMP and phospholipid derived messengers in coupling mechanisms of insulin secretion. *Physiol. Rev.*, 67: 1185–1248.

Rohner-Jeanrenaud, F. and Jeanrenaud, B. (1985) Involvement of the cholinergic system in insulin and glucagon oversecretion of genetic preobesity. *Endocrinology*, 116: 830–834.

Russell, R.C.G., Thomson, J.P.S. and Bloom, S.R. (1974) The effect of truncal and selective vagotomy on the release of pancreatic glucagon, insulin and enteroglucagon. *Br. J. Surg.*, 61: 821–824.

Sakaguchi, T. and Tamaguchi, K. (1980) Effects of vagal stimulation, vagotomy and adrenalectomy on release of insulin in the rat. *J. Endocr.*, 85: 131–136.

Sánchez-Andrés, J.V., Ripoll, C. and Soria, B. (1988) Evidence that muscarinic potentiation of insulin release is initiated by an early transient calcium entry. *FEBS Lett.*, 231: 143–147.

Schusdziarra, V., Bender, H., Torres, A. and Pfeiffer, E.F. (1983) Cholinergic mechanisms in intestinal phase insulin secretion in rats. *Regul. Pept.*, 6: 81–87.

Schwartz, T.W., Holst, J.J., Fahrenkrug, J., Jensen, S.L., Nielsen, O.V., Rehfeld J.F., Schaffalitzky de Muckadell, O.B. and Stadil, F. (1978) Vagal cholinergic regulation of pancreatic polypeptide secretion. *J. Clin. Invest.*, 61: 781–789.

Sehlin, J. and Täljedal, I.B. (1975) Glucose-induced decrease in Rb^+ permeability in pancreatic β-cells. *Nature*, 253: 635–636.

Sergeyeva, M.A. (1940) Microscopic changes in the islands of Langerhans produced by sympathetic and parasympathetic stimulation in the cat. *Anat. Rec.*, 77: 297–317.

Simon, C., Schlienger, J.L., Sapin, R. and Imler, M. (1986) Cephalic phase insulin secretion in relation to food presentation in normal and overweight subjects. *Phys. Behav.*, 36: 465–469.

Sjöström, L., Garellick, G., Krotkiewski, M. and Luyckx, A. (1980) Peripheral insulin in response to the sight and smell of food. *Metabolism*, 29: 901–909.

Skoglund, G., Lundquist, I. and Ahrén, B. (1988) Selective α_2-adrenoceptor activation by clonidine: effects on $^{45}Ca^{2+}$ efflux and insulin secretion from isolated rat islets. *Acta Physiol. Scand.*, 132: 289–296.

Smith, P.H. and Porte Jr, D. (1976) Neuropharmacology of the pancreatic islets. *Annu. Rev. Pharmacol. Toxicol.*, 16: 269–285.

Stagner, J.I. and Samols, E. (1986) Modulation of insulin secretion by pancreatic ganglionic nicotinic receptors. *Diabetes*, 35: 849–854.

Steffens, A.B. and Strubbe, J.H. (1983) CNS regulation of glucagon secretion. In A.J. Szabo (Ed.); *Advances in Metabolic Disorders*, vol. 10, Academic Press, New York, pp. 221–257.

Uvnäs-Wallensten, K. and Nilsson, G. (1978) A quantitative study of the insulin release induced by vagal stimulation in anesthetized cats. *Acta Physiol. Scand.*, 102: 137–142.

Wollheim, C.B., Siegel, E.G. and Sharp G.W.G. (1980) Dependency of acetylcholine-induced insulin release on Ca^{++} uptake by rat pancreatic islets. *Endocrinology*, 107: 924–929.

Zawalich, W.S. and Zawalich, K.C. (1988) Phosphoinositide hydrolysis and insulin release from isolated perifused rat islets. Studies with glucose. *Diabetes*, 37: 1294–1300.

S.-M. Aquilonius and P.-G. Gillberg (Eds.)
Progress in Brain Research, Vol. 84
© 1990 Elsevier Science Publishers B.V. (Biomedical Division)

CHAPTER 24

Prejunctional control of cholinergic nerves in airway smooth muscle exerted by muscarinic, purinergic and glutamergic receptors

Pål Aas

Norwegian Defence Research Establishment, Division for Environmental Toxicology, PO Box 25, N-2007 Kjeller, Norway

Introduction

The cholinergic parasympathetic nervous system exerts the dominant control of the airway smooth muscle. During the last few years it has been shown that the release of ACh from cholinergic nerve terminals in the airways is modulated by several different receptor mechanisms. Stimulation of some receptors reduces the release of ACh, while stimulation of other receptors enhances the neurotransmitter release (Aas, 1987).

There is at present good evidence for the existence of muscarinic autoreceptors on cholinergic nerves in airways in several species. In vitro experiments on bronchial smooth muscle from rat, where the transmitter output was measured directly, have revealed presynaptic muscarinic receptors, since oxotremorine reduced and scopolamine enhanced the release of ACh (Aas and Fonnum, 1986). Results from in vivo experiments in guinea pig and cat show that these autoreceptors are of the M_2 subtype (Fryer and Maclagan, 1984; Blaber et al., 1985). The evidence for the presence of these receptors was obtained in in vivo experiments using the selective cardiac muscarinic antagonist gallamine. Gallamine increased the transmitter output and thereby potentiated the effect of vagal stimulation. Gallamine had only small effects on the postjunctional constrictor response to injected ACh. Another new

M_2-specific antagonist, methoctramine, has recently been shown to display selectivity towards the cardiac M_2 muscarinic receptor (Melchiorre et al., 1987), but has not until now been used in experiments on airway smooth muscle.

Adenosine has been shown to decrease the release of many neurotransmitters both in the central and in the peripheral nervous system (for review see Snyder, 1985; Fredholm and Dunwiddie, 1988). There is general agreement that there are at least two types of receptor for adenosine. The receptors can be differentiated on the basis of the relative potency of a series of agonists (Londos et al., 1980). R-PIA (N^6-phenylisopropyladenosine) and CHA (chloroadenosine) are the most potent A_1 receptor agonists, whereas NECA (5′-N-ethyl-carboxamidoadenosine) is a more potent agonist for the A_2 receptor subtype.

The excitatory amino acids glutamate and aspartate function as important neurotransmitters in the mammalian central nervous system (CNS) (Curtis et al., 1960; Fonnum, 1984). Whether receptors for excitatory amino acids also exist in the peripheral nervous system in mammals is still a matter of discussion, but one recent report shows that NMDA receptors exist in the myenteric plexus (Moroni et al., 1986) and another that receptors for L-Glu are present in the respiratory system (Aas et al., 1989). Neuronal presynaptic receptors for excitatory amino acids in the peripheral nervous system have only been shown in the airway smooth muscle (Aas et al., 1989).

Material and Methods

Animals

Male Wistar rats (200–250 g) were used. The animals were given a standard laboratory diet and water ad libitum.

Physiological methods

Determination of bronchial smooth muscle contraction

The left and right bronchi were mounted in parallel as circular preparations on hooks made from cannulas (Aas and Helle, 1982). The organ bath contained Krebs-Henseleit buffer (50 ml, 37°C) of the following composition (final concentrations in mM): NaCl 118.4, KCl 4.7, $NaHCO_3$ 25.0, KH_2PO_4 1.16, $MgSO_4$ $7H_2O$ 1.19, $CaCl_2$ 2.6, glucose 11.1. The buffer was gassed with 95% O_2 and 5% CO_2 (pH = 7.4). For electrical stimulations the bronchi were mounted between platinum electrodes. The stimulation parameters were 20 Hz and 1.0 ms (supramaximal voltage) for 3 s at 40 s intervals. The preparations were given a preload of 1.0 g and were equilibrated for 60 min before the start of the experiments.

Determination of tracheal smooth muscle contraction

The rats were anaesthetized with urethane (1.5 $g \cdot kg^{-1}$ i.p.). The trachea was removed, tied into a tube, filled with Krebs-Henseleit buffer. The solution was gassed with 95% O_2 and 5% CO_2 (pH 7.4) and maintained at 37°C according to the method of Blackman and McCaig (1983). One platinum electrode was placed inside the tracheal tube and one outside for transmural stimulation. The stimulation parameters were 30 V (giving maximal response) for 5 s at 40 s intervals, 0.2 ms and 30 Hz. The preparations were equilibrated for 60 min before the start of the experiments. Contractions of the trachealis muscle were recorded with a Statham (P23AC) transducer as increases in internal tube pressure. Hexamethonium (50 μM) and indomethacin (1 μM) were present throughout the experiments. All drugs were added in a cumulative manner.

Determination of ACh release

Following decapitation the two primary bronchi were cut into pieces of approximately 1 mg wet wt. The smooth muscle tissue was superfused and stimulated by 51 mM potassium after previous incubation in 1.1 μM [^{3}H]choline chloride (10 $Ci \cdot mmol^{-1}$) for 60 min according to the method of Aas and Fonnum (1986). The release of [^{3}H]ACh was induced by raising the potassium concentration for 5 min. The concentration of sodium was reduced accordingly to keep the ionic strength constant. The superfusion medium had the following composition (in mM): NaCl 140.0, KCl 5.1, $CaCl_2$ 2.0, $MgSO_4$ 1.0, Na_2HPO_4 1.2, Tris-HCl 15.0, glucose 5.0. The media were continuously gassed with 100% O_2 (pH 7.4, 25°C). The radioactivity in the superfusion media were counted in 5 ml scintillation cocktail (Instagel).

Chemicals

Methoctramine was a gift from Dr. C. Melchiorre, Dept. of Chemical Sciences, University of Camerino, Italy. [*methyl*-^{3}H]Choline chloride, 80.0 Ci/mmol, was from New England Nuclear. All other chemicals were commercially available and of analytical reagent grade.

Statistics

Means and standard error of the mean (SEM) were calculated for all data. Student's *t*-test was applied to the results to determine significant differences between data groups.

Results

Muscarinic receptors

The muscarinic agonist oxotremorine (0.5 μM) reduced the Ca^{2+}-sensitive potassium (51 mM) evoked release of [^{3}H]ACh from cholinergic nerves in bronchial smooth muscle by approximately 20% (Table I). The antagonist scopolamine (0.3 μM), on the other hand, enhanced the release by about 33% (Table I). Neither of the drugs had any effects on the spontaneous release of [^{3}H]ACh.

The muscarinic M_2 antagonists gallamine and methoctramine enhanced the transmural nerve stimulation induced contraction of tracheal smooth muscle (Fig. 1). The two antagonists were approximately equipotent at a concentration of 0.6 μM. The muscarinic receptor was more sensitive

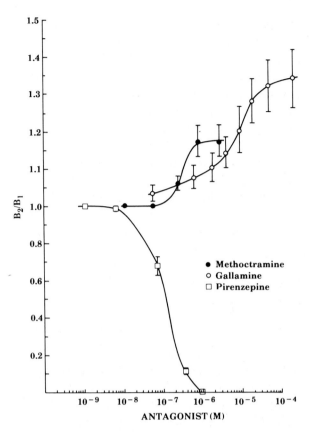

Fig. 1. The effect of gallamine, methoctramine and pirenzepine on the prejunctional transmural stimulation of the parasympathetic nerves in rat tracheal smooth muscle. The prejunctional effect is shown as an increase or decrease in the ratio B_2/B_1 where B_2 is the response after exposure to the muscarinic antagonists. Control responses (B_1, mmH$_2$O) to electrical stimulations were 104.4 $\pm$ 8.4 mmH$_2$O) for gallamine, 72.2 $\pm$ 11.5 mmH$_2$O for methoctramine and 73.7 $\pm$ 4.8 mmH$_2$O for pirenzepine. Results are expressed as the mean result $\pm$ SEM ($n = 5$).

TABLE I

The modulation of potassium evoked release of [^{3}H]ACh from cholinergic nerves in the rat primary bronchi.

Expt.	Potassium stimulation			
	1	2	3	n
A	100	80.3 $\pm$ 5.9 *	106.2 $\pm$ 5.5 ns	9
B	100	133.2 $\pm$ 11.3 ***	115.1 $\pm$ 11.6 ns	10
C	100	71.9 $\pm$ 5.2 **	84.3 $\pm$ 8.9 ns	7
D	100	44.6 $\pm$ 8.7 ***	122.1 $\pm$ 4.9 ns	10
E	100	102.1 $\pm$ 8.0 ns	108.2 $\pm$ 4.6 ns	8
F	100	131.0 $\pm$ 3.5 ***	161.0 $\pm$ 4.5 ***	12
G	100	154.0 $\pm$ 6.5 ***	173.0 $\pm$ 6.5 ***	6
H	100	116.0 $\pm$ 8.0 ns	123.0 $\pm$ 8.0 ns	9
I	100	99.2 $\pm$ 2.8 ns	105.4 $\pm$ 3.5 ns	9

The bronchial smooth muscle was stimulated three times consecutively, 40 (stimulation 1), 80 (stimulation 2) and 120 (stimulation 3) min after start of superfusion. The drugs were added 5 min before stimulation with potassium (51 mM, stimulation 2). A: Oxotremorine (0.5 μM); B: Scopolamine (0.3 μM); C: Adenosine (32 μM); D: Adenosine (100 μM); E: Adenosine (100 μM) in the presence of 8-phenyltheophylline (8-PT) (10 μM); F: NECA (50 nM); G: NECA (5 μM); H: NECA (5 μM) in the presence of 8-PT (50 μM); I: R-PIA (50 nM). The data in experiments A–E are extracted from Aas and Fonnum (1986). The responses are given in per cent $\pm$ SEM of the control stimulation with potassium (51 mM, stimulation 1), and corrected for the decline in [^{3}H] release with successive stimulations. Stimulations 1 and 3 are control stimulations with potassium (51 mM) only. *** $p < 0.01$, ** $p < 0.02$, * $p < 0.05$, $^{ns} p > 0.05$.

to inhibition by methoctramine than gallamine, but gallamine enhanced the transmural nerve stimulation to a higher extent (Fig. 1). The M_1-antagonist pirenzepine, on the other hand, reduced the contraction induced by electrical stimulation completely at a concentration of 1.0 μM (ID$_{50}$ = 0.1 μM) (Fig. 1). The muscarinic agonist pilocarpine reduced the nerve evoked contraction by more than 50% at a concentration of 10 μM (not shown).

Purinergic receptors

Adenosine and the A_2 receptor agonist 5'-(N-ethylcarboxyamido)adenosine (NECA) both had substantial effects on the release of [^{3}H]ACh. Adenosine reduced the release in a concentration-dependent manner and the effect was inhibited by 8-phenyltheophylline (Table I). NECA, on the other hand, enhanced the release of [^{3}H]ACh, and the release was concentration-dependent (Table I). The effect of NECA was also abolished by 8-phenyltheophylline. This inhibition was only seen in the presence of 8-phenyltheophylline, since a potentiation was observed during the third stimulation with potassium in the absence of the antagonist (Table I). R-PIA, on the other hand, had no effect on the potassium evoked release of [^{3}]ACh (Table I).

Glutamergic receptors

Previously, electrical stimulation was shown to induce release of ACh from the cholinergic nerves in the airways (Aas and Helle, 1982; Aas et al., 1986; 1988). L-Glutamate (L-Glu) specifically enhanced the electrically evoked contraction of bronchial smooth muscle (Fig. 2). The maximal increase in contraction by L-Glu was 104%. The concentration of L-Glu that induced a half-maximal response (ED_{50}) was 3.5 ± 0.1 mM ($n = 30$). Higher concentrations (> 22 mM), however, inhibited the electrical-field-induced contractions. L-Glu, in concentrations having presynaptic activity (< 22 mM), had no effect on the contraction induced by exogenous ACh. The concentration inducing half-maximal contraction (ED_{50}) and the intrinsic activity (α) of ACh were not changed (Table II). Atropine (1.1 μM) reduced the presynaptic effect of L-Glu by 32% ($n = 7$). The effect of L-Glu was not a result of enhanced levels of ACh due to inhibition of the acetylcholinesterase activity (not shown).

D-Glutamate (D-Glu), L-aspartate (L-Asp) and L-α-amino adipate (L-α-AA), however, reduced the electrical-field-induced contraction (Fig. 2). The reduction of contraction was 50% at 31 mM of D-Glu.

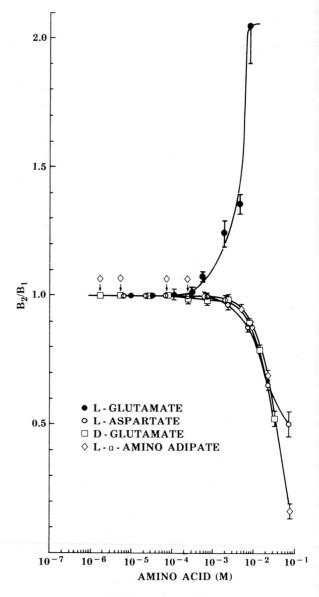

Fig. 2. The effect of L-glutamate, D-glutamate, L-aspartate and L-α-amino adipate on prejunctional transmural stimulation of the parasympathetic nerves in rat bronchial smooth muscle. The prejunctional effect is shown as an increase or decrease in the ratio B_2/B_1 where B_2 is the response after exposure to the amino acid. Results are expressed as the mean result $\pm$ SEM of 23, 10, 4 and 3 experiments respectively.

Neither of the antagonists L-glutamic acid diethyl ester (L-GDEE) (1.0 mM, $n = 6$) and 2-amino-5-phosphonovalerate (DL-APV) (20 μM and 1.0 mM, $n = 6$) had any effects on L-Glu-en-

TABLE II

Apparent affinity (ED_{50}) and intrinsic activity (α) of ACh in the absence and presence of L-glutamate (L-Glu)

	ED_{50} (μM)	α
Control	63 ± 35	1.00
L-Glu (8.6 mM)	69 ± 35 ns	1.12 ± 0.08 ns
L-Glu (62.0 mM)	85 ± 42 ns	1.21 ± 0.08 *

The results are expressed as the mean $\pm$ SEM of 6 experiments. * $p < 0.05$; [ns] $p > 0.05$.

hanced or L-Asp-reduced electrical-field-induced contraction. The apparent affinity (ED_{50}) and intrinsic activity (α) of L-Glu was not changed (not shown). NMDA, kainate and quisqualate had no effects on the bronchial smooth muscle or on the electrically induced contractions in concentrations up to 1–10 mM (not shown).

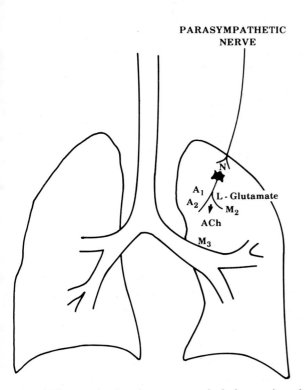

PARASYMPATHETIC
NERVE

A_1
A_2
L-Glutamate
M_2
ACh
M_3

Fig. 3. Diagram showing the parasympathetic innervation of the airways including possible receptors of importance for regulation of the cholinergic nerves in the airway smooth muscle.

Discussion

The present paper gives evidence for specific prejunctional receptors on cholinergic nerve terminals in the airway smooth muscle, which modulate the release of ACh. Muscarinic M_2, purinergic A_1 and A_2 and specific L-Glu receptors are functional receptors present on the nerve terminals, as illustrated in Fig. 3.

Muscarinic receptors

Presynaptic muscarinic receptors have been shown to be present in guinea pig myenteric plexus (Kilbinger and Wessler, 1980; Alberts et al., 1982), rat hippocampus (Nordström and Bartfai, 1980) as well as in rat airway smooth muscle (Aas and Fonnum, 1986) by the use of non-specific agonists and antagonists, such as oxotremorine and scopolamine, respectively. The classification of the muscarinic receptors has been complicated by the fact that there are no drugs which are specific for the presynaptic muscarinic receptor with no effect on the postsynaptic muscarinic receptor. The M_2 muscarinic receptor antagonist gallamine has, however, been shown to inhibit prejunctional muscarinic receptors in lung in vivo at doses which are several-fold lower than for postjunctional muscarinic receptors (Fryer and Maclagan, 1984; Blaber et al., 1985; Faulkner et al., 1986). The in vitro potentiation of the electrically evoked smooth muscle contraction by gallamine might be due to blockade of prejunctional M_2 receptors and thereby enhancement of the release of ACh. Similar results were obtained in rat airways (this paper) with the newly synthesized M_2-antagonist methoctramine, which was shown to be potent in myocardium in functional studies (Melchiorre et al., 1987) as well as in receptor binding studies (Michel and Whiting, 1988). The muscarinic agonist pilocarpine, which reduced the field-evoked contraction, provided further evidence for the presynaptic muscarinic receptor in agreement with previous reports (Blaber et al., 1985; Faulkner et al., 1986).

The results of the experiments in which the M_1 muscarinic antagonist pirenzepine inhibited the electrically evoked contraction instead of enhancing the contraction illustrates that it is not M_1, but M_2 receptors which are present on the cholinergic nerve terminals.

Purinergic receptors

The presynaptic effects of adenosine and NECA on the potassium-evoked release of $[^3H]ACh$ suggest that there are both A_1 and A_2 8-phenyltheophylline sensitive receptors on the cholinergic nerve terminals in airway smooth muscle. Previous studies have also shown the presynaptic effect of adenosine in other tissues (Fredholm and Hedquist, 1980), but the existence of presynaptic A_2 receptors which enhance the release of ACh upon stimulation has not previously been described. R-PIA, however, did not reveal the presence of an A_1 presynaptic receptor as described in other tissues in earlier work (for review see Fredholm and Dunwiddie, 1988). In spite of this lack of effect by R-PIA, the inhibition of $[^3H]ACh$ potassium-evoked release by adenosine in the airway smooth muscle has to be due to stimulation of a prejunctional receptor different from the A_2 receptor, since the A_2 agonist NECA potentiated the release of $[^3H]ACh$. It is interesting to note that adenosine and NECA have opposite effects. Whether this is of significant physiological importance is not clear, but the results might be of importance in the context of developing specific drugs which reduce the release of ACh and thereby the symptoms of obstructive lung diseases induced by ACh.

Glutamergic receptors

The results reported here provide evidence for a specific effect of L-Glu on peripheral cholinergic nerves. Although receptors for excitatory amino acids have been proposed to exist in the guinea pig myenteric plexus (Moroni et al., 1986), these receptors are of the NMDA type and not specific for L-Glu, as was seen in rat bronchial smooth muscle. The bronchial L-Glu receptor was not antagonized by the NMDA antagonist APV or the quisqualate receptor antagonist GDEE, which gives evidence that the receptor is different from the NMDA receptor in the guinea pig.

The stereoselectivity of the L-Glu receptor was shown by the fact that only L-Glu, and not the stereoisomer D-Glu, potentiated the electrical-field-induced contractions. Such a specificity has previously not been described for the L-Glu receptor. Furthermore, L-aspartate and L-α-amino adipate, which gave the opposite effect to L-Glu and reduced the release of ACh, provided further evidence for a specific excitatory receptor for L-Glu. The prejunctional location of this receptor was shown in experiments in which L-Glu had no effect on the application of exogenous ACh.

The possible involvement of this receptor in the "Chinese Restaurant Syndrome" is of particular interest, since the dose of glutamate that causes asthmatic symptoms in humans, 1.5–12 g per os (Schaumburg et al., 1969), corresponds to a systemic concentration of 0.1–1.0 mM glutamate. This is close to the concentrations of L-Glu that caused contraction in our experiments. Furthermore, Schaumburg reported that it was only the L-form that induced symptoms in their subjects, which is also in agreement with the present experiments. The symptoms of this syndrome could therefore well be explained by the effect of L-Glu.

Conclusions

The nerve terminals of the parasympathetic nerves innervating the airway smooth muscle are regulated by ACh, adenosine and by the excitatory amino acid L-Glu. Modulation of the ACh release by the prejunctional receptor mechanisms for these neurotransmitters may therefore alter the release of ACh and thereby the tonus of the airway smooth muscle. Alterations of these physiological regulatory mechanisms might have important implications in several diseases of the respiratory system.

References

Aas, P. (1987) Modulation of the cholinergic mechanisms in bronchial smooth muscle. In M.J. Dowdall and J.N. Hawthorne (Eds.), *Cellular and Molecular Basis for Cholinergic Function,* Ellis Horwood Ltd., Chichester, U.K., pp. 180–187.

Aas, P. and Fonnum, F. (1986) Presynaptic inhibition of acetylcholine release. *Acta Physiol. Scand.,* 127: 335–342.

Aas, P. and Helle, K.B. (1982) Neurotensin receptors in the rat bronchi. *Regul. Peptides,* 3: 405–413.

Aas, P., Veiteberg, T. and Fonnum, F. (1986) In vitro effects of soman on bronchial smooth muscle. *Biochem. Pharmacol.,* 35, 11, 1793–1799.

Aas, P., Malmei, T. and Fonnum, F. (1987) The effect of soman on potassium evoked [^{3}H]acetylcholine release in the isolated rat bronchi. *Pharmacol. Toxicol.,* 60, 206–209.

Aas, P., Walday, P., Tansø, R. and Fonnum, F. (1988) The effect of acetylcholinesterase-inhibition on the tonus of guinea-pig bronchial smooth muscle. *Biochem. Pharmacol.,* 37, 21, 4211–4216.

Aas, P., Tansø, R. and Fonnum, F. (1989) Stimulation of peripheral cholinergic nerves by glutamate indicates a new peripheral glutamate receptor. *Eur. J. Pharmacol.,* 164, 93–102.

Alberts, P., Bartfai, T. and Stjärne, L. (1982) The effects of atropine on [^{3}H]acetylcholine secretion from guinea pig myenteric plexus evoked electrically or by high potassium. *J. Physiol.,* 329, 93–112.

Blaber, L.C., Fryer, A.D. and Maclagan, J. (1985) Neuronal muscarinic receptors attenuate vagally-induced contraction of feline bronchial smooth muscle. *Br. J. Pharmacol.,* 86: 723–728.

Blackman, J.G. and McCaig, D.J. (1983) Studies on an isolated innervated preparation of guinea-pig trachea. *Br. J. Pharmacol.,* 80: 703–710.

Curtis, D.R., Phillis, J.W. and Watkins, J.C. (1960) The chemical excitation of spinal neurons by certain acidic amino acids. *J. Physiol.,* 150: 656–682.

Faulkner, D., Fryer, A.D. and Maclagan, J. (1986) Postganglionic muscarinic inhibitory receptors in pulmonary para-sympathetic nerves in the guinea pig. *Br. J. Pharmacol.,* 88: 181–187.

Fonnum, F. (1984) Glutamate: a neurotransmitter in the mammalian brain. *J. Neurochem.,* 42: 1–11.

Fredholm, B.B. and Dunwiddie, T.V. (1988) How does adenosine inhibit transmitter release? *Trends Pharmacol. Sci.,* 9: 130–134.

Fredholm, B.B. and Hedquist, P. (1980) Modulation of neurotransmission by purine nucleotides and nucleosides. *Biochem. Pharmacol.,* 29: 1635–1643.

Fryer, A.D. and Maclagan, J. (1984) Muscarinic inhibitory receptors in pulmonary parasympathetic nerves in the guinea pig. *Br. J. Pharmacol.,* 83: 973–978.

Kilbinger, H. and Wessler, I. (1980) Pre- and postsynaptic effects of muscarinic agonists in the guinea pig ileum. *Naunyn Schmiedeberg's Arch. Pharmacol.,* 314: 259–266.

Londos, C., Cooper, D.M.F. and Wolff, J. (1980) Subclasses of external adenosine receptors. *Proc. Natl. Acad. Sci. USA,* 77: 5, 2551–2554.

Melchiorre, C., Angeli, P., Lambrecht, G., Mutschler, E., Picchio, M.T. and Wess, M.T. (1987) Antimuscarinic action of methoctramine, a new cardioselective M-2 muscarinic antagonist, alone and in combination with atropine and gallamine. *Eur. J. Pharmacol.,* 144: 117–124.

Mitchel, A.D. and Whiting, R.L. (1988) Methoctramine, a polymethylene tetramine, differentiates three subtypes of muscarinic receptor in direct binding studies. *Eur. J. Pharmacol.,* 145: 61–66.

Moroni, F., Luzzi, S., Franchi-Micheli, S. and Zilletti, L. (1986) The presence of N-methyl-D-aspartate type receptors for glutamic acid in the guinea pig myenteric plexus. *Neurosci. Lett.,* 68: 57–62.

Nordström, Ö. and Bartfai, T. (1980) Muscarinic autoreceptors regulates acetylcholine release in rat hippocampus: in vitro evidence. *Acta Physiol. Scand.,* 108, 347–353.

Schaumburg, H.H., Byck, R., Gerstl, B.R. and Mashman, J.H. (1969) Monosodium L-glutamate: its pharmacology and role in the Chinese restaurant syndrome. *Science,* 163, 826–828.

Snyder, S.H. (1985) Adenosine as a neuromodulator. *Annu. Rev. Neurosci.,* 8, 103–124.

S.-M. Aquilonius and P.-G. Gillberg (Eds.)
Progress in Brain Research, Vol. 84
© 1990 Elsevier Science Publishers B.V. (Biomedical Division)

CHAPTER 25

Future prospects in muscarinic cholinergic pharmacology. Outstanding problems and promises

Tamas Bartfai [1] and Herbert Ladinsky [2]

[1] *Department of Biochemistry, Arrhenius Laboratories, University of Stockholm, S-106 91 Stockholm, Sweden, and* [2] *Department of Biochemistry, Istituto De Angeli, Boehringer Ingelheim Italia, 20139 Milan, Italy*

Introduction

The coming years will witness the refinement of existing drug therapies and implementation of new ones utilizing cholinergic agents and/or agents that affect cholinergic neurotransmission. The main reasons for this optimism lie in three types of discovery made in recent years.

I. Several subtypes of muscarinic receptor have been discovered with promise of more to come.

II. Different effector systems which are controlled by cholinergic receptors are being identified and the mode of their cholinergic control is being elucidated.

III. The coexistence of acetylcholine with different cotransmitters, mainly peptides, throughout the CNS and PNS is continually being discovered, so that co-storage of neurotransmitters in nerve terminals will soon be the rule rather than the exception. Undoubtedly these advances can be used in the development of specific and efficacious drugs with fewer side effects than those of today.

The realm of genetic engineering and the possibilities and disadvantages of gene therapies will not be discussed here.

Recent developments

I. The impact of the identification of subtypes of muscarinic receptors on cholinergic pharmacology is easily understandable in view of the widespread nature of the cholinergic innervation in the CNS and PNS. The distribution of the five known muscarinic receptor subtype clones in central and peripheral tissue, potential targets for selective drug action, is shown in Table I. The distinction between, for example, heart specific, glandular type muscarinic and brain muscarinic receptors will certainly improve cholinergic pharmacology of cardiovascular and exocrine control and treatment of certain movement disorders (cf. Chapter 21 of this volume). It can easily be envisaged that challenge of tissue membranes with the currently

TABLE I

Tissue distribution of mRNAs for the m_1–m_5 muscarinic cholinergic receptor subtypes determined by Nothern blot hybridization analysis

Tissue	mAChR subtype				
	m_1	m_2	m_3	m_4	m_5
Brain	+	+	+	+	−
G.I. smooth muscle	+	+	+	−	
Heart	−	+	−	−	−
Exocrine glands	+	−	+	−	−
Trachea	−	+	+	−	
Urinary bladder	−	+	+	−	

The data for m_1–m_4 subtypes were taken from Maeda et al. (1988) and for the m_5 subtype from Bonner et al. (1988). Although the m_5 was not detected in brain by Northern blot hybridization, it has been found in certain brain nuclei by in situ hybridization (Weiner and Brann, 1989).

available selective agents will unmask novel muscarinic receptor subtypes.

The ligands used today to distinguish between these receptors are all antagonists, and agonists with the same clear-cut profile have not yet been found with corresponding subtype specificities. It should also be noted that the allosteric binding site which, for example, binds galamine is not subject to the study it merits in terms of subtype specificity although it would undoubtedly make a good drug target. It is in fact reasonable to consider that neurotransmitter action at the receptor site could be modified allosterically by drugs acting at another point in the tertiary structure, thus modifying the conformation of the active site; in this way one can hope to modify agonist action by exogenous agents only at the location where the action is desired.

II. Identification of the cholinergic receptor-controlled effector systems and elucidation of the coupling mechanisms.

The muscarinic response appears to be mediated by the involvement of G_i or G_o type GTP binding proteins as transducing units between the agonist-occupied receptor and the effector systems. These transducers may couple the receptor to adenylate cyclase, to phospholipase C or to K^+ channels in different cell types. Several cell types exhibit muscarinic control of more than one of these effector systems and most of these muscarinic effects involve mobilization of Ca^{2+} from extracellular or intracellular sources and also a concomitant increase in cellular cGMP levels.

The tentative link between M_2 receptors and muscarinic agonist-mediated adenylate cyclase inhibition suggests that some degree of specificity of coupling of a given receptor subtype to a given effector system exists. This issue is, however, far from being resolved and some of the current approaches using stably transfected cells expressing only one subtype of muscarinic receptor may not provide unequivocal answers to which effector system this receptor subtype couples. Indeed, the number and type of G proteins present in the transfected cells, together with the specific phospholipid composition of their plasma membrane, may influence the coupling of the receptors to the effector system(s).

The more the information accumulates concerning the coupling mechanisms and the effector systems influenced by muscarinic receptors, the easier it becomes to mimic or to potentiate muscarinic actions by directly affecting these effector molecules.

The specificity of these pharmacological interventions is of course dependent on the uniqueness of the muscarinic control over the given effector in the given cellular response.

III. Coexistence of neurotransmitters. These approaches together with use of coexisting neurotransmitters mimicking agents may be useful while specific (and subtype specific) muscarinic ligands of agonist type are found. The approaches affecting effector systems will then be used together with methods to enhance the effects of the endogenous ACh by the employment of cholinesterase inhibitors and to enhance the effects of exogenous agonists by allosterically acting co-stored mimetics to regulate the muscarinic receptor.

The developments described above, although impressive, have evaded certain key issues of cholinergic neurobiology which will be restated here lest we forget them. More importantly these issues may bear on the next developments in cholinergic pharmacology and thus should be listed here as part of an attempt to review what may lie in front of us in the immediate future.

Outstanding problems

(1) The issue of presynaptic versus postsynaptic cholinergic receptors and the neuronal functions they mediate has not been investigated in depth by either pharmacological or molecular biological methods recently.

(2) Development of tolerance to chronic administration of muscarinic agonists, and development of supersensitivity upon chronic administration of cholinergic antagonists, although very important characteristics of the muscarinic cholinergic neu-

rotransmission, are not dealt with by current studies in molecular terms.

(3) The possibilities in the utilization of cotransmittors to acetylcholine at the muscarinic synapses are poorly understood and not studied in sufficient detail.

(4) The cDNA sequence information on receptor subtypes and the subsequent assignment of residues in the binding domain is only beginning to be used for predicting the ligand binding site and to assist in the design of drugs.

Conclusion

The establishment of cDNA sequences of the major cholinergic receptor types, of the cholin-esterases and of choline acetyltransferase does not close the chapter of cholinergic neurobiology and neuropharmacology, rather it provides a new start.

References

Bonner, T.I., Young, A.C., Brann, M.R. and Buckley, N.J. (1988) Cloning and expression of the human and rat m5 muscarinic acetylcholine receptor genes. Neuron, 1: 403–410.

Maeda, A., Kubo, T., Mishina, M. and Numa, S. (1988) Tissue distribution of mRNAs encoding muscarinic acetylcholine receptor subtypes. FEBS Lett., 239: 339–342.

Welner, D.M. and Brann, M.R. (1989) Distribution of m1-m5 muscarinic receptor mRNAs in rat brain. In R.R. Levine and E: Mutchler (Eds.). Subtypes of Muscarinic Receptors, The Fourth International Symposium, TIPS Suppl.

Cholinergic Mechanisms in the Central Nervous System

S.-M. Aquilonius and P.-G. Gillberg (Eds.)
Progress in Brain Research, Vol. 84
© 1990 Elsevier Science Publishers B.V. (Biomedical Division)

CHAPTER 26

Human brain cholinergic pathways

M.-Marsel Mesulam

*Bullard and Denny-Brown Laboratories, Division of Neuroscience and Behavioral Neurology, Harvard Neurology Department
and the Dana Research Institute of the Beth Israel Hospital, Boston, MA 02215, U.S.A.*

Introduction

The past decade has witnessed considerable advances in unravelling the organization of central cholinergic pathways. The availability of new anatomical methodology and the observation that cortical cholinergic innervation is markedly depleted in Alzheimer's disease constitute two important factors that have catalysed much of the recent progress in this field.

Acetylcholine is one of the most ubiquitous neurotransmitters in the mammalian central nervous system. Neuroanatomical experiments indicate that the cholinergic innervation of a given brain structure can be intrinsic or extrinsic. The innervation of the striatum, for example, is almost exclusively intrinsic and arises from cholinergic interneurons. In contrast, the cholinergic innervation of limbic structures, neocortex, thalamus and superior colliculus is predominantly extrinsic.

In the rodent, as much as a third of presynaptic cholinergic markers in the cerebral cortex originates from choline acetyltransferase (ChAT)-positive interneurons. Such putatively cholinergic interneurons may also exist in the fetal primate brain but apparently not during adulthood (Hendry et al, 1987). In the adult primate, it appears that the cortical cholinergic innervation is exclusively extrinsic.

The major cholinergic innervation for limbic structures and neocortex arises from four groups of cholinergic neurons in the basal forebrain; for

the thalamus from two cholinergic cell groups in the pontomesencephalic brainstem; for the interpeduncular nucleus (at least in part) from the medial habenula; and for the superior colliculus from the parabigeminal nucleus. In addition to these major pathways, there are also lesser cholinergic projections from the basal forebrain to the striatum, thalamus (especially the reticular and mediodorsal nuclei), and the interpeduncular nucleus; from the pontomesencephalic cell groups to the cerebral cortex and the superior colliculus; and from the parabigeminal nucleus to the thalamus.

The cholinergic cells that provide the major ascending projections to the cerebral cortex and thalamic nuclei are not entirely confined within traditional nuclear groups and they are also frequently intermingled with noncholinergic neurons. We therefore proposed an alternative designation of Ch1–Ch8 in order to specifically designate the major groups of cholinergic projection neurons (Fig. 1). According to this nomenclature, Ch1–Ch4 designate the cholinergic cell groups centered around the general area of the medial septal nucleus (Ch1), nucleus of the diagonal band of Broca (Ch2), nucleus of the horizontal band of Broca (Ch3) and the nucleus basalis of Meynert (Ch4); Ch5 and Ch6 designate the cholinergic cells centered around the pedunculopontine and laterodorsal nuclei, respectively; Ch7 designates the cholinergic cells in the medial habenula and Ch8 designates the cholinergic neurons in the

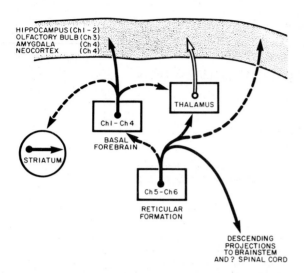

Fig. 1. Diagrammatic representation of some cholinergic pathways. The solid arrows indicate major pathways and the broken arrows minor pathways. The open circle and arrow indicate that the thalamocortical pathway is non-cholinergic.

parabigeminal nucleus. Ch1 and Ch2 are major sources of cholinergic projections to the hippocampus, Ch3 to the olfactory bulb, Ch4 to the amygdala and the cerebral cortex, Ch5–Ch6 to the thalamic nuclei, Ch7 to the interpeduncular nucleus and Ch8 to the superior colliculus. The Ch4, Ch5, Ch6 cell groups are particularly extensive in the primate brain. These three cell groups contain a compact center and also interstitial elements that extend into adjacent fiber bundles and nuclei.

The density of cholinergic fibers in neocortex and in thalamic nuclei shows major regional variations. For example, limbic and paralimbic areas of the cerebral cortex contain a far denser concentration of presynaptic cholinergic markers than immediately adjacent sensory association areas. These limbic and paralimbic areas also seem to be the only parts of the cerebral cortex that have substantial projections back into the basal forebrain cholinergic cell groups.

Of all the cholinergic cell groups in the primate brain, the Ch4 cell group, located predominantly within the nucleus basalis of Meynert, is the largest. This is in keeping with the marked cortical development in the primate line of evolution. On morphological grounds, the Ch4 complex in the monkey brain has been subdivided into anteromedial (Ch4am), anterolateral (Ch4al), intermediate (Ch4i) and posterior (Ch4p) sectors. The corticopetal projections from Ch4 display considerable overlap. However, each part of the cerebral cortex appears to receive its major cholinergic innervation from specific subsectors of Ch4. In that sense, the ascending projections from Ch4 to the cortical surface are topographically organized.

This information on the organization of cholinergic pathways has been obtained in laboratory animals and has been reviewed elsewhere (Mesulam, 1988). Recent observations are indicating that much of this organization is also shared in the human brain (Mesulam et al., 1983; Pearson et al., 1983; Nagai et al., 1983; Hedreen et al., 1984; Saper and Chelimsky, 1984; German et al., 1985; Mizukawa et al., 1986; Mesulam and Geula, 1988; Mesulam et al., 1989). The purpose of this report is to concentrate on the information that has been derived in the human brain, especially on the Ch4, Ch5 and Ch6 cell groups.

Human chemical neuroanatomy

Initial experiments with monoclonal antibodies to ChAT did not yield satisfactory immunostaining in the human basal forebrain. Subsequent immunohistochemical preparations based on a polyclonal antibody have demonstrated the existence of numerous ChAT-rich neurons in this region (Mesulam and Geula, 1988). We recently studied the constellation of cholinergic neurons centered around the nucleus basalis of Meynert (Fig. 2). In keeping with the nomenclature that we proposed for the monkey brain, these cholinergic neurons were designated as Ch4.

Concurrent histochemical and immunological staining demonstrated that all ChAT-positive Ch4 neurons also contained AChE. However, there is a small number of AChE-rich magnocellular cell bodies in the region of the nucleus basalis of

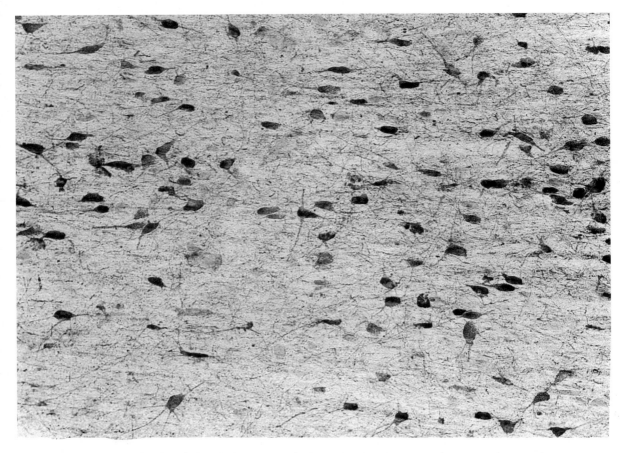

Fig. 2. ChAT-immunoreactive (i.e. cholinergic) neurons of the human nucleus basalis (Ch4). From a 76-year-old man. Polyclonal antibody, gift of L. Hersh. Magnification ×150 (From Mesulam and Geula, 1988).

Meynert which appeared ChAT-negative. Our observations show that approximately 90% of the magnocellular hyperchromic neurons in the human nucleus basalis are ChAT-positive and therefore belong to Ch4. The Ch4 complex of the human brain has a compact part that overlaps with the nucleus basalis of Meynert and numerous additional interstitial elements embedded within the adjacent fiber bundles such as the anterior commissure, inferior thalamic peduncle, ansa peduncularis, diagonal band of Broca, and the internal capsule.

On morphological grounds, the compact part of the human Ch4 complex could be divided into anteromedial (Ch4am), anterolateral (Ch4al), anterointermediate (Ch4ai), intermediate (Ch4i) and posterior (Ch4p) sectors. In addition to its larger size, it also appeared that the human Ch4 displays a greater level of differentiation than the Ch4 complex in the monkey brain. Previous observations had already noted that the nucleus basalis of Meynert shows a gradual increase in size and differentiation in the course of phylogenetic evolution (Gorry, 1963). Each hemisphere of the human brain contains approximately 200,000 magnocellular basal forebrain neurons, most of which belong to Ch4 (Arendt et al., 1985).

The human basal forebrain is cytochemically heterogeneous. For example, ChAT-containing Ch4 neurons of the nucleus basalis are intermingled with noncholinergic but NADPHd-positive neurons (Mesulam et al., 1989). Our observations show that some nucleus basalis neurons (e.g. those that are ChAT-negative and NADPHd-positive) do not belong to Ch4 and that some Ch4 neurons (e.g. interstitial ChAT-positive neurons embedded within the internal capsule) are located outside the traditional boundaries of the nucleus basalis. This cytochemical heterogeneity and the lack of confinement within cytoarchitectonic boundaries provide two of the most important justifications for the alternative Ch terminology.

Immunohistochemical observations in the reticular formation of the human pontomesencephalic region have revealed the presence of many ChAT-rich neurons. These neurons form two major complexes with a morphological organization very similar to the one described for the Ch5 and Ch6 cell groups in the brain of rodents and nonhuman primates (Mesulam et al., 1989). One of these cholinergic cell groups, corresponding to the Ch5 complex of other animals, reaches its peak density within the compact pedunculopontine nucleus of the human brain but also extends into the regions through which the superior cerebellar peduncle and central tegmental tract course (Fig. 3). The second constellation, designated Ch6, is centered on the laterodorsal tegmental nucleus

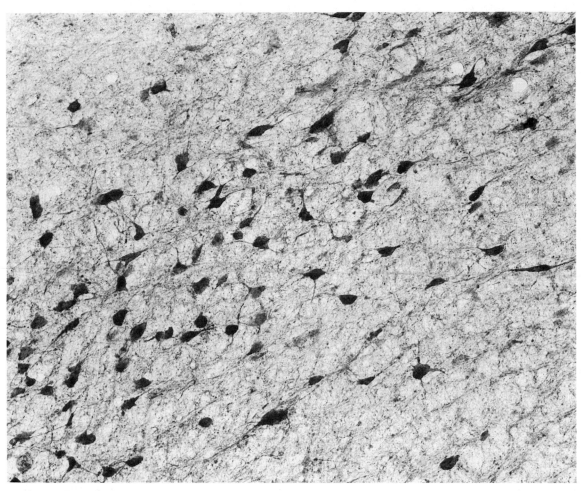

Fig. 3. ChAT immunoreactive neurons in the human pedunculopontine nucleus (Ch5). Same brain and same antibody as in Fig. 2. Magnification ×175. (From Mesulam et al, 1989).

and spreads into the central gray and medial longitudinal fasciculus. The two groups are related to each other in the form of partially overlapping constellations rather than discrete nuclei with firm boundaries. The Ch5 and Ch6 groups display a compact central core within the traditional nuclear boundaries of the pedunculopontine nucleus (pars compacta) and the laterodorsal tegmental nucleus, respectively. Both cholinergic cell groups also have interstitial elements that extend into surrounding fiber bundles. As in the case of Ch4, cytochemical heterogeneity is evident. For example, there is considerable intermingling of cholinergic Ch6 neurons with adjacent catecholaminergic neurons of the nucleus locus coeruleus complex. As in the basal forebrain, the lack of confinement within conventional nuclear boundaries and the cytochemical heterogeneity provide the justification for the Ch designation of these cholinergic cell groups. The majority of the basal forebrain and brainstem cholinergic cells are magnocellular and hyperchromic. However, the Ch4 neurons are considerably larger than those in Ch5 and Ch6.

The Ch4, Ch5 and Ch6 cell groups fit the description of "open" nuclei since their constituent neurons display considerable cytological heteromorphism, overlapping and isodendritic branching patterns and a propensity for extending into adjacent fiber bundles in the form of interstitial elements. These properties, shared by other cell groups of the reticular formation, support the suggestion of Ramon-Moliner and Nauta that the magnocellular cells of the basal forebrain (corresponding to the nucleus basalis and its cholinergic elements) represent a telencephalic extension of the brainstem isodendritic reticular core (Ramon-Moliner and Nauta, 1966).

The brainstem and forebrain cholinergic cell groups in the human brain share the cytochemical feature of being AChE-rich. However, there are also differences in the cytochemical signature of the individual cholinergic cell groups. For example, Ch5 and Ch6 but not Ch4 neurons are NADPHd-rich. Furthermore, all Ch4 neurons contain receptors for nerve growth factor (NGFr)

whereas Ch5 and Ch6 neurons do not contain immunohistochemically detectable NGFr. The NGFr is synthesized by the Ch4 perikarya and is transported anterogradely into the cholinergic axons that innervate the cerebral cortex. It is thought that Ch4 neurons require the trophic effect of NGF for survival (Hefti et al., 1986). This growth factor is synthesized by cortical neurons and binds to the NGF receptor molecules in cholinergic axons. The NGF-NGFr complex is then transported retrogradely to Ch4 cell bodies in the basal forebrain. The Ch5–Ch6 neurons display cytological features that are identical to those of Ch4 but do not require the trophic effect of NGF. The cholinergic neurons of Ch4, Ch5 and Ch6 also contain a number of neuropeptides. It appears that atriopeptin is present in almost all Ch5 and Ch6 neurons (at least in the rat) while calbindin and galanin are present in Ch4 neurons, at least in the monkey (Celio and Norman, 1985; Standaert et al., 1986; Walker et al., 1987). These overall differences in cytochemical signature probably influence the selective vulnerability of each cholinergic cell group to various physiological and degenerative processes.

Two kinds of experiments have been used to chart the anatomical organization of ascending cholinergic projections in experimental animals. One is based on the concurrent demonstration of choline acetyltransferase and retrogradely transported horseradish peroxidase. In another group of experiments, lesions in various cholinergic cell groups have been combined with subsequent histochemical and biochemical determinations of cholinergic markers at the target sites of ascending projections.

These approaches are not applicable to the human brain. However, some relatively indirect observations provide pertinent information. For example, patients with Alzheimer's disease show a profound depletion of presynaptic cortical cholinergic markers and also a loss of cell bodies in Ch4. There is a significant positive correlation between the extent of loss in cortical presynaptic markers and the extent of cell loss in Ch4. This indirectly supports the notion that Ch4 cells are the source of the corticopetal cholinergic innervation (Etienne et al., 1986).

In many cases of Alzheimer's disease, the depletion of cortical cholinergic markers is very widespread and uniformly severe. Such cases are not very useful for studying the topography of corticopetal projections from Ch4. However, in some patients, the loss of presynaptic cholinergic markers is relatively selective. In such cases, it becomes possible to match the topography of cholinergic depletion in the cerebral cortex with the topography of cell loss in Ch4. For example, we described two cases in whom the cell loss in Ch4 was unevenly distributed (Mesulam and Geula, 1988). In these patients, the cell loss in Ch4 was greatest (80–88%) in the posterior sector of Ch4 (Ch4p) and least (20–54%) in its anterior sector (Ch4a). Experiments based on retrograde transport combined with ChAT immunohistochemistry in the monkey had shown that Ch4p provides the major cholinergic innervation for the superior temporal gyrus and temporopolar cortex, whereas Ch4a provides the major cholinergic input for frontoparietal opercular cortex, the amygdala, and medial frontoparietal cortex (Mesulam et al., 1983; 1986b). Of these regions, sections from temporopolar and opercular cortex were available in these two cases of Alzheimer's disease and were stained with a sensitive acetylcholinesterase histochemical method that allowed us to count cortical AChE-rich (putatively cholinergic) axons. When compared to brains from age-matched, non-demented individuals, cholinergic axons in both cases of Alzheimer's disease were dramatically depleted in temporopolar cortex but virtually unaltered in the opercular cortex. These observations provide indirect support for the notion that the major cholinergic innervation of temporopolar cortex in the human brain is likely to emanate from Ch4p rather than from Ch4a, a conclusion consistent with the anatomical relationships that had been shown with experimental methods in the rhesus monkey. Many additional cases with relatively selective loss of corti-

cal cholinergic innervation will need to be studied in order to determine how closely the organization of ascending cholinergic projections from Ch4 in the human parallels the overall organization determined in the monkey brain. Brains of patients who have suffered structural damage to portions of Ch4 (as a consequence of stroke, tumor and so on) can also provide very useful information.

Ascending cholinergic projections from Ch5–Ch6 to thalamic nuclei have been demonstrated conclusively in several subprimate species with the help of retrograde tracing methods combined with immunohistochemistry (e.g. Hallanger et al., 1987). We assume that analogous projections exist in the primate brain but a definitive demonstration is yet to be published in either monkey or man.

There are major regional variations in the distribution of cholinergic projections to cortical areas and thalamic nuclei. Recent observations, based mostly on AChE histochemistry, have demonstrated that the regional variations described in

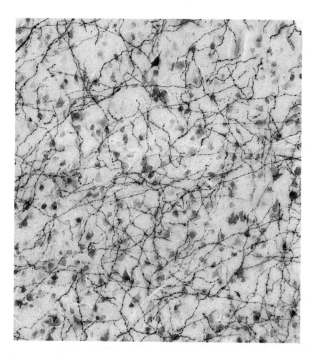

Fig. 4. AChE-rich (putatively cholinergic) axons in paralimbic temporopolar cortex in a 91-year-old man. Magnification ×162. (From Mesulam and Geula, 1988).

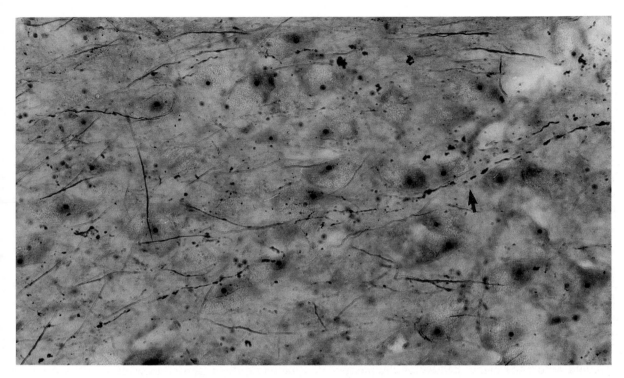

Fig. 5. This patient had a stroke which also damaged the uncus and amygdala. The brain was then processed with the Nauta method for the selective impregnation of degenerated fibers. The photomicrograph shows degenerated fibers (arrow) within the nucleus basalis, demonstrating the presence of a neural projection from the damaged uncal-amygdaloid area to the nucleus basalis.

the monkey brain also exist in the human (Mesulam and Geula, 1988). Our histochemical preparations in the neurologically normal human brain show that paralimbic areas such as the caudal orbitofrontal cortex, insula, temporopolar cortex, entorhinal cortex, and parts of the cingulate gyrus contain a more intense concentration of presynaptic cholinergic markers than immediately adjacent sensory association areas (Fig. 4). Core limbic areas such as the hippocampus and amygdala also display a very high intensity of cholinergic markers.

Experiments based on the anterograde transport of tritiated amino acids in monkeys, indicate that the major cortical input to the Ch4 region originates from a very limited set of regions, almost all of which belong to the limbic-paralimbic group of areas (Mesulam and Mufson, 1984; Russchen et al., 1985). It is unknown whether a simi-

lar organization exists in the human brain. We have examined the brains of two patients, one with a surgical lesion in the cingulate area and the other with a vascular lesion in the uncus and amygdala. In these brains, we detected anterograde degeneration (revealed with the Nauta method) in the region of Ch4. These observations, subject to all the caveats that are associated with axonal degeneration methods, indicate that the human Ch4 may also receive limbic and paralimbic input (Fig. 5). Many additional cases are needed, however, to determine if the type of selectivity demonstrated in the monkey is also present in the human brain.

Behavioral implications

Experimental observations in several species of animals have implicated central cholinergic pathways in the regulation of many behaviors including extrapyramidal motor control, arousal, sleep, mood, and especially memory. The relationship to memory and learning has attracted a great deal of interest. In humans, cholinergic antagonists cause a disruption of memory capacity (Drachman and Leavitt, 1974). In laboratory animals, basal forebrain lesions which deplete cortical cholinergic innervation cause memory impairments that can be reversed by the administration of cholinomimetic drugs (Flicker et al., 1983; Ridley et al., 1986).

The importance of cholinergic innervation to learning and memory may reflect several mechanisms. One possibility is that acetylcholine plays a special role in the cellular events that underly learning. For example, cholinergic transmission appears to play a direct role in the establishment of hippocampal long term potentiation (Tanaka et al., 1989). Alternatively, the influence upon memory could reflect the higher density of cholinergic pathways within limbic and paralimbic areas. Because of this selective concentration, cholinergic agonists may have a relatively greater impact on limbic and paralimbic parts of the brain, areas which are known to play a major role in the organization of memory and learning.

Based on an analysis of regional variations in cholinergic innervation, we made the suggestion that cortical cholinergic pathways could gate sensory information into and out of the limbic system (Mesulam et al., 1986). Many lines of investigation have shown that the transfer of information from sensory association cortex to limbic structures plays a pivotal role in memory and learning. Lesions that directly disrupt corticopetal cholinergic pathways, systemically administered cholinergic antagonists or disease conditions that involve basal forebrain cholinergic neurons may each interfere with memory and learning by disrupting this putative sensory-limbic gating mechanism.

The existence of a major cortical cholinergic depletion in Alzheimer's disease is well known (Bowen et al., 1976; Davies and Maloney, 1976).

Conceivably, cortical cholinergic fibers may have a special vulnerability to the pathology of Alzheimer's disease but it is unlikely that the cholinergic lesion is a prime mover in the pathophysiology of this complex degenerative condition (Mesulam, 1986). In addition to the cholinergic depletion, Alzheimer's disease is also associated with major neuronal and axonal degeneration in many limbic and association areas. These additional lesions can also underlie many of the behavioral changes seen in these patients. While the loss of cholinergic innervation undoubtedly contributes to the amnesias and other mental state deficits seen in Alzheimer's disease, it is not likely to constitute their primary anatomical substrate.

The ascending cholinergic innervation from Ch4 to cortex appears to be affected early and very severely in Alzheimer's disease. However, there is no evidence to favor a transmitter-specific vulnerability. For example, other cholinergic projections (including the intrinsic innervation in the striatum and the ascending projection from Ch5–Ch6 to thalamus) appear to be relatively spared. Furthermore, cholinergic innervation is only one of several corticopetal pharmacosystems involved in Alzheimer's disease. Just about every other widespread transmitter system that innervates cortex (e.g. serotonergic, norepinephrinergic) is also depleted, albeit to a lesser extent and probably not as early in the course of the disease (Mann et al., 1982). These are some of the reasons for suggesting that the prime mover in the pathology of this complex disease may originate in cortex and then cause retrograde alterations in cell groups that have widespread corticopetal projections. If there is a special relationship between Alzheimer's disease and the basal forebrain cholinergic neurons, this relationship may reflect the very widespread projections of these neurons to cerebral cortex, and perhaps their special dependency on cortically synthesized NGF.

The relationship of age to the cholinergic innervation of cortex is complex. Some investigators have reported a decline of cholinergic markers in the cortex of aging animals. Others have failed to confirm these observations. Some reports, including a few in the human brain, describe an age-related decrease in the number of Ch4 neurons while others suggest that the major alteration takes the form of a decrease in perikaryal volume rather than a loss in the number of Ch4 neurons (see Mesulam et al., 1987 for review).

We performed a semiquantitative study of AChE-rich (putatively cholinergic) axons in three cytoarchitectonic subregions of the human brain (Geula and Mesulam, 1989). There was an overall age-related decline in the density of these cholinergic axons but this was both modest and regionally selective. When we compared the density of these cholinergic axons from the second to the ninth decade of life, we found that the greatest loss did not exceed 20–25%. This contrasts sharply with the 80–90% loss that occurs in Alzheimer's disease. There was also some regional specificity to the age-related changes. For example, the changes in cingulate cortex were of much lesser intensity than those in entorhinal and inferotemporal cortex.

Aging is frequently associated with modest but clearly measurable deficits in memory function. Drachman and Leavitt (1974) showed that the administration of anticholinergic agents to young volunteers elicited memory impairments similar to those that arise during normal aging. These observations suggest that age-related memory changes may be caused by a depletion of cholinergic innervation. The very severe cholinergic depletion in Alzheimer's disease, the basal forebrain neuronal loss and the additional non-cholinergic degenerative changes (e.g. plaques, tangles), make it unlikely that cholinergic therapies alone will have a major impact in treating the mental changes. However, the situation may be quite different in normal aging where the cortical cholinergic depletion is modest, the basal forebrain cell loss probably absent and the additional degenerative changes relatively inconspicuous. These considerations suggest that cholinomimetic therapies may well reverse (or even pervent) age-related alterations of memory and learning.

Anatomical experiments show that the cortical input into Ch4 originates from limbic and paralimbic areas but not from other motor, sensory and association areas. Thus, most cortical areas have no direct feedback control over the cholinergic input that they receive whereas a handful of limbic-paralimbic areas are in a position to exert substantial monosynaptic control over their own cholinergic input and also over the cholinergic input directed to all other parts of the cerebral cortex. Because of this arrangement, the Ch4 group can act as a pivotal cholinergic relay for rapidly switching the physiological state of the entire neocortex in a way that primarily reflects the internal emotional and motivational state of the organism as encoded by limbic and paralimbic areas. This limited corticofugal control of widespread corticopetal projections is also a feature of other subcortical nuclei such as the nucleus locus coeruleus and the brainstem raphe nuclei. This skewed organization appears to be a key feature of brain structures that regulate behavioral states such as mood, arousal and attention (Mesulam, 1987).

While much has been learned about the organization of cholinergic pathways, much remains to be discovered. The human brain has a unique anatomy that underlies a behavioral repertoire not found in other species. So far our observations show that the overall plan of organization for ascending cholinergic pathways in the human brain displays many similarities to that of other primates. However, it is important to realize that the cholinergic pathways in the human brain may also possess distinctive and unique features. Much of the research in trying to reveal these finer details of human cholinergic neuroanatomy will depend on the fortuitous availability of appropriate cases, will not be as clear cut as animal experiments and will take a much longer time to conduct. Nonetheless, it is essential to obtain this information in order to understand further how this pharmacosystem is organized in the human brain, how it differs from the organization of cholinergic pathways in other animals and in what way these differences contribute to the unique behavioral repertoire of the human brain.

Acknowledgements

We thank Leah Christie, Kristin Loud and Annemarie Dineen for expert secretarial and technical assistance. Supported in part by the McKnight Foundation, Javits Neuroscience Investigator Award (NS20285), an Alzheimer's Disease Research Center Grant (AG05134) and the Alzheimer's Disease and Related Disorders Association (ADRDA).

References

Arendt, T., Bigl, V., Tennstedt, A. and Arendt, A. (1985) Neuronal loss in different parts of the nucleus basalis is related to neuritic plaque formation in cortical target areas in Alzheimer's disease. *Neuroscience,* 14: 1–14.

Bowen, D.M., Smith, C.B., White, P. and Davison, A.N. (1976) Neurotransmitter-related enzymes and indices of hypoxia in senile dementia and other abiotrophies. *Brain,* 99: 459–496.

Celio, M.R. and Norman, A.W. (1985) Nucleus basalis Meynert neurons· contain the vitamin D-induced calcium-binding protein calbindin-D 28. *Anat. Embryol.,* 173: 143–148.

Davies, P. and Maloney, A.J.F. (1976) Selective loss of central cholinergic neurons in Alzheimer's disease. *Lancet,* 2: 1403.

Drachman, D.A. and Leavitt, J. (1974) Human memory and the cholinergic system—A relationship to aging? *Arch. Neurol. Psychiatry* 30: 113–121.

Etienne, P., Robitaille, Y., Wood, P., Gauthier, S., Nair, N.P.V. and Quirion, R. (1986) Nucleus basalis neuronal loss, neuritic plaques and choline acetyltransferase activity in advanced Alzheimer's disease. *J. Neurosci.* 19: 1279–1291.

Flicker, C., Dean, R.L., Watkins, D.L., Fisher, S.K. and Bartus, R.T. (1983) Behavioral and neurochemical effects following neurotoxic lesions of a major cholinergic input to the cerebral cortex in the rat. *Pharmacol. Biochem. Behav.* 18: 973–981.

German, D.C., Bruce, G. and Hersh, L.B. (1985) Immunohistochemical staining of cholinergic neurons in the human brain using a polyclonal antibody to human choline acetyltransferase. *Neurosci. Lett.,* 61: 1–5.

Geula, C.G. and Mesulam, M-M. (1989) Cortical cholinergic fibers in aging and Alzheimer's disease: A morphometric study. *Neuroscience,* 33: 469–481.

Gorry, J.D. (1963) Studies of the comparative anatomy of the ganglion basale of Meynert. *Acta. Anat.* 55: 51–104.

Hallanger, A.E., Levey, A.I., Lee, H.J., Rye, D.B. and Wainer, B.H. (1987) The origins of cholinergic and other subcortical afferents to the thalamus in the rat. *J. Comp. Neurol.* 262: 105–124.

Hedreen, J.C., Struble, R.G., Whitehouse, P.J. and Price, D.L. (1984) Topography of the magnocellular basal forebrain system in human brain. *J. Neuropathol. Exp. Neurol.* 43: 1–21.

Hefti, F., Hartikka, J., Salvaterra, A., Weiner, W.J. and Mash, D.C. (1986) Localization of nerve growth factor receptors in cholinergic neurons of the human basal forebrain. *Neurosci. Lett.* 69: 37–41.

Hendry, S.H., Jones, E.G., Killackey, H.P. and Chalupa, L.M. (1987) Choline acetyltransferase-immunoreactive neurons in fetal monkey cerebral cortex. *Brain Res.,* 465: 313–317.

Mann, D.A., Yates, P.O. and Hawkes, J. (1982) The noradrenergic system in Alzheimer's disease. *J. Neurol. Neurosurg. Psychiat.,* 45: 115–119.

Mesulam, M-M. (1986) Alzheimer plaques and cortical cholinergic innervation. *Neuroscience,* 17: 275–276.

Mesulam, M-M. (1987) Asymmetry of neural feedback in the organization of behavioral states. *Science,* 237: 537–538.

Mesulam, M-M. (1988) Central cholinergic pathways: Neuroanatomy and some behavioral implications. In M. Avoli, T.A. Reader, R.W. Dykes and P. Gloor, (Eds.), *Neurotransmitters and Cortical Function,* Chapter 15, Plenum, New York, pp. 237–260.

Mesulam, M-M. and Geula, C. (1988) Nucleus basalis (Ch4) and cortical cholinergic innervation in the human brain: Observations based on the distribution of acetylcholinesterase and choline acetyltransferase. *J. Comp. Neurol.,* 275: 216–240.

Mesulam, M-M., Geula, C., Bothwell, M.A. and Hersh, L.B. (1989) Human reticular formation: Cholinergic neurons of the pedunculopontine and laterodorsal tegmental nuclei an some cytochemical comparisons to forebrain cholinergic neurons. *J. Comp. Neurol.,* 283: 611–633.

Mesulam, M-M. and Mufson, E.J. (1984) Neural inputs into the nucleus basalis of the substantia innominata (Ch4) in the rhesus monkey. *Brain,* 107: 253–274.

Mesulam, M-M., Mufson, E.J., Levey, A.I. and Wainer, B.H. (1983) Cholinergic innervation of cortex by the basal forebrain: Cytochemistry and cortical connections of the septal area, diagonal band nuclei, nucleus basalis (substantia innominata) and hypothalamus in the rhesus monkey. *J. Comp. Neurol.,* 214: 170–197.

Mesulam, M-M., Mufson, E.J. and Wainer, B.H. (1986a) Three-dimensional representation and cortical projection topography of the nucleus basalis (Ch4) in the macaque: Concurrent demonstration of choline acetyltransferase and retrograde transport with a stabilized tetramethylbenzidine method for HRP. *Brain Res.,* 367: 301–308.

Mesulam, M-M., Volicer, L. Marquis, J.K. Mufson, E.J. and Green, R.C. (1986b) Systematic regional differences in the cholinergic innervation of the primate cerebral cortex: Distribution of enzyme activities and some behavioral implications. *Ann. Neurol.* 19: 144–151.

Nagai, T., McGeer, P.L., Peng, J.H., McGeer, E.G. and Dolman, C.E. (1983) Choline acetyltransferase immunohistochemistry in brains of Alzheimer's disease patients and controls. *Neurosci. Lett.,* 36: 195–199.

Pearson, R.C.A., Sofroniew, M.V., Cuello, A.C., Powell, T.P.S., Eckenstein, F. Esiri, M.M. and Wilcock G.K. (1983) Persistence of cholinergic neurons in the basal nucleus in a brain with senile dementia of the Alzheimer's type demonstrated by immunohistochemical staining for choline acetyltransferase. *Brain Res.,* 289: 375–379.

Ramon-Moliner, E., and Nauta, W.J.H. (1966) The isodendritic core of the brainstem. J. Comp. Neurol., 126: 311–336.

Ridley, R.M., Murray, T.K., Johnson, J.A. and Baker, H.F. (1986) Learning impairment following lesion of the basal nucleus of Meynert in the marmoset: modification by cholinergic drugs. *Brain Res.,* 376: 108–116.

Russchen, F.T., Amaral, D.G. and Price, J.L. (1985) The afferent connections of the substantia innominata in the monkey. Macaca fascicularis. *J. Comp. Neurol.,* 24: 1–27.

Saper, C.B. and Chelimsky, T.C. (1984) A cytoarchitectonic and histochemical study of nucleus basalis and associated cell groups in the normal human brain. *Neuroscience,* 13: 1023–1037.

Standaert, D.G., Saper, C.B., Rye, D.C. and Wainer, B.H. (1986) Colocalization of atriopeptin-like immunoreactivity with choline acetyltransferase- and substance P-like immunoreactivity in the pedunculopontine and laterodorsal tegmental nuclei in the rat. *Brain Res.,* 382: 163–168.

Tanaka, Y., Sakurai, M. and Hayashi, S. (1989) Effect of scopolamine and HP 029, a cholinesterase inhibitor, on long-term potentiation in hippocampal slices of the guinea pig. *Neurosci. Lett.,* 98: 179–183.

Walker, L.C., Koliatsos, V.E., Kitt, C.A., Richardson, R.T. and Price, D.L. (1987) Galanin-containing somata in the nucleus basalis/diagonal band complex. *Soc. Neurosci. Abstr.* 13: 995.

S.-M. Aquilonius and P.-G. Gillberg (Eds.)
Progress in Brain Research, Vol. 84
© 1990 Elsevier Science Publishers B.V. (Biomedical Division)

CHAPTER 27

Cholinergic receptors in the rat and human brain: microscopic visualization

J.M. Palacios [1], G. Mengod [1], M.T. Vilaró [1], K.H. Wiederhold [1], H. Boddeke [1], F.J. Alvarez [1,*], G. Chinaglia [2] and A. Probst [2]

[1] Preclinical Research, Sandoz Ltd., CH-4002 Basle, and [2] Institute of Pathology, Department of Neuropathology, University of Basle, CH-4003 Basle, Switzerland

Introduction

More than 50 years ago Otto Loewi and Henry Dale received in the city of Stockholm the Nobel Prize awarded for their work on acetylcholine. Since then our understanding of the biology of cholinergic transmission has considerably advanced. The molecular characteristics of many pre- and postsynaptic components of the cholinergic synapse have been elucidated. The presence of all the elements of the cholinergic synapses in the human brain is well proved. Drugs acting on cholinergic pre- or postsynaptic mechanisms are known to affect human behavior. Alterations of cholinergic neurotransmission in the human brain have been correlated with a number of diseases including movement disorders, affective disorders and demential syndromes.

Dale published in 1914 his classic paper on "The action of certain esters and ethers of choline and their relation to muscarine" (Dale, 1914), describing the muscarine- and nicotine-like cholinergic responses. Although Dale was not familiar with the concept of the neurotransmitter receptor this work is the first description of the existence of

multiple cholinergic receptors: nicotinic and muscarinic. The research on these important sites has culminated in the recent past with the molecular cloning of the genes for several nicotinic and muscarinic receptor proteins (Peralta et al., 1987a,b; Kubo et al., 1986a,b; Bonner et al., 1987). These results have shown the cholinergic transmission to be much more complex than previously thought by the pioneers in the field.

In this paper we would like to review the advances in our understanding of the distribution of the cholinergic receptors in the human brain. We have used pharmacological and autoradiographical techniques to examine the anatomical and microscopical localization of cholinergic receptors and their alterations in the human brain. The main focus will be put on the muscarinic receptors. However, for the sake of completeness we will also review the available information on nicotinic receptors in the human brain.

Nicotinic cholinergic receptors in human brain

The nicotinic receptor (nAChR) was the first neurotransmitter receptor protein to be isolated, physically characterized, cloned and sequenced (Hucho, 1986). There is a wealth of pharmacological and electrophysiological evidence for the existence of multiple nAChRs. Ligand binding auto-

---

* Permanent address: Departamento de Farmacología Terapéutica, Facultad de Medicina, Universidad de Valladolid, E-47005 Valladolid, Spain.

radiography and the cloning of the genes of the different subunits of mammalian nAChR have confirmed these assumptions.

Initially, nAChRs were labelled with the toxin α-bungarotoxin (BTX) (Hunt and Schmidt, 1978). The development of other ligands, particularly [^{3}H]nicotine and [^{3}H]acetylcholine, has shown that the sites labelled by BTX in the brain are different from those labelled by nicotine and acetylcholine, suggesting that subtypes of nAChRs could exist. Autoradiographic studies in the rat brain have shown quite different localizations of the sites recognized by the toxin as compared to those recognized by nicotine and acetylcholine (Rainbow et al., 1984; Clarke et al., 1985; London et al., 1985). Furthermore, immunohistochemical studies with antibodies raised against different nAChRs have confirmed the existence of different nAChRs in the rat brain and their localization in distinct brain areas (Deutch et al., 1987; Swanson et al., 1987). Finally in situ hybridization studies using probes derived from the sequences of the mammalian nAChR have shown that the mRNAs coding for these receptors are expressed in different brain areas (Boulter et al., 1986; Goldman et al., 1986, 1987; Wada et al., 1988). In the rat brain weak signals for the α2 mRNA are visualized in the diencephalon contrasting with much higher expression of α3 and α4 transcripts in thalamic nuclei, especially in the medial habenula. Such studies have not yet been performed in human brain.

In the human central nervous system (CNS) the distribution of nAChR has been investigated using receptor ligand autoradiography with acetylcholine, nicotine and BTX as ligands (Lang and Henke, 1983; Gillberg et al., 1988; Adem et al., 1989). Adem and collaborators (1989) have used large cryosections of human brain to localize nAChR, using [^{3}H]nicotine as ligand. The areas containing high concentrations of nAChRs were the periaqueductal gray, putamen, substantia nigra pars compacta, cerebellum, occipital cortex and the dentate gyrus of the hippocampus. Lower levels of nicotine binding were observed in other cortical areas and in the caudate nucleus, in the pyramidal layer of the hippocampus and in the nucleus basalis of Meynert. Whitehouse et al. (1988) have reported that nAChR binding is reduced in Alzheimer's disease and Parkinson's disease. Using autoradiography these authors have found an important decrease of nAChRs in all layers of the frontal, temporal and occipital cortex. A loss of nAChRs in the nucleus basalis of Meynert has also been reported (Shimohama et al., 1986). These data are interpreted as an indication that nAChRs could be presynaptically located on the cortical afferents of the nucleus basalis. Thus, although the information on nAChRs in human brain is still incomplete, more and more data are accumulating, suggesting that these receptors could play an important role in the function of the cholinergic system in normal and pathological human brains.

Muscarinic cholinergic receptors

The mammalian brain is enriched in muscarinic cholinergic receptors (mAChR). Like the nicotinic receptors, mAChRs also constitute a family of related proteins. Initially the postulation of multiple mAChRs was based upon pharmacological experiments with compounds such as gallamine or the "atypical" agonist McN A 343 (see Palacios and Spiegel, 1986, for a review). These compounds presented selective effects on the heart or on the sympathetic ganglia without affecting other muscarinic responses. The presence of different mAChR subtypes was definitively established by the development of the tricyclic compound pirenzepine, a muscarinic antagonist able to block gastric acid secretion but without effects on the cardiovascular system (Hirschowitz et al., 1984). The results of radioligand binding investigations further supported the concept of multiple mAChRs which were classified as M_1: those exhibiting high sensitivity to pirenzepine, and as M_2: those showing low sensitivity to this non classical antagonist. The synthesis of new selective antagonists led to the postulation of further subdivisions of the muscarinic M_2 class ($M_{2\alpha}$, $M_{2\beta}$,

M_2/M_3) (Lambrecht et al., 1988; Doods et al., 1987). The existence of multiple homologous proteins corresponding to different mAChRs was definitively established by the cloning of cDNAs and genes encoding mAChRs (Kubo et al., 1986a,b; Peralta et al., 1987a,b; Bonner et al., 1987). Until now five different mAChRs have been cloned and sequenced from the human and rat genome (named m1 to m5). m1, m2 and m3 correspond to the pharmacologically defined M_1 (pirenzepine sensitive, enriched in the brain), M_2 (cardiac mAChR, with low sensitivity to pirenzepine) and M_3 (ileal receptor with intermediate sensitivity to pirenzepine, but also to other selective antagonists). There is no pharmacological correlate for the cloned m4 and m5 receptors at the present time. Using several approaches we have examined the regional distribution of the mRNAs coding for these receptors and the pharmacological characteristics of mAChR binding sites in different brain areas.

Regional expression of the mRNAs coding for the mAChRs

Synthetic oligonucleotide probes complementary to selected regions of the mAChR mRNAs have been used to analyse the presence of transcripts for these receptors using Northern analysis and in situ hybridization histochemistry. m1 mAChR transcripts were especially abundant in the neocortex and the hippocampal formation. Significant densities were also seen in the caudate-putamen. m3 and m4 mRNAs were found in the neocortex and in the hippocampus. While m3 transcripts were not detected in the caudate, m1 and m4 mRNAs were relatively abundant in this nucleus. m2 mRNA was particularly enriched in the pons and less abundant in other brain regions. More detailed information has been obtained by in situ hybridization histochemistry. Fig. 1 illustrates the presence of transcripts for the m1, m2, m3 and m4 mAChRs in coronal sections of the rat brain as visualized by this technique. We and others (Brann et al., 1988, Buckley et al., 1988; Vilaró et al., 1989) have shown that mAChR

mRNAs are present throughout the rat brain although differentially distributed. In the hippocampus high levels of hybridization signals were seen with probes for the m1 mRNA in the pyramidal and granule cell layers of the dentate gyrus. m3 and m4 mRNAs were also present in the pyramidal cell layer of the hippocampus but were less abundant in the granule cell layer. m2 transcripts were also detected in the rostral hippocampal formation.

Regional pharmacology of mAChRs in rat and human brain

We have used receptor autoradiography to examine the correspondence between the regional expression of mAChR mRNAs and the pharmacological characteristics of mAChR binding sites. Fig. 1 shows the sensitivity of N-[^{3}H]methylscopolamine ([^{3}H]NMS) binding to several muscarinic antagonists selective for different mAChR subtypes. [^{3}H]NMS binding to the hippocampal formation was blocked preferentially by compounds such as pirenzepine, hexahydrosiladifenidol (HHSD) and 4-diphenylacetoxy-N-methylpiperidine methbromide (4-DAMP) but less sensitive to the selective M_2 compound AF DX 116. In contrast as shown in Fig. 1, muscarinic binding to the superficial layer of the superior colliculus was readily blocked by AF DX 116 and HHSD but less affected by pirenzepine and 4-DAMP. In order to evaluate the affinities of these compounds more precisely full displacement curves were constructed by incubating serial consecutive microtome sections in the presence of the radioligand and different displacers at increasing concentrations. Autoradiograms were generated and quantified microdensitometrically. Such an analysis is illustrated in Fig. 2. The results showed that [^{3}H]NMS binds to sites presenting the characteristics of the M_1 receptor in CA1 area of the hippocampus while those in the superior colliculus showed properties of both M_2 and M_3 receptors.

In general the results of the regional pharmacological analysis are in good agreement with the

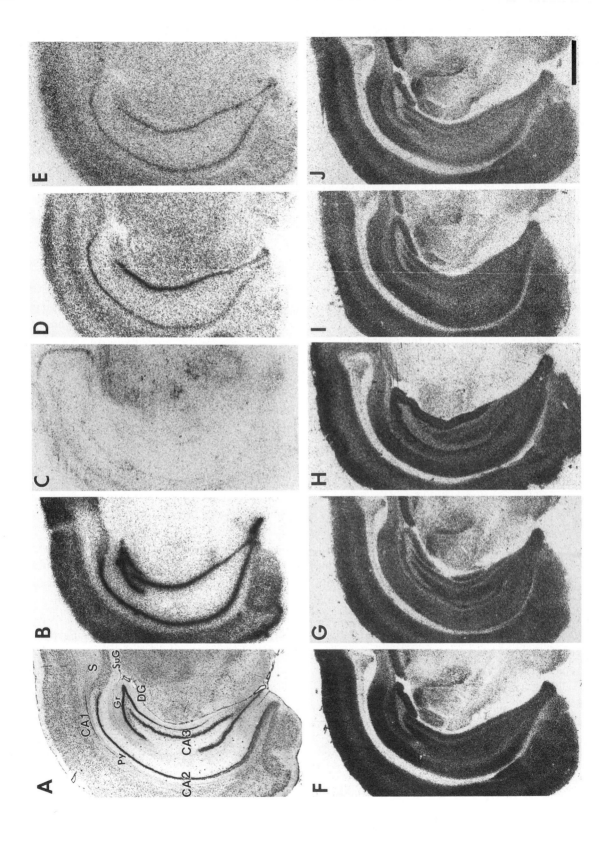

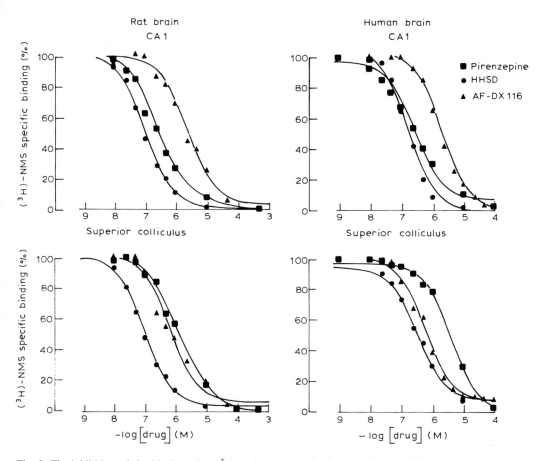

Fig. 2. The inhibition of the binding of N-[^{3}H]methylscopolamine by several muscarinic antagonists in two regions of the rat and human brain. The curves were generated from microdensitometric determinations of the competitions of [^{3}H]NMS binding by pirenzepine, AF DX 116 and hexahydrosiladifenidol. Note the reversed potencies of pirenzepine and AF DX 116 in CA1 field of hippocampus and in the superior colliculus in both rat and human.

Fig. 1. Visualization of the cells containing mRNAs for the different muscarinic cholinergic receptors subtypes in the rat hippocampus by in situ hybridization histochemistry and correlation with the distribution of muscarinic cholinergic receptor binding. (A) photomicrograph of cresyl violet stained tissue sections depicting the distribution of cell bodies in the rat hippocampus. S: subiculum. Py: pyramidal cell layer. Gr: granule cell layer. DG: dentate gyrus. SuG: Superficial grey layer of the superior colliculus. CA1, CA2, CA3: fields of the Ammon's horn. (B), (C), (D) and (E) illustrate the distribution of hybridization signal obtained with probes for the mRNA coding for m1, m2, m3 and m4 receptors respectively. (F) to (J) are photomicrographs from autoradiograms showing the distribution of muscarinic cholinergic receptor binding in tissue sections close to those used in the hybridization studies. (F) is from a section incubated with N-[^{3}H]methylscopolamine and illustrates binding to all types of muscarinic receptors. (G) shows the effects of pirenzepine (at 5×10^{-7} M concentration). Note the decrease in binding in the hippocampus but not in the SuG and other midbrain areas. (H) shows the effects of AF DX 116 (10^{-6} M), a preferential M_2 ligand. While binding to the hippocampus is little affected by AF DX 116 the binding in the SuG and midbrain is markedly reduced. (I) is from a section incubated with the radioligand in the presence of hexahydrosiladifenidol (10^{-7} M) which blocks binding in both the hippocampus and the superior colliculus, suggesting the presence of M_3 sites in the SuG. (J) shows the effects of 4-DAMP (10^{-8} M), which like pirenzepine preferentially blocked hippocampal binding. Bar, 2 mm.

distribution of transcripts for the different receptor mRNAs. The agreement is, however, not complete throughout the brain. For example, while the pyramidal cells of the rat hippocampus express the mRNAs for m1, m3 and m4 and, although at low abundance, for the m2 receptors, the properties of the sites labelled by [³H]NMS are consistent with a nearly homogeneous population of M_1 sites.

In the human brain Northern analysis has shown the presence of transcripts for m1, m2, m3 and m4 receptors. Pharmacological analysis of the characteristics of [³H]NMS binding in human brain tissue sections in the presence of selective displacers, such as pirenzepine, AF DX 116 and HHSD (Fig. 2) showed the presence of mAChR binding sites with the properties expected from M_1, M_2 and M_3 receptors. All these results taken together clearly indicate that four and probably five different mAChRs are expressed in the mammalian brain, including human brain. The regional distribution of these receptors in the human brain suggests that acetylcholine could regulate the functions of the different brain systems by acting on specific mAChR subtypes.

The distribution of muscarinic cholinergic receptors in the human brain and their alterations in neurological diseases

We have used quantitative receptor autoradiography to study the properties and distribution mAChR subtypes in the human brain (Cortés et al., 1984, 1986a, 1987; Palacios et al., 1986). In our initial studies we demonstrated that the properties of mAChRs in the human brain were comparable to those of the rat brain mAChRs (Cortés et al., 1986b). Because of the recent definition of further subtypes of the mAChRs the initial division into M_1 and M_2 receptors is no longer valid. The M_2 receptor population as defined by low affinity for pirenzepine can enclose other receptor subtypes. Thus, the previous studies do in fact encompass the distribution of M_1 and "non-M_1" mAChRs.

The highest densities of muscarinic M_1 sites were found in the basal ganglia, hippocampus,

substantia nigra and layers 2 and 3 of the neocortex. On cortical layers 4 and 6 the proportion of "non-M_1" sites was larger than that of M_1. The hypothalamus, substantia innominata and the substantia gelatinosa of the spinal trigeminal nucleus presented similar densities of M_1 and "non-M_1" sites. Finally, the thalamus, cerebellum and most nuclei of the brainstem contained receptors belonging predominantly to the "non-M_1" class. The distribution of the M_1 mAChR site has been confirmed using [³H]pirenzepine (Cortés et al., 1986b).

Receptor autoradiography is well suited for the analysis of pathological tissues, because it allows study of receptor and histopathological changes in the same tissue at the resolution of the light microscope. Receptor autoradiography has been applied to the study of mAChR alterations in human neuropathology.

Amyotrophic lateral sclerosis

mAChRs were first investigated in amyotrophic lateral sclerosis (ALS). Whitehouse and collaborators (1983) examined the binding of several ligands in the spinal cord of such patients. Of the receptors examined [³H]NMS binding showed the most dramatic change. The binding was substantially decreased in the ventral horn, especially in Rexed lamina IX which contains large motor cells. Reductions were noted in other laminae as well particularly in laminae II and III. Studies using carbachol to displace [³H]NMS from the "non-M_1" sites indicated that changes in ALS only concern the high affinity agonist mAChR sites. The loss of receptor binding was highly correlated with the degree of motoneuron loss. While a decrease of 75–80% in these neurons was found, the receptors were not decreased to that extent, i.e. reductions in mAChR were of 67%. The losses of receptors in ALS have been interpreted as a consequence of the death of motoneurons. Interestingly mAChR losses were also found in the dorsal horn (Whitehouse et al., 1983).

Senile dementia of the Alzheimer type

A loss of cholinergic innervation of the neocortex and hippocampus has been amply confirmed in Alzheimer's disease (SDAT). For this reason cholinergic receptors, both nAChR and mAChR, have been extensively investigated in SDAT. As the hippocampus is the most affected area in SDAT, the initial receptor studies were concentrated in this structure. The first autoradiographic studies revealed only weak alterations of mAChR densities in SDAT if any. Furthermore, no obvious correlation between the amount of receptors and the amount of senile plaques could be found. Receptor density over the plaques was comparable to that found in the surrounding neuropil (Palacios, 1982; Lang and Henke, 1983).

In a more detailed study, Probst et al. (1988) examined the correlation between mAChR density and the number of hippocampal pyramidal cells in a larger cohort of SDAT patients. The number of pyramidal cells per mm^2 in the CA1 sector was significantly decreased in SDAT cases as compared to controls, although there were large variations among cases. The most marked reductions in cell counts were observed in patients with a history of severe dementia. In contrast, the densities of muscarinic receptors, as well as the proportions of M_1 and "non-M_1" sites, were not significantly decreased. Furthermore, the ratio of muscarinic receptors per CA1 pyramidal cell was significantly increased in SDAT patients. This might indicate a possible upregulatory mechanism for muscarinic receptors in the population of remaining neurons in SDAT. However, there was a marked decrease in the concentration of mAChRs in few patients, without alterations of the M_1/"non-M_1" proportion. These patients had frequent extracellular remnants of neurofibrillary tangles (ghost tangles), but scarce neuritic plaques, and were those with most severe losses of pyramidal cells. These results suggest that compensatory mechanisms are no longer possible in cases with very severe neuronal loss.

Mash et al. (1985) found a selective reduction of M_2 ("non-M_1") receptors in the hippocampus in SDAT. This has been proposed to support a presynaptical localization of the M_2 subtype receptors on the terminals of cholinergic neurons.

Aubert et al. (1989), using [^{3}H]acetylcholine to label M_2 receptors have found a reduction of M_2 in SDAT. It should be mentioned that the density of M_2 receptors is extremely low, compared to the total density of mAChRs. M_2 sites account for about 30 fmol/mg of protein, while the total density of mAChRs is of about 500 fmol/mg of protein in the human hippocampus.

Huntington's chorea

Alterations on the density of mAChR have also been examined by autoradiography in several diseases affecting the human basal ganglia. In Huntington's chorea (HD) biochemical and autoradiographic studies have shown a marked loss (over 50%) of muscarinic binding in the caudate and putamen nuclei (Hiley and Bird, 1974; Wastek et al., 1976; Penney and Young, 1982; Whitehouse et al., 1985; Joyce et al., 1988). We have examined several cases of HD grade 2 and 3 and found decreased mAChR binding sites in the head of caudate and in the anterior putamen more so in the dorsal part (Fig. 3). Similar decreases were found in grade 2 and 3 (Fig. 4). In contrast, mAChR binding in the pallidum was not altered in grade 2 but significantly decreased in grade 3. The results obtained in the neostriatum suggest that a subpopulation of mAChRs is localized on striatal cells which degenerate in HD. However, as the loss of the mAChR is not in proportion with the degeneration of nearly 95% of the striatal neurons in grade 3 (Vonsattel et al., 1985), we have to admit that another subpopulation of these receptors are located on cells not affected by this process. In this sense it is interesting to mention that there is a selective survival of two populations of aspiny interneurons in HD, one containing somatostatin and neuropeptide Y and the other staining for acetylcholinesterase (Kowall et al., 1987). In schizophrenic patients chronically treated with neuroleptics the density of mAChRs in the basal ganglia has been found to be comparable to control patients. Thus, the neuroleptics are unlikely to exert any influence on this receptor type in HD.

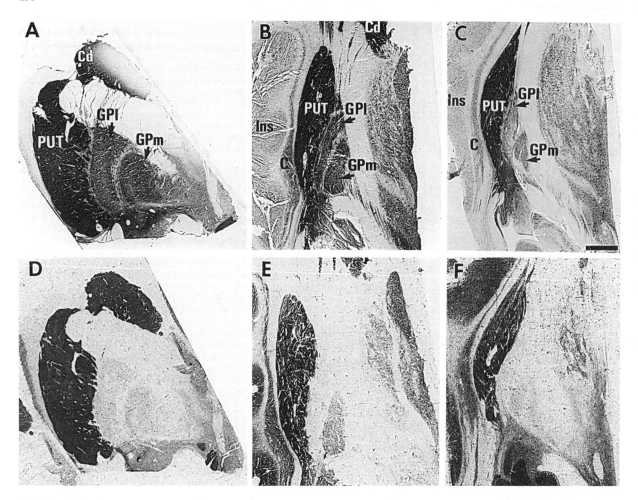

Fig. 3. Muscarinic cholinergic receptors in Huntington's chorea. (A), (B) and (C) are photographs from acetylcholinesterase stained sections from a control (A), a Huntington's Chorea grade 2 (B) and a grade 3 (C) case. (D), (E) and (F) are autoradiograms illustrating the distribution of muscarinic cholinergic receptor binding in sections adjacent to those shown in (A), (B) and (C) respectively. Note the decrease in muscarinic binding in the caudate (Cd) and putamen (PUT) in the Huntington's cases, and the preservation of this binding in the medial (GPm) and lateral (GPl) globus pallidus in the grade 2, and the decrease in grade 3. C: claustrum. Ins: insular cortex. Bar, 5 mm.

Parkinson's and Progressive Supranuclear Palsy diseases

In Parkinson's disease (PD) we did not observe alterations in the density of mAChRs in the striatum (Fig. 4). However, a significant increase in [³H]NMS binding was observed in the medial part of the globus pallidus. Interestingly, mAChRs were decreased significantly (Fig. 4) in caudate and putamen of patients dying from Progressive Supranuclear Palsy (PSP), a disease characterized, like PD, by decreased dopaminergic innervation.

In PSP the medial part of globus pallidus also showed increased binding of [³H]NMS. In this context it is worth mentioning that decreased numbers of cholinergic interneurons have been found by choline acetyltransferase (ChAT) immunocytochemistry in the neostriatum of the PSP, thus contrasting with normal ChAT reactive neurons in PD (Hirsch et al., 1989). The lack of cellular resolution of the autoradiographic technique does not allow for the identification of the striatal cells expressing mAChRs. Future studies

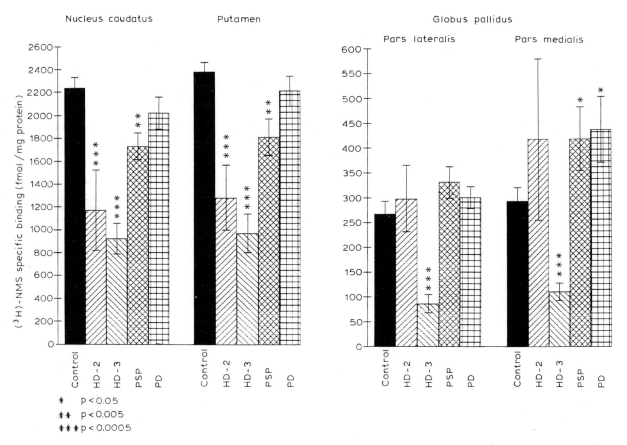

Fig. 4. Quantitative autoradiographic determination of the alterations in the density of muscarinic cholinergic binding in Huntington's disease grade 2 (HD-2), grade 3 (HD-3), Progressive Supranuclear Palsy (PSP) and Parkinson's disease (PD).

using in situ hybridization histochemistry or immunohistochemistry, once antibodies against these receptors are available, will be necessary to clarify this issue.

In conclusion, cholinergic receptors are well represented in the human brain with highly diversified regional distributions. Both nicotinic and muscarinic receptors are in fact families of several different receptor proteins. The heterogeneity of these receptors is much larger than previously suspected. Both nAChRs and mAChRs are involved in several diseases of the CNS. These results strongly support an involvement of the different cholinergic receptors in the function of specific brain areas. In the future it will be necessary to clearly establish the cellular localization of these receptors in the human brain. For that, the development of more selective ligands, of probes for the visualization of the mRNA coding for the different receptor subtypes and of antibodies, specific for the different receptor proteins, will be necessary. All these tools should provide the ways to clarify the distribution, localization and modification of cholinergic receptors at the cellular level. However, because most of the studies described until now have been carried out in postmortem materials, the understanding of modifications of cholinergic receptors in the human brain will require the development of ligands for the use of non invasive techniques, such as positron emission tomography, for the longitudinal study of receptor changes with the progression of diseases of the human brain.

References

Adem, A., Nordberg, A., Jossan, S.S., Sara, V. and Gillberg, P.G. (1989) Quantitative autoradiography of nicotinic receptors in large cryosections of human brain hemispheres. *Neurosci. Lett.,* 101: 247–252.

Aubert, I., Araujo, D.M., Gauthier, S. and Quirion, R. (1989) Muscarinic receptor alterations in human cognitive disorders. In, Subtypes of Muscarinic Receptors. The fourth international symposium. Wiesbaden, W. Germany. *Abstract* n° 4.

Bonner, T.I., Buckley, N.J., Young, A.C. and Brann, M.R. (1987) Identification of a family of muscarinic acetylcholine receptor genes. *Science,* 237: 527–532.

Boulter, J., Evans, K., Goldman, D., Martin, G., Treco, D., Heinemann, S. and Patrick, J. (1986) Isolation of a cDNA clone coding for a possible neural nicotinic acetylcholine receptor α-subunit. *Nature,* 319: 368–374.

Brann, M.R., Buckley, N.J. and Bonner, T.I. (1988) The striatum and cerebral cortex express different muscarinic receptor mRNAs. *FEBS Lett.,* 230: 90–94.

Buckley, N.J., Bonner, T.I. and Brann, M.R. (1988) Localization of a family of muscarinic receptor mRNAs in rat brain. *J. Neurosci.,* 8: 4646–4652.

Clarke, P.B.S., Schwartz, R.D., Paul, S.M., Pert, C.B. and Pert, A. (1985) Nicotine binding in rat brain: autoradiographic comparison of [³H]acetylcholine, [³H]nicotine, and [¹²⁵I]-α-bungarotoxin. *J. Neurosci.,* 5: 1307–1315.

Cortés, R., Probst, A. and Palacios, J.M. (1984) Quantitative light microscopic autoradiographic localization of cholinergic muscarinic receptors in the human brain: brainstem. *Neuroscience,* 12: 1003–1026.

Cortés, R., Probst, A., Tobler, H.J. and Palacios, J.M. (1986a) Muscarinic cholinergic receptor subtypes in the human brain. II. Quantitative autoradiographic studies. *Brain Res.,* 362: 239–253.

Cortés, R. and Palacios, J.M. (1986b) Muscarinic cholinergic receptor subtypes in the rat brain. I. Quantitative autoradiographic studies. *Brain Res.,* 362: 227–238.

Cortés, R., Probst, A. and Palacios, J.M. (1987) Quantitative light microscopic autoradiographic localization of cholinergic muscarinic receptors in the human brain: forebrain. *Neuroscience,* 20: 65–107.

Dale, H.H. (1914) The action of certain esters and ethers of choline, and their relation to muscarine. *J. Pharm. Exp. Ther.,* 68: 147–190.

Deutch, A.Y., Holliday, J., Roth, R.H., Chun, L.L.Y. and Hawrot, E. (1987) Immunohistochemical localization of a neuronal nicotinic acetylcholine receptor in mammalian brain. *Proc. Natl. Acad. Sci. U.S.A.,* 84: 8697–8701.

Doods, H.N., Mathy, M.J., Davidesko, D., Van Charldorp, K.J., De Jonge, A. and Van Zwieten, P.A. (1987) Selectivity of muscarinic antagonists in radioligand and in vivo experiments for the putative m1, m2 and m3 receptors. *J. Pharmacol. Exp. Ther.,* 242: 257–262.

Gillberg, P.G., d'Argy R. and Aquilonius S.M. (1988) Autoradiographic distribution of [³H]acetylcholine binding sites in the cervical spinal cord of man and some other species. *Neurosci. Lett.,* 90: 197–202.

Goldman, D., Simmon, D., Swanson, L.W., Patrick, J. and Heinemann, S. (1986) Mapping of brain areas expressing RNA homologous to two different acetylcholine receptor α-subunit cDNAs. *Proc. Natl. Acad. Sci. U.S.A.,* 83: 4076–4080.

Goldman, D., Deneris, E., Luyten, W., Kochhar, A., Patrick, J. and Heinemann, S. (1987) Members of a nicotinic acetylcholine receptor gene family are expressed in different regions of the mammalian central nervous system. Cell, 48: 965–973.

Hiley, C.R., Bird, E.D. (1974) Decreased muscarinic receptor concentration in post-mortem brain in Huntington's chorea. *Brain Res.,* 80: 355–358.

Hirsch, E.C., Graybiel, A.M., Hersh, L.B., Duyckaerts, C. and Agid, Y. (1989). Striosomes and extrastriosomal matrix contain different amount of immunoreactive choline acetyltransferase in the human striatum. *Neurosci. Lett.,* 96: 145–150.

Hirschowitz, B.I., Hammer, R., Giachetti, A., Keirns, J.J. and Levine, R.R. (1984) Subtypes of muscarinic receptor: proceedings of the international symposium on subtypes of muscarinic receptors. *TIPS,* Suppl. 1, January 1984.

Hucho, F. (1986) The nicotinic acetylcholine receptor and its ion channel. *Eur. J. Biochem.,* 158: 211–226.

Hunt, S. and Schmidt, J. (1978) Some observations on the binding pattern of α-bungarotoxin in the central nervous system of the rat. *Brain Res.,* 157: 213–232.

Joyce, J.N., Lexow, N., Bird, E. and Winokur, A. (1988) Organization of dopamine D1 and D2 receptors in human striatum: receptor autoradiographic studies in Huntington's disease and schizophrenia. *Synapse,* 2: 546–557.

Kowall, N.W., Ferrante, R.J. and Martin, J.B. (1987) Patterns of cell loss in Huntington's disease. *TINS,* 10: 24–29

Kubo, T., Fukuda, K., Mikami, A., Maeda, II., Takahashi, H., Mishina, M., Haga, T., Haga, K., Ichiyama, A., Kangawa, K., Kojima, M., Matsuo, H., Hirose, T. and Numa, S. (1986a) Cloning, sequencing and expression of complementary DNA encoding the muscarinic acetylcholine receptor. *Nature,* 323: 411–416.

Kubo, T., Maeda, A., Sugimoto, K., Akiba, I., Mikami, A., Takahashi, H., Haga, T., Haga, K., Ichiyama, A., Kangawa, K., Matsuo, H., Hirose, T. and Numa, S. (1986b) Primary structure of porcine cardiac muscarinic acetylcholine receptor deduced from the cDNA sequence. *FEBS lett.,* 209: 367–372.

Lambrecht, G., Moser, U., Wagner, M., Wess, J., Gmelin, G., Raseiner, K., Strohmann, C., Tacke, R. and Mutschler, E. (1988) Pharmacological and electrophysiological evidence for muscarinic m1 and m2 receptor heterogeneity. In R.R. Levine, N.J.M. Birsdall, R.A. North., M. Holman, A. Watanabe and L.L. Iversen (Eds.), Subtypes of Muscarinic

Receptors III, *TIPS, Suppl.,* February, Elsevier, Cambridge, pp.82.

Lang, W. and Henke, H. (1983) Cholinergic receptor binding and autoradiography in brains of non-neurological and senile dementia of Alzheimer type patients. *Brain Res.,* 267: 271–280.

London, E.D., Waller, S.B. and Wamsley, J.K. (1985) Autoradiographic localization of ^{3}H-nicotine binding sites in rat brain. *Neurosci. Lett.,* 53: 179–184.

Mash, D.C., Flynn, D.D. and Potter, L.T. (1985) Loss of m2 muscarinic receptors in the cerebral cortex in Alzheimer's disease and experimental cholinergic denervation. *Science,* 228: 1115–1117.

Palacios, J.M. (1982) Autoradiographic localization of muscarinic cholinergic receptors in the hippocampus of patients with senile dementia. *Brain Res.,* 23: 173–175.

Palacios, J.M. and Spiegel, R. (1986) Muscarinic cholinergic agonists: pharmacological and clinical perspectives. In D.F. Swaab, E. Fliers, M. Mirmiran, W.A. Van Gool and F. Van Haaren (Eds.). *Progress in Brain Research, Vol 70,* Elsevier, Amsterdam, pp. 485–498.

Palacios, J.M., Cortés, R., Probst, A. and Karobath, M. (1986) Mapping of subtypes of muscarinic receptors in the human brain with receptor autoradiographic techniques. *TIPS, suppl.1,* February, 1–5.

Penney, J.B. and Young, A.B. (1982) Quantitative autoradiography of neurotransmitter receptors in Huntington disease. *Neurology,* 32: 1391–1395.

Peralta, E.G., Ashkenazi, A., Winslow J.W., Smith, D.H., Ramachandran, J. and Capon, D.J. (1987a) Distinct primary structures, ligand-binding properties and tissue specific expression of four human muscarinic acetylcholine receptors. *EMBO J.,* 6: 3923–3929.

Peralta, E.G., Winslow J.W., Peterson, G.L., Smith, D.H., Ashkenazi, A., Ramachandran, J., Schimerlick M.I. and Capon D.J. (1987b) Primary structure and biochemical properties of an m2 muscarinic receptor. *Science* 236: 600–605.

Probst, A., Cortes, R., Ulrich, J. and Palacios J.M. (1988) Differential modification of muscarinic cholinergic receptors in the hippocampus of patients with Alzheimer's disease: an autoradiographic study. *Brain Res.,* 450: 190–201.

Rainbow, T.C., Schwartz, R.D., Parsons, B. and Kellar, K.J. (1984) Quantitative autoradiography of nicotine [^{3}H]acetylcholine binding sites in rat brain. *Neurosci. Lett.,* 50: 193–196.

Shimohama, S., Taniguchi, T., Fujiwara, M. and Kameyama, M. (1986) Changes in nicotinic and muscarinic cholinergic receptors in Alzheimer-type dementia. *J. Neurochem.,* 46: 288–293.

Swanson, L.W., Simmons, D.M., Whiting, P.J. and Lindstrom, J. (1987) Immunohistochemical localization of neuronal nicotinic receptors in the rodent central nervous system. *J. Neurosci.,* 7: 3334–3342.

Vilaró, M.T., Boddeke, H.W.G.M., Wiederhold, K.-H., Kischka, U., Mengod, G. and Palacios, J.M. (1989) Regional expression of muscarinic receptor (MChR) subtypes in rat brain: an in situ hybridization/receptor autoradiograhy study. In, Subtypes of Muscarinic Receptors. The fourth international symposium. Wiesbaden, W. Germany. Abstract n° 68.

Vonsattel, J.P., Myers, R.H., Stevens, T.J., Ferrante, R.J., Bird, E. and Richardson, E.P. (1985) Neuropathological classification of Huntington's disease. *J. Neuropathol. Exp. Neurol.,* 44: 559–577.

Wada, K., Ballivet, M., Boulter, J., Connolly, J., Wada, E., Deneris, E.S., Swanson, L.W., Heinemann, S. and Patrick, J. (1988) Functional expression of a new pharmacological subtype of brain nicotinic acetyl-choline receptor. *Science,* 240: 330–334.

Wastek, G.J., Stern, L.Z., Johnson, P.C. and Yamamura, H.I. (1976) Huntington's disease: regional alteration in muscarinic cholinergic receptor binding in human brain. *Life Sci.,* 19: 1033–1040.

Whitehouse, P.J., Wamsley, J.K., Zarbin, M.A., Price, D.L., Tourtelotte, W.W. and Kuhar, M.J. (1983). Amyotrophic lateral sclerosis: alterations in neurotransmitter receptors. *Ann. Neurol.,* 14: 8–16.

Whitehouse, P.J., Trifiletti, R.R., Jones, B.E., Folstein, S., Price, D.L., Snyder, S.H. and Kuhar, M.J. (1985) Neurotransmitter receptor alterations in Huntington's disease: autoradiographic and homogenate studies with special reference to benzodiazepine receptor complexes. *Ann. Neurol.,* 18: 202–210.

Whitehouse, P.J., Martino, A.M., Wagster, M.V., Price, D.L., Mayeux, R., Atack, J.R. and Kellar, K.J. (1988) Reductions in [^{3}H]nicotinic acetylcholine binding in Alzheimer's disease and Parkinson's disease: an autoradiographic study. Neurology, 38: 720–723.

S.-M. Aquilonius and P.-G. Gillberg (Eds.)
Progress in Brain Research, Vol. 84
© 1990 Elsevier Science Publishers B.V. (Biomedical Division)

CHAPTER 28

Physiological mechanisms of cholinergic action in the hippocampus

J.V. Halliwell

Department of Physiology, Royal Free Hospital School of Medicine, University of London, Rowland Hill Street, London NW3 2PF, U.K.

Introduction

The hippocampus contains high levels of acetylcholine (ACh). Most of this is contained in the terminals of afferent fibres originating in the septal/diagonal band nuclear complex of the ventral forebrain (Wainer et al., 1985; see Chapter 26 of this volume). Although this input is generally referred to as a cholinergic pathway, it is clear that the fibres can contain other neuroactive substances, such as galanin (see Chapter 30 of this volume). Mingled amongst the principal cells of the hippocampus are a small proportion of ACh-containing cells (Frotscher and Leranth, 1985). Neurochemical studies have reported release of ACh from the hippocampus following septal stimulation (Smith, 1974; Dudar, 1975). Taken together with the identification of high levels of the enzymes for ACh synthesis [cholineacetyltransferase (ChAT)] and degradation [acetylcholinesterase (AChE)] (Lewis and Shute, 1967; Fonnum, 1970; Storm-Mathisen, 1977), these observations fulfill the accepted criteria for identifying ACh as a neurotransmitter in the hippocampus.

In this chapter I shall identify the physiological mechanisms in the hippocampus that are targets for modulation and control by released ACh. I shall restrict the scope of this review to consider the electrophysiological processes that govern the excitability and firing patterns of neurones or populations of neurones and how cholinergic ac-

tions affect these processes. For consideration of higher mental functions involving cholinergic mechanisms in the hippocampus, such as behaviour, learning and memory, the reader is referred to other chapters in this volume.

Electrophysiology of the hippocampus

Classical experiments performed in mammals in vivo over the last two or three decades by Kandel et al. (1961), Eccles and his colleagues (see Eccles, 1969) and Andersen and associates (1971a,b) have revealed much about the repertoire of single hippocampal neurones, the existence of excitatory and inhibitory pathways and the organization of these connections into physiological lamina transversely orientated to the long axis of the hippocampus. These findings reported in vivo have been repeated in vitro in the hippocampal slice preparation, which was elaborated initially by Skrede and Westgaard (1971); this engenders confidence in the validity of in vitro preparations and that the basic physiological mechanisms in the hippocampus remain unscathed following isolation. Stability of recording, control of ionic environment and the employment of further cell dissociation and culture techniques have extended investigations to the level of specific membrane ionic conductances operating in hippocampal neurones. As may be seen below, these approaches have been invaluable in analyzing cholinergic action in the hippocampus.

The hippocampal slice

Since most of the recent findings concerning cholinergic action have been accomplished using hippocampal slices, it is useful to outline briefly the constituents of this preparation and the responses from it that are observable under control conditions. Moreover, consideration of the effects

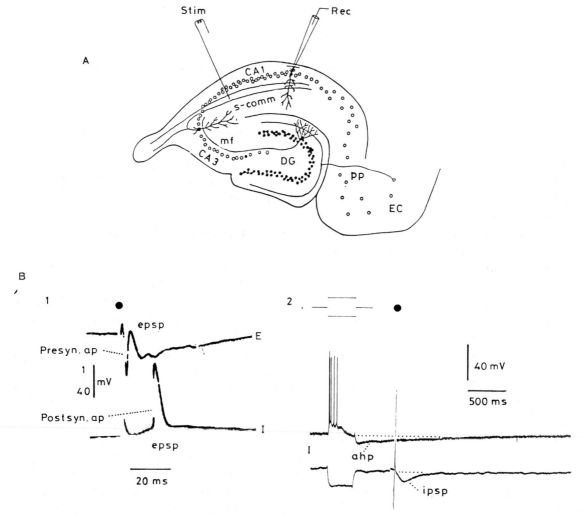

Fig. 1. A: Schematic diagram of a transverse hippocampal slice showing pyramidal cell layers (CA1, CA3) and granule cell layer (DG) and the positions of the fibre pathways that form the chain of excitatory connections linking entorhinal cortex (EC) to the dentate gyrus (perforant path: pp), the dentate to CA3 (mossy fibres: mf) and CA3 with CA1 (Schaffer collaterals: s-com). Mingled with the Schaffer collateral fibres are the commissural fibres originating in the contralateral hippocampus. The positions of an intrasomatic recording electrode in CA1 and a stimulating electrode amongst the afferent fibres are also indicated.
B: Electrophysiological responses in the hippocampal slice. 1: simultaneous extracellular (E) and intracellular (I) records from, respectively, the dendritic regions (at the level of s-com afferents) and an intrasomatic electrode in area CA1. Resting potential of the neurone was −68 mV, recorded with a 4 M K acetate-filled electrode. The stimulus was delivered at the time indicated (●). 2: intracellular records from another CA1 cell impaled with a 4 M K acetate-filled electrode, displayed on a longer time-scale than in 1 showing neuronal respones to ±0.3 nA injected directly into the soma through the electrode and the slower i.p.s.p. following the excitation caused by stimulation of s-com. Note the accommodation of firing in the face of continued current injection and the long afterhyperpolarization (AHP) associated with the cessation of repetitive firing.

of ACh and analogues upon these responses is a useful way of illustrating cholinergic mechanisms in the hippocampus.

Fig. 1A shows the two interlocking populations of principal neurones included in a transverse slice of mammalian hippocampus: the dentate gyrus [DG] consists of granule cells and the hippocampus proper CA1–CA3 of pyramidal neurones. Depending on the exact orientation of the transverse cut in relation to the long axis of the structure, the sequence of excitatory synapses characterizing a physiological lamina (Andersen et al., 1971) will be preserved to a greater or lesser extent. These run from the entorhinal cortex [EC] to synapse with DG (the perforant path [pp]), from DG to CA3 (via the mossy fibres [mf]) and from CA3 to CA1 (the Schaffer collaterals). The excitatory connections project onto specific regions of the dendrites of the cell groups: in the DG the lateral pp and medial pp occupy the outer and middle third of the molecular layer while the innermost third contains commissural afferents; in CA3 mf terminates mainly on proximal portions of apical dendrites, the distal portions receive some pp fibres whilst the remaining apical dendrites and basal dendrites receive commissural and other afferents; in CA1, commissural fibres are mingled with the Schaffer collaterals [s-com] onto spines on the extended portions of apical dendrites known as stratum radiatum, the pp terminates on the distalmost portions of apical dendrites and commissural and other afferents terminate on the basal arbours. Within or just basal to the principal cells are interneurones that stain positively for glutamic acid decarboxylase (GAD) (Storm-Mathisen, 1977; Ribak et al., 1978). These are inhibitory GABAergic interneurones and are of two broad types: one with a limited dendritic spread collecting input from the immediate principal cell population to subserve recurrent inhibition and another with dendrites that are contacted by the same excitatory afferents as the principal cells to mediate feed-forward inhibition (Alger, 1985). To put this into the context of cholinergic transmission, septal afferents terminate in all parts of the hippocampal formation (Frotscher and Leranth, 1985) but are more numerous in DG and CA3; they distribute to proximal dendritic regions of the cell populations and match muscarinic binding sites that are present (see Chapters 26 and 27 of this volume). There is some innervation of presumed interneurones and commissural neurones (Leranth and Frotscher, 1987). A lower density of muscarinic sites occurs in more distal dendritic regions which, of course also contain terminals of afferent fibres.

Evoked electrical activity in hippocampal slices

Stimulation of the mixed afferents contained within stratum radiatum of CA1 in a 500 μm slice evokes electrical activity in the neuronal population (Fig. 1B). Indication of the numbers of afferents stimulated is given by the magnitude of the di- or triphasic compound action potential which is the initial complex of the potential waveform recorded by an extracellular electrode positioned in stratum radiatum; evidence for the origin of this potential in the terminals and preterminals of the afferents includes (between threshold and maximal values) a dependence on stimulus strength, a latency distribution consistent with propagation in non- or lightly myelinated fibres orthogonal to pyramidal cell dendrites and resistance to manoeuvres that block synaptic transmission (see e.g. Andersen et al., 1978). The action potential volley is followed in the extracellular record from the dendrites by a slower, negative potential which is synaptic in origin, being blocked by removal of Ca from the medium (Andersen et al., 1978; Dingledine and Somjen, 1980), and results from the depolarization of pyramidal cell dendrites by released transmitter (glutamate or aspartate or a related compound: Storm-Mathisen, 1977) since it matches the occurrence of intrasomatically-recorded e.p.s.p.s that exceed firing threshold and trigger spikes in pyramidal neurones (Fig. 1B). Synchronous activity of pyramidal neurones generates extracellular current flow that is opposite in direction to that produced by synaptic input to the apical dendrites and causes positive notches to appear superimposed on the extracellularly-recorded dendritic synaptic wave. Consistent with profound depolarization as their origin, these are manifest as negative spikes (population spikes) when extracellular recordings are made from cell body regions; the magnitude of the population spike is related to the number of discharging neurones (Andersen et al., 1971a). Activity in pyramidal neurones produces a convergent excitation of inhibitory interneurones, which in turn feed their inhibitory influence back to the pyramids. This generates the i.p.s.p. that is seen in the longer time-course records in Fig. 1B. Two components of the i.p.s.p. are frequently seen: an initial component reflecting a chloride conductance increase due to the activation of $GABA_a$ receptors (Alger, 1985) and a much longer (up to 1s) component caused by an increased conductance to K^+ following activation of $GABA_b$ receptors (Dutar and Nicoll, 1988a).

In addition to exciting hippocampal neurones by activating synaptic input, these cells can be fired by injecting depolarizing current through the recording electrode. When suprathreshold currents of long duration (> 300 ms) are employed, only a few action potentials are generated at the start of the pulse, in spite of maintained current. This accommodation of firing is typical pyramidal cell behaviour and is also shown in Fig. 1B It can be seen that the cessation of firing coincides with a marked hyperpolarization of the cell, even during the passage of depolarizing current. The hyperpolarization outlasts the current pulse by up to 2 s and is one of three activity-dependent afterhyperpolarizations (AHPs) that obtain in hippocampal neurones (see Storm, 1989). A rapid AHP following a directly activated single spike and the AHP mentioned above are both caused by Ca-influx through voltage-operated Ca-channels opened during the action potential(s); they reflect Ca-dependent K^+-channels with different voltage and pharmacological sensitivities (see Storm, 1987). A medium-duration AHP which is Ca-independent can be demonstrated during blockade of the very long-lasting AHP (Storm, 1989). As described be-

low, this too reflects a mechanism that influences accommodation of neuronal firing; furthermore, we shall see that both are influenced by the consequences of muscarinic receptor stimulation and are therefore targets for cholinergic action.

Cholinergic responses in the hippocampus

Application of ACh or its stable analogues has long been known to accelerate the firing rate of forebrain neurones (including those in hippocampus: Biscoe and Straughn, 1966) in an atropine-sensitive manner. In pioneering experiments recording intracellularly from neocortical neurones Krnjevic and colleagues (1971) described a depolarizing response to ionophoresed ACh that

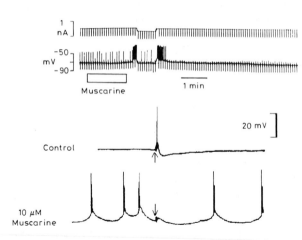

Fig. 2. Responses of CA1 neurone in a guinea-pig hippocampal slice bathed with medium containing 10 μM muscarine. The top panel shows a voltage recording from an intrasomatic K acetate-filled electrode and also the output from the circuit monitoring current injected into the cell through the recording electrode. The negative deflections on the voltage trace are electrotonic potentials caused by injection of 0.5 nA of hyperpolarizing current every 5 s to assess neuronal input resistance. The positive deflections are spontaneous or evoked action potentials, truncated by the slow frequency response of the chart recorder. During the depolarization caused by muscarine the cell was hyperpolarized to its control potential by the passage of steady direct current. Note the resistance increase associated with muscarinic action. The lower panel depicts expanded records taken from epoques before (control) and during the response to muscarine; synaptic stimuli were delivered as indicated by the arrows. The i.p.s.p. is suppressed on this occasion.

was accompanied by an increase in the cells' input resistance and suggested that a decrease in K^+-conductance was the underlying mechanism. The same conclusion was reached by Dodd et al. (1981) who were first systematically to investigate effects of ACh in the hippocampal slice with intracellular recording. Fig. 2 shows the depolarization, increased firing rate and membrane resistance increase induced by bath application of 10 μM muscarine (the selective agonist at the muscarinic subtype of AChR) to a guinea-pig CA1 pyramidal cell; it also shows that while the neurone is depolarized and presumably, as indicated by enhanced firing, experiencing increased excitability, inhibitory responses to stimulation of Schaffer-commissural afferents are diminished.

Cholinergic effects observable on synaptic transmission

Cholinergic reduction of inhibition has been described in the intact hippocampus in vivo (Ben-Ari et al., 1981) and in vitro, in the slice (Haas, 1982) and in cultured neurones (Segal, 1983). Disinhibition, of course, can contribute to the excitation caused by cholinergic activation and arise in several ways: first, the output of inhibitory transmitter could be diminished (Segal, 1983); second, the excitatory drive to inhibitory pathways could be reduced; third, inhibitory interneurones could themselves be inhibited, directly or indirectly. The third possibility may be discounted since Benardo and Prince (1982) observed in a proportion of CA1 neurones a rapid bicuculline-sensitive inhibition that preceded the more common slow excitation (cf. Fig. 2) when microdrops of ACh solution were applied to the exposed cut surface of a slice; an exactly parallel situation obtains in neocortex in vitro (McCormick and Prince, 1985), where presumed interneurones are directly and rapidly excited by ACh through a subtype of muscarinic receptor that is relatively insensitive to the selective antagonist pirenzepine (see below). Consistent with the idea that GABAergic interneurones can be excited directly by cholinergic activation is the

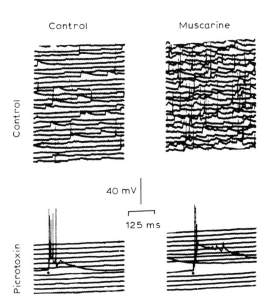

Fig. 3. Muscarinic activation can increase inhibition in the hippocampus. The four panels show raster-type displays of spontaneous synaptic activity recorded in a guinea-pig CA1 neurone with an electrode filled with 3 M KCl. A brief bath application of 10 μM muscarine causes, prior to suppression of excitatory transmission (see text), an increase in spontaneous synaptic activity. In the presence of 10 μM picrotoxin the spontaneous activity and its potentiation by muscarine are both blocked (lower panels). Synaptic responses are also shown in the presence of picrotoxin. Average resting potential −72 mV.

increase in spontaneously occurring depolarizing potentials observed when CA1 neurones are impaled with Cl^--containing electrodes and exposed to muscarinic agonists (Fig. 3). These potentials are sensitive to GABA$_a$ antagonists picrotoxin (Fig. 3) or bicuculline and are i.p.s.p.s which have a positively shifted reversal potential due to Cl^--loading (Alger and Nicoll, 1980). The direct nature of the cholinergic effect (cf. Leranth and Frotscher, 1987) on inhibitory neurones can be gleaned from the observation that increases in spontaneous i.p.s.p.s can occur when excitatory pathways are intact, as in Fig. 3, or when another *presynaptic* cholinergic action is operating to suppress transmitter release from excitatory terminals in the hippocampus and disrupt the circuitry nec-

260

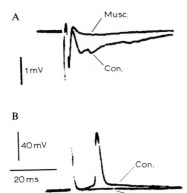

Fig. 4. Presynaptic depression of excitatory transmission by muscarine. Simultaneous extracellular (A) and intracellular records (B) are shown and comprise superimposed oscilloscope sweeps taken before (con) and during (musc) the (somatic) excitatory response to bath application of 10 μM muscarine in the same guinea-pig CA1 neurone as that depicted in Fig. 2. The presynaptic fibre volley is unaffected (A) but both the cellular and population e.p.s.p. are almost entirely abolished. In B the cell was manually clamped at the control resting potential, -72 mV, by passage of steady current.

essary for activating interneurones indirectly (see Fig. 4).

The presynaptic depression of excitatory transmitter release by ACh was first described by Yamamoto and Kawai (1967) in the dentate gyrus. Hounsgaard (1978) and Valentino and Dingledine (1981) reported similar diminution of evoked e.p.s.p.s recorded extracellularly and intracellularly in CA1 by ACh ionophoretically applied to dendritic regions close to the synaptic area. These cholinergic effects were muscarinic since they could be blocked with 0.01–0.1 μM atropine. No concomitant reduction or, indeed, a slight increase (Hounsgaard, 1978) in the presynaptic volley was observed and the blockade of e.p.s.p.s could not be ascribed to marked somatic conductance changes or alteration of postsynaptic sensitivity to excitatory amino acids (Valentino and Dingledine, 1981). Similar experiments in our own laboratory using bath-applied agonists muscarine and carbachol have given similar results (Fig. 4).

No change in the presynaptic volley was observed, even during complete suppression of the e.p.s.p.; the IC_{50} for blockade of the e.p.s.p. by

muscarine was 3–5 μM and blockade was completely antagonized by 0.1 μM atropine. Involvement of $GABA_a$-mediated inhibitory activity was ruled out by the failure of 10 μM bicuculline to have an effect on the muscarinic suppression of synaptic transmission. Recently, Dutar and Nicoll (1988c) have described an antagonism of carbachol-induced depression of e.p.s.p.s by concentrations of the cardiac muscarinic receptor antagonist gallamine which spared postsynaptic depolarizations, indicating heterogeneous receptors mediating pre- and postsynaptic cholinergic actions.

Direct cholinergic actions on hippocampal neurones

In view of mixed effects of ACh and other muscarinic agonists on synaptic transmission, it is clear that the excitation observed intracellularly cannot result wholly from an interference with tonic inhibition; consequently, we must look to direct cholinergic actions on the membrane properties of pyramidal neurones to explain the excitatory events. There are several aspects to the excitation of hippocampal neurones by cholinergic activation and its consequences: (i) Depolarization; by bringing the membrane potential closer to firing threshold, there could be an increased chance of impinging excitatory drive triggering action potentials. (ii) Resistance increase; the effectiveness of synaptic current delivered into neurones will strengthen as a result of the concomitant increase in length constant. (iii) Prolongation of firing. As mentioned above, accommodation of firing is normally pronounced in hippocampal neurones; muscarinic activation reduces accommodation regardless of whether Ca-entry is allowed or prevented (Benardo and Prince, 1982; Cole and Nicoll, 1984; Madison and Nicoll, 1984). Firing that is established following muscarinic stimulation is therefore prolonged because of the regulation of these accommodating mechanisms. The ionic basis of the direct actions of cholinergic agents on hippocampal neurones is considered in the next section.

Cholinergic modulation of ionic conductance

Ionic basis for depolarization and resistance increase

(1) Inward currents

Membrane responses of hippocampal neurones are non-linear; this is most obvious from the occurrence of both Na and Ca dependent action potentials (see e.g. Schwartzkroin and Slawsky, 1978) which are regenerative events. A fast class of TTX-sensitive Na-channels (Sah et al., 1988) and up to three classes of Ca-currents (Halliwell, 1983; Blaxter et al., 1989; Brown and Griffith, 1983b; Yaari et al., 1986), possibly representing different channel types (Fox et al., 1987), are responsible for these action potentials. In addition, instability of hippocampal cell behaviour is conferred by non-inactivating Na-channels which are also TTX-sensitive (French and Gage, 1985; see Fig. 5). Fig. 5 represents an extreme example of the expression of non-inactivating Na-current in a

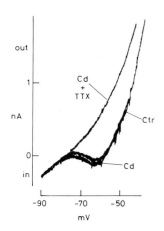

Fig. 5. Non-linear membrane characteristics of CA1 neurones. Membrane current responses are shown in graphical form recorded from a voltage-clamped rat CA1 cell subject to a ramp voltage command from −90 to −40 mV at 10 mV s⁻¹. Three traces are shown superimposed: a control, a record in the presence of 300 μM Cd (to block Ca-channels) and a record in the presence of Cd and with additional 0.5 μM TTX. TTX clearly blocks an inward current component activating negative to about −70 mV. In the presence of TTX an outward current activating at about −60 mV is revealed. Zero current level taken from resting potential, −74 mV. Recording electrode containing 3 M KCl.

voltage-clamped CA1 cell, possibly as a result of a deficit in other conductance(s). Nonetheless, it illustrates the existence of a net inward current in a subthreshold range of membrane potential that is resistant to the Ca-channel blocker Cd. The significance of this current is that, if unopposed by the presence of outward current, it will lead to spontaneous cell depolarization if the membrane potential is deflected into a voltage range where the current is activated. Furthermore, depolarization, whether spontaneous, manipulated, or drug-induced, will be accompanied by an apparent resistance increase; this phenomenon ("inward rectification") was noted by Hotson et al. (1979), who reported further that it was TTX-sensitive. Inward rectification was reported to be potentiated by ACh by Benardo and Prince (1982). The persistent Na-current could be a contributing factor to depolarization of hippocampal neurones by ACh and account in part for the voltage sensitivity that has been noted in behaviourally unrestrained neurones (Dodd et al., 1981; Benardo and Prince, 1982; Gahwiler and Dreifuss, 1982). Ca-spikes are enhanced by application of ACh (Gahwiler, 1985) but it is likely that this effect is secondary to suppression of outward current since there are reports of cholinergic suppression of Ca-currents in hippocampus (Gahwiler and Brown, 1987; Toselli and Lux, 1989).

(2) Outward currents

Fig. 5 also shows that when Na-conductance is blocked with TTX, an outward current, which is Cd-insensitive and therefore not Ca-dependent, develops positive to ~ −60 mV. This is due to the activation of a time- and voltage-dependent K⁺-conductance that shows no inactivation and contributes a component of steady-state membrane conductance at potentials positive to its activation threshold (−60 mV). This conductance was first described in bullfrog sympathetic ganglionic neurones by Brown and Adams (1980) and subsequently in hippocampal neurones by Halliwell and Adams (1982); it was dubbed the M-current (I_m) because of its blockade by *MUSCARINIC* receptor activation. When a persistent outward current is blocked in a neurone, the cell will depolarize, or, if under voltage clamp, show an inward shift in holding current required to maintain the membrane potential; testing for membrane conductance will indicate a reduction. Fig. 6A shows voltage-clamp records from a CA1 cell bathed in medium containing 0.5 μM TTX depicting responses to muscarine at two membrane potentials;

at the cell's resting potential (~ −70 mV) a large (50 μM) dose of muscarine elicits very little alteration in holding current and no obvious conductance change, whereas at −45 mV at which potential appreciable outward M-current is activated, 10 μM muscarine causes about 200 pA inward current by suppressing this conductance. Evidence for the latter is a decrease in the instantaneous conductance as measured by current deflections to

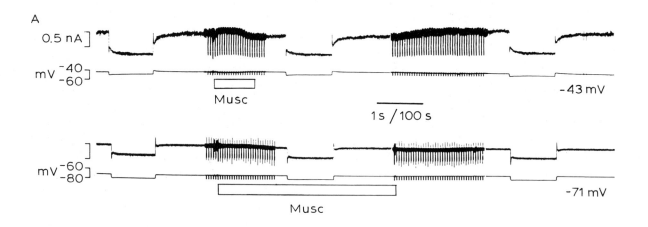

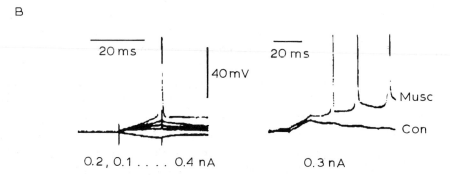

Fig. 6. M-current suppression by muscarine. A: Comparison of current responses to muscarine in a voltage-clamped guinea-pig CA1 neurone at two different holding potentials (−43 and −71 mV). The traces shown are of current (upper of pair) and voltage (lower) and are continuous, being expanded ×100 before during and after muscarine to show more detail. One second hyperpolarizing clamp steps were superimposed every 5 s to test cell membrane conductance. 10 μM muscarine was applied for 1 min when the cell was held at −43 mV; 50 μM muscarine was applied for 2 min at the −71 mV holding potential. The medium bathing the slice contained 0.5 μM TTX. B: Responses of the same neurone as in A to short current pulses before administration of TTX and voltage-clamping. The left panel shows responses to the indicated current injections which defined threshold current for exciting the cell as between 0.3 and 0.4 nA. The right panel shows superimposed cell responses to 0.3 nA before (CON) and during exposure to 10 μM muscarine; initial resting potential was −72 mV and no manual clamp was applied.

small negative voltage jumps, and a clear decrease in the time-dependent relaxations that stepwise hyperpolarization induces: the inward relaxations reflect the closure of M-channels following the step to a less positive potential and the outward relaxations indicate reopening upon the return to the holding potential (Brown and Adams, 1980). Since activation and deactivation kinetics of I_m are rather slow at positive potentials (tau = ~ 90 ms at −45 mV at 30°C) (Halliwell and Adams, 1982), this conductance does not contribute to spike repolarization. However, in quiescent neurones having rather negative resting potentials (−65−−70 mV), muscarinic activation causes a change in responsiveness to current stimulation that can be observed in the absence of marked alterations of membrane potential or conductance (Fig. 6A,B). Functionally speaking, this is a lowering of threshold as defined in terms of afferent input required to fire the cell; it is consistent with the voltage-sensitivity of M-current suppression. When resting potential of a hippocampal neurone lies within the voltage-range for the activation of I_m, suppression of this conductance will, as mentioned above, produce depolarization, which will also reduce the functional threshold for excitatory input. The role, therefore, of the M-current can be seen as a stabilizing mechanism that opposes depolarization, controlling, in particular the unstable membrane behaviour conferred by persistent inward currents (see above; Gahwiler, 1985).

There are recent reports that, in addition to the M-current, muscarinic agonists also suppress a voltage-insensitive "leak" K^+-conductance (Madison et al., 1987; Benson et al., 1988). This effect is antagonized by atropine and pirenzepine (Benson et al., 1988; Dutar and Nicoll, 1988c) and appears to be more potent than the action on the M-current (Madison et al., 1987). Suppression of leak conductance leads to depolarization of neurones having membrane potentials positive to E_K and a simple increase in cell input resistance will potentiate the amplitude of synaptic potentials. A change in leak conductance will also determine inter alia the potential at which spontaneous de-polarization due the non-inactivating Na-current starts. Reduction in leak conductance could have more powerfully excitatory effects than at first anticipated from the alteration of a linear conductance. The earliest voltage clamp studies (Halliwell and Adams, 1982) made no report of marked inward currents induced by muscarinic agonists at voltages negative to the M-current activation range; this discrepancy is difficult to resolve but may reflect heterogeneity in the balance between different membrane conductances operating in individual neurones.

Repetitive activity potentiated by cholinergic agonists

In contrast to the mechanisms of cholinergic action described above, which place a hippocampal neurone in a state of readiness to give a brisker response when an excitatory input arrives, there is also a muscarinic modulation of ongoing activity. The marked accommodation observed during long current injections is abolished by low (micromolar) doses of carbachol; likewise the AHP that accompanies accommodation is reduced by muscarinic agonists (Benardo and Prince, 1982; Cole and Nicoll, 1984b; Madison et al., 1987) (see Fig. 7). Lancaster and Adams (1986) identified the conductance responsible for the accommodation and the accompanying AHP as a K^+-conductance activated by aliquots of Ca entering the cell through voltage sensitive Ca-channels, opened during voltage excursion of individual action potentials. This conductance, called I_{AHP} declines slowly and independently of voltage. It is sensitive to blockade of Ca-channels (Hotson and Prince, 1980; Madison and Nicoll, 1982, 1984; Lancaster and Adams, 1986) and to buffering internal Ca with EGTA or BAPTA. It may be distinguished from other Ca-activated K^+-conductances by its resistance to TEA and Charybdotoxin (see Halliwell, 1990). I_{AHP} contributes no steady-state membrane conductance at −50 mV since holding currents at that potential do not shift when blocking doses of Cd are administered (Halliwell, unpublished); I_{AHP} has no role to play, therefore, in the

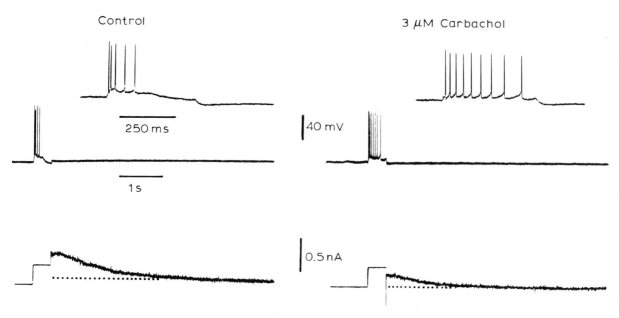

Fig. 7. Cholinergic suppression of I_{AHP} and accommodation in a rat CA1 neurone. Each panel shows: upper: cell voltage response to 0.3 nA current injected for 400 ms; middle: the same on a longer time-base, but with switch into-voltage clamp upon termination of current injection; lower: the current injected first to stimulate the neurone and then clamp it at -65 mV. Note the slow outward current responsible for the AHP and its inhibition by 3 μM carbachol in the bathing medium. Note also that carbachol does not reduce the interval between the first couple of action potentials in the train as might be predicted by an additional effect on the A-current (see text for further details).

cholinergic depolarizing response. Suppression of I_{AHP} changes the firing pattern of hippocampal neurones from phasic to tonic in nature.

When I_{AHP} is blocked by preventing Ca-influx with Ca-channel blockers such as Cd or verapamil, hippocampal neurones still display accommodation (Madison and Nicoll, 1984; Jones and Heinemann, 1988). Madison and Nicoll (1984) showed that under conditions of Ca-channel blockade, muscarinic activation still reduced the residual accommodation. Recently, Storm (1989) pointed out that an associated, medium duration AHP could be ascribed to M-current activation, since this was also sensitive to muscarinic agonists. The slow kinetics of the M-current can result in voltage-sensing of the *average* membrane potential during a spike train and the gradual activation of this K$^+$-conductance leads to a progressive slowing of discharge. With the M-current unavailable for activation, accommodation during a tonic discharge does not develop to such an extent.

Nakajima et al. (1986) have reported that muscarine inhibits yet another K$^+$-current, the A-current (I_A) in cultured hippocampal neurones. This is a conductance that is inactivated at -55 mV and potentials more positive, but hyperpolarization removes inactivation in a voltage-dependent manner to allow reactivation on subsequent depolarization past -60 mV (Gustafsson et al., 1982). The function of I_A is twofold (see Halliwell, 1990): first it controls threshold of firing from a negative resting potential (Segal at al., 1984) and second it contributes to the spacing of action potentials during repetitive activity (Connor and Stevens, 1971). Effects of cholinergic activation consistent with suppression of I_A have not been observed in slices of hippocampus in vitro (see Fig. 7) so that the findings of Nakajima et al., (1986) could represent a subtle cholinergic action only noticeable under the precise recording conditions available with whole-cell clamp or, alternatively, an anomalous link between receptors and channel modulators peculiar to development in tissue culture.

Cholinergic transmission in the hippocampus

The fibres of septal afferents course through stratum oriens and may be excited, but not selectively, by electrical stimuli in parts of CA1 and CA3. Cole and Nicoll (1983, 1984b) showed that single shocks elicited predominantly inhibitory potentials in CA1 neurones whereas larger shocks delivered in 20 Hz trains lead to a summation of hyperpolarizations that in turn gave way to a slow depolarization, a slow e.p.s.p. (see Fig. 8). The latter was associated with reduced membrane conductance, could last up to 2 min and was excitatory, increasing the rate neuronal firing. Similar effects of cholinergic fibre activation were reported by Segal (1988) for CA1 neurones and Muller and Misgeld (1986, 1989) in CA3 and DG cells. All these effects were blocked by atropine and mimicked by applied ACh; furthermore they were enhanced by AChE inhibitors. Collectively, they demonstrate a role for ACh in slow excitatory transmission in the hippocampus. In the absence of AChEs and with gentler stimulation, membrane potential effects are not always seen (Cole and Nicoll, 1984b); however, activation of cholinergic fibres occurs and can cause a reduction in accommodation, similar to that produced by muscarinic agonists. A concomitant reduction in the prolonged AHP occurs after repetitive cholinergic stimulation, suggesting that released ACh inhibits I_{AHP}. This indicates that, amongst the cholinergic actions enumerated above, inhibition of I_{AHP} is the most sensitive. This is born out by the study of Madison et al. (1987) in which the M-current was found to be ~ 10–100 times less sensitive to blockade by carbachol than I_{AHP}. Leak conductance was also more sensitive than I_m. Only when intense stimulation of stratum oriens was given in the presence of eserine was the M-current inhibited greatly. Taken together with the occurrence of slow e.p.s.p.s at potentials negative to the M-current activation range (Muller and Misgeld,

1986), these findings imply that I_{AHP} and the leak conductance are primary targets for inhibition by ACh released from terminals in the hippocampal slice. Furthermore, slow e.p.s.p.s can be elicited when I_{AHP} is blocked by other means (Madison et al., 1987), eliminating suppression of I_{AHP} as the mechanism whereby slow e.p.s.p.s are generated. The voltage sensitivity of slow e.p.s.p.s has yet to be satisfactorily determined: on occasion, they diminish in amplitude upon polarization to potentials well positive to E_K (Fig. 8; Cole and Nicoll, 1984; Muller et al., 1989) and on others show a reversal negative to E_K (Muller and Misgeld, 1986).

A different approach adopted by Gahwiler and Brown (1985a) has employed co-cultures of septal and hippocampal explants. In these preparations single stimuli to the septal cells evoke fast e.p.s.c.s mediated by an as-yet uncharacterized transmitter. Repetitive stimulation of the septal region elicits, in addition, a slow voltage-sensitive e.p.s.c. that is blocked by atropine, enhanced by eserine and mimicked by applications of ACh or muscarine. This slow e.p.s.c. can largely be attributed to M-current suppression.

Interactions with other neurotransmitter systems

The profile of cholinergic action in hippocampus suggests that different receptor subtypes mediate particular aspects of neuronal regulation. Other neurotransmitters converge on the same mechanisms that are modulated by ACh. Thus, activation of adenosine A_1 and $GABA_b$ receptors can have the same presynaptically depressant actions on transmitter release as the muscarinic effects described above (Dunwiddie and Hoffer, 1980; Lee et al., 1983; Lanthorn and Cotman, 1981). M-current is also inhibited by 5-HT (Colino and Halliwell, 1987). Leak K^+-conductance is reduced by noradrenaline and 5-HT (Madison and Nicoll, 1986a; Colino and Halliwell, 1987; Andrade and Nicoll, 1987). I_{AHP} is depressed by noradrenaline (Madison and Nicoll, 1982; Lancaster and Adams, 1986), histamine (Haas and Konnerth, 1983) 5-HT

266

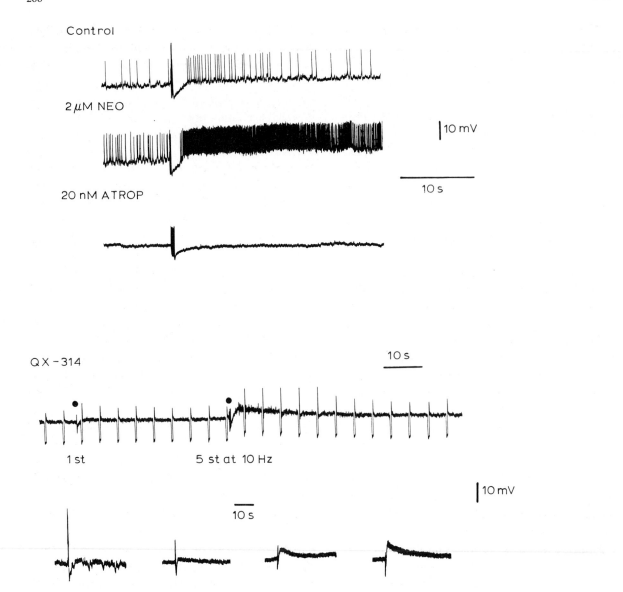

Fig. 8. Slow cholinergic excitatory actions in rat hippocampus. Top panel: delayed excitation of a CA1 neurone in response to 20 Hz, 0.5 s stimulation of fibres lying in stratum oriens of CA1, its potentiation by 2 μM neostigmine and abolition of both by 20 nM atropine. Membrane potential after atropine −67 mV; 3 M KCl-filled impaling electrode. Bottom panel: The slow e.p.s.p. persists after blockade of Na-channels with intracellular QX-314 (100mM in 3 M KCl filling solution of electrode) (Connors et al., 1982). In this cell at −45 mV membrane potential, 1 stimulus to stratum oriens produces a small slow e.p.s.p.; 5 stimuli at 10 Hz a larger e.p.s.p. with a conductance decrease (cf. Fig. 5). The lower traces show how e.p.s.p. amplitude varied with manipulated membrane potential (time scale compressed ×2.5 compared with upper trace). 2 μM neostigmine present in bathing medium.

(Colino and Halliwell, 1987; Andrade and Nicoll, 1987) and activators of adenylate cyclase (Madison and Nicoll, 1986b) or protein kinase C (PKC) (Baraban et al., 1986; Malenka et al., 1987). This convergence of neurotransmitter effects means that ongoing activation of receptors other than the muscarinic receptors mediating cholinergic actions can occlude the effects of ACh and vice versa.

There have been recent reports of hippocampal M-current being enhanced by somatostatin (Moore et al., 1988; Watson and Pitman, 1988). The long-duration AHP reflecting the activation of I_{AHP} can also be potentiated: namely, by adenosine receptor stimulation (Haas and Greene, 1984; Greene and Haas, 1985) which inhibits adenylate cyclase. The enhanced conductances, however, are still subject to inhibition by muscarinic action; in these instances the cell excitability changes brought about by cholinergic activation will be made more prominent by coincident activity at the other neurotransmitter receptors (e.g. Moore et al., 1988).

Ongoing activity in cholinergic pathways can affect hippocampal neuronal responses to other neurotransmitter candidates and not just by interactions described above. High-frequency stimulation of cholinergic fibres in stratum oriens reverses the inhibition of extracellularly recorded population spikes by applied adenosine and reduces the sensitivity of pyramidal cells to baclofen and adenosine (Worley et al., 1986). Baclofen, adenosine and 5-HT activate K^+-conductance through a pertussis toxin sensitive GTP-binding (G-) protein (Andrade et al., 1986; Trussell and Jackson, 1987; Nicoll, 1988) that is phosphorylated by protein kinase C (PKC) (Worley et al., 1986; see Nicoll, 1988). Potent muscarinic agonists that cause phosphatidyl inositol (PI) breakdown with the consequence of PKC activation following liberation of diacyl glycerol (DAG) are effective in suppressing the inhibitory effects of adenosine and baclofen, whereas partial agonists are ineffective or, indeed, antagonists (Worley et al., 1986). Cholinergic input to the hippocampus, therefore, can reduce the effectiveness of inhibitory pathways that use receptors linked to the K^+-conductance activator via

susceptible G-proteins (G_i or G_o); this is in addition to possible effects on inhibitory transmitter release discussed above.

Receptor subtypes and second messengers involved in cholinergic action in the hippocampus

Acetylcholine receptors

All the effects of ACh or cholinergic agonists described so far are atropine-sensitive. Although there are sites in the hippocampus that bind the nicotinic markers (see Clarke et al., 1985) and hippocampal cells express mRNA for combinations of nicotinic receptor subunits, which could be expressed on cell bodies (Wada et al., 1989), nicotinic responses are difficult to demonstrate. Cole and Nicoll (1984a) found *no* responses in the rat slice preparation that were attributable to the activation of nicotinic receptors; this is not a deficit of slice preparations per se since both presynaptic (Brown et al., 1984) and postsynaptic (Brown et al., 1983; Egan and North, 1985; McCormick and Prince, 1986) responses have been described in vitro. Rovira et al. (1983) reported nicotinic effects on field potentials in dendritic regions of CA1 in vivo, but since they are difficult to demonstrate in vitro, where the underlying mechanisms are more amenable to investigation, comment as to the physiological relevance is not possible.

The position regarding muscarinic receptor subtypes is presently in a state of flux. At least four mRNAs have been cloned for different muscarinic receptors (Bonner et al., 1987;) but the selectivity of available pharmacological antagonists does not discriminate between these. In classifying the subtype of receptor(s) involved in responses to ACh experimenters have relied on sensitivity to pirenzepine to classify muscarinic receptors into M_1 and M_2, the M_1 subtype being 10–100 times more sensitive than the non-M_1 (M_2) subtype (Hammer et al., 1980). To summarize a far from certain position, evidence exists that the presynaptic inhibitory action of ACh is relatively sensitive to the M_1-selective compound pirenzepine but is blocked by gallamine (Dutar and Nicoll, 1988c), which allosterically antagonizes ACh effects at the pirenzepine-resistant muscarinic M_2 sites in cardiac tissue. Pirenzepine potently antagonizes the depolarization and leak conductance decrease induced by carbachol (Muller and Misgeld, 1986; Benson et al., 1988) but opinion is divided about its effectiveness in discriminating between other physiological actions (Muller and Misgeld, 1986; Dutar and Nicoll, 1988c). Dutar and Nicoll (1988c) found that gallamine also antagonized the M-current suppression in accordance with similar findings in the olfactory cortex, another 3-layer cortex (Constanti and Sim, 1987a). Suppression of the AHP in olfactory cortex also seems to be M_2-mediated (Constanti and Sim, 1987b) in congruence with observations from Muller and Misgeld (1986), but full and partial agonists at non-M_1 sites appear equally effective in inhibiting the hippocampal I_{AHP} (Dutar and Nicoll, 1988c and J.V. Halliwell, unpublished). More selective drugs will be needed before all the physiological effects of ACh can be ascribed to particular receptor types, but it is likely that suppression of leak-conductance is an M_1-receptor event and that the presynaptic inhibition and the M-current inhibition are reliant on M_2-receptors.

Second messengers

In contrast to nicotinic responses studied in detail in the periphery which involve the direct gating of an ion-channel by the ligand and which are rapid (see Chapter 5 of this volume), the muscarinic actions are slow. This is taken to reflect the involvement of second messengers, generated as a result of receptor activation that have some intracellular site of action (see Nicoll, 1988). Activation of guanylate or adenylate cyclases does not appear to play a direct role in hippocampal cholinergic responses, at least in the electrophysiological actions described above (Cole and Nicoll, 1984a; Madison et al., 1987b; Nicoll, 1988). Attention has recently focussed on muscarinic receptor-activated PI turnover (see Nicoll, 1988) as a

second messenger pathway and two consequences of PI metabolism have been implicated in cholinergic effects on specific conductance mechanisms. First, inositol trisphosphate (IP_3), which is liberated intracellularly during PI breakdown, suppresses M-current when delivered to pyramidal neurones through the impaling electrode (Dutar and Nicoll, 1988a, 1988b). Second, activation of PKC, which occurs secondarily to the production of DAG from phospholipid breakdown mimics the action of muscarinic stimulation on both I_{AHP} and the $GABA_b$-dependent i.p.s.p. and K^+-conductance increase (Baraban et al., 1985; Worley et al., 1986; Malenka et al., 1987). These data are not proof of such mechanisms being responsible for some of the cholinergic actions observed in the hippocampus, but are certainly suggestive; experiments with appropriate inhibitors would add weight to the hypothesis. The suppression of I_m by intracellular IP_3 is unlike some other IP_3-mediated events (see Higashida and Brown, 1986) in that release of Ca from internal stores appears not to be involved (Dutar and Nicoll, 1988a,b) since buffering of internal Ca to a low level does not affect the response.

Conclusions

It is clear that cholinergic pathways can influence hippocampal function at several different levels to produce excitatory or inhibitory effects, and that the basal level of cell activity will determine the response to cholinergic stimulation. Thus, a quiescent hippocampal neurone might display no marked response at rest but, under direct cholinergic influence, be more susceptible to other afferent excitatory input and furthermore, once activated, show more prolonged firing; this could arise from suppression of the K-conductances described above. These mechanisms, then, influence threshold and cause a switch in neuronal firing behaviour from phasic to tonic. Neurones, individually or as populations can also be excited or inhibited by ACh changing the firing patterns of inhibitory interneurones which synaptically connect to them. Presynaptic cholinergic action can have the same consequences by depriving neurones of inhibitory or excitatory input following a reduction of transmitter release at the synapse. Postsynaptic cholinergic action can influence cell responses to other transmitters because of convergence onto the same target mechanisms and also by disrupting transduction between receptor activation and cellular events. The complexity of central cholinergic actions suggests that when a pathological deficit occurs, such as in Alzheimer's Disease, fine control of cortical function will be impaired at several levels. It is interesting that a drug tetrahydroaminoacridine (THA: tacrine) that ameliorates the condition of patients with Alzheimer's Disease (Summers et al., 1986) has actions that both potentiate and mimic the effects of ACh in several respects (Halliwell and Grove, 1989).

References

Alger, B.E. (1985) Hippocampus: Electrophysiological studies of epileptiform activity in vitro. In R. Dingledine (Ed.), *Brain Slices,* Plenum, New York, pp. 155–199.

Alger, B.E. and Nicoll, R.A. (1980) Spontaneous inhibitory post-synaptic potentials in the hippocampus: mechanism for tonic inhibition. *Brain Res.,* 200: 195–200.

Andersen, P., Bliss, T.V.P. and Skrede, K.K. (1971a) Unit analysis of hippocampal population spikes. *Exp. Brain Res.,* 13: 208–221.

Andersen, P. Bliss, T.V.P. and Skrede, K.K. (1971b) Lamellar organisation of hippocampal excitatory pathways. *Exp. Brain Res.,* 13: 222–238.

Andersen, P., Silfvenius, H., Sundberg, S.H., Sveen, O. and Wigstrom, H. (1978) Functional characteristics of unmyelinated fibres in the hippocampal cortex. *Brain Res.,* 144: 11–18.

Andrade, R., and Nicoll, R.A. (1987) Pharmacologically distinct actions of serotonin on single pyramidal neurones of the rat hippocampus recorded in vitro. *J. Physiol. (Lond.),* 394: 99–124.

Andrade, R., Malenka, R.C. and Nicoll, R.A. (1986) A G-protein couples serotonin and GABA$_B$ receptors to the same channels in hippocampus. *Science,* 234: 1261–1265.

Baraban, J.M., Snyder, S.H. and Alger, B.E. (1985) Protein kinase C regulates ionic conductance in hippocampal pyramidal neurons: Electrophysiological effects of phorbol esters. *Proc. Natl. Acad. Sci. USA,* 82: 2538–2542.

Benardo, L.S. and Drince, D.A. (1982) Cholinergic excitation of mmammalian hippocampal pyramidal cells. *Brain Res.,* 249: 315–331.

Ben-Ari, Y., Krnjevic, K. Reinhardt, W. and Ropert, N. (1981) Intracellular observations on the disinhibitory action of acetylcholine in the hippocampus. *Neuroscience,* 12: 2475–2484.

Benson, D.M., Blitzer, R.D., and Landau, E.M. (1988) An analysis of the depolarization produced in guinea-pig hippocampus by cholinergic receptor stimulation. *J. Physiol. (Lond.).,* 404: 479–496.

Biscoe, T.J. and Straughn, D.W. (1966) Microelectrophoretic studies of neurones in cat hippocampus. *J. Physiol. (Lond.),* 183: 341–359.

Blaxter, T.J., Carlen, P.L. and Niesen, C. (1989) Pharmacological and anatomical separation of calcium currents in rat dentate granule neurones in vitro. *J. Physiol. (Lond.),* 412: 93–112.

Bonner, T.I., Buckley, N.J., Young, A.C. and Brann, M.R. (1987) Identification of a family of muscarinic acetylcholine receptor genes. *Science,* 237: 527–532.

Brown, D.A. and Adams, P.R. (1980) Muscarinic suppression of a novel voltage-sensitive K$^+$-current in a vertebreate neurone. *Nature (Lond.),* 283: 673–676.

Brown, D.A. and Griffith, W.G. (1983) Persistent slow inward calcium current in voltage-clamped hippocampal neurones of the guinea-pig. *J. Physiol (Lond.),* 337: 303–320.

Brown, D.A., Docherty, R.J. and Halliwell, J.V. (1983) Chemical transmission in the rat interpeduncular nucleus in vitro. *J. Physiol. (Lond.),* 341: 655–670.

Brown, D.A., Docherty, R.J. and Halliwell, J.V. (1984) The action of cholinomimetic substances on impulse conduction in the habenulointerpeduncular pathway of the rat in vitro. *J. Physiol., (Lond.),* 353: 101–109.

Clarke, P.B.S., Schwartz, R.D., Paul, S.M., Pert, C.B. and Pert, A. (1985) Nicotinic binding in rat brain: Autoradiographic comparison of [3H] Acetylcholine, [3H] Nicotine and [125I]-alpha-Bungarotoxin. *J. Neurosci.,* 5: 1307–1315.

Cole, A.E. and Nicoll, R.A. (1983) Acetylcholine mediates a slow synaptic potential in hippocampal pyramidal cells. *Science,* 221: 1299–1301.

Cole, A.E. and Nicoll, R.A. (1984a) The pharmacology of cholinergic excitatory responses in hippocampal pyramidal cells. *Brain Res.,* 305: 283–290.

Cole, A.E. and Nicoll, R.A. (1984b) Characterization of a slow cholinergic postsynaptic potential recorded in vitro from rat hippocampal pyramidal cells. *J. Physiol. (Lond.),* 352: 173–188.

Colino, A. and Halliwell, J.V. (1987) Differential modulation of three separate K-conductances in hippocampal CA1 neurons by serotonin. *Nature (Lond.),* 328: 73–77.

Connor, J.A. and Stevens, C.F. (1971) Voltage-clamp studies of a transient outward membrane current in gastropod neural somata. *J. Physiol. (Lond.),* 223: 21–30.

Connors, B.W. and Prince, D.A. (1982) Effects of local anesthetic QX-314 on the membrane properties of hippocampal pyramidal neurons. *J. Pharmacol. Exp. Ther.,* 220: 476–481.

Constanti, A and Sim, J.A. (1987a) Calcium-dependent potassium conductance in guinea-pig olfactory cortex neurones in vitro. *J. Physiol. (Lond.)*, 387: 173–194.

Constanti, A. and Sim, J.A. (1987b) Muscarinic receptors mediating suppression of the M-current in guinea-pig olfactory neurones may be of the M_2-subtype. *Br. J. Pharmacol.*, 90: 3–5.

Dingledine, R. and Somjen, G. (1981) Calcium dependence of synaptic transmission in the hippocampal slice. *Brain Res.*, 207: 218–222.

Dodd, J., Dingledine, R. and Kelly, J.S. (1981) The excitatory action of acetylcholine on hippocampal neurones of the guinea pig and rat maintained in vitro. *Brain Res.*, 207: 109–177.

Dudar, J.D. (1975) The effect of septal nuclei stimulation on the release of acetylcholine from the rabbit hippocampus. *Brain Res.*, 83: 123–133.

Dunwiddie, T.V. and Hoffer, B.J. (1980) Adenine nucleotides and synaptic transmission in the in vitro rat hippocampus. *Br. J. Pharmacol.*, 69: 59–68.

Dutar, P. and Nicoll, R.A. (1988a) A physiological role for $GABA_b$ receptors in the central nervous system. *Nature*, 332: 156–158.

Dutar, P. and Nicoll, R.A. (1988b) Stimulation of posphatidylinositol (PI) turnover may mediate the muscarinic suppression of the M-current in hippocampal pyramidal cell. *Neurosci Lett.*, 85: 89–94.

Dutar, P and Nicoll, R.A. (1988c) Classification of muscarinic responses in hippocampus in terms of receptor subtypes and second-messenger systems: Electrophysiological studies in vitro. *J. Neurosci.*, 8: 4214–4224.

Eccles J.C. (1969) The Inhibitory Pathways of the Central Nervous System. Liverpool: Liverpool University Press.

Egan, T.M. and North, R.A. (1986a) Actions of acetylcholine and nicotine on rat locus coeruleus neurons in vitro. *Neuroscience*, 19: 565–571.

Egan, TM, and North RA (1986b) Acetylcholine acts on m_2-muscarinic receptors to excite rat locus coeruleus neurones. *Br. J. Pharmacol.*, 85: 733–735.

Fonnum, F. (1970) Topographical and subcellular localization of choline acetyltransferase in the rat hippocampal region. *J. Neurochem.*, 17: 1029–1037.

Fox AP, Nowycky MC, Tsien RW (1987) Single-channel recordings of three types of calcium channels in chick sensory neurones. *J Physiol (Lond)* 394: 173–200.

Frotscher, M. and Leranth, C. (1985) Cholinergic innervation of the hippocampus as revealed by choline acetyltransferase immunocytochemistry: a combined light and electron microscopic study. *J. Comp. Neurol.*, 239: 237–246.

French, C.R. and Gage, P.W. (1985) A threshold sodium current in pyramidal cells in rat hippocampus. *Neurosci. Letts*, 56: 289–293.

Gahwiler, B.H. (1984) Facilitation by acetylcholine of tetrodotoxin resistant spikes in rat hippocampal pyramidal cells. *Neuroscience*, 11: 382–388.

Gahwiler, B.H. and Brown, D.A. (1985) Functional innervation of cultured hippocampal neurones by cholinergic affer-

ents from co-cultured septal explants. *Nature (Lond.)*, 313: 577–579.

Gahwiler, B.H. and Brown, D.A. (1987) Muscarine affects calcium-currents in rat hippocampal pyramidal cells in vitro. *Neurosci. Lett.*, 76: 301–306.

Gahwiler, B.H. and Dreifuss, J.J. (1982) Multiple actions of acetylcholine on hippocampal pyramidal cells in organotypic explant cultures. *Neuroscience*, 7: 1243–1256.

Greene, R.W. and Haas, H.L. (1985) Adenosine actions on CA1 pyramidal neurones in rat hippocampal slices. *J. Physiol. (Lond.)*, 366: 119–127.

Gustafsson, B., Galvan, M., Grafe, P. and Wigstrom, H. (1982) A transient outward current in a mammalian central neurone blocked by 4-aminopyridine. *Nature (Lond.)*, 299: 252–254.

Haas, H.L. (1982) Cholinergic disinhibition in hippocampal slices of the rat. *Brain Res.*, 233: 200–204.

Haas, H.L. and Greene, R.W. (1984) Adenosine enhances afterhyperpolarization and accommodation in hippocampal pyramidal cells. *Pflugers Arch.*, 402: 244–247.

Haas, H.L. and Greene, R.W. (1986) Effects of histamine on hippocampal pyramidal cells of the rat in vitro. *Exp. Brain Res.*, 62: 123–130.

Haas, H.L. and Konnerth, A. (1983) Histamine and noradrenaline decrease calcium-activated potassium conductance in hippocampal pyramidal cells. *Nature (Lond.)*, 302: 432–434.

Halliwell, J.V. (1983) Caesium-loading reveals two distinct Ca-currents in voltage-clamped guinea-pig hippocampal neurones in vitro. *J. Physiol. (Lond.)*, 341: 10P.

Halliwell, J.V. (1990) K^+ Channels in the central nervous system. in N.S. Cook (Ed.), *Potassium Channels: Structure, Classification, Function and Therapeutic Potential*, Chichester: Ellis Horwood, pp. 348–381.

Halliwell, J.V. and Adams, P.R. (1982) Voltage-clamp analysis of muscarinic excitation in hippocampal neurones. *Brain Res.* 250: 71–92.

Halliwell, J.V. and Grove, E.A. (1989) 9-amino-1,2,3,4-tetrahydroacridine (THA) blocks agonist-induced potassium conductance in rat hippocampal neurones. *Eur. J. Pharmacol.*, 163: 369–372.

Hammer, R., Berrie, E.P. Birdsall, N.J.M., Burgen, A.S.V. and Hulme, E.C. (1980) Pirenzepine distinguishes between different subclasses of muscarinic receptors. *Nature*, 283: 90–292.

Higashida, H. and Brown, D.A. (1986) Two polyphosphatidylinositide metabolites control two K^+-currents in a neuronal cell. *Nature*, 323: 333–335.

Hotson, J.R. and Prince, D.A. (1980) A calcium-activated hyperpolarization follows repetitive firing in hippocampal neurons. *J. Neurophysiol.*, 43: 409–419.

Hotson, J.R., Prince, D.A. and Schwartzkroin, P.A. (1979) Anomalous inward rectification in hippocampal neurons. *J. Neurophysiol.*, 42: 889–895.

Hounsgaard, J. (1978) Presynaptic inhibitory action of acetylcholine in area CA1 of the hippocampus. *Exp. Neurol.*, 62: 787–797.

Jones, R.S.G. and Heinemann, U. (1988) Verapamil blocks the afterhyperpolarization but not the spike frequency accommodation of rat CA1 pyramidal cells in vitro. *Brain Res.,* 462: 367–371.

Kandel, E.R., Spencer, W.A. and Brinley, F.J. (1961) Electrophysiology of hippocampal neurons. I. Sequential invasion and synaptic organization. *J. Neurophysiol.,* 24: 225–252.

Krnjevic, K., Pumain, R. and Renaud, L. (1971) The mechanism of excitation by acetylcholine in the cerebral cortex. *J. Physiol. (Lond.),* 215: 447–465.

Lancaster, B. and Adams, P.R. (1986) Calcium-dependent current generating the afterhyperpolarization of hippocampal neurons. *J. Neurophysiol,* 55: 1268–1282.

Lanthorn, T.H. and Cotman, C.W. (1981) Baclofen selectively inhibits excitatory synaptic transmission in the hippocampus. *Brain Res.,* 225: 171–178.

Lee, K.S., Schubert, P., Reddington, M. and Kreutzberg, G.W. (1983) Adenosine receptor density and the depression of evoked electrical activity in the rat hippocampus in vitro. *Neurosci. Lett.,* 37: 81–85.

Leranth, C. and Frotscher, M. (1987) Cholinergic innervation of hippocampal GAD and somatostatin-immunoreactive commissural neurons. *J. Comp. Neurol.,* 261: 33–47.

Lewis, P.R. and Shute, C.C.D. (1967) The cholinergic limbic system: projection to hippocampal formation, medial cortex, nuclei of the ascending cholinergic reticular system and the subfornical organ and supraoptic crest. *Brain,* 90: 521–540.

McCormick, D.A. and Prince, D.A. (1985) Two types of muscarinic response to acetylcholine in mammalian cortical neurons. *Proc Natl. Acad. Sci. USA,* 82: 6344–6348.

McCormick, D.A. and Prince, D.A. (1986) Mechanisms of action of acetylcholine in the guinea-pig cerebral cortex in vitro. *J. Physiol. (Lond),* 375: 169–194.

McCormick D.A. and Prince, D.A. (1987) Acetylcholine causes rapid nicotinic excitation in the medial habenular nucleus of guinea pig in vitro. *J. Neurosci.,* 7: 742–752.

Madison, D.V. and Nicoll, R.A. (1982) Noradrenaline blocks accommodation of pyramidal cell discharge in the hippocampus. *Nature (Lond.),* 299: 636–638.

Madison, D.V. and Nicoll, R.A. (1984) Control of repetitive discharge of rat CA1 pyramidal neurones in vitro. *J. Physiol. (Lond.),* 354: 319–331.

Madison, D.V. and Nicoll, R.A. (1986a) Actions of noradrenaline recorded intracellularly in rat hippocampal CA1 pyramidal neurones, in vitro. *J. Physiol. (Lond.),* 372: 221–244.

Madison, D.V. and Nicoll, R.A. (1986b) Cyclic adenosine 3′, 5′-monophosphate mediates beta-receptor actions of noradrenaline in rat hippocampal pyramidal cells. *J. Physiol.,* 372: 245–259.

Madison, D.V., Lancaster, B. and Nicoll, R.A. (1987) Voltage-clamp analysis of cholinergic action in the hippocampus. *J. Neurosci.,* 7: 733–741.

Malenka, R.C., Madison, D.V., Andrade, R. and Nicoll, R.A. (1986) Phorbol esters mimic some cholinergic actions in hippocampal pyramidal neurons. *J. Neurosci.,* 6: 475–480.

Misgeld, U., Muller, W and Polder, H.R. (1989) Potentiation and suppression by eserine of muscarinic synaptic transmission in the guinea-pig hippocampal slice. *J. Physiol. (Lond.),* 409: 191–206.

Moore, S.D., Madamba, S.G., Joels, M. and Siggins, G.R. (1988) Somatostatin augments the M-current in hippocampal neurons. *Science,* 239: 278–280.

Muller, W. and Misgeld, U. (1986) Slow cholinergic excitation of guinea-pig hippocampal neurons is mediated by two muscarinic receptor subtypes. *Neurosci. Lett.,* 67: 107–112.

Nakajima, Y., Nakajima S, Leonard RJ, Yamaguchi K (1986) Acetylcholine raises excitability by inhibiting the fast transient potassium current in cultured hippocamal neurones. *Proc Natl. Acad Sci (USA)* 83: 3022–3026.

Nicoll, R.A. (1988) The coupling of neurotransmitter receptors to ion channels in the brain. *Science* 241: 545–551.

Ribak, C.E., Vaughn, J.E. and Saito, K. (1978) Immunocytochemical localization of glutamic acid decarboxylase in neuronal somata following colchicine inhibition of axonal transport. *Brain Res.,* 150: 315–332.

Rovira, C., Cherubini, E. and Ben-Ari, Y. (1982) Opposite actions of muscarinic and nicotinic agents on hippocampal dendritic negative fields recorded in rats. *Neuropharmacology,* 21: 933–936.

Sah, P., French, C.R. and Gage, P.W. (1985) Effects of noradrenaline on some potassium currents in CA1 neurones in rat hippocampal slices. *Neurosci. Lett.,* 60: 295–300.

Sah, P., Gibb, A.J. and Gage, P.W. (1988) The sodium current underlying action potentials in guinea-pig hippocampal CA1 neurons. *J. Gen. Physiol.,* 91: 373–398.

Schwartzkroin, P.A. (1976) Further characteristics of hippocampal CA1 cells in vitro. *Brain Res.,* 128: 53–68.

Schwartzkroin, P.A. and Slawsky, M. (1977) Probable calcium spikes in hippocampal neurons. *Brain Res.,* 135: 157–161.

Segal, M. (1982) Multiple actions of acetylcholine at a muscarinic receptor studied in the rat hippocampal slice. *Brain Res.,* 246: 77–87.

Segal. M. (1983) Rat hippocampal neurons in culture: responses to electrical and chemical stimuli. *J. Neurophysiol.,* 50: 1249–1264.

Segal, M. (1988) Synaptic activation of a cholinergic receptor in rat hippocampus. *Brain Res.,* 452: 79–86.

Segal, M., Rogawski, M.A. and Barker, J.L. (1984) A transient potassium conductance regulates the excitability of cultured hippocampal and spinal neurons. *J. Neurosci.,* 4: 604–609.

Skrede, K.K., and Westgaard, R.H. (1971) The transverse hippocampal slice: a well-defined cortical structure maintained in vitro. *Brain Res.,* 35: 589–593.

Smith, C.M. (1974) Acetylcholine release from the cholinergic septohippocampal pathway, *Life Sci.,* 14: 2159–2166.

Storm, J.F. (1987) Action potential repolarization and a fast after-hyperpolarization in rat hippocampal pyramidal cells. *J. Physiol. (Lond),* 385: 733–759.

Storm, J.F. (1989) An after-hyperpolarization of medium duration in rat hippocampal pyramidal cells. *J. Physiol. (Lond.),* 409: 171–190.

Storm-Mathisen, J. (1977) Localization of transmitter candidates in the brain: The hippocampal formation as a model. *Prog. Neurobiol.*, 8: 119–181.

Summers, W.K., Majovsky, L.V.. Marsh, G.M., Takichi, K. and Kling, K. (1986) Oral tetrahydroaminoacridine in long-term treatment of senile dementia, Alzheimer type. *N. Engl. J. Med.*, 315: 1241–1287.

Toselli, M. and Lux, H.D. (1989) GTP-binding protein mediates acetylcholine inhibition of voltage-dependent calcium channels in hippocampal neurons. *Pflueger's Arch.*, 413: 319–321.

Trussell, L.O. and Jackson, M.B. (1987) Dependence of an adenosine-activated potassium current on a GTP-binding protein in mammalian central neurons. *J. Neurosci.*, 7: 3306–3316.

Valentino, R. and Dingledine, R. (1981) Presynaptic inhibitory effect of acetylcholine in the hippocampus, *J. Neurosci.*, 1: 784–792.

Wada, E., Wada, K., Boulter, J.., Deneris, E., Heinemann, S. Patrick, J. and Swanson, L.W. (1989) The distribution of alpha2, alpha3, alpha4 and beta2 neuronal nicotine receptor subunit mRNAs in the central nervous system. A hybridization histochemical study in the rat. *J. Comp. Neurol.*, 284: 314–355.

Wainer, B.H., Levey, A.I., Rye, D.B.. Mesulam, M-M. and Mufson, E.J. (1985) Cholinergic and non-cholinergic septo-hippocampal pathways. *Neurosci. Lett.*, 54: 45–52.

Watson, T.W.J. and Pitman,, Q.J. (1988) Pharmacological evidence that somatostatin activates the M-current in hippocampal pyramidal neurones. *Neurosci. Lett.*, 91: 172–176.

Worley, P.F., Baraban, J.M., McCarren, M., Snyder, S.H. and Alger, B.E. (1987) Cholinergic phosphatidylinositol modulation of inhibitory, G protein-linked, neurotransmitter actions: Electrophysiological studies in rat hippocampus. *Proc. Natl. Acad. Sci. USA*, 84: 3467–3471.

Yaari, Y., Hamon, B. and Lux, H.D. (1987) Development of two types of calcium channels in cultured mammalian hippocampal neurons. *Science*, 235: 80–82.

Yamamoto, C. and Kawai, N. (1967) Presynaptic action of acetylcholine in thin sections from the guinea pig dentate gyrus in vitro. *Exp. Neurol.*, 19: 176–187.

S.-M. Aquilonius and P.-G. Gillberg (Eds.)
Progress in Brain Research, Vol. 84
© 1990 Elsevier Science Publishers B.V. (Biomedical Division)

CHAPTER 29

Principal aspects of the regulation of acetylcholine release in the brain

G. Pepeu, F. Casamenti, M.G. Giovannini, M.G. Vannucchi and F. Pedata

Department of Preclinical and Clinical Pharmacology, University of Florence, Viale Morgagni 65, 50134 Florence, Italy

Introduction

The study of acetylcholine (ACh) release coupled with the recording of neuronal activity and, whenever possible, the investigation of behavior, is the most direct approach for understanding the role of central cholinergic neurons and identifying metabolic conditions, neurotransmitters and drugs which may modify their activity. However, while it is relatively easy to correlate ACh release and electrical activity in peripheral nerves in which either all or the majority of the fibres are cholinergic in nature, such as in the motor nerves (Thesleff, 1988), the correlation is difficult in the CNS. Here the cholinergic neurons and their fibres are always mixed with non-cholinergic neurons. Since ACh release from many nerve endings must be collected in order to quantify it, relatively large brain regions, also containing many non cholinergic nerve endings, are needed, irrespective of the procedure used for measuring ACh release. Thus, correlations between electrical activity of specific neuronal pathways and ACh release become approximate. Similarly approximate is the correlation between ACh release and behavior.

In spite of these limitations, important information on the role and function of the cholinergic neurons has been obtained from release studies. In this short review the conditions influencing ACh release in the brain will be illustrated by examples taken from in vivo and in vitro investigations.

Methods for investigating ACh release in the brain

The methods which can be used for investigating ACh release in the brain are listed in Table I. Detailed descriptions of the advantages and limitations, and the methodological details of in vivo techniques can be found in Marsden (1984). The perfusion of the cerebral ventricles has been a source of useful information (Feldberg, 1963), but was abandoned because of the need for large animals and the difficulties in identifying the cholinergic pathways involved in the release.

The use of brain slices for investigating the cholinergic synapse has been described by Weiler et al. (1982). Spontaneous and evoked release can be measured, the latter elicited by potassium depolarization, pharmacological and electrical stimulations. A review of the papers investigating the mechanisms of ACh release in synaptosomes was made by Gibson and Blass (1982). The use of cultured neuronal cells for ACh release investigation is still limited and mostly confined to PC12

TABLE I

Methods for investigating ACh release in the brain

In vivo	In vitro
Perfusion of cerebral ventricles	Brain slices or prisms
Perfusion of the spinal cord	Synaptosomes
Push pull cannula	Neuronal cultures
Cortical cups	
Intracranial microdialysis	

TABLE II

Mechanisms regulating acetylcholine release in the CNS

Postsynaptic stimulation and inhibition of cholinergic neuron
  firing
ACh synthesis:
  enzyme activity
  precursor availability
Presynaptic influence on the release mechanisms
Presynaptic auto and heteroreceptors

---

pheochromocytoma cells (Melega and Howard, 1984).

The presence of acetylcholinesterase (AChE) inhibitors in the incubation or superfusing medium is always necessary for measuring a reliable and constant release of endogenous ACh. In order to overcome the artifacts due to AChE inhibition, in vitro preparations may be loaded with radioactive choline (Ch) and its evoked labeled Ch release can be taken as an indication of ACh release (Hertting et al., 1980). The similarities and differences between the two approaches have been investigated by Beani et al. (1984).

Regulation of acetylcholine release

Table II lists the mechanisms regulating brain ACh release.

Postsynaptic stimulation and inhibition of cholinergic neuron firing

Evoked ACh release in vitro (Hertting et al., 1980) and spontaneous ACh in vivo (Damsma et al., 1988) are blocked by tetrodotoxin and therefore depend on propagated electrical activity. A direct relationship has also been demonstrated in vitro (Pedata et al., 1983) and in vivo (see ref. in Pepeu, 1973) between stimulation frequency, i.e. firing activity, and ACh release. Consequently, the increase in cortical electrical activity during arousal is associated with a larger ACh release than the reduced neuronal firing occurring during slow waves sleep, as repeatedly demonstrated with the cortical cup technique (see ref. in Pepeu, 1973; Moroni and Pepeu, 1984). Direct stimulation or inhibition of the cholinergic neurons of the nucleus basalis is accompanied by an increase or decrease in ACh release from the cerebral cortex (Casamenti et al., 1986).

The activity of the cholinergic neurons is influenced by many neurotransmitter-neuromodulators acting on postsynaptic receptors located on neuronal somata and dendrites. Differences in the types of postsynaptic receptors involved exist between different regions, as shown in Table III.

The use of the microdialysis technique has surprisingly not confirmed the well established concept of the dopaminergic-cholinergic balance in the striatum (Lehman and Langer, 1983). Using this technique, the administration of amphetamine is followed by a transient increase in striatal ACh (Pepeu et al., 1989) instead of the expected decrease (Cantrill et al., 1983). Similarly, contrasting results on ACh release have been obtained by

TABLE III

Postsynaptic receptors influencing ACh release

Region	Type of receptor	Method used	Effect on release	References
Striatum	D$_2$	slices,	inhibition	Lehman and Langer, 1983
		push-pull cannula	inhibition	Lehman and Langer, 1983
	NMDA	slices	stimulation	Scatton and Lehman, 1982
Forebrain	D$_2$	cortical cup	stimulation	Casamenti et al., 1986
	CCK	cortical cup	stimulation/ inhibition	Magnani et al., 1984
	GABA	cortical cup	inhibition	Casamenti et al., 1986
	opioid	cup	inhibition	Pepeu, 1973
	5HT	cup	inhibition	Bianchi et al., 1986

Westerink et al. (1989) with the administration of dopaminergic antagonists. The possibility that the presence of cholinesterase inhibitors in the perfusing fluid may mask the response to dopaminergic agonists and antagonists needs to be investigated.

ACh synthesis

The amount and the duration of ACh release from the nerve endings depends on ACh store and synthesis. Since choline acetyltransferase (ChAT) activity in the cholinergic neurons is not rate-limiting, the rate of synthesis depends on the availability of the two precursors, Ch and acetylCoA (Tucek, 1988). In this review only a few recent works investigating directly the role of precursors on ACh release will be mentioned. In vivo direct administration of a large dose of Ch brings about only a small increase in ACh release as recently confirmed by the microdialysis technique in the striatum (De Boer et al., 1989). On the contrary inhibition of Ch uptake by intracerebroventricular administration is followed by a marked decrease in striatal ACh release (Consolo et al., 1987). In vitro Ch addition to the superfusing fluid strongly enhances basal and evoked ACh release (Ulus et al., 1989). It may be assumed that in vivo, under physiological conditions, a sufficient extracellular Ch concentration is maintained by different Ch sources including phospholipids.

The dependence of ACh synthesis on glucose metabolism and acetylCoa formation has been well demonstrated (Tucek, 1978). Whether it is possible to stimulate ACh release in vivo by enhancing acetylCoa formation needs to be demonstrated.

The sensitivity of ACh release to hypoxia has been demonstrated in brain slices (Gibson and Peterson, 1982) and synaptosomes (Sanchez-Prieto, 1987). The low pH occurring during hypoxia could be an important contributory factor.

An age-dependent decrease in ACh release has been shown in vivo (Wu et al., 1988) and in vitro (Pedata et al., 1983). The decrease in ACh release results from a reduction in ACh synthesis (Van-

nucchi and Pepeu, 1987). The cause of the reduction has not yet been identified since no consistent decrease in ChAT activity has been shown in normal aging (see ref. in Wu, 1988).

Presynaptic influence on the release mechanisms

Since evoked ACh release is strictly calcium-dependent in vitro (Hertting et al., 1980 and in vivo (Consolo et al., 1987) drugs which inhibit or enhance calcium penetration in the nerve endings during depolarization decrease or increase, respectively, ACh release. Examples are offered by the parallel decrease in calcium uptake and evoked ACh release brought about by quinacrine in cortical synaptosomes (Baba et al., 1983), and by the increase in ACh release induced in cortical slices by calcium ionophores (Casamenti et al., 1978), and in vivo by 4-aminopyridine (Casamenti et al., 1982) which promote voltage-dependent calcium influx.

Further biochemical events involved in the evoked ACh release from cholinergic nerve endings are the inhibition of Na^+ K^+-activated adenosine triphosphatase (Vizi, 1979) and activation of protein kinase C (Allgaier et al., 1988). The complete chain of events leading to the mobilization of the vesicular and cytoplasmatic ACh stores and their efflux in the synaptic cleft is still open to investigation. Each of the events may be the target of neurotransmitters or drugs modulating ACh release.

Presynaptic auto- and heteroreceptors

Table IV lists presynaptic receptors whose effects on ACh release have been clearly demonstrated in vitro and/or in vivo. The list is by no means complete and is intended only as an indication of the complexity of the modulation taking place at presynaptic level. In each brain area the cholinergic nerve endings are equipped with qualitatively and/or quantitatively different sets of presynaptic receptors, making possible a differential regional modulation. For instance, Marchi et al. (1983) demonstrated that the activation of striatal muscarinic autoreceptors is less

TABLE IV

Presynaptic auto- and heteroreceptors modulating ACh release

Region	Type of receptors	Method used	Effect on release	References
Striatum	M_1	slices	decrease	Hadhazy and Szerb, 1977
		dialysis	decrease	Consolo et al., 1987
	5HT	slices	decrease	Gillet et al., 1985
	A_1	slices	decrease	Harms et al., 1979
	opioid	slices	decrease	Mulder et al., 1984
Hippocampus	M_1	slices	decrease	Hadhazy and Szerb, 1977
	GABA	synaptosomes	increase	Bonanno and Raiteri, 1986
	A_1	slices	decrease	Jackisch et al., 1984
		synaptosomes	decrease	Pedata et al., 1986
Cortex	M_1	cup	decrease	Pepeu, 1973
		slices	decrease	Hadhazy and Szerb, 1977
	α_2	slices	decrease	Vizi, 1979
		cup	decrease	Beani et al., 1978
	A_1	slices	decrease	Pedata et al., 1983
		synaptosomes	decrease	Pedata et al., 1986
	GABA	slices	decrease	Bianchi et al., 1982

effective in reducing ACh release in the striatum than in the cortex and hippocampus. Similarly, adenosine inhibition of ACh release is more effective in the hippocampus than in the cerebral cortex (Pedata et al., 1986). Comparison of Tables III and IV reveals that the cholinergic neurons can be both stimulated and inhibited by neurotransmitters/neuromodulators acting postsynaptically. In contrast, with a single exception, all presynaptic receptors inhibit ACh release. However, this inhibition is never complete but only reduces by approximately 50% the release as shown, for example, for the muscarinic autoreceptors and the A_1 (Pedata et al., 1986) and D_2 (Hertting et al., 1980) receptors. The concurrent activation of two inhibitory receptors does not necessarily result in a summation of effects (Pedata et al., 1986). Conversely, their blockade may be followed by a large increase in neurotrasmitter release (Pepeu, 1973; Hertting et al., 1980). The physiological role of this multiple, discrete inhibitory control of ACh release needs further clarification.

Conclusions

The aim of this review was to present the principles, not to cover all the facets of ACh release.

The limits of space are the main reason for the many omissions which can be found. Release of ACh has been investigated in other brain regions, besides those mentioned; the effects of peptides such as TRH, enkephalins and galanine (see Chapter 30 of this volume) have not been described. The central cholinergic neurons are involved in many functions, including cognitive processes and motor regulation. The large number of mechanisms modulating their activity is indirect evidence of their critical role and opens the way to effective pharmacological interventions.

References

Allgaier, C., Daschmann, B., Huang, H.Y. and Hertting, G. (1988) Protein kinase C and presynaptic modulation of acetylcholine release in rabbit hippocampus. *Br. J. Pharmacol.* 93: 525–534.

Baba, A., Ohta, A. and Iwata, H. (1983) Inhibition by quinacrine of depolarization-induced acetylcholine release and calcium influx in rat brain cortical synaptosomes. *J. Neurochemistry* 40: 1758–1761.

Beani, L., Bianchi, C., Giacomelli, A. and Tamberi, F. (1978) Noradrenaline inhibition of acetylcholine release from guinea-pig brain. *Eur. J. Pharmacol.* 48: 179–183.

Beani, L., Bianchi, C., Siniscalchi, A., Sivilotti, L., Tanganelli, S. and Veratti, E. (1984) Different approaches to study endogenous acetylcholine release: endogenous ACh versus tritium efflux. *Naunyn-Schmiedeberg's Arch. Pharmacol.* 328: 119–126.

Bianchi, C., Tanganelli, S., Marzola, G. and Beani, L. (1982) GABA-induced changes in acetylcholine release from slices of guinea-pig brain. *Naunyn Schmiedeberg's Arch. Pharmacol.* 318: 253–258.

Bianchi, C., Siniscalchi, A. and Beani, L. (1986) The influence of 5-hydroxytryptamine on the release of acetylcholine from guinea-pig brain ex vivo and in vitro. *Neuropharmacology* 25: 1043–1049.

Bonanno, G. and Raiteri, M. (1986) GABA enhances acetylcholine release from hippocampal nerve endings through a mechanisms blocked by a GABA uptake inhibitor. *Neurosci. Lett.* 70: 360–363.

Cantrill R.C., Arbilla, S. and Langer S.Z. (1983) Inhibition by d-amphetamine of the electrically evoked release of [^{3}H]acetylcholine from slices of rat striatum: involvement of dopamine receptors. *Eur. J. Pharmacol.* 87: 167–168.

Casamenti, F., Mantovani, P. and Pepeu, G. (1978) Stimulation of acetylcholine output from brain slices caused by the ionophores BrX 537A and A 23187. *Br. J. Pharmacol.* 63: 259–265.

Casamenti, F., Corradetti, R., Loffelholz, K., Mantovani, P. and Pepeu, G. (1982) Effects of 4-aminopyridine on acetylcholine output from the cerebral cortex of the rat in vivo. *Br. J. Pharmacol.* 76: 439–445.

Casamenti, F., Deffenu, G., Abbamondi A.L. and Pepeu, G. (1986) Changes in cortical acetylcholine output induced by modulation of the nucleus basalis. *Brain Res. Bull.* 16: 689–695.

Consolo, S., Wu, C.F., Fiorentini, F., Ladinsky, H. and Vezzani, A. (1987) Determination of endogenous acetylcholine release in freely moving rats by transstriatal dialysis coupled to a radioenzymatic assay: effect of drugs. *J. Neurochemistry* 48: 1459–1465.

Damsma, G., Westerink, B.H.C., de Boer, P., de Vries, J.B. and Horn, A.S. (1988) Basal acetylcholine release in freely moving rats detected by online trans-striatal dialysis: pharmacological aspects. *Life Sci.* 1161–1168.

de Boer, P., Westerink, B.H.C., Damsma, G. and Horn, A.S. (1989) Microdialysis of acetylcholine from the striatum of awake rats: behavioral and pharmacological aspects. In *Basal Ganglia 89*, International Basal Ganglia Society, Third Triennial Meeting, Capo Boi, June 1989, Abstract Book, p. 52.

Feldberg, W. (1963) *A Pharmacological Approach to the Brain from its Inner and Outer Surface*, Arnold (Publishers), London, pp. 1–128.

Gibson, G. and Blass J.P. (1982) Synaptomes. In I. Hanin and A.M. Goldberg (Eds.), *Progress in Cholinergic Biology: Model Cholinergic Synapses*, Raven Press, New York, pp. 271–288.

Gibson, G. and Peterson C. (1982) Decreases in the release of acetylcholine in vitro with low oxigen. *Biochem. Pharmacol.* 31: 111–115.

Gillet, G., Ammor, S. and Fillon, G. (1985) Serotonin inhibits acetylcholine release from rat striatum slices: evidence for a presynaptic receptor-mediated effect. *J. Neurochem.* 45: 1687–91.

Hadhazy, P. and Szerb, J.C. (1977) The effect of cholinergic drugs on [^{3}H]acetylcholine release from slices of rat hippocampus, striatum and cortex. *Brain Res.* 123: 311–322.

Harms, H.H., Wardeh, G. and Mulder, A.H. (1979) Effects of adenosine on depolarization-induced release of various radiolabelled neurotransmitters from slices of rat corpus striatum. *Neuropharmacology* 18: 577–580.

Hertting, G., Zumstein, A., Jackisch, R., Hoffmann, I. and Starke, K. (1980) Modulation by endogenous dopamine of the release of acetylcholine in the caudate nucleus of the rabbit. *Naunyn-Schmiedeberg's Arch. Pharmacol.* 315: 111–117.

Jackisch, R., Strittmatter, H., Kasakov, L. and Hertting, G. (1984) Endogenous adenosine as a modulator of hippocampal acetylcholine release. *Naunyn Schmiedeberg's Arch. Pharmacol.* 327: 319–326.

Lehman, J. and Langer S.Z. (1983) The striatal cholinergic interneuron: synaptic target of dopaminergic terminals? *Neuroscience* 10: 1105–1120.

Magnani, M., Mantovani, P. and Pepeu, G. (1984) Effect of cholecystokinin octapeptide and ceruletide on the release of acetylcholine from cerebral cortex of the rat in vivo. *Neuropharmacology* 23: 1305–1309.

Marchi, M., Paudice, P., Caviglia, A.M. and Raiteri, M. (1983) Is acetylcholine release from striatal nerve endings regulated by muscarinic autoreceptors? *Eur. J. Pharmacol.* 91: 63–68.

Marsden, C.A. (Ed.) (1984) *Measurement of Neurotransmitter Release In vivo*, John Wiley, Chichester, pp. 1–233.

Melega, W.P. and Howard B.D. (1984) Biochemical evidence that vesicles are the source of the acetylcholine released from stimulated PC12 cells. *Proc. Natl. Acad. Sci. USA* 81: 6535–6538.

Moroni, F. and Pepeu, G. (1984) The cortical cup technique. In C.A. Marsden (Ed.), *Measurement of Neurotransmitter Release In vivo*, John Wiley, Chichester, pp. 63–80.

Mulder, A.H., Wardeh, G. Hogenboom, F. and Frankhuizen A.L. (1984) K- and delta-opioid receptor agonists differentially inhibit striatal dopamine and acetylcholine release. *Nature* 308: 278–280.

Pedata, F., Antonelli, T., Lambertini, L., Beani, L. and Pepeu G. (1983) Effect of adenosine, adenosine triphosphate, adenosine deaminase, dipyridamole and aminophylline on acetylcholine release from electrically-stimulated brain slices. *Neuropharmacology* 22: 609–614.

Pedata, F., Slavikova, J., Kotas, A. and Pepeu, G. (1983) Acetylcholine release from rat cortical slices during postnatal development and aging. *Neurobiol. Aging* 4: 31–35.

Pedata, F., Giovannelli, L, De Sarno, P. and Pepeu, G. (1986) Effect of adenosine, adenosine derivatives, and caffeine on acetylcholine release from brain synaptosomes: interactions with muscarinic autoregulatory mechanisms. *J. Neurochem.* 46: 1593–1598.

Pepeu, G. (1973) The release of acetylcholine from the brain:

an approach to the study of the central cholinergic mechanisms. *Progr. Neurobiol.* 2: 257–288.

Pepeu, G., Casamenti, F., Giovannini, M.G. and Vannucchi, M.G. (1989) Microdialysis investigations of acetylcholine release: drug effects on aging rats. In Kewitz, H. (Ed.), *Pharmacological Interventions on Central Cholinergic Mechanisms in Senile Dementia (Alzheimer's Disease)*, Zuckschwerdt Verlag, Munich, pp. 162–167.

Sanchez-Prieto, J., Harvey, S.A.K. and Clark, J.B. (1987) Effects of in vitro anoxia and low pH on acetylcholine release by rat brain synaptosomes. *J. Neurochemistry* 48: 1278–1284.

Scatton, B. and Lehman, J. (1982) *N*-Methyl-D-aspartate-type receptors mediate striatal ^{3}H-acetylcholine release evoked by excitatory aminoacids. *Nature* 297: 422–424.

Thesleff, S. (1988) Different kind of acetylcholine release from the motor nerve. *Int. Rev. Neurobiol.* 28: 59–88.

Tucek, S. (1978) *Acetylcholine synthesis in neurons.* Chapman and Hall, London.

Tucek, S. (1988) Choline acetyltransferase and the synthesis of acetylcholine. In Whittaker, V.P. (Ed.) *The Cholinergic Synapse. Handbook of Experimental Pharmacology,* Vol. 86, Springer Verlar, Berlin, pp. 125–165.

Ulus, I.H., Wurtman, R.J., Mauron, C. and Blusztajn J.K.

(1989) Choline increases acetylcholine release and protects against the stimulation-induced decrease in phosphatide levels within membranes of rat corpus striatum. *Brain Res.* 489: 217–227.

Vannucchi, M.G. and Pepeu, G. (1987) Effects of phosphatidylserine on acetylcholine release and content in cortical slices from aging rats. *Neurobiol. Aging* 8: 403–407.

Vizi, S. (1979) Presynaptic modulation of neurochemical transmission. *Prog. Neurobiol.* 12: 181–190.

Vizi, E.S. (1979) Na^+ K^+ activate adenosinetriphosphatase as a trigger in transmitter release. *Neuroscience* 3: 367–384.

Weiler, M.H., Misgeld, U. and Jenden D.J. (1982) Brain slices. In I. Hanin and A.M. Goldberg (Eds.), *Progress in Cholinergic Biology: Model Cholinergic Synapses,* Raven Press, New York, pp. 271–288.

Westerink, B.H.C., de Boer, P., Damsma, G., de Vries, J.B. and Horn A.S. (1989) In *Basal Ganglia 89*, International Basal Ganglia Society, Third Triennial Meeting, Capo Boi, June 1989, Abstract Book, p. 181.

Wu, C.F., Bertorelli, R., Sacconi, M., Pepeu, G. and Consolo, S. (1988) Decrease of brain acetylcholine release in aging freely moving rats detected by microdialysis. *Neurobiol. Aging* 9: 357–361.

S.-M. Aquilonius and P.-G. Gillberg (Eds.)
Progress in Brain Research, Vol. 84
© 1990 Elsevier Science Publishers B.V. (Biomedical Division)

CHAPTER 30

Functional aspects of acetylcholine-galanin coexistence in the brain

S. Consolo[1], E. Palazzi[1], R. Bertorelli[1], G. Fisone[1,2], J. Crawley[3], T. Hökfelt[4] and T. Bartfai[2]

[1] *Laboratory of Cholinergic Neuropharmacology, Istituto di Ricerche Farmacologiche "Mario Negri", Milan, Italy,* [2] *Department of Biochemistry, Arrhenius Laboratory, S-106 91 Stockholm, Sweden,* [3] *Unit of Behavioral Neuropharmacology, National Institute of Mental Health, Bethesda, MD 20892, U.S.A., and* [4] *Department of Histology, Karolinska Institute, S-104 05, Stockholm, Sweden*

Introduction

Galanin is a 29-amino-acid peptide isolated in 1983 from the upper small intestine of pigs on the basis of its C-terminal amide (Tatemoto et al., 1983). The peptide derived its name from the N-terminal and C-terminal residues, glycine and alanine respectively (Fig. 1). Since its discovery, galanin has been shown to have a number of physiological and pharmacological actions, including inhibition of acetylcholine (ACh) stimulated contraction of small intestine, of glucose-stimulated release of insulin, of dopamine release from rat median eminence, of ACh release from guinea pig *Taenia coli* and enhancement of growth hormone and prolactin release (Rokaeus, 1987).

Antisera have been raised against the porcine peptide, and radioimmunoassay and immunohistochemical mapping have revealed extensive galanin immunoreactivity in neurons of the central (Rokaeus et al., 1984; Skofitsch and Jacobowitz, 1985; Melander et al., 1986a) and peripheral (Melander et al., 1985a) nervous systems. Autoradiography of [^{125}I]galanin binding indicated the

presence of putative galanin receptors in several brain regions (Skofitsch et al., 1986).

In the mammalian brain, galanin-like immunoreactivity appears to coexist with other peptides or neurotransmitters, including vasopressin in the paraventricular parvocellular and magnocellular nuclei, cholecystokinin in spinothalamic neurons (Ju et al., 1987), norepinephrine in the locus coeruleus (Melander et al., 1986a,b; Holets et al., 1988), dopamine in the median eminence (Nordstrom et al., 1987), histamine in the arcuate nucleus (Kohler et al., 1986). It is colocalized with GABA in the hypothalamus and with choline acetyltransferase (ChAT), a marker of the cholinergic system, in a large population of cholinergic neurons of the medial septal and diagonal band

PORCINE GALANIN 1-29

GLY-TRP-THR-LEU-ASN-SER-ALA-GLY-TYR-LEU-
LEU-GLY-PRO-HIS-ALA-ILE-ASP-ASN-HIS-ARG-
SER-PHE-HIS-ASP-LYS-TYR-GLY-LEU-ALA-NH2

RAT GALANIN 1-29

GLY-TRP-THR-LEU-ASN-SER-ALA-GLY-TYR-LEU-
LEU-GLY-PRO-HIS-ALA-ILE-ASP-ASN-HIS-ARG-
SER-PHE-SER-ASP-LYS-HIS-GLY-LEU-THR-NH2

Fig. 1. Amino acid sequences of porcine (A) and rat (B) galanin.

Correspondence to: Dr. Silvana Consolo, Istituto di Ricerche Farmacologiche "Mario Negri", via Eritrea 62, 20157 Milan, Italy.

nuclei of rat. In the owl monkey (Melander and Staines, 1986), baboon (Flint Beal et al., 1988) and human (Chan-Palay, 1988a,b; Kowall and Flint Beal, 1989) galanin appears to coexist with ChAT in the nucleus basalis of Meynert, too. The coexistence of galanin and ACh has been extensively studied because of the basal forebrain neurons' important role in higher brain functions such as memory and learning. Interestingly, galanin is the only neuropeptide known to coexist with ACh in these systems.

Melander et al. (1985b), employing a retrograde tracing technique combined with ChAT and galanin immunohistochemistry, showed that the cell bodies of the medial septal and diagonal band nuclei containing ChAT and galanin project to the hippocampus, almost entirely to the ventral part (Melander et al., 1986b). Accordingly, Fisone et al. (1989) found that the concentration of the high-affinity binding sites for $[^{125}I]$galanin in the ventral part (107 ± 15 fmol/mg protein) was double that in the dorsal part (52 ± 17 fmol/mg protein). The specific binding of $[^{125}I]$galanin to membranes from the ventral hippocampus was significantly reduced by GTP and by pertussis toxin-catalysed ADP-ribosylation, suggesting that the galanin receptor is coupled to an inhibitory G protein. Autoradiographic studies indicated a similar distribution of the galanin receptors in the hippocampus (Skofitsch et al., 1986; Fisone et al., 1987); these were done with a subsaturating concentration of the labeled ligand.

Lesion of the septum and fimbria markedly reduced the density of galanin binding sites in the ventral hippocampus as determined by receptor autoradiography (Fisone et al., 1987). This indicates that a large proportion of the putative galanin receptors are localized on the septal cholinergic afferents to this region.

Galanin's effect on in vitro and in vivo ACh release

On the basis of the above findings and results showing that galanin reduces classical transmitter release in some systems (Ekblad et al., 1985; Yau

et al., 1986; Nordstrom et al., 1987) a possible presynaptic regulatory effect of galanin on ACh in the ventral hippocampus seemed possible. To test this we examined whether galanin modulates ACh release in vivo and in vitro from the ventral and dorsal parts of the hippocampus.

Galanin used in these studies was purified from pig intestine (Bachem, Bubendorf, Switzerland). Recently, rat galanin has been cloned and sequenced (Vrontakis et al., 1987; Kaplan et al., 1988). The primary sequence of the rat and pig peptides differs at residues 23, 26, 29 (Fig. 1) but the affinities of the two peptides for $[^{125}I]$galanin are the same (Fisone et al., 1989).

$[^3H]$ACh release from hippocampal slices was measured by preloading the tissue with $[^3H]$choline, during an incubation of 45 min, at 37°C in Krebs-Ringer buffer, according to the previously described method (Fisone et al., 1987). Depolarization of the slices by 25 mM K$^+$ evoked $[^3H]$ACh release from the ventral and dorsal parts to the same extent (Table I). Addition of 1 μM galanin to the medium lowered K$^+$-evoked $[^3H]$ACh release from the ventral hippocampal slices but had no effect on the dorsal part (Table I). Galanin's effect was concentration-dependent (Fisone et al., 1987). Reduction of the evoked release was maximal (39%) with 500 nM galanin. Galanin's inhibitory effects are probably exerted at high-affinity receptors, since reduction of ACh release was half-maximal at 50 nM galanin. The

TABLE I

Effect of 1 μM galanin on the 25 mM K$^+$-evoked release of $[^3H]$ACh and $[^3H]$choline from slices of the rat dorsal and ventral hippocampus

Tissue slice	Fractional release of $[^3H]$ACh and $[^3H]$choline	
	No galanin	Galanin
Dorsal hippocampus	0.075 ± 0.003	0.073 ± 0.004
Ventral hippocampus	0.074 ± 0.004	0.059 ± 0.003 [a]

The data are the means $\pm$ S.E. of six animals.
[a] $p < 0.05$, galanin vs. no galanin group by Student's t-test.

affinity is probably even higher, considering the limited permeability of tissue slices to the peptide.

Reduction of ACh release by galanin from the ventral but not the dorsal hippocampus was demonstrated in vivo using the microdialysis technique coupled with a specific and sensitive radioenzymatic method (Consolo et al., 1987; Wu et al., 1988). A thin dialysis tube (220 μm internal and 310 external diameter, molecular weight cut-off > 15,000) was inserted transversally through both dorsal hippocampi with the following coordinates: A, −3.6 mm from Bregma and V, 3.6 mm from occipital bone. In other rats a dialysis probe (CMA 10, Carnegie Medicine AB, Stockholm, Sweden) was implanted vertically (coordinates: −5 mm posterior to Bregma; 2.5 mm lateral to midline and 6.8 mm below surface of dura mater) into the ventral hippocampus of one side. The experiments were done the day after implantation.

Release of endogenous ACh from the hippocampus was evoked by subcutaneous administration of the muscarinic antagonist scopolamine (0.5 mg/kg). This caused a time-dependent increase in ACh outflow from the dorsal (data not shown) and ventral hippocampus (Fig. 2). Galanin by itself, injected intracerebroventricularly at the dose of 10 μg/15μl, did not affect basal ACh release from the ventral part but when it was given before scopolamine it fully prevented the evoked release of ACh (Fig. 2). Galanin, at half the above dose, 5 μg, still reduced scopolamine-stimulated ACh release although not as strongly as before (Fig. 2). In the dorsal hippocampus galanin did not affect either basal or scopolamine-stimulated ACh release (Fisone et al., 1987).

The reduction of ACh release by galanin is not due to its acting directly at muscarinic receptors because galanin up to 100 μM had no effect on the specific binding of [³H]QNB to membranes of either ventral or dorsal hippocampus. This is in accordance with the fact that galanin had no effect on scopolamine-induced ACh release from the dorsal hippocampus, whose concentration of muscarinic receptors is similar to that in the ventral part.

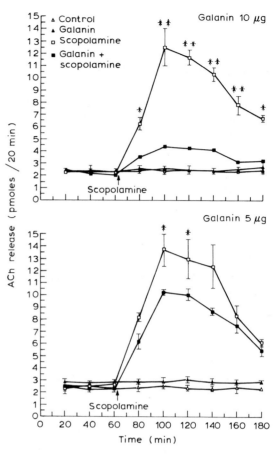

Fig. 2. Effect of galanin (GAL) (10 μg/15 μl, i.c.v.) on scopolamine-induced (0.5 mg/kg, s.c.) ACh release as a function of time in ventral hippocampus. GAL was injected 2 min before scopolamine. The Ringer perfusion solution contained 10 μM physostigmine sulfate; the perfusion rate was 2 μl min⁻¹. Perfusate was collected for 1 h (three 20-min fractions) before injection of GAL and/or scopolamine. The data are the means ± S.E. of 3–4 animals. Interaction between GAL and scopolamine: *p < 0.05 and **p < 0.01; ANOVA (2×2) and Tukey's test for unconfounded means.

The data taken together suggest that galanin acts as an inhibitory modulator of the coexisting neurotransmitter ACh in the ventral hippocampus. Consistent with this conclusion are recent electrophysiological findings that galanin dramatically depresses the slow cholinergic excitatory post-synaptic potential induced by the release of endogenous ACh on the pyramidal neurons of the rat ventral hippocampus (Dutar et al., 1989).

Galanin's action on transmembrane signal transduction

ACh, acting at muscarinic receptors in the hippocampus, inhibits adenylate cyclase activity (Olianas et al.,1983), stimulates cGMP synthesis (Nordstrom and Bartfai, 1981) and elicits phosphoinositide (PI) breakdown (Brown et al., 1984). The latter reaction, particularly the hydrolysis of phosphatidylinositol-4,5-bisphosphate (PIP_2) by phospholipase C, leads to the generation of two second messengers, inositol-1,4,5-trisphosphate (IP_3), which releases Ca^{2+} from intracellular non-mitochondrial stores, and 1,2-diacylglycerol, which activates proteinkinase C.

We examined the cAMP and cGMP generating systems and PI system as possible second messengers of the inhibitory action of galanin on ACh release in the rat ventral hippocampus. Table II shows that $1\mu M$ galanin applied to tissue miniprisms from the ventral hippocampus did not affect basal cAMP and cGMP levels and did not

TABLE II

Effect of galanin on cAMP and cGMP synthesis in slices from rat ventral hippocampus

	cAMP		cGMP	
	Vehicle	Galanin	Vehicle	Galanin
Control	100 ± 7	98 ± 9	100 ± 5	112 ± 6
Forskolin (1 μM)	184 ± 12 [a]	233 ± 51 [a]	–	–
K^+ (25 mM)	–	–	178 ± 12 [a]	184 ± 33 [a]

Porcine galanin was employed at a 1 μM concentration. The data are the means $\pm$ S.E. of 3–6 rats and are expressed as percentages of the respective control values.

[a] $p < 0.01$ vs. respective control groups by Student's t-test.

prevent the rises in cAMP stimulated by forskolin or in cGMP provoked by K^+ depolarization (Bartfai et al., 1988). However, the peptide did influence the effect of the muscarinic agonist carbachol (CARB) on PI turnover in the ventral hippocampus (Fig. 3). CARB ($10^{-6}-10^{-3}M$) stimulated accumulation of [^{3}H]inositol phosphates ([^{3}H]InsPs) in a concentration-dependent

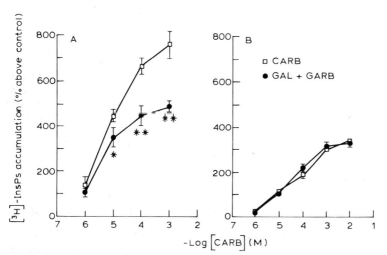

Fig. 3. Effect of galanin (GAL) ($1\mu M$) on carbachol (CARB)-stimulated [^{3}H]inositol phosphate ([^{3}H]InsPs) accumulation in miniprisms from the ventral (A) and dorsal (B) hippocampi. Miniprisms were labeled for 30 min with 0.3 μM myo-[2-^{3}H]inositol then incubated for 45 min with the different concentrations of CARB in the presence of 5 mM LiCl. GAL was added 2 min before CARB. [^{3}H]InsPs accumulation was analysed as described by Brown et al. (1984). Values are percentages above control (3808 $\pm$ 295 cpm/21.600 cpm in lipids). GAL did not significantly influence basal [^{3}H]InsPs accumulation. Significance of GAL/CARB interactions was: 10^{-5} M CARB, $F_{1/31} = 5.9$, *$p < 0.05$; 10^{-4} M CARB, $F_{1/30} = 16.3$, **$p < 0.01$; 10^{-3} M CARB, $F_{1/31} = 14.1$ **$p < 0.01$. Two-way ANOVA (2×2) and Tukey's test for unconfounded means. The EC_{50} was determined by an Allfit program, using a four-parameter logistic function $p = 0.029$.

manner in this part of the hippocampus with an EC_{50} of 6.4 μM (Fig. 3A). This action was completely prevented by 1 μM atropine, attesting to the specific involvement of muscarinic receptors in CARB's effect (data not shown). Galanin added to the incubation medium at a concentration of 1 μM, did not alter basal [^{3}H]InsPs accumulation but it reduced the stimulation induced by 10^{-3} M and 10^{-4} M CARB by about 35% (Fig. 3A); at 10^{-5} M CARB galanin caused a smaller but still significant reduction (22%). At a lower agonist concentration, galanin had no effect. The EC_{50} of CARB, in the presence of galanin, was 22 μM. The inhibitory effect of galanin on 10^{-4} M CARB-stimulated PI breakdown in the ventral hippocampus was concentration-dependent from 0.03 up to 1 μM (data not shown).

In the dorsal hippocampus, CARB-stimulated PI turnover was also concentration-dependent but the maximal increase was less than 400% at 10^{-2} M CARB, half of the maximal effect in the ventral part. The EC_{50} was 70 μM. Galanin did not prevent stimulation with any concentration of CARB (Fig. 3B).

The inhibitory effect of galanin on signal transduction in the ventral hippocampus appears to be specific for muscarinic receptor-mediated PI breakdown. Among the neurotransmitters which appear to use PI breakdown for transmembrane signalling in the hippocampus, neither the effects of noradrenaline (400% vs. control at 10^{-4} M), acting at α_1-adrenergic receptors (Kendall et al., 1985) nor those of 5-hydroxytryptamine (150% vs. control at 10^{-4} M), acting at 5-HT type 2 receptors (Kendall and Nahorski, 1985) were reduced by galanin.

It thus appears that galanin antagonized the ability of CARB to stimulate [^{3}H]InsPs accumulation, specifically in the ventral hippocampus.

Role of Ca^{2+} channels in the inhibitory effects of galanin on PI turnover

Recent evidence indicates that in tissues with ligand gated channels permeable to Ca^{2+}, or in excitable tissues, two distinct mechanisms exist for phospholipase C activation: direct receptor coupling (probably through a GTP-binding protein) to phospholipase C; or activation induced by a rise in cytosolic Ca^{2+} (Eberhard and Holz, 1988). The findings that galanin either does not directly interfere with the muscarinic receptor sites in the ventral hippocampus or does not reduce by itself basal [^{3}H]InsPs accumulation rule out the possibility that the peptide directly modifies phospholipase C. In addition in the hippocampus galanin does not change cAMP production, which could have influenced indirectly PI turnover through an unknown cascade of events. In the light of these observations we investigated whether galanin inhibits phospholipase C by lowering Ca^{2+} influx.

Tissue miniprisms from ventral hippocampus were depolarized by raising the K^+ concentration from 6 to 18 mM. In the medium with the highest K^+ concentration, CARB's action on PI turnover was enhanced, as already reported (Eva and Costa, 1986), but galanin had no effect (Fig. 4). Thus, extracellular Ca^{2+} and its influx across the mem-

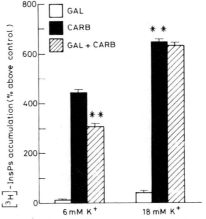

Fig. 4. Effect of 18 mM K^+ on CARB (10^{-4} M) stimulated [^{3}H]InsPs accumulation in the absence and presence of 1 μM galanin (GAL). GAL and 18 mM K^+ did not significantly influence basal [^{3}H]InsPs accumulation. Each bar represents the mean $\pm$ S.E. of three experiments done in triplicate. Interaction: GAL + CARB vs. CARB $F_{1/30} = 18.5$, **$p < 0.01$, GAL + CARB + K^+ vs. CARB $F_{1/30} = 22.7$, **$p < 0.01$. Two-way ANOVA (2×2) and Tukey's test for unconfounded means.

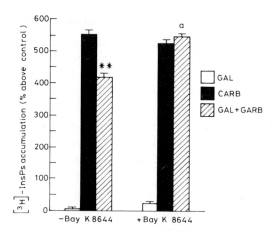

Fig. 5. Effect of 1 μM BAY K 8644 on CARB-stimulated $(10^{-4}$ M) [^{3}H]InsPs accumulation in the absence and presence of 1 μM galanin (GAL). GAL and BAY K 8644 did not significantly influence basal [^{3}H]InsPs accumulation. Each bar represents the mean $\pm$ S.E. of three experiments done in triplicate. Interaction: GAL + CARB vs. CARB $F_{1/32} = 12.44$ **p < 0.01, BAY K 8644 + GAL + CARB vs. GAL + CARB $F_{1/32}$ = 10.60 **p < 0.01. Two-way ANOVA (2 × 2) and Tukey's test for unconfounded means.

brane may play a role in the inhibitory effect of galanin on PI turnover.

This hypothesis was supported by the following experiments in which internal Ca^{2+} concentration $((Ca^{2+})_i)$ was modified by either adding BAY K 8644, a dihydropyridine (DHP) analogue which activates the L-type of voltage-dependent Ca^{2+} channels (VSCC) allowing Ca^{2+} to flow into the neurons, or by pre-exposing hippocampal mini-prisms to the inorganic ion Cd^{2+}, known to prevent the entry of extracellular Ca^{2+} through VSCC. BAY K 8644, added at the concentration of 1 μM did not by itself affect 10^{-4} M CARB stimulation of PI breakdown but when added before galanin (1 μM) it completely prevented the inhibitory effect of the peptide (Fig. 5). Cd^{2+} ion, at the concentration of 200 μM, known to block all three VSCC (Miller, 1987), reduced CARB-induced [^{3}H]InsPs accumulation by 50% (Table III). Galanin, in the presence of Cd^{2+}, had no further effect. At one tenth this concentration, 20 μM, Cd^{2+} still prevented the activity of galanin (data not shown). The data indicate that galanin pre-

vents Ca^{2+} influx triggered by VSCC and this effect is reflected in the reduction of PI turnover stimulated by the muscarinic agonist CARB.

In neurons, the main mechanism for Ca^{2+} entry across the membrane is through VSCC, which are believed to comprise at least three groups of molecules, the T, N and L types (Tsien et al., 1988), each with its own unique properties and pharmacology. Interestingly, the distribution of these channels in different cells varies widely, but all three types are found in hippocampal pyramidal cells. In order to investigate further whether VSCC are involved in the inhibitory action of galanin on PI turnover we used selective VSCC antagonists. The DHP compound nifedipine (NIF) (1 μM), an L-type selective blocker of VSCC, did not by itself affect the 10^{-4} M CARB stimulation of [^{3}H]InsPs accumulation but potentiated the action of galanin (1 μM). Inhibition by galanin, in the presence of NIF, amounted to about 50%, significantly higher than galanin alone (30%) (Table III). Thus galanin may reduce Ca^{2+} influx by acting on different channels from NIF. When all three types of VSCC are blocked by Cd^{2+}, the maximum inhibition of CARB-stimulated PI turnover was 50%, the same as produced by galanin and NIF together. Therefore, the two drugs probably do not act on the same channel (the L-type)

TABLE III

Effect of Cd^{2+}, NIF and ω-CTx on CARB-stimulated [^{3}H]InsPs accumulation in the presence and absence of galanin

	CARB	Gal + CARB	Drug	Drug + CARB
Cd^{2+} 200 μM	100 $\pm$ 2	74 $\pm$ 3 [a]	46 $\pm$ 7 [a]	46 $\pm$ 7
NIF 1 μM	100 $\pm$ 4	72 $\pm$ 2 [a]	97 $\pm$ 3	53 $\pm$ 2 [b]
ω-CT 2 μM	100 $\pm$ 2	68 $\pm$ 2	75 $\pm$ 2 [a]	67 $\pm$ 4

Results are percentages of the increase in [^{3}H]InsPs accumulation induced by 10^{-4} M CARB (taken as 100%). Control values (3808 $\pm$ 295 cpm/21 600 cpm in lipids) are considered as 0%. The CARB's effect was 682 $\pm$ 56% above control values. Cd^{2+}, ω-CT 2 and Gal (1 μM) were added respectively 5, 15 and 2 min before CARB; NIF was added together with CARB. The results are the means $\pm$ S.E. of three experiments performed in triplicate.
[a] p < 0.01 vs. CARB, [b] p < 0.01 vs. Gal + CARB.

in a synergistic manner because if they did, the inhibition would be lower than 50%. Therefore, as NIF acts selectively on the L-type channel, galanin must act on one or both of the other types (N and T channels).

To clarify this point further we examined the action of galanin in the presence of omega conotoxin (ω-CT). This novel peptide toxin irreversibly blocks N and L type calcium channels in chick dorsal root ganglion neurons (McCleskey et al., 1987) and has potent action on calcium channels in neuronal cells (Oyama et al., 1987; Suzuki and Yoshioka, 1987). ω-CT, at the maximal concentration of 2 μM, reduced CARB's effect about 25% by itself (Table III). When it was added before galanin, there was no summation of the individual maximal inhibitory effects. The data taken together suggest that the VSCC involved in the inhibitory action of galanin is NIF insensitive, Cd^{2+}-sensitive and ω-CT sensitive and inactivated by prior K^+ depolarization. In the light of these properties it can be deduced that galanin may act on the N-type VSCC in its inhibitory action of CARB-stimulated PI turnover.

Galanin inhibition on Ca^{2+} influx could be direct, through an action on VSCC, or indirectly mediated by an effect on K^+ channels. The possibility exists that galanin, hyperpolarizing the hippocampal cells by activation of K^+ channels, lowers Ca^{2+} influx through VSCC and, in this way, reduces the activity of phospholipase C.

Behavioral effects of galanin

Behavioral effects of galanin in the brain have been investigated using learning and memory paradigms mediated by the septo-hippocampal pathway in the rat. In an animal model of Alzheimer's disease, rats with ibotenic acid lesions of the nucleus basalis–medial septal area were tested on an appetitive T-maze task, after microinjection of galanin, ACh, galanin + ACh, or saline into the lateral ventricles or into the ventral hippocampus (Mastropaolo et al., 1988). In this paradigm, sham-operated rats reach the criterion of nine or

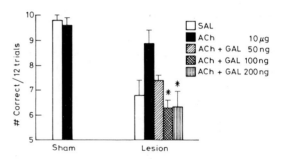

Fig. 6. Galanin reduces ACh-induced improvement in choice accuracy on a food-reinforced T-maze delayed alternation task, in rats with ibotenic acid lesions of the nucleus basalis and medial septal area. Data are expressed as means $\pm$ S.E. ($n = 6$–10) for each treatment group, $*p < 0.01$ as compared to ACh.

more correct choices out of twelve consecutive trials, where the food-rewarded choice is the arm of the T-maze opposite to the arm that was rewarded in the last trial, with a 90 second interval between trials. Rats with lesions of the ventral forebrain fail to reach this criterion, performing at chance levels of six correct out of twelve consecutive trials. Galanin, administered intraventricularly at doses of 100, 200, 500, or 1000 ng/5 μl, neither reduced choice accuracy in the sham-operated control rats nor increased choice accuracy in the lesioned rats. ACh, 7.5 or 10 μg/5 μl intraventricularly, or 1 μg/0.5 μl into the ventral hippocampus, significantly improved choice accuracy in the lesioned rats. Galanin given in combination with ACh significantly attenuated the ability of ACh to improve choice accuracy, both intraventricularly at doses of 100–500 ng galanin in combination with 10 μg ACh, and intrahippocampally at the dose of 200 ng galanin with 1 μg ACh (Fig. 6). These findings suggest that galanin acts as an inhibitory modulator of ACh in this paradigm of working memory having no effect alone, but attenuating the actions of ACh.

In another spatial navigation task, the Morris swim maze, galanin 1 μg and 5 μg i.c.v. impeded acquisition of the task, but had no effect on retention (Sundstrom et al., 1988). Thus galanin appears to have inhibitory effects on learning. It is interesting to note that higher doses of galanin were used in this study than in the one described before. The finding that higher doses had direct inhibitory effects in normal rats while lower doses had modulatory inhibitory effects in lesioned rats may indicate a greater sensitivity to galanin after ventral forebrain lesions.

Conclusions

All experimental evidence to date indicates that specifically in the ventral hippocampus galanin acts as an inhibitory modulator of ACh, the neurotransmitter with which it coexists. Presynaptically the peptide reduces the ACh release evoked by K^+ depolarization or by blockade of muscarinic autoreceptors which normally inhibit ACh release. In this context an important point that needs clarification is whether galanin is released and/or co-released with ACh from the septo-hippocampal terminals. At the postsynaptic level galanin inhibits the PI breakdown induced by muscarinic receptor stimulation. The inhibitory effect of galanin on phospholipase C is mediated by a lowering of Ca^{2+} influx activated by VSCC.

Behavioral findings are consistent with the interpretation that galanin may contribute to an inhibitory feedback process in brain regions critical to learning and memory.

References

Bartfai, T., Bertorelli, R., Consolo, S., Diaz-Arnesto, L., Fisone G., Hokfelt, T., Iverfeldt, K., Palazzi, E. and Ogren, S.O. (1988) Acute and chronic studies on functional aspects of coexistence. *J. Physiol.*, 83: 37–47.

Brown, E., Kendall, D.A. and Nahorski, S.R. (1984) Inositol phospholipid hydrolysis in rat cerebral cortical slices: I. Receptor characterisation. *J. Neurochem.*, 42: 1379–1387.

Chan-Palay, V. (1988a) Neurons with galanin innervate cholinergic cells in the human basal forebrain and galanin and acetylcholine coexist. *Brain Res. Bull.*, 21: 465–472.

Chan-Palay, V. (1988b) Galanin hyperinnervates surviving neurons of the human basal nucleus of Meynert in dementias of Alzheimer's and Parkinson's disease: a hypothesis for the role of galanin in accentuating cholinergic dysfunction in dementia. *J. Comp. Neurol.*, 273: 543–557.

Consolo, S., Wu, C.F., Fiorentini, F., Ladinsky, H. and Vezzani, A. (1987) Determination of endogenous acetylcholine release in freely moving rats by transstriatal dialysis coupled to a radioenzymatic assay: effect of drugs. *J. Neurochem.*, 48: 1459–1465.

Dutar, P., Lamour, Y. and Nicoll, R.A. (1989) Galanin blocks the slow cholinergic EPSP in CA 1 pyramidal neurons from ventral hippocampus. *Eur. J. Pharmacol.*, 164: 355–360.

Eberhard, D.A. and Holz, R.W. (1988) Intracellular Ca^{2+} activates phospholipase C. *Trends Neurosci.*, 11: 517–521.

Ekblad, E., Hakanson, R., Sundler, F. and Wahlestedt, C. (1985) Galanin: Neuromodulatory and direct contractile effects on smooth muscle preparations. *Br. J. Pharmacol.*, 86: 241–246.

Eva, C. and Costa, E. (1986) Potassium ion facilitation of phosphoinositide turnover activation by muscarinic receptor agonists in rat brain. *J. Neurochem.*, 46: 1429–1435.

Fisone G., Wu, C.F., Consolo, S., Nordstrom, O., Brynne, N., Bartfai, T., Melander, T. and Hokfelt, T. (1987) Galanin inhibits acetylcholine release in the ventral hippocampus of the rat: histochemical, autoradiographic, in vivo and in vitro studies. *Proc. Natl. Acad. Sci. USA*, 84: 7339–7343.

Fisone G., Langel, U., Carlquist, M., Bergman, T., Consolo, S., Hokfelt, T., Unden, A., Andell, S. and Bartfai, T. (1989) Galanin receptor and its ligands in the rat hippocampus. *Eur. J. Biochem.*, 181: 269–276.

Flint Beal, M., Clevens, R.A., Chattha, G.K., MacGarvey, U.M., Mazurek, M.F. and Gabriel, S.M. (1988) Galanin-like immunoreactivity is unchanged in Alzheimer's disease and Parkinson's disease dementia cerberal cortex. *J. Neurochem.*, 51: 1935–1941.

Holets, V.R., Hokfelt, T., Rokaeus, A., Terenius, L. and Goldstein, M. (1988) Locus coeruleus neurons in the rat containing neuropeptide Y, tyrosine hydroxylase or galanin and their efferent projections to the spinal cord, cerebral cortex and hypothalamus. *Neuroscience*, 24: 893–906.

Ju, G., Melander, T., Ceccatelli, S., Hokfelt, T. and Frey, P. (1987) Immunohistochemical evidence for a spinothalamic pathway co-containing cholecystokinin- and galanin-like immunoreactivities in the rat. *Neuroscience*, 20: 439–456.

Kaplan, L.M., Spindel, E.R., Isselbacher, K.J. and Chin, W.W. (1988) Tissue-specific expression of the rat galanin gene. *Proc. Natl. Acad. Sci. USA*, 85: 1065–1069.

Kendall, D.A. and Nahorski, S.R. (1985) 5-Hydroxytryptamine-stimulated inositol phospholipid hydrolysis in rat cerebral cortex slices: Pharmacological characterization and effects of antidepressants. *J. Pharmacol. Exp. Ther.*, 233: 473–479.

Kendall, D.A., Brown, E. and Nahorski, S.R. (1985) α_1-Adrenoceptor-mediated inositol phospholipid hydrolysis in rat cerebral cortex: relationship between receptor occupancy and response and effect of denervation. *Eur. J. Pharmacol.*, 114: 41–52.

Kohler, C., Ericson, H., Watanabe, T., Polak, J., Palay, S.L., Palay, V. and Chan-Palay, V. (1986) Galanin immunoreactivity in hypothalamic neurons: further evidence for multiple chemical messengers in the tuberomammillary nucleus. *J. Comp. Neurol.*, 250: 58–64.

Kowall, N.W. and Flint Beal M. (1989) Galanin-like immunoreactivity is present in human substantia innominata and in senile plaques in Alzheimer's disease. *Neurosci. Lett.,* 98: 118–123.

Mastropaolo, J., Nadi, N.S., Ostrowski, N.L. and Crawley, J.N. (1988) Galanin antagonizes acetylcholine on a memory task in basal forebrain-lesioned rats: *Proc. Natl. Acad. Sci. USA,* 85: 9841–9845.

McCleskey, E.W., Fox, A.P., Feldman, D.H., Cruz, L.J., Olivera, B.M., Tsien, R.W. and Yoshikami, D. (1987) ω-Conotoxin: direct and persistent blockade of specific types of calcium channels in neurons but not muscle. *Proc. Natl. Acad. Sci. USA,* 84: 4327–4331.

Melander, T. and Staines, W.A. (1986) A galanin-like peptide coexists in putative cholinergic somata of the septum-basal forebrain complex and in acetylcholinesterase-containing fibers and varicosities within the hippocampus in the owl monkey (Aotus Trivirgatus). *Neurosci. Lett.,* 68: 17–22.

Melander, T., Hokfelt, T. and Rokaeus, A., Fahrenkrug, J., Tatemoto, K. and Mutt, V. (1985a) Distribution of galanin-like immunoreactivity in the gastro-intestinal tract of several mammalian species. *Cell Tissue Res.,* 239: 253–270.

Melander, T., Staines, W.A., Hokfelt, T., Rokaeus, A., Eckenstein, F., Salvaterra, P.M. and Wainer, B.H. (1985b) Galanin-like immunoreactivity in cholinergic neurons of the septum-basal forebrain complex projecting to the hippocampus of the rat. *Brain Res.,* 360: 130–138.

Melander, T., Hokfelt, T. and Rokaeus, A. (1986a) Distribution of galanin-like immunoreactivity in the rat central nervous system. *J. Comp. Neurol.,* 248: 475–517.

Melander, T., Staines, W. and Rokaeus, A., (1986b) Galanin-like immunoreactivity in hippocampal afferents in the rat, with special reference to cholinergic and noradrenergic inputs. *Neuroscience,* 19: 223–240.

Miller, R.J. (1987) Multiple calcium channels and neuronal function. *Science,* 235: 46–52.

Nordstrom, O. and T., Bartfai, T. (1981) 8-Br-cyclic GMP mimics activation of muscarinic autoreceptor and inhibits acetylcholine release from rat hippocampal slices. *Brain Res.,* 213: 467–471.

Nordstrom, O., Melander, T., Hokfelt, T., Bartfai, T. and Goldstein, M. (1987) Evidence for an inhibitory effect of the peptide galanin on dopamine release from the rat median eminence. *Neurosci. Lett.,* 73: 21–26.

Olianas, M.C., Onali, P., Neff, N.H. and Costa, E. (1983) Adenylate cyclase activity of synaptic membranes from rat striatum. Inhibition by muscarinic receptor agonists. *Mol. Pharmacol.,* 23: 393–398.

Oyama, Y., Tsuda, Y., Sakakibara, S. and Akaike, N. (1987) Synthetic ω-conotoxin: a potent calcium channel blocking neurotoxin. *Brain Res.* 424: 58–64.

Rokaeus, A. (1987) Galanin: a newly isolated biologically active neuropeptide. *Trends Neurosci.,* 10: 158–164.

Rokaeus, A., Melander, T., Hokfelt, T., Lundberg, J.M., Tatemoto, K., Carlquist, M. and Mutt, V. (1984) A galanin-like peptide in the central nervous system and intestine of the rat. *Neurosci. Lett.,* 47: 161–166.

Skofitsch, G. and Jacobowitz, D.M. (1985) Immunohistochemical mapping of galanin-like neurons in the rat central nervous system. *Peptides,* 6: 509–546.

Skofitsch, G., Sills, M. and Jacobowitz, D.M. (1986) Autoradiographic distribution of ^{125}I-galanin binding sites in the rat central nervous system. *Peptides,* 7: 1029–1042.

Sundstrom, E., Archer, T., Melander, T., Hokfelt, T. (1988) Galanin impairs acquisition but not retrieval of spatial memory in rats studied in the Morris swim maze. *Neurosci. Lett.,* 88: 331–335.

Suzuki, N. and Yoshioka, T. (1987) Differential blocking action of synthetic omega-conotoxin on components of Ca^{2+} channel current in clonal GH3 cells. *Neurosci. Lett.,* 75: 235–239.

Tatemoto, K., Rokaeus, A., Jornvall, H., McDonald, T.J. and Mutt, V. (1983) Galanin — a novel biologically active peptide from porcine intestine. *FEBS Lett.,* 164: 124–128.

Tsien, R.W., Lipscombe, D., Madison, D.V., Bley, K.R. and Fox, A.P. (1988) Multiple types of neuronal clacium channels and their selective modulation. *Trends Neurosci.,* 11: 431–438.

Vrontakis, M.E., Peden, L.M., Duckworth, M.L. and Friesen, H.G. (1987) Isolation and characterization of a complementary DNA (galanin) clone from estrogen-induced pituitary tumor messenger RNA. *J. Biol. Chem.,* 262: 16755–16758.

Wu, C.F., Bertorelli, R., Sacconi, M., Pepeu, G. and Consolo, S. (1988) Decrease of acetylcholine release in aging freely moving rats detected by microdialysis. *Neurobiol. Aging* 9: 357–361.

Yau, W.M., Dorsett, J.A. and Youther, M.L. (1986) Evidence for galanin as an inhibitory neuropeptide on myenteric cholinergic neurons in the guinea pig small intestine. *Neurosci. Lett.,* 72: 305–308.

S.-M. Aquilonius and P.-G. Gillberg (Eds.)
Progress in Brain Research, Vol. 84
© 1990 Elsevier Science Publishers B.V. (Biomedical Division)

CHAPTER 31

AF64A-induced cholinergic hypofunction

Israel Hanin

Department of Pharmacology and Experimental Therapeutics, Loyola University of Chicago School of Medicine, 2160 South First Avenue, Maywood, IL 60153, U.S.A.

Introduction

Availability of a specific neurotoxin provides the investigator with a powerful tool. By studying the consequences of selectively perturbing a particular neurotransmitter system in vivo, researchers can better understand the essential regulatory mechanisms for that system. Moreover, by mimicking selective deficits of specific neurotransmitters known to be diminished in particular disease states using neurotransmitter-selective neurotoxic agents, one could conceivably develop a potential animal model of the disease state.

Progress in the development of cholinergic neurotoxins ("cholinotoxins") has lagged behind that of the other neurotransmitter-specific neurotoxins. This may be because the rate of breakdown and resynthesis of acetylcholine in vivo is extremely rapid (milliseconds), making it difficult to study factors involved in acetylcholine regulation with conventional techniques. Mechanisms regulating the other neurotransmitter systems are more amenable to exploration, have been studied more extensively, and thus are better understood. A selective "cholinotoxin" would, however, be very useful in developing a potential animal model of Alzheimer's disease, since a cholinergic deficit has been strongly associated with dementia in this disease state (Coyle et al., 1983; Perry et al., 1978).

This paper concerns the potential use of ethylcholine aziridinium (referred to in our laboratory as AF64A; also referred to by others as ECMA) as a neurotoxin specific for the cholinergic system in

vivo. Several critical reviews about this substance have been published to date (Fisher and Hanin, 1980; Hanin et al.; 1987). This paper, therefore, will serve as an overview, in order to focus on the current status of knowledge regarding this interesting agent.

Results and Discussion

AF64A is structurally similar to choline (see Fig. 1), except that two of the methyl groups on the quaternary nitrogen have been converted to the aziridinium moiety, and the third methyl group has been elongated to the ethyl structure. These structural modifications, while not noticeably altering the compound's three-dimensional similarity to choline (Fisher and Hanin, 1980; Mistry et al., 1986), impart cytotoxic properties. Conceivably, it is this combination of structural features in the molecule (i.e., the structural similarity to choline on the one hand, and the cytotoxic aziridinium component on the other) that first allows it to be preferentially recognized by choline uptake sites, then causes it to exert a destructive

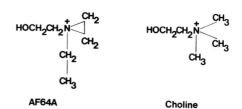

Fig. 1. Structural representation of AF64A and choline.

TABLE I

Neurotransmitter and enzyme-related effects of AF64A administration: a general overview

Parameter studied	Effect		References
	In vivo	In vitro	
Cholinergic effects			
Acetylcholine levels	↓↓↓	*	9, 42, **43**[+], 54, 58, 84
Acetylcholine release	*	↓↓↓	42, 54, 55, 64, 73
Acetylcoenzyme A levels	↓	*	42
Choline levels	0	0	92
Choline acetyltransferase activity	↓↓↓	0	6, **7**, 9, 11, 15, 42, 45, 47, 50, 54, 57, 65, 66, 67, 72, 75, 76, 82, 89, **90**
Acetylcholinesterase activity	↓↓↓	0	3, 21, 32, 50, 54, 64, 67, 76
High-affinity transport of choline	↓↓↓	↓↓↓	11, **18**, 55, 58, 59, 64, 67, 71, **74**, 87, **90**
Low-affinity transport of choline	↓↓	↓↓	54
Quinuclidynyl benzilate binding	0	0	20, 21, 27, 33, 88
cis-Methyl-dioxolane binding	0	*	88
Nicotine binding	↑↑↑	*	42
Pirenzepine binding	0	↓	20, 33, 88
Hemicholinium binding	↓↓↓	*	20, 33, 64, 88
Choline dehydrogenase activity	*	↓↓	7
Choline kinase activity	*	↓↓	76
Phosphatidylcholine levels	*	0 or ↓↓	7, 76
Phosphatidylethanolamine levels	*	↓↓	76
Phosphatidylserine levels	*	↓↓	76
Dopaminergic effects			
Dopamine levels	∪ or ↓↓↓	*	15, 36, 50, **56**, 92
Dihydroxyphenylacetic acid levels	∪	*	15, 36, 92
Homovanillic acid levels	∪	*	36, 92
Tyrosine hydroxylase activity	∪	*	75
Dopamine uptake	0	0	47, 50, 67
SCH 22390 binding	0	*	20
Sulpiride binding	↓↓↓	*	20
Noradrenergic effects			
Norepinephrine levels	∪ or 0	*	15, 29, 36, 92
Norepinephrine-induced phosphoinositide metabolism	*	↑↑↑	**22**
Norepinephrine uptake	*	0	50
MAO-B activity	↑↑↑	*	47
MAO-A activity	0	*	47
GABAergic effects			
GABA levels	0	*	21, 75
Glutamate decarboxylase activity	0 or ∪, ↓↓	*	64, 75, 89, **90**
GABA uptake	0 or ∪	*	67, 75, **90**
Serotonergic effects			
Serotonin levels	0 or ∪	*	15, 29, 37, 92
5-Hydroxyindoleacetic acid levels	0 or ∩	*	15, 37, 92
Serotonin uptake	0	0	50, 59

TABLE I (continued)

Parameter studied	Effect		References
	In vivo	In vitro	
Effects on other neurotransmitter systems			
Somatostatin-immunoreactive retinal cells	*	0	62
Glycinergic retinal cells	0	*	62
Enkephalinergic retinal cells	0	*	62
Somatostatin levels	0 or ∪	*	39
Neuropeptide Y levels	0 or ∩	*	39
Aspartate uptake	0	*	89
Effects on other enzyme systems			
Lactate dehydrogenase	*	0	76
Chymotripsinogen	*	0	76
Carboxypeptidase A	*	0	76
Alcohol dehydrogenase	*	0	76
Other effects			
Aluminum accumulation in hippocampus and parietal cortex	↑↑↑	*	83

GABA, gamma-aminobutyric acid;
*, not measured;
0, no effect;
∪, transient decrease;
∩, transient increase;
3, Arst et al., 1983
6, Bailey et al., 1986
7, Barlow and Marchbanks, 1984
9, Blaker and Goodwin, 1987
11, Casamenti et al., 1986
15, Chrobak et al., 1988
18, Curti and Marchbanks, 1984
20, Dawson et al., 1987
21, Estrada et al., 1988
22, Eva et al., 1987
27, Fisher et al., 1987
29, Gaal et al., 1986
32, Gower et al., 1986
33, Gulya et al., 1986
36, Hortnagel et al., 1987a
37, Hortnagel et al., 1987b
39, Hortnagel et al., 1990
42, Ishii et al., 1987
43, Jarrard et al., 1984
45, Johnson et al., 1988
47, Jossan et al., 1989
50, Kozlowski and Arbogast, 1986
54, Leventer et al., 1985
55, Leventer et al., 1987

↓, intermediary effect;
↓↓, reduction only at high concentrations;
↓↓↓, significant reduction;
↑↑↑, significant increase.
Bold references do not show cholinospecificity of AF64A.
56, Levy et al., 1984
57, Mantione et al., 1981
58, Mantione et al., 1983a
59, Mantione et al., 1983b
60, McArdle and Hanin, 1986
62, Millar et al., 1987
64, Mouton et al., 1988
65, Nakahara et al., 1988a
66, Nakahara et al., 1988b
67, Nakamura et al., 1988
71, Pittel et al., 1987
72, Pope et al., 1985
73, Potter et al., 1986
74, Rylett and Colhoun, 1980
75, Sandberg et al., 1984
76, Sandberg et al., 1985
82, Stwertka and Olson, 1986
83, Szerdahelyi and Kasa, 1988
84, Tateishi et al., 1987
87, Uney and Marchbanks, 1987
88, Vickroy et al., 1986
89, Villani et al., 1986
90, Villani et al., 1988
92, Walsh et al., 1984

effect, after covalent binding to the cholinoreactive site.

Over the past few years, information has been accumulating regarding the effects of AF64A administration, from the molecular level to the level of the intact animal. Several comprehensive reviews have been written summarizing the existing state of knowledge of the mode of action of AF64A (Fisher and Hanin, 1986a,b; Hanin et al., 1987, and others). Tables I–IV outline, in very general terms, the findings obtained to date using AF64A at the neuropharmacological, electrophysiological, behavioral and cell-culture levels, respectively. For brevity, these tables do not discriminate between results obtained with different doses, or sites of administration of AF64A (see below). Rather, they just list the effects which have been observed following administration of the compound to experimental animals.

These results provide considerable information suggesting that AF64A may induce a selective cholinotoxicity in animals. Moreover, AF64A treatment results in memory and learning deficits in experimental animals which are reversed by cholinergic agonists (Table III), providing further support for the cholinospecificity of AF64A.

There have, however, been several claims that AF64A may actually exert its effects through non-selective, noncholinergic means (Allen et al., 1988; Asante et al., 1983; Colhoun and Rylett, 1986;

Eva et al., 1987; Jarrard et al., 1984; Lamour and Dutar, 1986; Levy et al., 1984; McGurk et al., 1987; Spencer et al., 1985; Stwertka and Olson, 1985; Villani et al., 1986; but see Villani et al., 1988). These claims are based on observations of significant tissue destruction produced by AF64A at and around the site of its administration in the brain. An explanation for this discrepancy may be inherent in the nature of endogenous factors that control the disposition of choline in vivo. Choline normally participates in both a low-affinity and a high-affinity system in vivo. The high-affinity system is responsible for the uptake of choline into the cholinergic nerve terminal and its subsequent conversion into acetylcholine. The low-affinity system involves choline incorporation into phospholipids and other components of the cell membrane, and thus is more generalized and not necessarily cholinospecific (Freeman and Jenden, 1976; Jenden, 1979; Jope, 1979). This divergence in the handling of choline in vivo could explain the discordant observations reported for AF64A. Specifically, if the dose of AF64A used is low enough, it would selectively be used by the high-

TABLE II

Neurophysiological effects of AF64A administration: a general overview

Effects observed	References
Inhibition of presynaptic function in the cat superior cervical ganglion in vivo	Mantione et al., 1983a
Increase in REM latency and slow wave sleep; plus shortened sleep time in rats	Lehr et al., 1984
Reduction in number of quanta released from mouse soleus nerve preparation	McArdle and Hanin, 1985
Blockade of axonal transport of acetylcholinesterase	Kasa and Hanin, 1985
Shortening of mean antidromic latency of neurons of the medial septum-nucleus of the diagonal band of Broca	Lamour et al., 1986a [a]
Disappearance of a subpopulation of septo-hippocampal neurons after icv administration of AF64A in the rat	Lamour et al., 1986a [a]
Impairment of cholinergic neuromuscular transmission in guinea pig ileum and urinary bladder	Hoyl et al., 1986
Impairment of cholinergic neuromodulation in the enteric nervous system of guinea pig distal colon	Hoyl et al., 1986
No effect on RSA (rhythmical slow activity) in the hippocampus	Stewart et al., 1987

[a] This reference does not show cholinospecificity of AF64A.

affinity uptake system and would thus be cholinospecific. If, on the other hand, the dose of AF64A is high enough to also affect the low-affinity system, then nonspecific destructive effects on the membrane would readily occur in the vicinity of the toxin. The concentration zone distinguishing specific from nonspecific effects is relatively narrow: the effective K_is of low- and high-affinity concentrations of choline differ by a factor of only 17 (Mantione et al., 1983b).

The dose-dependent cholinoselective function of AF64A is demonstrated by its concurrent effects on central cholinergic, serotonergic and adrenergic mechanisms. We recently found that

TABLE III

Behavioral effects of AF64A administration: a general overview

Effect observed	References
After icv administration:	
Impairment in passive avoidance behavior	10, **11** *, 13, 23, **43**, 64, 65, 66, 68, 72, 77, 92 (but see **12**, 32)
improved with physostigmine treatment	10, 66, 68
improved with AF102B treatment	23, 65
Impairment in radial maze performance	10, 14, 15, 23, 32, **43**, 92
improved with AF102B treatment	23
Longer escape latencies in Morris water maze test	10, 23, 30, 32, 78
improved with AF102A and AF102B treatment	23
Impairment in T-maze performance	13, 14, 23, 32, 66
improved with AF102B treatment	23
Improved with physostigmine treatment	66
Impairment in active avoidance behavior	68, 85 (but see 77)
reversed by physostigmine treatment	68
Hyperactivity in postnatally treated rat pups	77
After intrastriatal administration:	
Impairment in passive avoidance behavior	75
Increase in spontaneous nocturnal but not day time locomotor activity	75
No change in sensitivity to electrical shock	75
Robust ipsilateral rotation in response to amphetamine and apomorphine	82
After intrahippocampal administration:	
Impairment in passive avoidance behavior	6
Impairment in two-way active avoidance in a shuttle box paradigm	6
Impairment in eight-arm radial maze performance	91
Deficit in food-reinforced lever press schedule	9
Deficit in retention but not in acquisition of memory using the Thompson-Bryant box	34
Shortening of step-down latencies	84
After basal forebrain administration:	
Impairment in habituation to a novel environment	**79**
Impairment in passive or ative avoidance behavior	**79**
Longer escape latencies in water maze test	67, **79**
Impairment in T-maze test	67

TABLE III (continued)

Effect observed	References
After medial septal administration:	
No effect on habituation to a novel environment	**79**
No effect on passive or active avoidance behavior	**79**
Longer escape latencies in water maze test	**79**
Reversal learning deficit	**79**
After intracortical infusion:	
Marked retention deficits in passive avoidance testing	64

Bold references do not show cholinospecificity of AF64A.

10, Brandeis et al., 1986
12, Caulfield et al., 1983
13, Cherkin et al., 1986
14, Chroback et al., 1987
23, Fisher and Hanin, 1980
30, Gobert et al., 1987
34, Gurkliss et al., 1986
68, Ogura et al., 1987

77, Speiser et al., 1988
78, Spencer et al., 1987
79, Spencer et al., 1985
85, Tedford et al., 1988
91, Walsh and Hanin, 1986
For other references see Table I.

when doses of up to 2 nmol AF64A were administered bilaterally into the cerebral ventricles of rats, there was a significant and permanent attenuation of cholinergic activity as well as a transient secondary effect on central serotonergic and noradrenergic function, which returned to normal within 7 days. When higher doses of AF64A were given the inhibitory effect on cholinergic function was, again, significant and permanent. However, attenuation of serotonergic and adrenergic function

TABLE IV

Effects of AF64A administration in tissue culture

System used	Effect of AF64A	References
Cholinergic neuroblastoma X glioma cell line, NG108-15	Rapid decrease in cellular choline acetyltransferase activity	Sandberg et al., 1985
Chick embryo (8 day) neuron enriched cultures	Dose-dependent (10^5–10^{-3} M) selective cholinotoxicity; glial cells remain intact	Davies et al., 1986
Neonatal rat neuron-enriched primary brain cell culture	Inhibition of synthesis of acetylcholine at ≤ 30 μM without affecting choline acetyltransferase activity	Koppenaal et al., 1986
Fetal rat primary culture of whole brain, septum, midbrain;	Selective reduction in acetylcholinesterase staining, and no effect on uptake or release in dopaminergic cells; at ≤ 22.5 μM	Amir et al., 1988
Fetal rat reaggregate culture of whole brain	Selective cholinergic damage at ≥ 12.5 μM	Pillar et al., 1988
LAN2 cholinergic neuroblastoma and A1235 noncholinergic neuroglioma cell lines	Preferential DNA strand breakage in the cholinergic cell line	Barnes et al., 1988
Fetal rat reaggregate culture of whole brain	No recovery of ChAT activity following NGF or TRH	Atterwill et al., 1989

was no longer transient; it lasted for the duration of the experiment (28 days). The latter effect has been attributed to a nonselective influence of AF64A on brain tissue (possibly via the low-affinity system), while the former has been attributed to a selective cholinotoxic influence via the high-affinity choline transport system (Hortnagl et al., 1987a,b).

TABLE V

CNS site of AF64A administration, dose and effect

Site of administration	Dose (nmol)	Effect		References
		Specific	Nonspecific	
Cortex	4×1.0	×		64
	6×2.0	×		80
Lateral ventricle				
Bilaterally	1.5		×	43
Bilaterally	≤ 3.0	×		85
Unilaterally	≤ 10.0	×		73
Dorsal hippocampus	1.0	×		9, 91
	2.0	×		59, 86
	4.0	×		91
	5.0	×		6
	10.0	×		84
	50.0	×		84
Nucleus basalis	0.02	×	×	(50) (61)
	0.05	×	×	(50) (61)
	≥ 0.1	×	×	(50) (61)
	1.0	×	×	(67) (79)
Corpus striatum	0.02		×	61
	0.05		×	61
	0.1		×	61
	0.2		×	1
	1.0		×	82
	8.0	×		75
Medial septum	1.0		×	79
Substantia innominata	0.073		×	4
Substantia nigra	3.0		×	56
Interpeduncular nucleus	1.0		×	90

1, Allen et al., 1988
4, Asante et al., 1983
61, McGurk et al., 1987
80, Stephens et al., 1987
86, Tonnaer et al., 1986
For other references see Tables I and III.

Further support for this concept is also evident in several recent reports by other investigators using neurochemical, electrophysiological, and cell culture approaches (see Tables I, II and IV and references therein), who demonstrated that AF64A does indeed produce specific cholinergic lesions in vivo. However, the dose range for this effect is quite narrow and has to be determined experimentally for each specific application.

The dose dependency of selectivity of AF64A also appears to be region-specific in the brain. Different loci of administration are differentially sensitive to the effect of the compound (Hanin et al., 1987; Table V). Higher doses of AF64A can be tolerated, with cholinoselectivity evident following intracerebroventricular, intrahippocampal or intracortical administration of the compound. Other brain regions appear, however, to be very sensitive to the toxic effect of AF64A, and hence susceptible to nonspecific destruction at very low concentrations (Table V).

The purity of the compound is also important. Traces of the bis-mustard analogue of AF64A generated during the synthesis of the mono-mustard precursor of AF64A, if not isolated from the final product, are highly toxic and nonselective in their destructive effects. Incomplete cyclization of the mustard precursor of AF64A in the process of its conversion to the aziridinium product would result, on the other hand, in a solution that is less potent than expected. In the presence of water, AF64A may also be converted to inactive piperazinium analogues (Fisher et al., 1982; Goldstein et al., 1988; Hortnagl et al., 1988). These conditions must all be avoided by adherence to careful and reproducible preparatory procedures.

What would be important studies to conduct with AF64A in the immediate future? Studies employing the appropriate dose of the compound and using definitive histochemical approaches have not yet been conducted in a comprehensive and systematic manner. These studies would demonstrate the selective effect of AF64A administration at the level of the cholinergic nerve terminal membrane.

Another important question to investigate is the study of various pharmacological manipulations on the neurochemical and behavioral consequences of AF64A administration. Strategic use of specific pharmacological agonists and antagonists of individual neurotransmitter systems would allow us to gain further insight into the selectivity of action of AF64A.

Much is known about the mode of action of the catecholamine- and indoleamine-related neurotoxins because they have been available for a longer period of time than has AF64A. On the other hand, many unanswered questions about the mode of action of AF64A, as well as the suitability of the substance as a cholinotoxin in vivo, still remain. It is hoped that, with time and further investigations, the answers to these questions will also become known.

Acknowledgements

The work reported in this paper has been supported by National Institute of Mental Health Grant No. MH42572, by the UCB s.a. Pharmaceutical Sector (Brussels), and by the Max Kade Foundation. The author also wishes to acknowledge his many collaborators whose scientific contributions have been referred to in this overview.

References

Allen, Y.S., Marchbanks, R.M. and Sinden, J.D. (1988) Nonspecific effects of the putative cholinergic neurotoxin ethylcholine mustard aziridinium ion in the rat brain examined by autoradiography, immunocytochemistry and gel electrophoresis. Neurosci. Lett., 95: 69–74.

Amir, A., Pittel, Z., Shahar, A., Fisher, A. and Heldman, E. (1988) Cholinotoxicity of the ethylcholine aziridinium ion in primary cultures from rat central nervous system. Brain Res., 454: 298–307.

Arst, D.S., Berger, T.W., Fisher, A. and Hanin, I. (1983) AF64A reduces acetylcholinesterase (AChE) staining, and uncovers AChE-positive cell bodies in rat hippocampus, in vivo. Fed. Proc., 42: 657.

Asante, J.W., Cross, A.J., Deakin, J.F.W., Johnson, J.A. and Slater, H.R. (1983) Evaluation of ethylcholine mustard aziridinium ion (ECMA) as a specific neurotoxin of brain cholinergic neurones. Br. J. Pharmacol., 573P.

Atterwill, C.K., Collins, P., Meakin, J., Pillar, A.M. and Prince, A.K. (1989) Effect of nerve growth factor and thyrotropin releasing hormone on cholinergic neurones in developing rat brain reaggregate cultures lesioned with ethylcholine mustard aziridinium. Biochem. Pharmacol., 38: 1631–1638.

Bailey, E.L., Overstreet, D.H. and Croker, A.D. (1986) Effects of intrahippocampal injections of the cholinergic neurotoxin AF64A on open field activity and avoidance learning in the rat. Behav. Neural. Biol., 45: 263–274.

Barlow, P. and Marchbanks, R.M. (1984) Effect of ethylcholine mustard on choline dehydrogenase and other enzymes of choline metabolism. J. Neurochem., 43: 1568–1573.

Barnes, D.M., Hanin, I. and Erickson, L.C. (1988) Cytotoxic and DNA-damaging effects of AF64A in cholinergic and non-cholinergic human cell lines. Fed. Proc., 47: 1749.

Blaker, W.D. and Goodwin, S.D. (1987) Biochemical and behavioral effects of intrahippocampal AF64A in rats. Pharmacol. Biochem. Behav., 28: 157–163.

Brandeis, R., Pittel, Z., Lachman, C., Heldman, E., Luz, S., Dachir, S., Levy, A., Hanin, I. and Fisher, A. (1986) AF64A-induced cholinotoxicity: Behavioral and biochemical correlates. In A. Fisher, I. Hanin and C. Lachman (Eds.), Alzheimer's and Parkinson's Diseases. Strategies for Research and Development, Plenum Press, New York, pp. 469–477.

Casamenti, F., Bracco, L., Pedata, F. and Pepeu, G (1986) Biochemical and behavioral effects of ethylcholine mustard aziridinium ion. In I. Hanin (Ed.), Dynamics of Cholinergic Function, Plenum Press, New York, pp. 1137–1143.

Caulfield, M.P., May, P.J., Pedder, E.K. and Prince, A.K. (1983) Behavioral studies with ethylcholine mustard aziridinium (ECMA). Br. J. Pharmacol., 79: 287.

Cherkin, A., Smith, G.E. and Flood, J.F. (1986) Learning in mice is altered by ethylcholine aziridinium ion: A model for amnestic syndromes. Soc. Neurosci. Abstr., 12: 711.

Chrobak, J.J., Hanin, I. and Walsh, T.J. (1987) AF64A (ethylcholine aziridinium ion), a cholinergic neurotoxin, selectively impairs working memory in a multiple component T-maze task. Brain Res., 414: 15–21.

Chrobak, J.J., Hanin, I., Schmechel, D.E. and Walsh, T.J. (1988) AF64A-induced memory impairment: behavioral, neurochemical and histological correlates. Brain Res., 463: 107–117.

Colhoun, E.H. and Rylett, R.J. (1986) Nitrogen mustard analogues of choline: Potential for use and misuse. Trends Pharmacol. Sci., 78: 55–58.

Coyle, J.T., Price, D.L. and DeLong, M.R. (1983) Alzheimer's disease: A disorder of cortical cholinergic innervation. Science, 219: 1184–1190.

Curti, D. and Marchbanks, R.M. (1984) Kinetics of irreversible inhibition of choline transport in synaptosomes by ethylcholine mustard aziridinium. J. Membr. Biol., 82: 259–268.

Davies, D.L., Sakellaridis, N., Valcana, T. and Vernadakis, A. (1986) Cholinergic neurotoxicity induced by ethylcholine aziridinium (AF64A) in neuron-enriched cultures. Brain Res., 378: 251–261.

Dawson, V.L., Wamsley, J.K., Filloux, F.M. and Dawson, T.M. (1987) Alterations in muscarinic M-2 and dopamine

D-2 receptors in the rat brain following intrastriatal injection of the cholinotoxin, AF64A: An autoradiographic study. *Soc. Neurosci. Abstr.,* 13: 1198.

Estrada, C., Triguero, D., del Rio, R.F. and Ramos, P.G. (1988) Biochemical and histological modifications of the rat retina induced by the cholinergic neurotoxin AF64A. *Brain Res.,* 439: 107–115.

Eva, C., Fabrazzo, M. and Costa, E. (1987) Changes of cholinergic, noradrenergic and serotonergic synaptic transmission indices elicited by ethylcholine aziridinium ion (AF64A) infused intraventricularly. *J. Pharmacol. Exp. Ther.,* 241: 181–186.

Fisher, A. and Hanin, I. (1980) Minireview: Choline analogs as potential tools in developing sensitive animal models of central cholinergic hypofunction. *Life Sci.,* 27: 1615–1634.

Fisher, A. and Hanin, I. (1986a) The AF64A-treated rat as an experimental model for Alzheimer's disease (AD): A critical evaluation. In A. Fisher, I. Hanin, and C. Lachman (Eds.), *Alzheimer's and Parkinson's disease. Strategies for Research and Development,* Plenum Press, New York, pp. 427–445.

Fisher, A. and Hanin, I. (1986b) Potential animal models for senile dementia of Alzheimer's type, with emphasis on AF64A-induced cholinotoxicity. *Annu. Rev. Pharmacol. Toxicol.,* 26: 161–181.

Fisher, A., Mantione, C.R., Abraham, D.J. and Hanin, I. (1982) Long-term cholinergic hypofunction induced in mice by ethylcholine mustard aziridinium ion (AF64A) in vivo. *J. Pharmacol. Exp. Ther.,* 222: 140–145.

Fisher, A. Brandeis, R., Pittel, Z., Karton, I., Sapir, M., Dachir, S., and Levy, A. (1987) AF102B: a new M1 agonist with potential application in Alzheimer's disease (AD). *Soc. Neurosci. Abstr.,* 13: 657.

Freeman, J.J. and Jenden, D.J. (1976) Minireview: The source of choline for acetylcholine synthesis in brain. *Life Sci.,* 19: 949–962.

Gaal, Gy, Potter, P.E., Hanin, I., Kakucska, I. and Vizi, E.S. (1986) Effects of intracerebroventricular AF64A administration on cholinergic, serotoninergic and catecholaminergic circuitry in rat dorsal hippocampus. *Neuroscience,* 19: 1197–1205.

Gobert, J.G., Gower, A.J., Hanin, I., Jamsin, P., Rousseau, D. and Wulfert, E. (1987) AF64A induces impairment of Morris Water Maze and hyperactivity in the rat at doses which do not cause widespread necrosis. *Br. J. Pharmacol.,* 91: 448P.

Goldstein, S., Grimee, R., Hanin, I. and Wulfert, E. (1988) Formation and degradation of 1-(ethyl)-1-(2-hydroxyethyl) aziridinium chloride in aqueous media – a comparative NMR study. *J. Neurosci. Methods,* 23: 101–105.

Gower, A.J., Rousseau, D., Jamsin, P., Gobert, J., Hanin, I. and Wulfert, E. (1989) Behavioural, biochemical and histological effects of low concentrations of AF64A administered intracerebroventricularly in the rat. *Eur. J. Pharmacol* 166: 271–281.

Gulya, K., Fisher, A., Hanin, I. and Yamamura, H.I. (1986) Studies on [^{3}H] hemicholinium-3 ([^{3}H]HC-3), [^{3}H]pirenzepine ([^{3}H]PZ) and [^{3}H] (-) quinuclidinyl benzilate ([^{3}H](−)QNB) binding with choline and acetylcholine analogues (AF30, AF64, AF64A). *Fed. Proc.,* 45: 921.

Gurkliss, J., Leventer, S. and Hanin, I. (1986) AF64A (ethylcholine mustard aziridinium) impairs memory retention in rats. *Fed. Proc.,* 45: 923.

Hanin, I., Fisher, A., Hortnagl, H., Leventer, S.M., Potter, P.E. and Walsh, T.J. (1987) Ethylcholine aziridinium (AF64A; ECMA) and other potential cholinergic neuron-specific neurotoxins. In H.Y. Meltzer (Ed.), *Psychopharmacology: The Third Generation of Progress,* Raven Press, New York, pp. 341–349.

Hortnagl, H., Potter, P.E. and Hanin, I. (1987a) Effect of cholinergic deficit induced by ethylcholine aziridinium (AF64A) on noradrenergic and dopaminergic parameters in rat brain. *Brain Res.,* 421: 75–84.

Hortnagl, H., Potter, P.E. and Hanin, I. (1987b) Effect of cholinergic deficit induced by ethylcholine aziridinium on serotonergic parameters in rat brain. *Neuroscience,* 22: 203–213.

Hortnagl, H., Potter, P.E., Happe, K., Goldstein, S., Leventer, S., Wulfert, E. and Hanin, I. (1988) Role of aziridinium moiety in the in vivo cholinotoxicity of ethylcholine aziridinium ion (AF64A). *J. Neurosci. Methods,* 23: 107–113.

Hortnagl, H., Sperk, G., Sobal, G. and Maas, D. (1990) Cholinergic deficit induced by ethylcholine aziridinium ion (AF64A) transiently affects somatostatin and neuropeptide Y levels in rat brain *J. Neurochem.,* 54: 1608–1613.

Hoyle, C.H.V., Moss, H.E. and Burnstock, G. (1986) Ethylcholine mustard aziridinium ion (AF64A) impairs cholinergic neuromuscular transmission in the guinea-pig ileum and urinary bladder, and cholinergic neuromodulation in the guinea-pig distal colon. *Gen. Pharmacol.,* 17: 543–548.

Ikegami, S., Nihonmatsu, I., Hatanaka, H., Takei, N. and Kawamura, H. (1989) Recovery of hippocampal cholinergic activity by transplantation of septal neurons in AF64A treated rats. *Neurosci. Lett.,* 101: 17–22.

Ishii, T., Nishio, H., Hata, F. and Yagasaki, O. (1987) Neurochemical study on the effect of AF64A administered intraperitoneally on cholinergic nerve activity in rat brain. *Jpn. J. Pharmacol.,* 43: 134P.

Jarrard, L.E., Kent, G.J., Meyerhoff, J.L. and Levy, A. (1984) Behavioral and neurochemical effects of intraventricular AF64A administration in rats. *Pharmacol. Biochem. Behav.,* 21: 273–280.

Jenden, D.J. (1979) An overview of choline and acetylcholine metabolism in relation to the therapeutic uses of choline. In A. Barbeau, J.H. Growdon and R.J. Wurtman (Eds.), *Nutrition and the Brain. Choline and Lecithin in Brain Disorders,* Raven Press, New York, pp. 13–24.

Johnson, G.V.W., Simonato, M. and Jope, R.S. (1988) Dose- and time-dependent hippocampal cholinergic lesions induced by ethylcholine mustard aziridinium ion: effects of nerve growth factor, GM1 ganglioside, and vitamin E. *Neurochem. Res.,* 8: 685–692.

Jope, R.S. (1979) High affinity choline transport and acetyl CoA production in brain and their roles in the regulation of acetylcholine in rat brain. *Brain Res. Rev.,* 1: 313–344.

Jossan, S.S., Hiraga, Y. and Oreland, L. (1989) The cholinergic neurotoxin ethylcholine mustard aziridinium (AF64A) induces an increase in MAO-B activity in the rat brain. *Brain Res.*, 476: 291–297.

Kasa, P. and Hanin, I. (1985) Ethylcholine mustard aziridinium blocks the axoplasmic transport of acetylcholinesterase in cholinergic nerve fibers of the rat. *Histochemistry*, 83: 343–345.

Koppenaal, D.W., Raizada, M.K., Momol, E.A., Morgan, E. and Meyer, E.M. (1986) Effects of AF64A on [^{3}H]acetylcholine synthesis in neuron-enriched primary brain cell cultures. *Dev. Brain Res.*, 30: 110–113.

Kozlowski, M.R. and Arbogast, R.E. (1986) Specific toxic effects of ethylcholine nitrogen mustard on cholinergic neurons of the nucleus basalis of Meynert. *Brain Res.*, 372: 45–54.

Lamour, Y. and Dutar, P. (1986) Central cholinergic systems in the rat: An electrophysiological approach in young and aged animals. In A. Bes (Ed.), *Senile Dementias: Early Detection,* John Libbey Eurotext., pp. 223–228.

Lamour, Y., Dutar, P., Rascol, O. and Jobert, A. (1986) Septohippocampal neurons after intraventricular AF64A administration in rats: an electrophysiological study. *Exp. Neurol.*, 92: 413–420.

Lehr, E., Kuhn, F.-J. and Hinzen, D.H. (1984) AF64A neurotoxicity: Behavioral and electrophysiological alterations in rats. *Soc. Neurosci. Abstr.*, 10: 775.

Leventer, S., McKeag, D., Clancy, M., Wulfert, E. and Hanin, I. (1985) Intracerebroventricular AF64A reduces ACh release from rat hippocampal slices. *Neuropharmacology*, 24: 453–459.

Leventer, S.M., Wulfert, E. and Hanin, I. (1987) Time course of ethylcholine mustard aziridinium ion (AF64A)-induced cholinotoxicity in vivo. *Neuropharmacology*, 26: 361–365.

Levy, A., Kant, G.J., Meyerhoff, J.L. and Jarrard, L.E. (1984) Non-cholinergic neurotoxic effects of AF64A in the substantia nigra. *Brain Res.*, 305: 169–172.

Mantione, C.R., Fisher, A. and Hanin, I. (1981) the AF64A treated mouse: Possible model for central cholinergic hypofunction. *Science*, 213: 579–580.

Mantione, C.R., DeGroat, W.C., Fisher, A. and Hanin, I. (1983a) Selective inhibition of peripheral cholinergic transmission in the cat produced by AF64A. *J. Pharmacol. Exp. Ther.*, 225: 616–622.

Mantione, C.R., Zigmond, M.J., Fisher, A. and Hanin, I. (1983b) Selective presynaptic cholinergic neurotoxicity following intrahippocampal AF64A injection in rats. *J. Neurochem.*, 41: 251–255.

McArdle, J.J. and Hanin, I. (1986) Acute in vivo exposure to ethylcholine aziridinium (AF64A) depresses the secretion of quanta from motor nerve terminals. *Eur. J. Pharmacol.*, 131: 119–121.

McGurk, S.R., Hartgraves, S.L., Kelly, P.H., Gordon, M.N. and Butcher, L.L. (1987) Is ethylcholine mustard aziridinium ion a specific cholinergic neurotoxin? *Neuroscience*, 22: 215–224.

Millar, T.J., Ishimoto, I., Boelen, M., Epstein, M.L., Johnson, C.D. and Morgan, I.G. (1987) The toxic effects of ethyl-

choline mustard aziridinium ion on cholinergic cells in the chicken retina. *J. Neurosci.*, 7: 343–356.

Mistry, J.S., Abraham, D.J. and Hanin, I. (1986) Neurochemistry of aging: I. Toxins for an animal model of Alzheimer's disease. *J. Med. Chem.*, 29: 376–380.

Mouton, P.R. Meyer, E.M., Dunn, A.J., Millard, W. and Arendash, G.W. (1988) Induction of cortical cholinergic hypofunction and memory retention deficits through intracortical AF64A infusions. *Brain Res.*, 444: 104–118.

Nakahara, N., Iga, Y., Mizobe, F. and Kawanishi, G. (1988a) Amelioration of experimental amnesia (passive avoidance failure) in rodents by the selective M_1 agonist AF102B. *Jpn. J. Pharmacol.*, 48: 502–506.

Nakahara, N., Iga, Y., Mizobe, F. and Kawanishi, G. (1988b) Effects of intracerebroventricular injection of AF64A on learning behaviors in rats. *Jpn. J. Pharmacol.*, 48: 121–130.

Nakamura, S., Nakagawa, Y., Kawai, M., Tohyama, M. and Ishihara, T. (1988) AF64A (ethylcholine aziridinium ion)-induced basal forebrain lesion impairs maze performance. *Behav. Brain Res.*, 29: 119–126.

Ogura, H., Yamanishi, Y. and Yamatsu, K. (1987) Effects of physostigmine on AF64A-induced impairment of learning acquisition in rats. *Jpn. J. Pharmacol.*, 44: 498–501.

Perry, E.K., Tomlinson, B.E., Blessed, G., Bergmann, K., Gibson, P.H. and Perry, R.H. (1978) Correlation of cholinergic abnormalities with senile plaques and mental test scores in senile dementia. *Br. Med. J.*, 2: 1457–1459.

Pillar, A.M., Prince, A.K. and Atterwill, C.K. (1988) The neurotoxicity of ethylcholine mustard aziridinium (ECMA) in rat brain reaggregate cultures. *Toxicology*, 49: 115–119.

Pittel, Z., Fisher, A. and Heldman, E. (1987) Reversible and irreversible inhibition of high-affinity choline transport caused by ethylcholine aziridinium ion. *J. Neurochem.*, 49: 468–474.

Pope, C.N., Englert, L.F. and Ho, B.T. (1985) Passive avoidance deficits in mice following ethylcholine aziridinium chloride treatment. *Pharmacol. Biochem. Behav.*, 22: 297–299.

Potter, P.E., Harsing, L.G., Jr., Kakucska, I., Gaal, Gy and Vizi, E.S. (1986) Selective impairment of acetylcholine release and content in the central nervous system following intracerebroventricular administration of ethylcholine mustard aziridinium ion (AF64A) in the rat. *Neurochem. Int.*, 8: 199–206.

Rylett, R.J. and Colhoun, E.H. (1980) Kinetic data on the inhibition of high-affinity choline transport into rat forebrain synaptosomes by choline-like compounds and nitrogen mustard analogues. *J. Neurochem.*, 34: 713–719.

Sandberg, K., Sanberg, P.R., Hanin, I., Fisher, A. and Coyle, J.T. (1984) Cholinergic lesion of the striatum impairs acquisition and retention of a passive avoidance response. *Behav. Neurosci.*, 98: 162–165.

Sandberg, K., Schnaar, R.L., McKinney, M., Hanin, I., Fisher, A. and Coyle, J.T. (1985) AF64A: an active site directed irreversible inhibitor of choline acetyltransferase. *J. Neurochem.*, 44: 439–445.

Speiser, Z., Amitzi-Sonder, J., Gitter, S. and Cohen, S. (1988) Behavioral differences in the developing rat following postnatal anoxia or postnatally injected AF64A, a cholinergic neurotoxin. *Behav. Brain Res.,* 30: 89–94.

Spencer, C.J., Moos, W.H., Davis, R.E., Schwarz, R.D., Kinsora, J. and Smith, M. E. (1987) Neurotoxin (AF64A) model of cholinergic hypofunction: An improved synthetic procedure for AF64A. *Soc. Neurosci. Abstr.,* 13: 487.

Spencer, D.G., Horvath, E., Luiten, P., Schuurman, T. and Traber, J. (1985) Novel approaches in the study of brain acetylcholine function: Neuropharmacology, neuroanatomy, and behavior. In J. Traber and W.H. Gispen (Eds.), *Senile Dementia of the Alzheimer Type,* Springer-Verlag, Berlin/Heidelberg, pp. 325–342.

Stephens, P.H., Tagari, P. and Cuello, A.C. (1987) Ethylcholine mustard aziridinium ion lesions of the rat cortex result in retrograde degeneration of basal cholinergic neurons: implications for animal models of neurodegenerative disease. *Neurochem. Res.,* 12: 613–618.

Stewart, D.J., Leventer, S.M., Hanin, I. and Vanderwolf, C.H. (1987) Hippocampal electrical activity in relation to behavior following ethylcholine aziridinium ion (AF64A) treatment. *Pharmacol. Biochem. Behav.,* 26: 357–364.

Stwertka, S.A. and Olson, G.L. (1986) Neuropathology and amphetamine-induced turning resulting from AF64A injections into the striatum of the rat. *Life Sci.,* 38: 1105–1110.

Szerdahelyi, P. and Kasa, P. (1988) Intraventricular administration of the cholinotoxin AF64A increases the accumulation of aluminium in the rat parietal cortex and hippocampus, but not in the frontal cortex. *Brain Res.,* 444: 356–360.

Tateishi, N., Takano, Y., Honda, K., Yamada, K., Kamiya, Y. and Kamiya, H-O. (1987) Effects of intrahippocampal injections of the cholinergic neurotoxin AF64A on presynaptic cholinergic markers and on passive avoidance response in the rat. *Clin. Exp. Pharmacol. Physiol.,* 14: 611–618.

Tedford, C.E., Corey, J.C., Leventer, S., Rosengarten, M.L., Lorens, S., Wulfert, E. and Hanin, I. (1988) Behavioral and neurochemical impairment in young and aged Fischer 344 rats after intracerebroventricular (I.C.V.) administration of AF64A. *Fed. Proc.,* 47: 2866.

Tonnaer, J.A.D.M., Lammers, A.J.J.C., Wieringa, J.H. and Steinbusch, H.W.M. (1986) Immunohistochemical evidence for degeneration of cholinergic neurons in the forebrain of the rat following injection of AF64A-picrylsulfonate into the dorsal hippocampus. *Brain Res.,* 370: 200–203.

Uney, J.B. and Marchbanks, R.M. (1987) Specificity of ethylcholine mustard aziridinium as an irreversible inhibitor of choline transport in cholinergic and noncholinergic tissue. *J. Neurochem.,* 48: 1673–1676.

Vickroy, T.W., Watson, M., Leventer, S.M., Roeske, W.R. and Hanin, I. (1986) Regional differences in ethylcholine mustard aziridinium (AF64A)-induced deficits in presynaptic cholinergic markers for the rat central nervous system. *J. Pharmacol. Exp. Ther.,* 231:577–582.

Villani. L., Contestabile, A., Migani, P., Poli, A. and Fonnum, F. (1986) Ultrastructural and neurochemical effects of the presumed cholinergic toxin AF64A in the rat interpeduncular nucleus. *Brain Res.,* 379: 223–231.

Villani, L. Bissoli, R., Garolini, S., Guarnieri, T., Battistini, S., Saverino, O. and Contestabile, A. (1988) Effect of AF64A on the cholinergic systems of the retina and optic tectum of goldfish. *Exp. Brain Res.,* 70: 455–462.

Walsh, T.J. and Hanin, I. (1986) A review of the behavioral effects of AF64A, a cholinergic neurotoxin. In A. Fisher, I. Hanin and C. Lachman (Eds.), *Alzheimer's and Parkinson's Diseases. Strategies for Research and Development,* Plenum Press, New York, pp. 461–467.

Walsh, T.J., Tilson, H.A., DeHaven, D.L., Mailman, R.B., Fisher, A. and Hanin, I. (1984) AF64A, a cholinergic neurotoxin, selectively depletes acetylcholine in hippocampus and cortex, and produces long-term passive avoidance and radial-arm maze deficits in the rat. *Brain Res.,* 321: 91–102.

S.-M. Aquilonius and P.-G. Gillberg (Eds.)
Progress in Brain Research, Vol. 84
© 1990 Elsevier Science Publishers B.V. (Biomedical Division)

CHAPTER 32

Injury and repair of central cholinergic neurons

A.C. Cuello, L. Garofalo, D. Maysinger, E.P. Pioro and A. Ribeiro Da Silva

Department of Pharmacology and Therapeutics, McGill University, 3655 Drummond Street, Montreal, Quebec, Canada H3G 1Y6

Introduction

Although acetylcholine has been the first substance to be recognized as a chemical transmitter, it has been only in the last decade that convincing morphological evidence has been gathered for the existence of specific cholinergic cell bodies and fibre projections in the central nervous system (for reviews see Fibiger, 1982; Butcher and Woolf, 1984; Cuello and Sofroniew, 1984; Mesulam, Chapter 26 of this volume). The knowledge of the existence of these cholinergic neurons has greatly facilitated research in other fields, including neuropathology. For example, the most rostrally located (forebrain) cholinergic neurons have been implicated in the pathology of Alzheimer's disease (Whitehouse et al., 1982). However, the involvement of forebrain cholinergic neurons in this disease is most likely a secondary consequence of a primary cortical pathology whereby a retrograde neuronal degeneration takes place for the cortically projecting cells of the nucleus basalis magnocellularis (NBM). In support of such a view is the evidence that in animal models extensive cortical infarctions result in the cell body shrinkage and loss of neurites with a concomitant depletion

of choline acetyltransferase activity (ChAT) in the NBM of the rat (Sofroniew et al., 1983; Stephens et al., 1985). The finding that basal forebrain neurons can specifically take up and transport nerve growth factor (NGF) (Schwab et al., 1979) and that injured septal-hippocampal cholinergic neurons respond positively to the NGF (Hefti et al., 1984; Hefti, 1986; Williams et al., 1986; Kromer, 1987; Cuello et al., 1989) administration has brought a new dimension to studies in brain plasticity and neuronal repair.

Forebrain cholinergic neurons contain NGF binding sites (Richardson et al., 1986; Raivich and Kreutzberg, 1987; Dawbarn et al., 1988; Riopelle et al., 1988) and their terminal targets produce the trophic factor which can be transported retrogradely to cell bodies of these neurons (Thoenen et al., 1987). Furthermore, β-NGF has also been found to affect forebrain cholinergic neurons in vitro (Hefti et al., 1985; Hatanaka and Tsukui, 1986).

Besides NGF, a number of other endogenous substances have been reported to display neurotrophic activity in a variety of experimental situations (for review see Varon et al., 1988). Of these substances, the ganglioside series of glycosphingolipids are of particular interest as they might resemble "bona fide" trophic factors in many ways (for reviews see Ledeen, 1985; Cuello, 1989).

Ceccarelli and coworkers (1976) provided the first evidence for reparative effects of gangliosides on peripheral cholinergic neurons and Wojcik and coworkers (1982) provided the first demonstration

---

Abbreviations: NGF, nerve growth factor; CNS, central nervous system; NBM, nucleus basalis magnocellularis; NGFR, nerve growth factor receptor; IR, immunoreactivity; ChAT, choline acetyltransferase; i.c.v., intracerebroventricular; MPTP, 1-methyl-4-phenyl-1,2,3,6-tetrahydropyridine; BSA, bovine serum albumin; HACU, high-affinity choline uptake.

of the in vivo effects of gangliosides on injured central cholinergic pathways in adult rats. Wojcik and collaborators (1982) have shown that the intramuscular application of a mix of gangliosides in rats with extensive lesions of the septal nucleus facilitated the recovery of hippocampal AChE and ChAT activities. In addition, the intraperitoneal (i.p.) daily administration of the ganglioside GM1 was shown to facilitate the biochemical recovery of cortical cholinergic markers following unilateral electrolytic lesions of the NBM (Pedata et al., 1984; Casamenti et al., 1985; Florian et al., 1987). Alternatively, Gradkowska and collaborators (1986) later demonstrated that GM1 can promote biochemical recovery of the hippocampal cholinergic system following fimbria-fornix transection.

Administration of GM1 also prevents the retrograde cell shrinkage of cholinergic neurons of the NBM which follows cortical infarction (Cuello et al., 1986) or cell death in the medial septum after unilateral hippocampal ablation (Sofroniew et al., 1986). The nature of these ganglioside effects on cholinergic neurons and their possible interactions with NGF remain to be established.

In this brief review we will discuss the localization of NGF-receptors in CNS cholinergic neurons, the effects of NGF on injured cholinergic neurons of the NBM and the actions of gangliosides alone or in combination with NGF over these neurons and their terminal projections following cortical devascularising lesions

NGF-receptor immunoreactive sites in forebrain cholinergic neurons

NGF has been shown to exert neurotrophic effects on neurons of the developing basal forebrain in vitro (Hartikka and Hefti, 1988: Hatanaka et al., 1988) and in vivo (Mobley et al., 1986). It is assumed that these effects can only occur in cells possessing the NGF receptor (NGFR), specifically its high affinity form (Hosang and Shooter, 1987; Hempstead et al., 1989). Radioautographic [^{125}I] NGF studies have demonstrated high-affinity binding sites on cholinergic neurons of the basal

forebrain, including those in the NBM (Richardson et al., 1986; Raivich and Kreutzberg, 1987). The development of monoclonal antibodies identifying the NGFR in rat (Chandler et al., 1984) and primate (Ross et al., 1984) has allowed the light microscopic characterization of NGFR-containing neurons and fibers in the NBM and other basal forebrain nuclei of these species (Gomez-Pinilla et al., 1987; Kiss et al., 1988; Kordower et al., 1988; Schatteman et al., 1988; Pioro and Cuello, 1989a; Woolf et al., 1989). Although it is not yet clear whether the anti-rat NGFR antibody, 192-IgG (Chandler et al., 1984), recognizes only the low-affinity NGFR (Chandler et al., 1984) or both its low- and high-affinity forms (Green and Greene, 1986), 192-IgG-positive neurons in the NBM appear to correspond to those possessing high-affinity NGF-binding sites (Richardson et al., 1986; Raivich and Kreutzberg, 1987). However, not all NGFR immunoreactive (IR) neurons in the basal forebrain are cholinergic, as revealed by acetylcholinesterase (AChE) histochemistry (Springer et al., 1987) and choline acetyltransferase (ChAT) immunocytochemistry (Dawbarn et al., 1988; Batchelor et al., 1989; Pioro and Cuello, 1989a). The reverse is also true, i.e. many forebrain cholinergic neurons are seemingly lacking NGFR sites. In the rat none of the cortical ChAT immunoreactive neurons are NGFR-bearing cells and only few cholinergic neurons of the neostriatum display NGFR. Furthermore, cholinergic neurons of the brainstem are in most cases devoid of a receptor for NGF (Pioro and Cuello, 1989b; Woolf et al., 1989). The topographic relationship between ChAT-immunoreactive and NGFR- immunoreactive neural systems is schematically represented in Fig. 1.

The similar morphological appearances of the ChAT- and NGFR-containing NBM neurons are shown (Fig. 2a,b). It is therefore not surprising that the distribution of ChAT and NGFR-IR fibers projecting from these neurons to their terminal fields in the neocortex and hippocampus is so similar (Gomez-Pinilla et al., 1987; Pioro and Cuello, 1989a; Woolf et al., 1989; Fig. 2c,d).

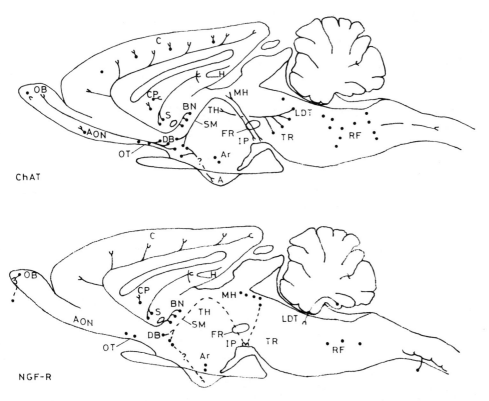

Fig. 1. Schematic representations of parasagittal adult rat brain sections displaying ChAT-IR (upper) and NGFR-IR (lower) neurons and fiber pathways. The overlap of neurons containing these two antigens is discussed in the text. Abbreviations: OB — olfactory bulb; AON — anterior olfactory nucleus; DB — nucleus of the diagonal band; S — septum; CP — caudate putamen; H — hippocampus; BN — nucleus basalis; A — amygdala; TH — thalamus; Ar — arcuate nucleus; TR — tegmental reticular system; LDT — lateral dorsal tegmental nucleus; RF — hindbrain reticular formation; C — cortex; IP — nucleus interpeduncularis; SM — stria medullaris; MH — medial habenula; OT — olfactory tubercle; FR — fasciculus retroflexus. For the sake of clarity, classical motor and autonomic preganglionic neurons are not represented.

We have recently examined the subcellular distribution of the NGFR reaction product in the somata and distal axons of putatively cholinergic neurons in the NBM. Identification of the sites of NGFR metabolism and internalization is pivotal in understanding how the receptor interacts with NGF. Immunoreactivity in the soma is most prominent along the plasma membrane (Fig. 2e). Intracellular sites of protein synthesis and modification containing reaction product include the rough endoplasmic reticulum (RER) and Golgi complex, respectively (Fig. 2e). Multivesicular bodies (secondary lysosomes), which are sites of protein catabolism, possess prominent NGFR-IR

(inset of Fig. 2e). Some coated vesicles, closely apposed to or contiguous with the cell membrane, can also be seen to contain reaction product (Fig. 2f). Cortically projecting axons of these neurons can be seen to contain NGFR immunoreactivity consistent with the transport of the receptor to NGF-producing regions (Fig. 2g).

The above observations are consistent with a functional role of NGF and its receptor in basal forebrain cholinergic neurons of the adult rat. Whether other CNS cholinergic and non-cholinergic neurons respond to NGF remains to be established. In this regard, it has been shown that NGF might modulate ChAT activity in the

304

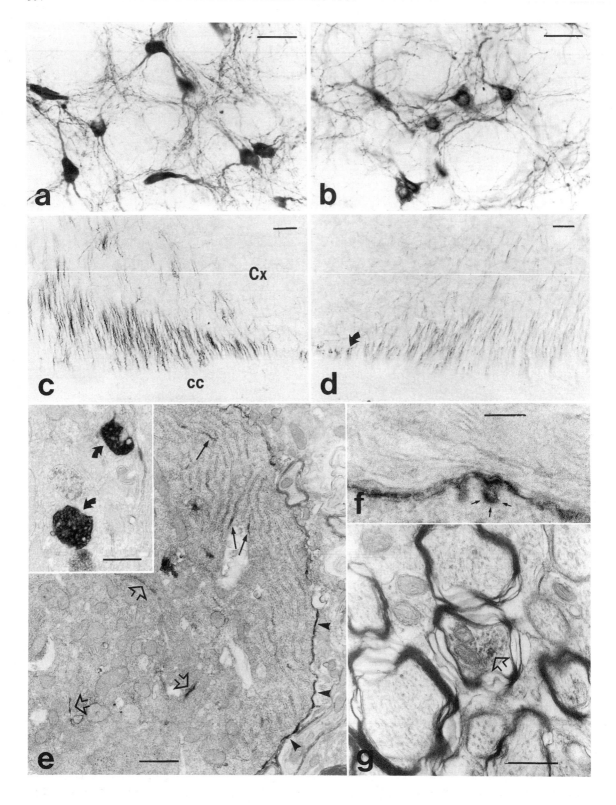

neostriatum (Mobley et al., 1985) and up-regulate its own receptor in the same region of the brain (Gage et al., 1989).

Nerve growth factor and gangliosides protect injured forebrain cholinergic neurons

In our own laboratory interest has centered on the NBM-to-cortex cholinergic pathway. We have observed that thirty days following unilateral cortical damage, induced by a devascularizing lesion, retrograde cholinergic cell shrinkage and neurite loss occur in the rat ipsilateral NBM (Sofroniew et al., 1983). Further to these immunohistochemical changes, a decrease in ChAT activity was noted in microdissected samples of the NBM (Stephens et al., 1985). Using this model, we have shown that NGF administered intracerebroventricularly (i.c.v.) via a minipump, beginning immediately post-lesion, at a dosage of 12 μg/day for 7 days, can prevent the biochemical (Fig. 3B) and morphological damage which occurs in the NBM following decortication (Cuello et al., 1989). Furthermore, this treatment produces an increase above control levels in both ChAT activity (Fig. 3A) and high-affinity choline uptake (HACU) in the remaining ipsilateral cortex of lesioned rats (Fig. 4A). A recovery in the activity of these two cholinergic markers after NGF treatment has been reported also following anterograde damage to the NBM (Haroutunian et al., 1986, Di Patre et al., 1989).

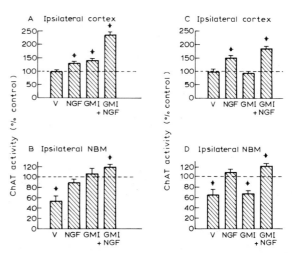

Fig. 3. Effect of NGF and/or GM1 on ChAT activity in the ipsilateral cortex (A and C) and NBM (B and D) of unilaterally decorticated rats. Animals received either: vehicle (V = PBS + 0.1% BSA), NGF (12 μg/day, 7 days) and/or GM1 (in A and B: 5 mg/kg/day, 7 days; in C and D: 0.5 mg/kg/day, 7 days). Factors were administered intracerebroventricularly via minipump (Alzet 2001), beginning immediately after lesioning. Animals were killed 30 days post-lesion (i.e., 23 days after treatment ended). ChAT activity was determined according to the Fonnum (1975) method and protein quantities were measured according to the Bradford (1976) method. $n = 5$–6 animals/group. Control values: (A) 35.81 ± 2.39 nmol/ACh/mg protein/hr; (B) 57.67 ± 3.86 nmol/ACh/mg protein/hr; (C) 39.20 ± 3.77 nmol/ACh/mg protein/hr; (D) 69.06 ± 4.67 nmol/ACh/mg protein/hr. *$p < 0.05$ Anova, post-hoc Newman-Keuls' test.

In addition to promoting biochemical recovery in vivo, the i.p. administration of GM1 was also shown to prevent morphological degeneration occurring in cholinergic neurons of the rat nucleus

---

Fig. 2. a,b: Similar light microscopic appearances of magnocellular neurons and fiber plexus in the rat NBM containing ChAT-immunoreactivity (a) and NGFR-immunoreactivity (b). Scale bar = 40 μm. c,d: High magnification light micrographs demonstrating very similar pattern of ChAT-IR (c) and NGFR-IR (d) fibers entering the cerebral cortex (Cx) from the corpus callosum (cc). The fields are arranged as "mirror images" with the midline in between to emphasize their correlation. The curved arrow in (d) indicates approximate location from where the electron micrograph of a NGFR-IR axon (shown in g) is taken. Scale bar = 40 μm. e: Low magnification electron micrograph showing subcellular NGFR reaction product distributed along the cell membrane (arrowheads), in rough endoplasmic reticulum (arrows) and scattered Golgi complexes (open arrows). Scale bar = 1 μm. Inset shows immunoreactive multivesicular bodies. Scale bar = 0.5 μm. f: High magnification view of two immunoreactive vesicles which are contiguous with the stained cell membrane. One (small arrows) may be coated suggesting endocytosis. Scale bar = 0.2 μm. g: High magnification appearance of transversely sectioned myelinated axons projecting into the neocortex from the corpus callosum (as indicated by curved arrow in d). NGFR reaction product is aggregated near the center of one axon (open arrow). Scale bar = 0.5 μm. (Pioro, Ribeiro da Silva and Cuello, unpublished.)

basalis and medial septum following unilateral decortication (Cuello et al., 1986) or unilateral removal of the hippocampus (Sofroniew et al., 1986), respectively. Furthermore, the i.c.v. administration of GM1 for shorter periods (7 days, via a minipump) and at lower doses (5 mg/kg/day) to unilaterally decorticated rats also prevents the fall in ChAT activity (Fig. 3B) and preserves the morphological appearance of cholinergic cells in the NBM (Cuello et al., 1987) in a manner comparable to that obtained with NGF. Such treatment also increased ChAT activity and the level of HACU in the ipsilateral remaining cortex (Fig. 4A) significantly over control values. In addition, we have observed in this brain area, from GM1-treated lesioned rats, an increase over control values in the ratio of stimulated over basal acetylcholine release recovered using the microdialysis technique (Maysinger et al., 1988, 1989; Fig. 5).

In view of the above evidence suggesting trophic roles for both GM1 and NGF in central cholinergic neurons, and the previously mentioned speculation that GM1 may depend on the presence of neuronotrophic factor(s) to exert its effects, our laboratory initiated studies to examine whether GM1 could modulate the actions of NGF in vivo. Several studies in which in vitro systems were used have suggested that this may be the case (Ferrari et al., 1983; Katoh-Semba et al., 1984; Leon et al., 1984; Doherty et al., 1985; Skaper et al., 1985; Schwartz et al., 1982). In initial studies in our laboratory (Cuello et al., 1987), NGF was administered i.c.v. via minipumps to unilaterally decorticated adult rats at doses of 12 μg/day for 7 days. Another group of rats received NGF at the same rate in combination with an effective GM1 dosage (5 mg/kg/day, 7 days i.c.v.). In contrast to levels measured in microdissected brain areas of lesioned rats treated solely with NGF or GM1, ChAT activity in the NBM of lesioned rats treated with both these factors simultaneously increased significantly over control values (Fig. 3B). Moreover, in the remaining ipsilateral cortex ChAT activity increased 100% over control values (Fig.

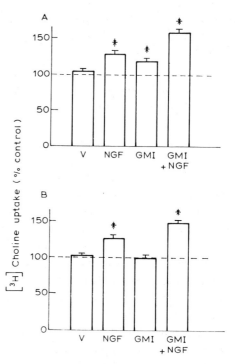

Fig. 4. High-affinity choline uptake (HACU) in the ipsilateral remaining cortex of adult rats, following unilateral decortication. Rats were treated with either: vehicle (V = artificial c.s.f. + 0.1% BSA), NGF (12 μg/day, 7 days) and/or GM1 (in A: 5 mg/kg/day, 7 days; in B: 0.5 mg/kg/day, 7 days) intracerebroventricularly via minipump (Alzet 2001). Rats were sacrificed 30 days post-lesion. HACU was determined according to the method of Simon et al. (1976). Protein content was determined according to the Bradford (1976) method. $n = 6$ animals/group. Control values: (A) 7.6 ± 0.8 pmol ^{3}H-choline/mg protein/4 min; (B) 8.3 ± 1.2 pmol ^{3}H-choline/mg protein/4 min. (Garofalo and Cuello, unpublished data.)

3A). Furthermore, we have also shown that treatment with NGF (dosage and mode of administration as described above) given concurrently with an ineffective GM1 dosage (0.5 mg/kg/day, 7 days i.c.v.) increased the activity of cholinergic markers in the NBM and ipsilateral remaining cortex over those measured in control or NGF only treated rats (Fig. 3C,D). Cortical levels of HACU measured in these rats showed a similar pattern (Fig. 4A,B), thus further reinforcing the notion that GM1 may modulate the actions of NGF in vivo. More recently, Di Patre and collaborators (1989) have also reported an in vivo potentiation by GM1 on NGF effects of central cholinergic neurons following anterograde lesioning of the NBM. Furthermore, this interaction between GM1 and NGF also appears to occur in vivo in the peripheral nervous system as well (Vantini et al., 1988).

Conclusions

Trophic responses to β-NGF by centrally located cholinergic neurons have been well substantiated for septal-hippocampal and basalis-cortical projections. From the cellular and subcellular analysis of NGFR immunoreactive sites it can be assumed that those responses are, in all probability, receptor mediated. The sequence of events that follow this receptor-ligand interaction may include induction of specific genes (Greenberg et al., 1985; Kruijer et al., 1985; Milbrandt, 1986; Leonard et al., 1987) and second messenger systems (Cremins et al., 1986; Hama et al., 1986) which result in the translation and/or modification of specific proteins involved in trophic responses. The interaction of gangliosides with β-NGF over central cholinergic neurons could occur at any of those levels. The possibility that this interaction occurs

at the level of the cell membrane should be primarily considered. Exogenous gangliosides are known to be incorporated into neural cell membranes (Toffano et al., 1980) and immobilized GM1 is capable of binding β-NGF with low affinity (Schwartz and Spirman, 1982). Therefore, it is possible that gangliosides could provide additional binding sites for growth factors or, alternatively, modify the state of the growth factor receptor. This is the case for the ganglioside GD2 and the vitronectin receptor in the plasma membrane of human melanoma cells (Cheresh et al., 1987).

The opportunity for a cooperative interaction between gangliosides and β-NGF in the in vivo cholinergic model is heightened by the occurrence of an increase in β-NGF levels in the target areas of basal forebrain cholinergic neurons following mechanical lesions (for review see Whittemore and Seiger, 1987). However, ganglioside actions on dopaminergic neurons (Agnati et al., 1983; Toffano et al., 1983) cannot be explained simply on this basis since NGF is apparently not a trophic agent for dopaminergic neurons (Schwab et al., 1979).

In our in vivo cholinergic model, the effects of β-NGF and/or GM1 on ChAT activity in the remaining neocortex may be due either to increased production of the biosynthetic enzyme or sprouting of terminals with resultant reorganization of cholinergic fibers. We favour the possibility that sprouting of cholinergic fibers occurs in cortically damaged rats which have been treated with gangliosides, as release of acetylcholine is enhanced from the remaining cortex (Maysinger et al., 1988) as well as the uptake of tritiated choline (Garofalo and Cuello, unpublished). Such animals also show an improved behavioural performance over lesioned-untreated animals in passive avoidance or Morris water maze tests (Elliott et al., 1989).

It has been found that in response to injury the brain produces low amounts of endogenous trophic factors immediately after the insult (for example Nieto-Sampedro et al., 1983). Therefore, in instances of extensive lesions of the nervous tissue,

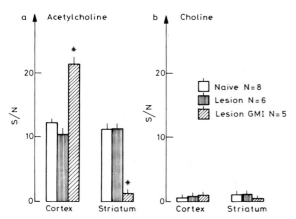

Fig. 5. Ratio of stimulated and non-stimulated (S/N) acetylcholine (A) and choline (B) levels measured in perfusates collected by microdialysis from the cortex and striatum of naive, saline-treated (lesion) and GM1-treated (lesion GM1) decorticated rats. Vertical lines show S.E.M. Comparisons have been tested with Student's t-test, *$p < 0.05$. (Maysinger et al., 1988.)

neurons are likely to be in an extremely vulnerable state which could result in irreversible anterograde and retrograde cellular damage. Central cholinergic neurons seem to be particularly vulnerable to losses of target sites and terminal networks. It might be speculated that such vulnerability is responsible for the cholinergic involvement in disease states affecting the hippocampus and cerebral cortex, such as in Alzheimer's disease (Appel, 1981; Hefti, 1983). It is therefore of importance that in experimental animals the retrograde degenerative changes can be partly reversed with the timely administration of β-NGF. Whether these observations are applicable to clinical states (e.g. Alzheimer's disease) is far from clear. In an optimistic scenario, it could be hoped that trophic factor therapy might salvage forebrain cholinergic neurons destined to degenerate or die. Such an effect should prevent further deterioration of higher functions which may depend on the integrity of the CNS cholinergic system (Bartus et al., 1982). However, factor therapy would probably not correct the primary cause of the disease. Furthermore, the application of trophic substances might also elicit undesirable sprouting of responding neurons, as has already been speculated (Geddes et al., 1985; Butcher and Woolf, 1989).

In our experiments it has been of interest to note that the application of gangliosides and nerve growth factor might show some parallels. However, much larger doses of glycosphingolipids are required to obtain similar results and the protective effects of exogenous gangliosides on cholinergic neurons in lesioned rats are absent in aged rats (Stephens et al., 1987). This could be explained by the fact that aging is accompanied by an apparent loss of β-NGF receptors (Koh and Loy, 1988), and a diminished production of endogenous factors after injury (Whittemore and Seiger, 1987). Further experimentation on the responsiveness of cholinergic and non-cholinergic neurons to trophic substances should provide a firmer framework to consider the potential values of these agents in the therapeutics of the injured, aged or diseased brain.

Acknowledgements

The authors would like to acknowledge support from the Medical Research Council of Canada, the office of the Dean, Faculty of Medicine (McGill University) and partial assistance from FIDIA Research Laboratories. The editorial and secretarial assistance of Diane Leggett and Mary Babineau, as well as the technical expertise of Alan Forster, is gratefully appreciated. Lorella Garofalo is the recipient of a studentship provided by Fonds de la Recherche Scientifique (Quebec).

References

Agnati, L.F., Fuxe, K., Calza, L., Benfenati, F., Cavicchioli, L., Toffano, G. and Goldstein, M. (1983) Gangliosides increase the survival of lesioned nigral dopamine neurons and favour the recovery of dopaminergic synaptic function in striatum of rats by collateral sprouting. *Acta Phys. Scand.,* 119: 374–363.

Appel, S.H. (1981) A unifying hypothesis for the cause of amyotrophic lateral sclerosis, Parkinsonism, and Alzheimer's disease. *Ann. Neurol.,* 10: 499–505.

Bartus, R.T., Dean, R.L.III, Beer, B., Lippa, A.S. (1982) The cholinergic hypothesis of geriatric memory dysfunction. *Science,* 217: 408–417.

Batchelor, P.E., Armstrong, D.M., Blaker, S.N. and Gage, F.H. (1989) Nerve growth factor receptor and choline acetyltransferase colocalization in neurons within the rat forebrain: response to fimbria-fornix transection. *J. Comp. Neurol.,* 284: 187–204.

Bradford, M.M. (1976) A rapid and sensitive method for the quantitation of microgram quantities of protein using the principle of dye binding. *Anal. Biochem.,* 72: 238–254.

Butcher, L.L. and Woolf, N.J. (1984) Histochemical distribution of acetylcholinesterase in the central nervous system: clues to the localization of cholinergic neurons. In: A. Björklund and T. Hökfelt (Eds.), *Handbook of Chemical Neuroanatomy, (Classical Transmitters and Transmitter Receptors in the CNS, Part II)* Vol. 3, Elsevier, Amsterdam, pp 1–50.

Butcher, L.L. and Woolf, N.J. (1989) Neurotrophic agents exacerbate the pathologic cascade of Alzheimer's disease. *Neurobiol. Aging,* 10: 557–570.

Casamenti, F., Bracco, L., Bartolini, L. and Pepeu, G. (1985). Effects of ganglioside treatment in rats with a lesion of the cholinergic forebrain nuclei. *Brain Res.,* 338: 45–52.

Ceccarelli, B., Aporti, F. and Finesso, M. (1976). Effects of brain gangliosides on functional recovery in experimental regeneration and reinnervation. In G. Porcellati, B. Ceccarelli, and G. Tattamanti (Eds.), *Ganglioside Function,* Plenum Press, New York, pp 275–293.

Chandler, C.E., Parsons, L.M., Hosang, M. and Shooter, E.M. (1984) A monoclonal antibody modulates the interaction of nerve growth factor with PC12 cells. *J. Biol. Chem.,* 259: 6882–6889.

Cheresh, D.A., Pytela, R., Pierschbacher, D., Klier, F.G., Ruoslahti, E. and Reisfeld, R.A. (1987) An Arg-Gly-Asp-directed receptor on the surface of human melanoma cells exists in a divalent cation-dependent functional complex with the disialoganglioside GD2. *J. Cell Biol.,* 105: 1163–1173.

Cremins, J., Wagner, J.A. and Halegouia, S. (1986) Nerve growth factor action is mediated by cyclic AMP and Ca^{+2}/phospholipid dependent protein kinases. *J. Cell. Biol.,* 103: 887–893.

Cuello, A.C. (1989) Glycosphingolipids that can regulate nerve growth and repair. In M.W. Anders, J.T. August, R. Murad and A.S. Nies (Eds.), *Advances in Pharmacology,* in press.

Cuello, A.C. and Sofroniew, M.V. (1984) The anatomy of the CNS cholinergic neurons. *Trends Neurosci.,* 7: 74–78.

Cuello, A.C., Stephens, P.H., Tagari, P.C., Sofroniew, M.V. and Pearson, R.C.A. (1986) Retrograde changes in the nucleus basalis of the rat, caused by cortical damage, are prevented by exogenous ganglioside GM1. *Brain Res.,* 376: 373–377.

Cuello, A.C., Maysinger, D., Garofalo, L., Tagari, P., Stephens, P.H., Pioro, E. and Piotte, M. (1987) Influence of gangliosides and nerve growth factor on plasticity of forebrain cholinergic neurons. In K. Fuxe and L.F. Agnati (Eds.), *Receptor-receptor Interactions 1987,* McMillan Press, London, pp 62–77.

Cuello, A.C., Garofalo, L., Kenigsberg, R.L. and Maysinger, D. (1989) Gangliosides potentiate in vivo and in vitro effects of nerve growth factor on central cholinergic neurons. *Proc. Natl. Acad. Sci. USA,* 86: 2056–2060.

Dawbarn, D., Allen, S.J. and Semenenko, F.M. (1988) Coexistence of choline acetyltransferase and nerve growth factor receptors in the rat basal forebrain. *Neurosci. Lett.,* 94: 138–144.

Di Patre, P.L., Casamenti, F., Cenni, A. and Pepeu, G. (1989) Interaction between nerve growth factor and GM1 monosialoganglioside in preventing cortical choline acetyl transferase and high affinity choline uptake decrease after lesion of the nucleus basalis. *Brain Res.,* 480: 219–224.

Doherty, P., Dickson, J.G., Flanigan, T.P. and Walsh, F.S. (1985) Ganglioside GM1 does not initiate but enhances neurite regeneration of nerve growth factor-dependent sensory neurones. *J. Neurochem.,* 44: 1259–1265.

Elliott, P.J., Garofalo, L. and Cuello, A.C. (1989) Limited neocortical devascularizing lesions causing deficits in memory retention and choline acetyltransferase activity — effects of the monosialoganglioside GM1. *Neuroscience,* 31: 63–76.

Ferrari, G., Fabris, M. and Gorio, A. (1983) Gangliosides enhance neurite outgrowth in PC12 cells. *Dev. Brain Res.,* 8: 215–22.

Fibiger, H.C. (1982) The organization and some projections of cholinergic neurons of the mammalian forebrain. *Brain Res. Rev.,* 4: 327–388.

Florian, A., Casamenti, F. and Pepeu, G. (1987) Recovery of cortical acetylcholine output after ganglioside treatment in rats with lesion of the nucleus basalis. *Neurosci. Lett.,* 75: 313–316.

Fonnum, F. (1975) A rapid radiochemical method for the determination of choline acetyltransferase. *J. Neurochem.,* 24 :407–409.

Gage, F.H., Batchelor, P., Chen, K.S., Chin, D., Higgins, G.A., Koh, S., Deputy, S., Rosenberg, M.B., Fischer, W. and Björklund, A. (1989) NGF receptor reexpression and NGF-mediated cholinergic neuronal hypertrophy in the damaged adult neostriatum. *Neuron,* 2: 1177–1184.

Geddes, J.W., Monaghan, D.T., Cotman, C.W., Lott, I.T., Kim, R.C. and Chin, H.C. (1985) Plasticity of hippocampal circuitry in Alzheimer's disease. *Science,* 230: 1179–81.

Gomez-Pinilla, F., Cotman, C.W. and Nieto-Sampedro, M. (1987) NGF receptor immunoreactivity in rat brain: topographical distribution and response to entorhinal ablation. *Neurosci. Lett.,* 82: 260–266.

Gradkowska, M., Skup, M., Kiedrowski, L., Clzolari, S. and Oderfeld-Nowak, B. (1986) The effect of GM1 ganglioside on cholinergic and serotoninergic system in the rat hippocampus following partial denervation is dependent on the degree of fiber degeneration. *Brain Res.,* 375: 417–422.

Green, S.H. and Greene, L.A. (1986) A single Mr = 103,000 ^{125}I-beta-nerve growth factor-affinity-labeled species represents both the low and high affinity forms of the nerve growth factor receptor. *J. Biol. Chem.,* 261: 15316–15326.

Greenberg, M.E., Greene, L.A., and Ziff, E.B. (1985) Nerve growth factor and epidermal growth factor induce rapid transient changes in proto-oncogene transcription in PC12 cells. *J. Biol. Chem.,* 260: 14101–14110.

Hama, T., Huang, d.-P. and Guroff, G. (1986) Protein kinase C as a component of a nerve growth factor sensitive phosphorylation system in PC12 cells. *Proc. Natl. Acad. Sci. USA,* 83: 2352–2357.

Haroutunian, V., Kanof, P. and Davis, K. (1986) Partial reversal of lesion-induced deficits in cortical cholinergic markers by nerve growth factor. *Brain Res.,* 386: 397–399.

Hartikka, J. and Hefti, F. (1988) Development of septal cholinergic neurons in culture: plating density and glial cells modulate effects of NGF on survival, fiber growth, and expression of transmitter-specific enzymes. *J. Neurosci.,* 8: 2967–2985.

Hatanaka, H. and Tsukui, H. (1986) Differential effects of nerve-growth factor and glioma-conditioned medium on neurons cultured from various regions of fetal rat central nervous system. *Dev. Brain Res.,* 30: 47–56.

Hatanaka, H., Tsukui, H. and Nihonmatsu, I. (1988) Developmental change in the nerve growth factor action from induction of choline acetyltransferase to promotion of cell survival in cultured basal forebrain cholinergic neurons from postnatal rats. *Dev. Brain Res.,* 39: 85–95.

Hefti, F. (1983) Is Alzheimer's disease caused by a lack of nerve growth factor? *Ann. Neurol.,* 13: 109–110.

Hefti, F. (1986) Nerve growth factor promotes survival of septal cholinergic neurons after fimbrial transections. *J. Neurosci.,* 6: 2155–2162.

Hefti, F., Dravid, A. and Hartikka, J. (1984) Chronic intraventricular injections of nerve growth factor elevate hippocampal choline acetyltransferase activity in adult rats with partial septo-hippocampal lesions. *Brain Res.*, 293: 305–311.

Hefti, F., Hartikka, J., Eckenstein, F., Gnahn, H., Heumann, R. and Schwab, M.E. (1985) Nerve growth factor increases choline acetyltransferase but not survival or fibre outgrowth of cultured foetal septal cholinergic neurones. *Neuroscience*, 14: 55–68.

Hempstead, B.L., Schleifer, L.S. and Chao, M.V. (1989) Expression of functional nerve growth factor receptors after gene transfer. *Science*, 243: 373–375.

Hosang, M. and Shooter, E.M. (1987) The internalization of nerve growth factor by high affinity receptors on pheochromocytoma PC12 cells. *EMBO J.*, 6: 1197–1202.

Katoh-Semba, R., Skaper, S.D. and Varon, S. (1984) Interaction of GM1 ganglioside with PC12 pheochromocytoma cells: serum and NGF-dependent effects on neuritic growth (and proliferation). *J. Neuroscience*, 12: 299–310.

Kiss, J., McGovern, J. and Patel, A.J. (1988) Immunohistochemical localization of cells containing nerve growth factor receptors in the different regions of the adult rat forebrain. *Neuroscience*, 27: 731–748.

Koh, S. and Loy, R. (1988) Age-related loss of nerve growth factor sensitivity in rat basal forebrain neurons. *Brain Res.*, 440: 396–401.

Kordower, J.H., Bothwell, M.A., Schattemann, G. and Gash, D.M. (1988) Nerve growth factor receptor immunoreactivity in the nonhuman primate (*Cebus apella*): distribution, morphology and localization with cholinergic enzymes. *J. Comp. Neurol.*, 277: 465–486.

Kromer, L. (1987) Nerve growth factor treatment after brain injury prevents neuronal death. *Science*, 235: 214–216.

Kruijer, W., Schubert, D. and Verma, I. (1985) Induction of the proto-oncogene *fos* by nerve growth factor. *Proc. Natl. Acad. Sci. USA*, 82: 7330–7334.

Ledeen, R. (1985) Gangliosides of the neuron. *Trends Neurosci.*, 8(4): 169–174.

Leon, A., Benvegnu, D., Daltoso, L., Presti D., Facci L., Giorgi D. and Toffano, G. (1984) Dorsal root ganglia and nerve growth factor: a model for understanding the mechanisms of GM1 effect on neuronal repair. *J. Neurosci. Res.*, 12: 277–288.

Leonard, D.G.B., Ziff, E.B. and Green, L.A. (1987) Identification and characterization of mRNAs regulated by nerve growth factor in PC2 cells. *Mol. Cell. Biol.*, 7: 3156–3167.

Maysinger, D., Herrera-Marschitz, M., Carlsson, A., Garofalo, L., Cuello, A.C. and Ungerstedt, U. (1988) Striatal and cortical acetylcholine release in vivo in rats with unilateral decortication: effects of treatment with monosialoganglioside GM1. *Brain Res.*, 461: 355–360.

Maysinger, D., Herrera-Marschitz, M., Ungerstedt, U. and Cuello, A.C. (1989) Acetylcholine release in vivo: effects of chronic treatment with monosialoganglioside GM1. *Neuropharmacology*, in press.

Milbrandt, J. (1986) Nerve growth factor rapidly induces c-*fos*

mRNA in PC12 rat pheochromocytoma cells. *Proc. Natl. Acad. Sci. USA*, 83: 4789–4793.

Mobley, W.C., Rutkowski, J.L., Tennekoon, G.I., Buchanan, K., and Johnston, M.V. (1985) Choline acetyltransferase activity in striatum of neonatal rats increased by nerve growth factor. *Science*, 229: 284–287.

Mobley, W.C., Rutkowski, J.L. Tennekoon, G.I., Gemski, J., Buchanan, K. and Johnston, M.V. (1986) Nerve growth factor increases choline acetyltransferase activity in developing basal forebrain neurons. *Mol. Brain Res.*, 1: 53–62.

Nieto-Sampedro, M., Manthorpe, M., Barbin, G., Varon, S. and Cotman, C.W. (1983) Injury-induced neuronotrophic activity in adult rat brain: correlation with survival of delayed implants in the wound cavity. *J. Neurosci.*, 3: 2219–2229.

Pedata, F., Giovanelli, L., Pepeu, G. (1984) GM1 ganglioside facilitates the recovery of high affinity choline uptake in the cerebral cortex of rats with a lesion of the nucleus basalis magnocellularis. *J. Neurosci. Res.*, 12: 421–427.

Pioro, E.P. and Cuello, A.C. (1990a) Distribution of nerve growth factor receptor immunoreactivity in the adult rat central nervous system. Effect of colchicine and correlation with the cholinergic system. I. Forebrain. *Neuroscience*, 34: 57–87.

Pioro, E.P. and Cuello, A.C. (1990b) Distribution of nerve growth factor receptor immunoreactivity in the adult rat central nervous system. Effect of colchicine and correlation with the cholinergic system. II. Brainstem, cerebellum and spinal cord. *Neuroscience*, 34: 89–110.

Raivich, G. and Kreutzberg, G.W. (1987) The localization and distribution of high affinity beta-nerve growth factor binding sites in the central nervous system of the adult rat. A light microscopic autoradiographic study using [^{125}I]beta-nerve growth factor. *Neuroscience*, 20: 23–36.

Richardson, P.M., Verge, V.M.K. and Riopelle, R.J. (1986) Distribution of neuronal receptors for nerve growth factor in the rat. *J. Neurosci.*, 6: 2312–2321.

Riopelle, R.J., Richardson, P.M. and Verge, V.M.K. (1988) Distribution and characteristics of nerve growth factor binding on cholinergic neurons of rat and monkey forebrain. *Neurosci. Lett.*, 94: 138–144.

Ross, A.H., Grob, M., Bothwell, M., Elder, D.E., Ernst, C.S., Marano, N., Ghrist, B.F.D., Slemp, C.C., Herlyn, M., Atkinson, B. and Koprowski, H. (1984) Characterization of nerve growth factor receptor in neural crest tumors using monoclonal antibodies. *Proc. Natl. Acad. Sci. USA*, 81: 6681–6685.

Schatteman, G.C., Gibbs, L., Lanahan, A.A., Claude, P. and Bothwell, M. (1988) Expression of NGF receptor in the developing and adult primate central nervous system. *J. Neurosci.*, 8: 860–873.

Schwab, M.E., Otten, U., Agid, Y. and Thoenen, H. (1979) Nerve growth factor (NGF) in the rats CNS: absence of specific retrograde axonal transport and tyrosine hydroxylase induction in the locus coeruleus and substantia nigra. *Brain Res.*, 168: 473–483.

Schwartz, M. and Spirman, N. (1982) Sprouting from chicken

embryo dorsal root ganglia induced by nerve growth factor is specifically inhibited by affinity purified antiganglioside antibodies. *Proc. Natl. Acad. Sci. USA,* 79: 6080–6083.

Simon, J.R., Atweh S., and Kuhar, M.J. (1976) Sodium dependent high affinity choline uptake: a regulatory step in the synthesis of acetylcholine. *J. Neurochem.,* 26: 909–922.

Skaper, S.D., Katoh-Semba, R. and Varon, S. (1985) GM1 ganglioside accelerates neurite outgrowth from primary peripheral and central neurons under selective culture conditions. *Dev. Brain Res.,* 23: 19–26.

Sofroniew, M.V., Pearson, R.C.A., Eckenstein, F., Cuello, A.C. and Powell, T.P.S. (1983) Retrograde changes in cholinergic neurons in the basal forebrain of the rat following cortical damage. *Brain Res.,* 289: 370–374.

Sofroniew, M.V., Pearson, R.C.A., Cuello, A.C., Tagari, P.C. and Stephens, P.H. (1986) Parenterally administered GM1 ganglioside prevents retrograde degeneration of cholinergic cells of the rat basal forebrain. *Brain Res.,* 398: 393–396.

Springer, J.E., Koh, S., Tayrien, M.W. and Loy R. (1987) Basal forebrain magnocellular neurons stain for nerve growth factor receptor: Correlation with cholinergic cell bodies and effects of axotomy. *J. Neurosci. Res.,* 17: 111–118.

Stephens, P.H., Cuello, A.C., Sofroniew, M.V., Pearson, R.C.A. and Tagari, P. (1985) The effects of unilateral decortication upon choline acetyltransferase and glutamate decarboxylase activities in the nucleus basalis and other areas of the rat brain. *J. Neurochem.,* 45: 1021–1026.

Stephens, P.H., Tagari, P.C., Garofalo, L., Maysinger, D., Piotte, M. and Cuello, A.C. (1987) Neural plasticity of basal forebrain cholinergic neurons: effects of gangliosides. *Neurosci. Lett.,* 80: 80–84.

Thoenen, H., Bandtlow, C. and Heumann, R. (1987) The physiological function of nerve growth factor in the central nervous system: comparsion with the periphery. *Rev. Physiol. Biochem. Pharmacol.,* 109: 145–178.

Toffano, G., Benvegnu, A., Bonetti, A., Facci, L., Leon, A., Orlando, F., Ghidoni, R. and Tettamanti, G. (1980) Inter-action of GM1 ganglioside with crude rat brain neuronal membranes. *J. Neurochem.,* 35: 861–866.

Toffano, G., Savoini, G., Moroni, F., Lombardi, G., Calza, L. and Agnati, L.F. (1983) GM1 ganglioside stimulates the regeneration of dopaminergic neurons in the cetral nervous system. *Brain Res.,* 261: 163–166.

Vantini, G., Fusco, M., Bigon, E. and Leon, A. (1988) GM1 ganglioside potentiates the effect of nerve growth factor in preventing vinblastine induced sympathectomy in new born rats. *Brain Res.,* 448: 252–258.

Varon, S., Manthorpe, M., Davis, G.E., Williams, L.R. and Skaper, S.D. (1988) Growth Factors. In S.G. Waxman (Ed.), *Advances in Neurology, Vol. 47: Functional Recovery in Neurological Disease 1988,* Raven Press, New York, pp 493–521.

Whitehouse P.J., Price D.L., Struble R.G., Clark A.W., Coyle J.T. and DeLong, M.R. (1982) Alzheimer's disease and senile dementia: loss of neurons in the basal forebrain. *Science,* 215: 1237–1239.

Whittemore, S.R. and Seiger, A. (1987) The expression, localization and functional significance of β nerve growth factor in the central nervous system. *Brain Res. Rev.,* 12: 439–464.

Williams, L., Varon, S., Peterson, G., Wictorin, K., Fischer, W., Björklund, A. and Gage, F. (1986) Continuous infusion of nerve growth factor prevents basal forebrain neuronal death after timbria fornix transection. *Proc. Natl. Acad. Sci. USA,* 83: 9231–9235.

Wojcik, M., Ulas, J. and Oderfeld-Nowak, B. (1982) The stimulating effect of ganglioside injections on the recovery of choline acetyltranserase and acetylcholinesterase activities in the hippocampus of the rat after septal lesions. *Neuroscience,* 7: 495–499.

Woolf, N.J., Gould, E. and Butcher, L.L. (1989) Nerve growth factor is associated with cholinergic neurons of the basal forebrain but not the pontomesencephalon. *Neuroscience,* 30: 143–152.

S.-M. Aquilonius and P.-G. Gillberg (Eds.)
Progress in Brain Research, Vol. 84
© 1990 Elsevier Science Publishers B.V. (Biomedical Division)

CHAPTER 33

New approaches to clinical and postmortem investigations of cholinergic mechanisms

Agneta Nordberg [1,6], Abdu Adem [1,6], Lena Nilsson-Håkansson [1], Gösta Bucht [4],
Per Hartvig [3], Irina Alafuzoff [5], Matti Viitanen [6], Bengt Långström [2]
and Bengt Winblad [6]

Departments of [1]Pharmacology and [2]Organic Chemistry, Uppsala University, [3]Hospital Pharmacy, University Hospital, Uppsala, [4]Department of Geriatric Medicine, Umeå University, and [5]Departments of Pathology and [6]Geriatric Medicine, Karolinska Institute, Stockholm, Sweden

Introduction

In contrast to the catecholaminergic systems (dopaminergic, noradrenergic serotonergic) where peripheral and central (CSF) markers have contributed to important knowledge about the pathophysiology and treatment of neurological and psychiatric diseases less is known about the cholinergic system in man. Clinical research on cholinergic mechanisms in the CNS of man have, thus, been hampered by the lack of appropriate methods and markers. The growing interest in the etiology and treatment of neurogenerative diseases such as Alzheimer's disease, senile dementia of the Alzheimer type (AD/SDAT) and related dementia disorders where the cholinergic system seems to play an important role has stimulated the efforts to find new research tools and approaches in clinical cholinergic research.

The different tissues and techniques used for cholinergic research in man are illustrated in Fig. 1. Data for the cholinergic system in human brain have mainly been obtained from neurochemical studies in autopsy brains but occasionally also from biopsied brains. The analysis has mostly been restricted to measurement of enzyme activities (acetylcholinesterase, choline acetyltransferase) and cholinergic receptor densities. Acetylcholine (ACh) is a labile compound which is difficult to measure since it is easily hydrolysed postmortem. New techniques using labelled isotopes will now enable us to measure in autopsy brain tissue dynamic, functional mechanisms such as regulations of transmitter activity (ACh synthesis/release) and second messenger response (Candy et al., 1984; Ohm et al., 1990). Positron emission tomography (PET) is a new technique for in vivo studies of central cholinergic activity in human brain. Some attempts to study cholinergic receptors have already been made. Great interest

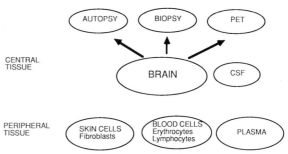

Fig. 1. Neural and nonneural tissue and techniques used in studies on cholinergic activity in man.

Correspondence to: Agneta Nordberg, MD. PhD., Department of Pharmacology, Box 591, S-751 24 Uppsala, Sweden.

has also been taken in whether nonneural peripheral elements such as plasma, blood cells, skin
cells (fibroblasts) can be used as model systems
for cholinergic transmission and activity. The advantage with these model systems is that they can
easily be obtained from patients and allow repeated measurements.

The aim of this chapter is to illustrate some
new clinical and post-mortem techniques and show
how they can be used in the study of cholinergic
mechanisms in man in normal and pathological
states.

Peripheral markers of cholinergic activity in man

The presence of acetylcholinesterase, cholinesterase, choline and cholinergic receptors in peripheral nonneural elements has stimulated research to find out whether peripheral tissues might
serve as a model for cholinergic activity in the
brain if a homology exists. In an attempt to use
acetylcholinesterase and cholinesterase as peripheral markers for cholinergic activity in dementia
diseases the outcome has been disappointing since
conflicting findings have been reported (Smith et
al., 1982; Chipperfield et al., 1981; Marquis et al.,
1984). Endogenous choline (Ch) content in plasma
has been measured in several studies. Although
findings are somewhat conflicting an elevated level
of Ch in plasma has been obtained in plasma of
elderly compared to young individuals (Sherman
et al., 1986). An enhanced temperature-dependent
accumulation of Ch has also been observed in red
blood cells from elderly compared to young
volunteers (Glen et al., 1981; Sherman et al., 1986).
Changes in plasma or red cell Ch content have
been investigated in diseases with a cholinergic
deficit such as Alzheimer's disease or in other
various neurological, psychiatric diseases (tardive
dyskinesia, mania, depression): the results have,
however, been conflicting (Blass et al., 1985;
Domino et al., 1985; Sherman et al., 1986).

The research on cholinergic receptors on peripheral blood cells seems more promising. The
presence of cholinergic muscarinic receptors

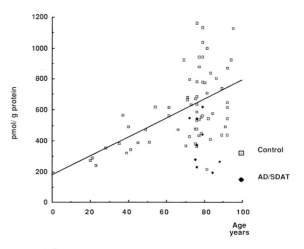

Fig. 2. [^{3}H]Nicotine (7 nM) binding to living lymphocytes
from healthy volunteers of various ages (20–100 years) and
AD/SDAT patients. None of the subjects were smokers.

(Strom et al., 1981; Adem et al., 1986a,b) and
nicotinic receptors (Adem et al., 1986a) has been
demonstrated on intact lymphocytes and lysed
lymphocyte membranes. Muscarinic receptors have
also been demonstrated on blood red cells
(Aronstam et al., 1977). Functional relevance for
the lymphocyte cholinergic receptors has been
claimed, since the muscarinic receptors, for example, can be modulated by GTP proteins (Bering et
al., 1987). The number of nicotinic lymphocyte
receptors increases with age. A significant increase
was seen when the binding of [^{3}H]nicotine was
measured in lymphocytes from healthy volunteers
of various ages (Fig. 2). A similar increase in the
number of muscarinic receptors with age is also
observed (data not shown). The observed changes
might be due to distinct changes of the cholinergic
receptors or a general membrane effect with
changes in e.g. lipid composition and membrane
fluidity.

A decrease in the number of muscarinic and
nicotinic binding sites has been observed in
lymphocytes obtained from patients with the clinical diagnosis of AD/SDAT (Adem et al., 1985,
1986a). [^{3}H]Nicotine binding in a group of institutionalized AD/SDAT patients compared to age-
matched controls is shown in Fig. 2. No signifi-

cant changes in either muscarinic or nicotinic receptors have been observed in lymphocytes from patients with multi-infarct dementia (MID) (Adem et al., 1986a). In lymphocytes from patients with Parkinson's disease the nicotinic but not the muscarinic binding sites were reduced (Adem et al., 1986a). Concerning the muscarinic receptors present observations have recently been confirmed by other groups (Rabey et al., 1986; Ravizza et al., 1988). We are now in a longitudinal study investigating a large population of both institutionalized and non-institutionalized AD/SDAT patients. Receptor changes are monitored and correlated with the severity and progression of the disease. The possibility that lymphocyte choliner-

gic receptors may act as an antemortem marker in dementia disorders and other forms of degenerative dieseases deserves further exploration.

Cholinergic mechanisms in human brain as studied by positron emission tomography (PET)

Positron emission tomography (PET) is a non-invasive in vivo imaging technique that gives cross-sectional images of the tissue radioactivity in brain following administration of short-lived positron-emitting radionuclides such as ^{18}F or ^{11}C to experimental animals or humans. The method has already been shown to have a great potential for psychopharmacological research. In order to study

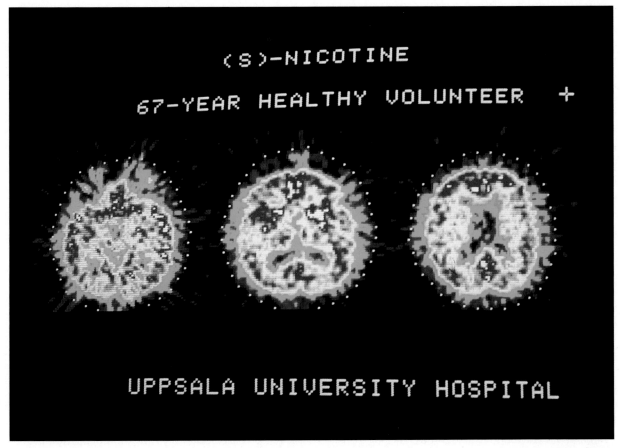

Fig. 3. Three positron emission tomography (PET) sections through the superiour cortical regions (right), the basal ganglia (middle) and the inferiour cortical regions, cerebellum (left) of the brain of a 67-year-old healthy volunteer receiving a tracer dose of $(-)(S)[^{11}C]$nicotine intravenously. The color scale indicates ^{11}C-radioactivity nCi/cm^3/dose × bw^{-1} during 30 min following intravenous injection: Red = high; Yellow = medium; Blue = low activity.

the cholinergic system in human brain in vivo PET studies using [¹¹C]choline ([¹¹C]Ch) were performed by Gauthier et al. (1985). Eckernäs et al. (1985) also studied the uptake of [¹¹C]Ch to monkey brain. The use of [¹¹C]Ch as radiolabelled marker for cholinergic activity in brain has, however, some disadvantages. A very small proportion of the [¹¹C]Ch compund is taken up by the brain following intravenous injection and Ch is metabolized not only to ACh but also to phosphorylcholine and betaine. Attempts have therefore been made to visualize muscarinic receptors in brain (Eckelmann et al., 1984; Holman et al., 1985). By using ¹²³I-3-quinuclidinyl-4-iodobenzilate and single photon emission tomography (SPECT) Holman et al., (1985) observed a relative preservation of the muscarinic binding sites in brain of an Alzheimer patient compared to a healthy age-matched control. Recently attempts have been made to measure nicotinic cholinergic receptors with [¹¹C]nicotine and the PET technique in monkey (Nordberg et al., 1989a) and human brains (Nybäck et al., 1989; Nordberg et al., 1990). When a tracer dose of (−)(S)[¹¹C]nicotine is injected intravenously to a human subject it quickly disappears from the arterial blood and the radioactivity is rapidly taken up and distributed to various parts of the brain, and peaks in brain within 5 min and then declines in 15–20 min. The regional distribution of (−)(S)[¹¹C]nicotine-derived radioactivity in the brain of a 67-year-old healthy volunteer is shown in Fig. 3. The uptake of ¹¹C-radioactivity is high in brain areas such as the thalamus, caudate nucleus, insula cortex, putamen, frontal cortex, temporal cortex and intermediate in the occipital cortex, cerebellum and low in white matter and the ventricles (Fig. 3). The regional distribution of [¹¹C]nicotine shows great similarities with results obtained from in vitro mapping of nicotinic receptors in human brain (Adem and Nordberg, 1988; Adem et al., 1988, 1989; Nordberg et al., 1988b).

Postmortem studies of AD/SDAT brains have revealed a deficit in the number of cortical nicotinic receptors (Nordberg and Winblad, 1986;

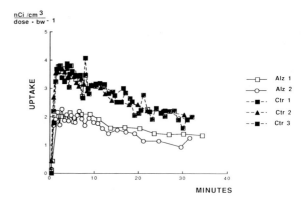

Fig. 4. Uptake and time course of ¹¹C-radioactivity in the temporal cortex following intravenous injection of (+)(R) [¹¹C]nicotine to two Alzheimer patients (age 63 and 65 years, duration of the disease 9 and 7 years respectively) and three age-matched controls.

Whitehouse et al., 1986). Furthermore a change in the proportion of high affinity to low affinity binding sites has been observed (Nordberg et al., 1988a). In order to visualize these receptor changes in vivo the (+)(R) and the (−)(S) isomer of [¹¹C]nicotine have been given to Alzheimer patients and age-matched controls. A lower uptake of both isomers was observed, especially the (+)(R) isomer in cortical areas in Alzheimer patients as compared to age-matched controls (Fig. 4). Studies using [¹¹C]butanol as a flow marker indicate that the difference in uptake of [¹¹C]nicotine between controls and Alzheimer patients might not solely be due to a difference in blood flow but probably also to differences in receptor density. Studies are now in progress to further clarify the significance of the underlying mechanisms for the difference in uptake of the [¹¹C]nicotine isomers by Alzheimer and control brains.

An increased number of nicotinic receptors has recently been reported in postmortem brains of smokers (Benwell et al., 1988). Animals that are exposed to repeated injections of nicotine also develop a tolerance and an enhanced number of nicotinic receptors in brain (Schwartz and Kellar, 1983; Larsson et al., 1986); especially of the high-affinity type (Romanelli et al., 1988). Smokers receiving an intravenous tracer dose of [^{11}C]nicotine show by PET a higher brain uptake of the radiolabelled compound than the nonsmokers (Nybäck et al., 1989). The uptake of $(-)(S)$ [^{11}C]nicotine was especially higher in smokers as compared to nonsmokers (Nybäck et al., 1989) The observation might indicate an enhanced density of high-affinity (desensititized?) nicotinic binding sites in smokers. The studies are encouraging for further research in understanding the underlying mechanisms for tobacco dependence.

Studies of functional cholinergic activity in post-mortem brain tissue

Neurotransmitter levels, neurotransmitter-related enzyme activities and radioligand binding densities were until recently the only measurable parameters in autopsy brain tissue. Metabolically and functional active preparations can now be obtained from human brain after considerable postmortem delays. By freezing the tissue slowly in an isotonic solution of sucrose, storing it at $-70°C$ and then on the experimental day rapidly thawing, metabolic active preparations can be prepared (Hardy and Dodd, 1983). The agonal state of the tissue is of utmost importance. If the subject has died suddenly viable preparations can be prepared from control brains up to 24 h post-

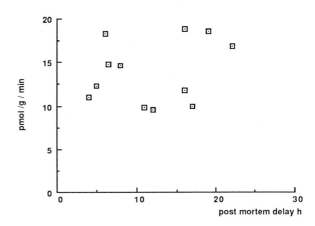

Fig. 6. Correlation between postmortem delay (hours) and [^{3}H]ACh release in human cortical tissue (pmol/g wet tissue/min). Each point represents data from one individual.

mortem. If the death has been slow, as often is the case in dementia diseases, the tissue respiration declines faster postmortem (Wester et al., 1985).

In order to study functional cholinergic activity in autopsy brain tissue an in vitro method has been developed (Nilsson et al., 1986). Methods for studies of the in vitro Ch uptake (Rylett et al., 1983) in postmortem brain tissue and ACh synthesis in microprisms of brain biopsies (Sim et al., 1980) have been described. To develop a technique where the regulation of ACh release and the influence of potential drugs could be studied in postmortem brain tissue would be preferable since neurosurgery seldom is carried out in the demented patients for example. A schematical description of the method is outlined in Fig. 5. Thin brain slices (0.4 mm thick) are prepared under oxygenation, incubated with labelled Ch ([^{3}H]Ch) at high (35 mM) and low (5 mM) potassium concentration and a calcium-dependent potassium evoked release of labelled ACh ([^{3}H]ACh) is measured (Nilsson et al., 1986). The ACh release in the tissue slices is stable for at least 60 min. No significant difference in the potassium evoked [^{3}H]ACh release from human frontal cortex has been observed when the postmortem delay was varied between 4 and 22 h (Fig. 6). A significant

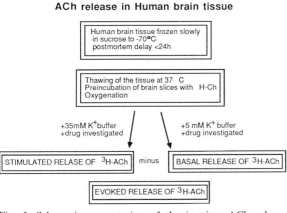

Fig. 5. Schematic presentation of the in vitro ACh release method using post-mortem brain tissue.

decrease in [^{3}H]ACh release with age has been noticed (data not shown). The potassium-evoked in vitro release of ACh positively correlates with the number of nicotinic and muscarinic receptors when measured in the same tissue sample (Nordberg et al., 1987; Nordberg and Nilsson, 1990). The advantage of this in vitro release technique is that the influence of drugs on dynamic transmitter events can be studied. The muscarinic receptor antagonist atropine significantly enhances the in vitro release of ACh in human cortical tissue (Nordberg et al., 1988c), while indirect muscarinic agonists such as the cholinesterase inhibitors physostigmine and tetrahydroaminoacridine (THA) decrease the release of ACh (Nilsson et al., 1986, 1987). The finding illustrates the fact that the feedback mechanisms via presynaptic muscarinic receptors are present and active in these autopsy brain tissue preparations.

The potassium-evoked release of ACh is markedly decreased in AD/SDAT cortical tissue as compared to tissue from control subjects (Nilsson et al., 1986). A decrease in the evoked release of ACh has also been observed in MID brains (Nordberg et al., 1989b). Opposite to control tissue, physostigmine and THA in AD/SDAT cortical tissue facilitate the ACh release and restore it to control level (Nilsson et al., 1986, 1987) (Fig.

7). This observation must be considered of potential interest since various cholinesterase inhibitors including physostigmine and THA are at present under clinical trial in AD/SDAT patients. In order to further evaluate the mechanism by which cholinesterase inhibitors facilitate the release of ACh in AD/SDAT cortical tissue, different nicotinic and muscarinic antagonists have been added to the testsystem. Nicotinic antagonists such as dihydro-β-erythroidine (DHBE) partially and mecamylamine fully counteract the effect of THA on ACh release in AD/SDAT tissue while they have no effect on the control tissue (Nordberg et al., 1988b, 1989c). Atropine fully antagonizes the facilatory effect of THA in AD/SDAT tissue (Nordberg et al., 1988b). The mechanism of THA in AD/SDAT tissue might thus directly or indirectly be mediated via both muscarinic and nicotinic receptors. Since the nicotinic receptor properties are changed in AD/SDAT brains (Nordberg et al., 1988a) an enhanced release of ACh via presynaptic active nicotinic receptors can not be excluded. These investigations illustrate the importance of using brain tissue obtained at autopsy from patients when developing new potential drugs against the diseases. It must be considered of the utmost importance for diseases such as AD/SDAT where an animal model does not exist.

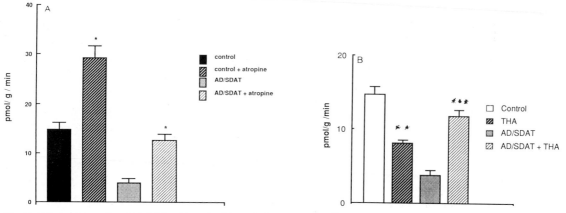

Fig. 7. Effect of atropine (10^{-5} M) (A) and THA (10^{-4} M) (B) on [^{3}H]ACh release in control and AD/SDAT cortical tissue. $*p < 0.05$; $**p < 0.01$; $***p < 0.001$.

Acknowledgements

The financial support of the Swedish Medical Research Council, The Swedish Tobacco Company, Loo and Hans Osterman's fund, and Stohne's fund is highly acknowledged.

References

Adem, A. and Nordberg, A. (1988) Nicotinic cholinergic receptor heterogeneity in mammalian brain. In M.J. Rand and K. Thurau (Eds.), *The Pharmacology of Nicotine*, IRL Press, Oxford, pp. 227–247.

Adem, A. Nordberg, A., Bucht, G. and Winblad, B. (1985) Comparison of nicotinic and muscarinic binding sites in lymphocytes from Alzheimer patients and age-matched controls. *Acta Physiol. Scand.*, 124, suppl. 542, 234.

Adem, A., Nordberg, A. Bucht, G. and Winblad, B. (1986a) Extraneural cholinergic markers in Alzheimer's and Parkinson's disease. *Prog. Neuro-Psychopharmacol. Biol Psychiat.*, 10: 247–257.

Adem, A., Nordberg, A. and Slanina, P. (1986b) A muscarinic receptor type in human lymphocytes: A comparison of ^{3}H-QNB binding to intact lymphocytes and lysed lymphocyte membranes. *Life Sci.*, 38: 1359–1368.

Adem, A., Sing Jossan, S., Brandt, I., Winblad, B. and Nordberg, A. (1988) Distribution of nicotinic receptors in human thalamus as visualized by ^{3}H-nicotine and ^{3}H-acetylcholine receptor autoradiography. *J. Neural Transm.*, 73: 77–83.

Adem, A., Nordberg, A., Jossan, S.S., Sara, V. and Gillberg, P.G. (1989) Quantitative autoradiography of nicotinic receptors in large cryosections of human brain hemispheres. *Neurosci. Lett.*, 101: 247–252.

Aronstam, R.S., Abood, L.G. and MacNeil, M.K. (1977) Muscarinic cholinergic binding in human erythrocyte membranes. *Life Sci.*, 20: 1175–1180.

Benwell, M.E.M., Balfour, D.J.K. and Anderson, J.M. (1988) Evidence that tobacco smoking increase the density of $(-)$-^{3}H-nicotine binding sites in human brain. *J. Neurochem.*, 50: 1243–1247.

Bering, B., Moises, H.W. and Muller, W.E. (1987) Muscarinic cholinergic receptors on intact human lymphocytes-properties and subclass characterization. *Biol. Psychiatry* 22: 1451–1458.

Blass, J.P., Hanin, I., Barclay, L., Kopp, U. and Reding, M.J. (1985) Elevated red cell to plasma choline ratios in Alzheimer's disease. In I. Hanin (Ed.) *Dynamic of Cholinergic Function, Advances in Behavioral Biology*, vol. 30, Plenum Press, New York, pp. 273–282.

Candy, J.M. Court, J.A., Perry, R.H. and Smith, C.J. (1984) Carbachol-stimulated phosphatidyl inositol hydrolysis in the cerebral cortex after freezing and postmortem delay. *Br. J. Pharmacol.*, 83: 356P.

Chipperfield, B., Newman, P.M. and Moyes, I.C.A. (1981) Decreased erythrocyte cholinesterase activity in dementia. *Lancet* ii: 199.

Dodd, P.R., Hambley, J.W., Cowburn, R.F. and Hardy, J. (1988) A comparison of methodologies for the study of functional transmitter neurochemistry in human brain. *J. Neurochem.*, 50: 1333–1345.

Domino, E.F., Mathews, B. and Tait, S. (1985) Plasma and red blood cell choline in aging: rat, monkey and man. In I. Hanin (Ed.) *Dynamics of Cholinergic Function, Advances in Behavioral Biology*, vol.30, Plenum Press, New York, pp. 283–290.

Eckelmann, W.E., Reba, R.C., Rzeszotarski, W.J. et al. (1984) External imaging of cerebral muscarinic acetylcholine receptors, *Science* 223: 291–293.

Eckernäs, S-Å., Aquilonius, S-M., Bergström, K., Hartvig, P., Lilja, A., Lindberg, B., Lundqvist, H., Långström, B., Malmborg, P., Moström, U. and Någren, K. (1985) The use of positron emission tomography for the evaluation of choline metabolism in the brain of the Rhesus monkey. In I. Hanin (Ed.) *Dynamics of Cholinergic Function, Advances in Behavioral Biology*, vol. 30, Plenum Press, New York, pp. 303–311,

Gauthier, S., Diksic, M., Yamamoto, L., Tyler, J. and Feindel, W. (1985) Positron emission tomography with ^{11}C-Choline in human subjects. *Can. J. Neurol. Sci.*, 12:214.

Glen, A.I.M., Yates, C.M., Simpson, J., Christie, J.E., Shering, A., Whalley, L.J. and Jellineh, E.H. (1981) Choline uptake in patients with Alzheimer pre-senile dementia. *Psychol. Med.*, 11:469–476.

Hardy, J. and Dodd, P.R. (1983) Metabolic and functional studies on post-mortem human brain. *Neurochem. Int.*, 5:253–266.

Holman, B.L., Gibson, R.E., Hill, T.C., Eckelman, W.C., Albert, M. and Rebz, R.C. (1985) Muscarinic acetylcholine receptors in Alzheimer's disease. In vivo imaging with iodine ^{123}I-labeled l-quinuclidinyl-4-iodobenzilate and emission tomography. *JAMA* 254:3063–3066.

Larsson, C., Nilsson, L., Hallen, A. and Nordberg, A. (1986) Subchronic treatment of rats with nicotine: effects on tolerance and ^{3}H-acetylcholine and ^{3}H-nicotine binding in the brain. *Alcohol Drug Depend.*, 17: 37–45.

Marquis, J.K., Vollicer, L., Direnfeld, L.K. and Freeman, M. (1984) Assay of cholinesterase in plasma, erythrocytes and cerebrospinal fluid (CSF) of SDAT patients and normal controls. In R.J. Wurtman, S.J. Corkin, J.H. Growdon (Eds) *Alzheimer's Disease: Advances in Basic Research and Therapies*. Springer Verlag, PP. 161–182.

Nilsson, L., Nordberg, A., Hardy, J., Wester, P. and Winblad, B. (1986) Physostigmine restores ^{3}H-acetylcholine efflux from Alzheimer brain slices to normal level. *J. Neural Transm.*, 67: 275–285.

Nilsson, L., Adem, A., Hardy, J., Winblad, B. and Nordberg, A. (1987) Do tetrahydroaminoacridine (THA) and physostigmine restore acetylcholine in AD/SDAT brains via nicotinic receptors? *J. Neural Transm.*, 70: 357–368.

Nordberg, A. and Nilsson-Håkansson, L. (1990) Modulation of cholinergic activity in Alzheimer brains by potential drugs. In W.E. Bunney, H. Hippius, G. Laakmann (Eds.), *Neuro-*

psychopharmacology, Proceedings of the XVI th CINP congress, Springer Verlag, in press.

Nordberg, A. and Winblad, B. (1986) Reduced number of ^{3}H-nicotine and ^{3}H-acetylcholine binding sites in the frontal cortex of Alzheimer brains. *Neurosci. Lett.,* 72: 115–119.

Nordberg, A., Adem, A., Nilsson, L. and Winblad, B. (1987) Cholinergic deficits in the CNS and peripheral non-neuronal tissue in Alzheimer dementia. In M. Dowdall, J. Hawthorne (Eds.), *Cellular and Molecular Basis of Cholinergic Function.* Ellis Horwood, Chichester, UK, pp 858–868.

Nordberg, A., Adem, A., Hardy, J. and Winblad, B. (1988a) Changes in nicotinic receptor subtypes in temporal cortex of Alzheimer brains. *Neurosci. Lett.,* 86:317–321.

Nordberg, A., Adem, A., Nilsson, L. and Winblad, B. (1988b) Nicotinic and muscarinic cholinergic receptor heterogeneity in the human brain at normal aging and dementia of Alzheimer type. In B. Tomlinson, G. Pepeu, C.M. Wischik (Eds.), *New Trends in Aging Research,* Fidia Series vol. 15, Liviana Press, Italy, pp. 27–36.

Nordberg, A., Nilsson, L., Adem, A., Hardy, J. and Winblad, B. (1988c) Effect of THA on acetylcholine release and cholinergic receptors in Alzheimer brains. In E. Giacobini, R. Becker (Eds.), *Current Research in Alzheimer Therapy: Cholinesterase Inhibitors.* Taylor and Francis, New York, pp. 247–257.

Nordberg, A., Hartvig, P., Lundqvist, H., Antoni, G., Ulin, J. and Långström, B. (1989a) Uptake and distribution of $(+)$-(R) and $(-)$ (S)-N-(methyl-^{11}C)-nicotine in the brain of Rhesus monkey-an attempt to, study nicotinic receptors in vivo. *J. Neural Transm.,* (P-D-Sect) 1: 195–205.

Nordberg, A., Nilsson-Håkansson, L., Adem, A., Hardy, J., Alafuzoff, I., Lai, Z., Herrera-Marschitz. M. and Winblad, B. (1989b) The role of nicotinic receptors in the pathophysiology of Alzheimer's disease. In A. Nordberg, K. Fuxe, B. Holmstedt, A. Sundwall (Eds.), *Nicotinic Receptors in the CNS – Their Role in Synaptic Transmission. Prog. Brain Res. vol. 79,* Elsevier, Amsterdam, pp. 353–362.

Nordberg, A., Nilsson. Håkansson, L., Adem, A., Lai, Z. and Winblad, B (1989c) Multiple actions of THA on cholinergic neurotransmission in Alzheimer brains. In H. Iqbal, H. Wiesnewski, B. Winblad (Eds.), *Alzheimer's Disease and Related Disorders.* Allan Liss, New York, pp. 1169–1178.

Nordberg, A., Hartvig, P., Lilja, A., Viitanen, M., Amberla, K., Lundqvist, H., Anderson, J., Nybäck, H., Ulin, J., Anderson, Y., Winblad, B. and Långström, B. (1990) Nicotinic receptors in brain of Alzheimer patients as studied by ^{11}C-nicotine and positron emission tomography (PET). Proceedings of the Vth symposium on the Medical Application of Cyclotrons, *Acta Radiol.,* in press.

Nybäck, H., Nordberg, A., Långström, B., Halldin, C., Hartvig, P., Åhlin, A., Schwan, C.G. and Sedvall, G. (1989) Attempts to visualize nicotinic receptors in the brain of monkey and man by positron emission tomography, In A. Nordberg, K. Fuxe, B. Holmstedt, A. Sundwall (Eds.),

Nicotinic Receptors in the CNS – Their Role in Synaptic Transmission, Prog. Brain Res., vol. 79, Elsevier, Amsterdam, pp. 313–319.

Ohm, T., Bohl, J., Steinmetz, H. and Lemmer, B. (1990) Reduced stimulated cyclase activity in postmortem hippocampus of demented patients. In W.E. Bunney, H. Hippius, G. Laakmann (Eds.), *Neuropsychopharmacology,* Proceedings of the XVIth CINP congress, Springer Verlag, in press.

Rabey, J.M., Shenkman, L. and Gilad, G.M. (1986) Cholinergic muscarinic binding by lymphocytes: changes with age, antagonist treatment and senile dementia. In A. Fisher, I. Hanin, C. Lachman (Eds.), *Alzheimer and Parkinson's Disease: Strategies in Research and Development.* Plenum Press, New York, pp. 345–353.

Ravizza, L., Ferrero, P., Eva, C., Rocca, P., Tarenzi, L. and Benna, P. (1988) Peripheral cholinergic changes and pharmacological aspects in Alzheimer's disease. In E. Giacobini, R. Becker (Eds.), *Current Research in Alzheimer Therapy – Cholinesterase Inhibitors,* Taylor and Francis, New York, pp. 355–363.

Romanelli, L., Öhman, B., Adem, A. and Nordberg, A. (1988) Subchronic treatment of of rats with nicotine: interconversion of nicotinic receptor subtypes in brain. *Eur. J. Pharmacol.,* 148: 289–291.

Rylett, R.J., Bull, M.J. and Colhoun, E.H. (1983) Evidence for high affinity choline transport in synaptosomes prepared from hippocampus and neocortex of patients with Alzheimer's disease. *Brain Res.,* 289: 169–175.

Schwartz, R.D and Kellar, K.J. (1983) Nicotinic cholinergic receptor binding sites in brain: in vivo regulation. *Science* 220: 214–216.

Sherman, K., Gibson, G.E. and Blass, J.P. (1986) Human red blood cells choline uptake with age and Alzheimer's disease. *Neurobiol. Aging* 7: 205–209.

Sim, N.R., Smith, C.C.T., Davison, A.N., Bowen, D.M., Flack, R.H.A. and Snowden, J.S. (1980) Glucose metabolism and acetylcholine synthesis in relation to neuronal activity in Alzheimer's disease. *Lancet* i: 333–336.

Smith, R.C., Ho, B.T., Hsu, L., Vroulis, G., Claghorn, J. and Schoolar, J. (1982) Cholinesterase enzymes in the blood of patients with Alzheimer's disease. *Life Sci.,* 30: 543–546.

Strom, T.B., Lane, M.A. and George, R. (1981) The parallel, time dependent, biomodal change in lymphocyte -mediated cytotoxicity after lymphocyte activation. *J. Immunol.,* 127: 705–710.

Wester, P., Bateman, D.E., Dodd, P.R., Edwardson, J.A., Hardy, J.A., Kidd, A.M., Perry, R.H. and Singh, G.B. (1985) Agonal status affects the metabolic activity of nerve endings isolated from postmortem human brain. *Neurochem. Pathol.,* 3: 169–180.

Whitehouse, P.J., Martino, A.M., Antuono, P.G., Lowenstein, P.R., Coyle, J.T., Price, D.L. and Kellar, K.J. (1986) Nicotinic acetylcholine binding sites in Alzheimer's disease. *Brain Res.,* 371: 146–151.

S.-M. Aquilonius and P.-G. Gillberg (Eds.)
Progress in Brain Research, Vol. 84
© 1990 Elsevier Science Publishers B.V. (Biomedical Division)

CHAPTER 34

The cholinergic system in Alzheimer disease

Ezio Giacobini

Department of Pharmacology, Southern Illinois University, School of Medicine, Springfield, IL 62794-9230, U.S.A.

Introduction

Cholinergic deficits in Alzheimer disease (AD) have been well documented. Choline acetyltransferase (ChAT), the synthetic enzyme for acetylcholine (ACh), is consistently reduced by 50–95% in cortex and hippocampus of AD patients compared to age-matched controls (Bowen et al., 1976; Davies, 1979; Perry et al., 1978; Reisine et al., 1978; Zubenko et al., 1989). Reductions are also observed in high-affinity choline uptake (HACU) (Rylett et al., 1983; Sims et al., 1983), in in vitro synthesis of ACh and release during depolarization (Blessed et al., 1968; Neary et al., 1986b), in presynaptic muscarinic and nicotinic receptor binding (Mash et al., 1985; Whitehouse, 1987; Kellar et al., 1987; Whitehouse et al., 1988; Giacobini et al., 1988a,b, 1989), in ACh and acetylcholinesterase (AChE) levels in cortex (Richter et al., 1980) and in cerebrospinal fluid (CSF) (Johns et al., 1983; Elble et al., 1987, 1989). The reduction of these presynaptic cholinergic markers is associated with a marked loss of cells in the nucleus basalis of Meynert which project to cortex (Whitehouse et al., 1982). By contrast, postsynaptic muscarinic receptor mechanisms appear to be relatively spared in AD patients (London and Coyle, 1978; Reisine

et al., 1978; Davies, 1979; Giacobini et al., 1988a, 1989). The reductions of cortical and CSF cholinergic markers are closely correlated with the extent of neuropathology (senile plaques) and with the severity of cognitive impairment (Bowen et al., 1976; Perry et al., 1978; Fuld et al., 1982; Johns et al., 1983; Francis et al., 1985; Neary et al., 1986a; Elble et al., 1987). We have described changes in ACh and Ch metabolism in aging animals (Giacobini et al., 1987) and in the CSF of AD patients which may be related to neuronal membrane breakdown and reduced uptake of Ch by cholinergic neurons (Elble et al., 1989).

Cortical deafferentation in Alzheimer disease

A diagram of the cholinergic systems most affected in AD is shown in Table I. The forebrain nuclei (mainly the basal nucleus), neocortical re-

Address correspondence to: Ezio Giacobini, M.D., Ph.D., Department of Pharmacology, SIU School of Medicine, P.O. Box 19230, Springfield, IL 62794-9230 USA.

TABLE I

Cholinergic pathology of Alzheimer disease

	Cholinergic representation	
	Neurons	Projections
1. Neocortex (front. par. temp)	+	+ +
2. Hippocampus	−	+ + +
3. Amygdala	−	+ +
4. Ventral striatum	+ +	−
5. Basal forebrain	+ + +	−
6. Locus coeruleus	−	+
7. Raphé	−	+

gions, hippocampus, ventral striatum and amygdala are characteristically affected by the disease.

Cortical deficits in AD patients can be interpreted as reflecting denervation phenomena related to major neurotransmitter systems, mainly cholinergic and noradrenergic. This denervation has been related to the severe reduction in number of neurons in the nucleus basalis and in the locus coeruleus (Whitehouse et al., 1982; Bondareff and Mountjoy, 1986; Zweig et al., 1988).

Cholinergic cortical denervation can be reproduced in the experimental animal. Downen et al. (1989), after applying unilateral ibotenic acid lesions of the basal forebrain in the rat, observed a 75% decrease in cortical ChAT activity and cortical ACh release two weeks after lesion. These changes were partially reversible (after six weeks) and were accompanied by decreases in presynaptic α and κ-bungarotoxin (BTX) binding.

In AD, the degree of cholinergic deafferentation is related to the extent of the cognitive impairment (Perry et al., 1978; Bird et al., 1983; Soininen et al., 1984). Sims et al. (1983) have used neocortical autopsies and biopsies to study presynaptic cholinergic nerve ending function. They showed that ACh synthesis, ChAT activity as well as Ch uptake correlated with the histopathological findings. Other authors studied ^{3}H-ACh release in AD cortical slices of autopsies and its regulation by nicotinic and muscarinic receptors (Nilsson et al., 1987). Receptor changes in AD probably reflect and are secondary to neuronal pathology. An understanding of receptor alterations is particularly important because it may lead to the development of new therapeutic approaches. A better understanding of cholinergic receptor deficits and their relationship to memory and cognitive function might improve our ability to design specific drugs of therapeutic value.

Cortical cholinergic projections: their interaction with the glutamate system

The basal forebrain cholinergic system is made up of a group of large cholinergic neurons which

extends from the medial septum, through the diagonal band of Broca to the nucleus basalis of Meynert (NBM) (Butcher and Woolf, 1986; Mesulam, 1988). The medial septum and the diagonal band provide the primary cholinergic innervation of the hippocampus, while the NBM innervates the cerebral cortex and the amygdaloid complex. Acetylcholine exerts a facilitatory effect on cortical and hippocampal neurons (McCormick and Prince, 1986; Cole and Nicoll, 1984). The modulatory effect of ACh is probably mediated indirectly through glutamate (NMDA) receptors (Metherate et al., 1988). This effect makes the cortical neurons more likely to discharge following excitatory glutamatergic inputs (Metherate et al., 1988). The facilitatory effect is a result of a prolonged decrease in a Ca^{2+}-activated K^+ current producing a change in K^+ conductance and consequently a decrease in after-hyperpolarization (Cole and Nicoll, 1984). Acetylcholine may be able to increase the response of hippocampal and cortical neurons transiently or more persistently. Nicotinic receptors may exist on glutamatergic terminals which may regulate glutamate release. Muscarinic inhibition of glutamate release in rat hippocampus has been demonstrated by Marchi et al. (1989) and the presence of both muscarinic and nicotinic receptors has been demonstrated with EM immunohistochemistry by Schroder et al. (1989) in pyramidal cells in rat and humans. It is, therefore, possible that ACh may play an important role in regulating glutamate release in cortex. These effects of ACh release on selective cortical neurons, due to changes in NBM activity, may be involved in processes of arousal and learning (Richardson and DeLong, 1988). Acetylcholine can also play a role in the long-term change in excitability of somatosensory cortical neurons that occurs following deafferentation (Lamour and Dykes, 1988). Thus, ACh may act as a permissive agent that can bring about enhancement of those neuronal responses, such as glutamate release, which most strongly excite a neuron (Lamour and Dykes, 1988). The association of pathological changes in the NBM and cognitive impairments in animal models in particular is important in order to understand the functional implications of the pathological process of AD. However, the complex situation of multi-transmitter involvement of the disease can be studied only in the human brain. There is a need for relating areas of interaction of cholinergic and non-cholinergic systems in cortex and their combined effect and influence on behavior and symptoms. Studies of nicotinic receptor systems represent a first step in trying to elucidate the role of cholinergic innervation in normal and pathological conditions. It is also important to characterize presynaptic receptor populations which relate to modulation of release mechanism in the cortex.

Changes in nicotinic receptors in Alzheimer disease

In Alzheimer and in other degenerative disease (Gerstmann-Straussler, Parkinson dementia of GUAM type and Dementia pugilistica), pathological and biochemical lesions in the cholinergic neuron are localized mainly to the presynaptic region. Alterations include biochemical and morphological changes in the structures storing, synthesizing and releasing ACh and possibly also in cholinergic receptors regulating ACh release. By comparing cholinergic terminals in the CNS of normally aged with AD patients, it is apparent that muscarinic and nicotinic receptors are not equally affected (Giacobini et al., 1988a, 1989; Zubenko et al., 1989; Rinne et al., 1989).

Surveys, including percent changes in nicotinic receptors in the frontal cortex of AD patients, reveal a striking difference from aging normal controls (Giacobini et al., 1988a, 1989). Nicotinic receptor binding studies are mainly from autopsies using three different ligands (nicotine (NIC), α-BTX and ACh). Out of eight autopsy studies (1981–1988), including one from our laboratory (DeSarno et al., 1988; Fig. 1), six show decreases from 44–65% and two show no difference. Using ^{3}H-QNB as ligand, we found no differences in specific binding in autopsy material but a signifi-

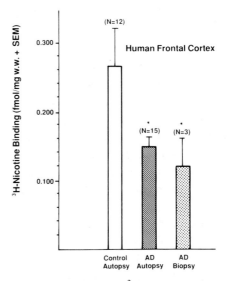

Fig. 1. Comparison of ^{3}H-nicotine binding (fmol/mg w.w. $\pm$ S.E.M.) in samples of human and frontal cortex from normal controls and Alzheimer patients (biopsies and autopsies). Significantly different from controls, $p < 0.05$.

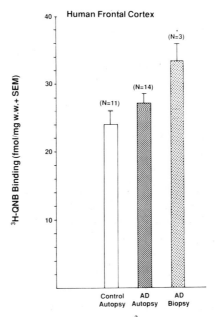

Fig. 2. Comparison of ^{3}H-QNB binding (fmol/mg w.w. $\pm$ S.E.M) in samples of human frontal cortex from normal controls and Alzheimer patients (biopsies and autopsies). Significantly different from controls, $p < 0.05$.

cant 39% increase in the biopsies (Fig. 2). Brain muscarinic receptors are differently affected by AD and Parkinson disease (PD). A decrease in M_2-receptor binding is seen in the hippocampus of AD patients while PD patients have unaltered binding (Rinne et al., 1989). Using ^{3}H-NIC as a ligand, we found a 44% decrease in the autopsies and a 55% decrease in the biopsies (Fig. 1). Preservation of the tissue might explain the differences between biopsy and autopsy material. However, in younger subjects it could reflect early changes in AD. These decreases in binding correlate to enzymatic (ChAT and AChE activity) changes (Davies, 1979; Rossor et al., 1982; Bird et al., 1983; Giacobini et al., 1988a,b, 1989), supporting a presynaptic localization of the lesion.

The agonists used in these studies are not selective for either pre- or postsynaptic cholinergic sites. Therefore, it is difficult to say whether presynaptic sites on cholinergic axons are preferentially affected or postsynaptic sites on cholinoceptive neurons are also involved.

A second effect of decreased cholinergic receptor function is regulation of ACh release and the effect of drugs on this release. Release of ^{3}H-ACh can be measured in frontal cortex slices from human autopsy after short post-mortem delay (Nordberg et al., 1987) and from biopsies (De-Sarno et al., 1988; Giacobini et al., 1988a). A significant reduction (50–70%) in the evoked release of ACh has been reported by both laboratories. A reduction in ACh release and in number of nicotinic binding sites in the frontal cortex of AD patients supports the hypothesis of a selective loss of presynaptic nicotinic receptors in AD (Giacobini et al., 1988a).

Although α-BTX has proved to be a useful cholinergic ligand in the peripheral nervous system, mainly at the neuromuscular junction, it is not suitable as a marker for the CNS (Morley et al., 1983). Experiments performed with iontophoretic techniques do not support the hypothesis that α-neurotoxins such as α-BTX bind to functional nicotine receptors in mammalian CNS (Morley and Kemp, 1981; Chiappinelli, 1985).

Consequently, characterization and quantitation of nicotinic cholinergic binding sites in the brain has met with difficulty. Recent studies have indicated differences between central and peripheral nicotinic receptors (Marks and Collins, 1982; Shimohama et al., 1985; Sugiyama and Yamashita, 1986). Chiappinelli (1985) and Wolf et al. (1987) have used a BTX which they named kappa-bungarotoxin (κ-BTX) to characterize central nicotinic receptors in the chicken and in the rat. Kappa-bungarotoxin has been recently isolated from snake venom (Chiappinelli, 1985). It was shown to be a potent and selective antagonist of neuronal nicotinic receptors (Chiappinelli, 1985), including CNS sites in the chicken optic lobe (Wolf et al., 1987). We have observed that using ^{3}H-NIC, ^{125}I-α-BTX and ^{125}I-κ-BTX, at least three putative categories of nicotinic receptor are present in the human brain. Our studies suggest that each type of these receptors may have different kinetics, distribution and localization. Kappa-bungarotoxin or neuronal BTX has been shown to block nicotinic synaptic transmission in a variety of neuronal preparations where α-BTX has no effect. Vidal and Changeux (1989) have demonstrated that the effect of NIC applied by iontophoresis to the prefrontal cortex of the rat is blocked by κ-BTX but not by other nicotinic antagonists. The agonistic actions of ACh in cerebellar neurons is also selectively blocked by κ-BTX (de la Garza et al., 1989).

Nicotinic receptor subtypes in human cortex: changes with Alzheimer disease

The existence of several subtypes of nicotinic cholinergic receptor in the brain would suggest specific anatomical localizations and functions. In situ hybridization techniques suggest the presence of three independent nicotinic receptor subtypes in the rat brain (Heinemann et al., 1988).

Combining ^{3}H-NIC, ^{125}I-α-BTX and ^{125}I-κ-BTX as ligands, several categories of nicotinic receptors can be postulated in the human brain (Giacobini et al., 1988b). We reported the kinetics, distribution and localization of three subtypes present in the human frontal cortex. We also described for the first time specific changes related to receptor subtypes in human cortex of AD patients (Giacobini et al., 1988b).

We used autopsy brains from healthy young controls (age 21–57 years), and healthy elderly controls (age 64–94 years) as well as from AD patients (age 67–78 years) from our Regional Alzheimer Center, for homogenate or slice in vitro assays of nicotinic binding. The right hemisphere was isolated and stored at −90°C for binding assays, the contralateral was fixed for histologically diagnosis.

Specific binding with increasing concentrations of ^{3}H-(−)-NIC, ^{125}I-α- or ^{125}I-κ-BTX to membranes of human frontal cortex was saturable. Scatchard plots were curvilinear and Hill coefficients far from unity, indicating the presence of multiple classes of binding sites for these three ligands.

There were significant decreases in the number (B_{max}) of high- (47%) and low- (50%) affinity binding sites of ^{3}H-(−)-NIC in AD patients as compared to elderly controls (Table II). Alzheimer patients showed a significant decrease of B_{max} in the low-affinity binding site of ^{125}I-κ-BTX but not in the high-affinity site, as compared to young (57%) and elderly (52%) controls. There was only a non-significant decrease in B_{max} in the low-affinity binding site of ^{125}I-α-BTX in AD patients, as compared to young and elderly controls (34.0% and 31.6%) (Table II).

TABLE II

Percent decrease in number of (−)-[^{3}H]nicotine, κ-[^{125}I]- or α-[^{125}I]-bungarotoxin binding sites in frontal cortex of Alzheimer patients as compared with elderly controls

	High affinity (% B_{max})	Low affinity (% B_{max})
(−)-[^{3}H]NIC	47	50 [a]
κ-[^{125}I]BTX	0	52 [a]
α-[^{125}I]BTX	0	32 [b]

$n = 6$–8; [a] significant, $p < 0.005$; [b] not significant.

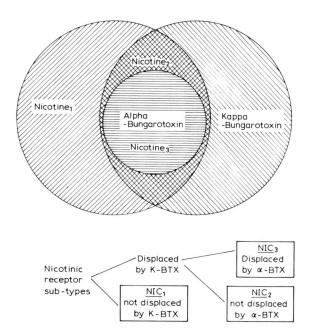

Fig. 3. Diagram of subtypes of nicotinic receptors in human frontal cortex demonstrated by using nicotine, α-bungarotoxin and κ-bungarotoxin as ligands. See text.

Autoradiographic analysis showed that ^{125}I-κ-BTX specific binding sites are concentrated mainly in the middle and deep cortical layers. The same localization has been observed by us in the monkey (*Macacus rhesus*). With autoradiography, a pronounced decrease in density of ^{125}I-κ-BTX binding sites was seen in AD patient vs. elderly controls.

The kinetic characteristics of these three binding sites were studied by means of competition experiments. These demonstrated the presence of two categories of nicotinic binding sites, one which was displaced by κ-BTX and one which was not displaced by this toxin (Fig. 3). We named the latter Nicotine$_1$ (Fig. 3). The binding site not displaced by κ-BTX could be subdivided into two subtypes, one which was displaced by α-BTX and one which was not. We named these two binding sites Nicotine$_2$ and Nicotine$_3$, respectively (Fig. 3).

A functional role of cortical nicotinic receptors can be demonstrated by the effect of BTXs on the evoked fractional release of ACh from rat frontal cortex slices. In these experiments, the first electrical stimulation (S$_1$, 20 mA, 1 Hz, 5 min) is a pre-drug testing control and the third electrical stimulation (S$_3$) is a post-drug testing control. The only significant decrease was seen in the S$_2$/S$_1$ ratio of ACh release following 1 μM κ-BTX but not after 1 μM α-BTX. The S$_3$/S$_1$ ratio did not change after the third stimulation. This shows that κ-BTX, but not α-BTX, decreases the electrically evoked release of ACh from rat frontal cortex slices and that this effect is reversible.

Mapping of nicotinic receptors in rodent brain, using various radiolabelled agonists (Clarke et al., 1985), in situ hybridization (Goldman et al., 1987) and immunohistochemistry (Swanson et al., 1987), has demonstrated the presence of a high number of ACh receptors in the neocortex. Our data on human brain autoradiography of κ-BTX binding sites also show the highest density in the cortex. We have seen variable regional distributions in the presence of ($-$)-NIC, α-BTX or κ-BTX. Receptor subtypes in human cortex have been previously suggested based on various ligands such as ^{3}H-ACh, [3]H-($-$)-nicotine and ^{125}I-α-BTX (Adem, 1987). The regional distribution and the pharmacology of agonists and antagonist binding sites suggest that these subtypes may be present in different neuronal populations in pre- and post-synaptic locations.

Our results show that two main categories of nicotinic receptors, one κ-BTX insensitive and the other one κ-BTX sensitive are present in human cortex (Fig. 3). Our experiments show that α-BTX displaces high- (100%) and low- (25%) affinity binding sites of κ-BTX but does not decrease the electrically evoked release of ACh. The κ-BTX-sensitive subtype has an α-BTX binding site which includes the high-affinity binding site of κ-BTX. The other subtype does not have an α-BTX binding site and modulates ACh release from rat frontal cortex through a κ-BTX-sensitive nicotinic receptor. Thus, our data are in agreement with the molecular biological data on receptor gene families in mammalian species (Heinemann et al., 1988; Lindstrom et al., 1988) suggesting that human cortex has at least three different subtypes of

nicotinic receptor, each showing specific kinetics, regional distribution and synaptic localization. These three subtypes are represented in the human frontal cortex. In addition, we have found that parietal, temporal lobe and hippocampus exhibit the same binding sites with a different receptor density and distribution. Hippocampal cortex (CA3) shows the highest density in κ-BTX binding sites.

The fact that κ-BTX, but not α-BTX, decreases the electrically evoked fractional release of ACh in rat brain is a strong indication for a presynaptic localization of κ-BTX binding site. This agrees with the finding of Vidal and Changeux (1989), who demonstrated an antagonism of κ-BTX (1.4 μM) to stimulation by iontophoretically applied NIC in slices of rat prefrontal cortex. In these experiments none of the classical nicotinic antagonists and α-BTX was found to have any effect on nicotinic responses.

Conclusion

In agreement with our previous data and the data found in the literature (cf. Giacobini et al., 1988a, 1989), with NIC, both high- and low-affinity binding sites were significantly decreased about 50% in AD patients as compared to elderly controls. With κ-BTX as a ligand, only low-affinity binding sites were decreased (-52%) while with α-BTX there were no significant changes. A decrease in nicotinic, but not muscarinic, receptors has been correlated to presynaptic changes including ChAT activity (Giacobini et al., 1988a, 1989) and loss of cells in the nucleus basalis of Meynert which project to cortex (Whitehouse et al., 1982; Coleman and Flood, 1989). In human biopsy studies we demonstrated the presence of evoked ACh release which is sensitive to the increase in ACh produced by AChE inhibition (Giacobini et al., 1988a). The effect of κ-BTX on ACh release seen by us in rat cortex and the changes in κ-BTX binding sites seen in AD cortex suggest the presence of a class of presynaptic nicotinic receptors

TABLE III

Putative cholinergic markers of Alzheimer

	Neural		Non-neural			
	Cortical biopsy or autopsy	CSF	Lymphocytes	Erythrocytes	Plasma	Serum
Nicotinic receptor binding	Decreased		Decreased			
Muscarinic (post syn.) receptor binding	No difference		Decreased			
ChAT activity	Decreased	Not measurable				
AChE activity	Decreased	Decreased	Decreased	Decreased but not specific	AChE increase; BuChE no difference or increase	
Release of ACh	Decreased	Measurable after ChEI				
Ach synthesis	Decreased					
High-affinity Ch uptake	Decreased	Increased Ch levels		Normal or increased Ch levels		
Altered Ch metabolism	Decreased	Increased Ch levels			No difference	
Cortisol					Increased	
Cortisol after cholinergic drugs					Increased	
Antibodies to cholinergic neurons		Present				Present
Anti-NGF antibodies		Present				Increased

References for these studies are found in the text.

which modulates ACh release and which is selectively reduced in AD.

Neural cholinergic markers in CSF

Table III summarizes the changes in cholinergic markers that correlate with a diagnosis of AD. The table collates results from several investigations. Neural markers are from biopsy or autopsy material, and extraneural markers are from CSF, lymphocytes, erythrocytes, plasma and serum. The CSF is the most accessible CNS compartment that can be exploited in the evaluation of the living patients and experimental animals. However, the use of CSF markers raises several questions regarding the origin of these markers and their relation to neuronal metabolism.

Acetylcholine

A review of CSF and ACh metabolism has been published recently (Giacobini, 1986). Levels of ACh ranging from 3 to 479 pmol/ml have been measured in human CSF. Judging from these data one may conclude that trace amounts (low picomole range) of ACh are probably present in normal human CSF. Following an i.c.v. (intracerebroventricular) injection of Phy (8 μg) producing 85% inhibition of cholinesterase (ChE) activity in CSF, we found an increase in CSF ACh from 0.9 nmol/ml to a peak value of 5 nmol/ml at 180 min (Giacobini et al., 1988c) (Fig. 2). At 360 min, CSF ACh levels were still elevated (4 nmol/ml) despite only 30% CSF ChE inhibition. Choline levels were stable, indicating that this precursor was not utilized to synthesize ACh in CSF.

We suggested that ACh may be released from the CNS into the CSF where its concentration is maintained at a high steady-state level because of the sustained ChE inhibition. Do ACh and Ch found in human CSF reflect closely extracellular fluid concentrations in the brain as suggested by animal experiments (Tucek, 1984)? If so, high and sustained cerebral ACh in CSF could be used as a marker of the effect of Phy. Such a marker would

be important in order to establish the central effect of ChE inhibitors during therapy for AD.

Choline levels and acetylcholinesterase activity

Choline is a precursor in the synthesis of ACh and of neuronal membrane phospholipids. Although the chief source of brain Ch is exogenous, some Ch synthesis is present in brain and may play a role in AD (Blusztajn and Wurtman, 1983). We measured multiple Ch levels and AChE activities in the CSF of 66 AD patients and 22 age-matched controls over a span of 24 months in order to study changes related to disease progression (Elble et al., 1989). We found a statistically significant reduction in AChE activity (Fig. 4) and an increase in Ch (Fig. 5) with advancing dementia (Fig. 3). These changes were not related to age (Figs. 6 and 7). We suggested that the rise in CSF Ch may be related to neuronal membrane breakdown and reduced uptake by cholinergic neurons. The reduction in CSF AChE activity is consistent with the depletion of cholinergic neurons in AD. In recent studies, we found that Ch levels, but not

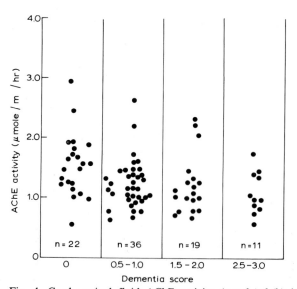

Fig. 4. Cerebrospinal fluid AChE activity (μmol/ml/h) in normal controls [clinical dementia rating (CDR) = 0] and patients with dementia of Alzheimer type (CDR 1, 2 and 3). *n* = number of patients (modified from Elble et al., 1989).

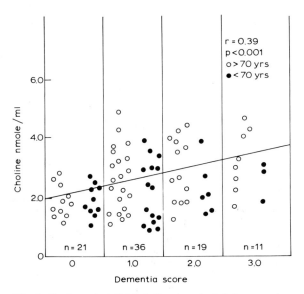

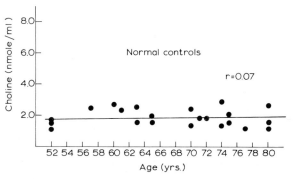

Fig. 7. Choline levels (nmol/ml) in CSF of normal controls of various ages.

Fig. 5. Cerebrospinal fluid choline (nmole/ml) in normal controls [clinical dementia rating (CDR) = 0] and patients with dementia of Alzheimer type (CDR 1, 2 and 3). *n* = number of patients (modified from Elble et al., 1989).

AChE activity, were significantly lower in patients with PD, cerebellar ataxia, and Huntington disease, compared with healthy controls (Table IV). In AD, levels of Ch were also significantly lower in familial patients than in non-familial patients, but there was no difference in AChE activity in these two groups (Kumar and Giacobini, 1988). It is noteworthy that Down's syndrome is the only other disease known to be associated with increased CSF Ch (Table IV) (Schapiro et al., 1989).

Therefore, increased Ch and decreased AChE activity in CSF in AD may be important biochemical markers of neuronal damage and cholinergic dysfunction. Of particular interest is the relation of the biochemical finding to the progression and severity of the disease seen in AD (Elble et al., 1989).

Choline acetyltransferase

Early studies (Johnson and Domino, 1971; Haber and Grossman, 1980) reported a significant activity of ChAT in the CSF, but Aquilonius and Eckernas (1976) reported later that most activity was non-enzymatic. DeKosky et al. (1989) measured ChAT activity of different CSF fractions using the specific inhibitor NVP. They found that normal human CSF does not contain ChAT and

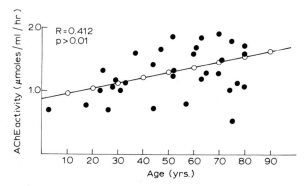

Fig. 6. Cerebrospinal fluid acetylcholinesterase (AChE) activity as function of age in 32 normal controls ($r = 0.412$, $p < 0.01$) (modified from Elble et al., 1987).

TABLE IV

Percent changes in levels in choline and acetylcholinesterase activity in the CSF of neurological patients as compared with normal controls

Disease	Choline	AChE activity
Alzheimer [a]	+60	−30
Down's Syndrome [e]	+28	no difference
Parkinson [b]	−56	no difference
Huntington [c]	−62	no difference
Cerebellar Ataxia [d]	−66	no difference

[a] Elble et al., 1988, 1989; [b] Manyam et al., 1990a; [c] Manyam et al., 1990b; [d] Manyam and Giacobini, 1989; [e] Schapiro et al., 1989.

that all ACh synthesis in CSF reflects non-enzymatically catalysed synthesis.

General conclusions

As summarized in Table III, several neural and non-neural markers of cholinergic function correlate with a diagnosis of AD. However, none of these markers is singularly diagnostic. In order of importance, we would rank first data from biopsy indicating a decrease in number of cholinergic receptors in cortex, particularly presynaptic nicotinic receptors, enzyme activities related to ACh synthesis (ChAT), hydrolysis (AChE) and release of ACh. In CSF, decreased AChE activity and increased levels of Ch are the only two indexes that correlate with the severity of dementia. Among several extraneuronal markers the presence of antibodies to cholinergic neurons, if confirmed, is of particular interest. In the future, new markers may be developed which might be more selective for presynaptic changes. These include new and more specific ligands for nicotinic receptors and the possibility of in vivo visualization of these receptors with PET-scanning.

Acknowledgements

The author wishes to thank Elizabeth Williams for technical assistance and Diana Smith for typing and editing the manuscript. Supported in part by National Institutes of Aging AG05416.

References

Adem, A. (1987) Characterization of muscarinic and nicotinic receptors in neural and non-neural tissue — changes in Alzheimer's disease. In *Comprehensive Summaries of Uppsala Dissertations from the Faculty of Pharmacy,* 32. Distributor: Almqvist and Wiksell Intl., Stockholm.

Aquilonius, S.M. and Eckernas, S.A. (1976) Choline acetyltransferase in human cerebrospinal fluid — non-enzymatically and enzymatically catalyzed acetylcholine synthesis. *J. Neurochem.,* 27: 317–318.

Bird, T.D., Stranahan, S., Sumi, S.M. and Raskind, M. (1983) Alzheimer's disease: choline acetyltransferase activity in brain tissue from clinical and pathological subgroups. *Ann. Neurol.,* 14: 284–293.

Blessed, G., Tomlinson, B.E. and Roth, M. (1968) The association between quantitative measures of dementia and of the senile change in the cerebral grey matter of elderly patients. *Br. J. Psychiat.,* 114: 797–811.

Blusztajn, J.K. and Wurtman, R.J. (1983) Choline and cholinergic neurons. *Science,* 221: 614–620.

Bondareff, W. and Mountjoy, C.Q. (1986) Number of neurons in nucleus locus coeruleus in demented and non-demented patients: rapid estimation and correlated paramters. *Neurobiol. Aging,* 7: 297–300.

Bowen, D.A., Smith, C.B., White, P. and Davison, A.M. (1976) Neurotransmitter related enzymes and indexes of hypoxia in senile dementia and other abiotrophies. *Brain,* 99: 459–496.

Butcher, L.L. and Woolf, N.J. (1986) Cholinergic systems in the brain and spinal cord: anatomic organization and overview of functions. In A. Fisher, I. Hanin and C. Lachman (Eds.), *Alzheimer and Parkinson Disease — Advances in Behavioral Biology,* Plenum Press, New York, pp. 5–16.

Chiappinelli, V.A. (1985) Actions of snake venom toxins on neuronal nicotinic receptors and other neuronal receptors. *Pharmac. Ther.,* 31: 1–32.

Clarke, P.B.S., Schwartz, R.D., Paul, S.M., Pert, C.B. and Pert, A. (1985) Nicotinic binding in rat brain — autoradiographic comparison of ^{3}H-nicotine and ^{125}I-α-bungarotoxin. *J. Neurosci.,* 5: 1307–1315.

Cole, A.E. and Nicoll, R.A. (1984) The pharmacology of cholinergic excitatory responses in hippocampal pyramidal cells. *Brain Res.,* 305: 283–290.

Coleman, P.D. and Flood, D.G. (1989) Neuron numbers and dendritic extent in normal aging and Alzheimer's disease. *Neurobiol. Aging,* 8: 521–545.

Davies, P. (1979) Neurotransmitter-related enzymes in senile dementia of the Alzheimer type. *Brain Res.,* 171: 319–327.

DeKosky, S.T., Scheff, S.W. and Hackney, C.G. (1989) Acetylcholine synthesis in human CSF: implications for study of central cholinergic metabolism. *Neurochem. Res.,* 14(2): 191–196.

de la Garza, R., Freedman, R. and Hoffer, B.J. (1989) κ-Bungarotoxin blockade of nicotine electrophysiological actions in cerebellar Purkinje neurons, *Neurosci. Lett.,* 99: 95–100.

DeSarno, P., Giacobini, E., McIlhany, M. and Clark, B. (1988) Nicotinic receptors in human CNS: a biopsy study. In A. Agnoli (Ed.), *Proceedings 2nd Intl. Symposium on Senile Dementias,* John Libbey Eurotext, Ltd., Montrouge, France, pp. 329–334.

Downen, M.D., Sugaya, K., Arneric, P. and Giacobini, E. (1989) Presynaptic markers of cholinergic function in cortex following ibotenic acid lesion of the basal forebrain. In E.M. Meyer, J. Simpkins and J. Yamamoto (Eds.), *Novel Treatments and Models for AD,* Plenum Press, New York (in press).

Elble, R., Giacobini, E. and Scarsella, G.F. (1987) Cholinesterases in cerebrospinal fluid. *Arch. Neurol.,* 44: 403–407.

Elble, R., Giacobini, E. and Higgins, C. (1989) Choline levels are increased in cerebrospinal fluid of Alzheimer patients. *Neurobiol. Aging,* 10: 45–50.

Francis, P.T., Palmer, A.M., Sims, N.R., Bowen, D.M., Davison, A.N., Esiri, N.M., Neary, D., Snowden, J.S. and Wilcock, G.K. (1985) Neurochemical studies of early onset. *N. Engl. J. Med.,* 313: 7–11.

Fuld, P.A., Katzman, R. and Davies, P. (1982) Intrusions as a sign of Alzheimer dementia, chemical and pathological verification. *Ann. Neurol.,* 11: 155–159.

Giacobini, E. (1986) Brain acetylcholine — a view from the cerebrospinal fluid (CSF). *Neurobiol. Aging,* 7(5):392–396.

Giacobini, E., Mattio, T. and Mussini, I. (1987) Aging of cholinergic synapses in the avian iris. Part I — biochemical studies. *Neurobiol. Aging,* 8: 123–129.

Giacobini, E., DeSarno, P., McIlhany, M. and Clark, B. (1988a) The cholinergic receptors system in the frontal lobe of Alzheimer patients. In F. Clementi, C. Gotti and E. Sher (Eds.), *Nicotinic Acetylcholine Receptors in the Nervous System — NATO ASI Series H,* Vol. H25, Springer-Verlag, Berlin, pp. 367–378.

Giacobini, E., Sugaya, K., DeSarno, P. and Chiappinelli, V. (1988b) Three subtypes of nicotinic receptors in human cortex. *Soc. Neurosci. Abstr.* p. 55.4.

Giacobini, E., Becker, R., McIlhany, M. and Kumar, V. (1988c) Introacerebro-ventricular administration of cholinergic drugs — preclinical trials and clinical experience in Alzheimer patients. In E. Giacobini and R. Becker (Eds.), *Current Research in Alzheimer Therapy,* Taylor & Francis, New York, pp. 113–122.

Giacobini, E., DeSarno, P., Clark, B. and McIlhany, M. (1989) The cholinergic receptor system of the human brain. Neurochemical and pharmacological aspects in aging and Alzheimer. In A. Nordberg (Ed.), *Progress in Brain Research, Vol. 79,* Elsevier, Amsterdam, pp. 335–343.

Goldman, D., Deneris, E., Luyten, W., Kochlar, A., Patrick, J. and Heinemann, S. (1987) Members of a nicotine acetylcholine receptor gene family are expressed in different regions of the mammalian central nervous system. *Cell,* 48: 965–973.

Haber, B. and Grossman, R.G. (1980) Acetylcholine metabolism in intracranial and lumbar cerebrospinal fluid and in blood. In J.H. Wood (Ed.), *Neurobiology of Cerebrospinal Fluid, Vol. 1,* Plenum Press, New York, pp. 345–350.

Heinemann, S., Boulter, J., Deneris, E., Connolly, J., Gardner, P., Wada, E., Ballivet, M., Swanson, L. and Patrick, J. (1988) The nicotinic acetylcholine receptor gene family. In F. Clementi, C. Gotti and E. Sher (Eds), *Nicotinic Acetylcholine Receptors in the Nervous System — NATO ASI Series H, Vol. H25,* Springer-Verlag, Berlin, pp. 173–191.

Johns, C.A., Levy, M.I., Greenwald, B.S., Rosen, W.G., Horvath, T.B., Davis, B.M., Mohs, R.C. and Davis, K.L. (1983) Studies of cholinergic mechanisms in Alzheimer's disease. In N. Katzman (Ed.), Banbury Report 15: *Biological Aspects of Alzheimer's Disease,* Cold Spring Harbor, pp. 435–449.

Johnson, S. and Domino, E.F. (1971) Cholinergic enzymatic activity of cerebrospinal fluid of patients with various neurological disease. *Clin. Chim. Acta,* 35: 421–428.

Kellar, K.J., Whitehouse, P.J., Martino-Barrows, A.M., Marcus, K. and Price, D.L. (1987) Muscarinic and nicotinic cholinergic binding sites in Alzheimer disease cerebral cortex. *Brain Res.,* 436: 62–68.

Kumar, V. and Giacobini, E. (1988) Cerebrospinal fluid choline, and acetylcholinesterase activity in familial vs. non-familial Alzheimer's disease patients. *Arch. Gerontol. Geriatr.,* 7: 111–117.

Lindstrom, J., Whiting,, P., Schoepfer, R., Luther, M. and Casey, B. (1988) Structure of neuronal nicotinic receptors. In F. Clementi, C. Gotti and E. Sher (Eds.), *Nicotinic Acetylcholine Receptors in the Nervous System — NATO ASI Series, Vol. H25,* Springer-Verlag, Berlin. pp. 159–172.

Lamour, Y. and Dykes, R.W. (1988) Somatosensory neurons in partially deafferented rat hindlimb granular cortex subsequent to transection of the sciatic nerve: effects of glutamate and acetylcholine. *Brain Res.,* 449: 18–33.

London, E. and Coyle, J.T. (1978) Pharmacological augmentation of acetylcholine levels in kainate-lesioned rat striatum. *Biochem. Pharmacol.,* 27: 2962–2965.

Manyam, B.V., Colliver, J.A. and Giacobini, E. (1990a) Cerebrospinal fluid choline levels are decreased in Parkinson's disease. *Ann. Neurol.,* 27: 683–685.

Manyam, B.V., Giacobini, E. and Colliver, J.A. (1990b) Cerebrospinal fluid acetylcholinesterase and choline measurements in Huntington's disease. *J. Neurol.,* (in press).

Marchi, M., Bocchieri, P., Garbarino, L. and Raiteri, M. (1989) Muscarinic inhibition of endogenous glutamate releae from rat hippocampus synaptosomes, *Neurosci. Lett.,* 96: 229–234.

Marks, H.J. and Collins, A.C. (1982) Characterization of nicotine binding in mouse brain and comparison with the binding of alpha-bungarotoxin and quinuclidinyl benzilate. *Mol. Pharmacol.,* 22: 554–564.

Mash, D.C., Flynn, D.D. and Potter, L.T. (1985) Loss of M_2 muscarine receptors in the cerebral cortex in Alzheimer's disease and experimental cholinergic denervation. *Science,* 228: 1115–1117.

Mesulam, M.-M. (1988) Central cholinergic pathways — neuroanatomy and some behavioral implications. In M. Avoli, T.A. Reader, R.W. Dykes and P. Gloor (Eds.), *Neurotransmitters and Cortical Function,* Plenum Press, New York, pp. 237–260.

Metherate, R., Tremblay, N. and Dykes, R.W. (1988) Transient and prolonged effects of acetylcholine on responsiveness of cat somatosensory cortical neurons. *J. Neurophysiol.,* 59(4):1253–1276.

McCormick, D. and Prince, D.A. (1986) Mechanisms of action of acetylcholine in the guinea-pig cerebral cortex in vitro. *J. Physiol.,* 375: 169–194.

Morley, B.J. and Kemp, G.E. (1981) Characterization of a putative nicotinic acetylcholine receptor in mammalian brain. *Brain Res. Rev.,* 3: 82–104.

Morley, B.J., Dwyer, D.S., Strang-Brown, P.F., Bradley, R.J. and Kemp, G.E. (1983) Evidence that certain peripheral anti-acetylcholine receptor antibodies do not interact with brain bungarotoxin binding sites. *Brain Res.,* 262: 109–116.

Neary, D., Snowden, J.S., Bowen, D.M., Sims, N.R., Mann, D.M.A., Benton, J.S., Northen, B., Yates, P.O. and Davison, A.N. (1986a) Neuropsychological syndromes in presenile dementia due to cerebral atrophy. *J. Neurol. Neurosurg. Psychiatr.,* 49: 163–174.

Neary, D., Snowden, J.S., Mann, D.M.A., Bowen, D.M., Sims, N.R., Northern, B., Yates, P.O. and Davison, A.N. (1986b) Alzheimer's disease: a correlative study. *J. Neurol. Neurosurg. Psychiatr.,* 49: 229–237.

Nilsson, L., Adem, A., Hardy, J., Winblad, B. and Nordberg, A. (1987) Do tetrahydroaminoacridine (THA) and physostigmine restore acetylcholine release in Alzheimer brains via nicotinic receptors? *J. Neural Transm.,* 70: 347–368.

Nordberg, A., Adem, A., Nilsson, L. and Winblad, B. (1987) Cholinergic deficits in CNS and peripheral non-neuronal tissue in Alzheimer dementia. In M.J. Dowdall, J.N. Hawthorne (Eds.), *Cellular and Molecular Basis of Cholinergic Function,* Ellis Horwood Publ., pp., 858–868.

Perry, E.K., Tomlinson, E., Blessed, G., Bergmann, K., Gibson, P.H. and Perry, R.H. (1978) Correlation of cholinergic abnormalities with senile plaques and mental test scores in senile dementia. *Br. J. Med.,* 42: 1457–1459.

Reisine, T., Yamamura, H.I., Bird, E.D., Spokes, E. and Enna, S.J. (1978) Pre- and postsynaptic neurochemical alterations in Alzheimer's disease. *Brain Res.,* 159: 477–481.

Richardson, R.T. and DeLong, M.R. (1988) A reappraisal of the functions of the nucleus basalis of Meynert. *Trends Neurosci.,* 11: 264–267.

Richter, J.A., Perry, E.K. and Tomlinson, B.E. (1980) Acetylcholine and choline levels in post-mortem human brain tissue: preliminary observations in Alzheimer's disease. *Life Sci.,* 26: 1683–1689.

Rinne, J.O., Lonnberg, P., Marjamaki, P. and Rinne, U.P. (1989) Brain muscarinic receptor subtypes are differently affected in Alzheimer's disease and Parkinson's diseases. *Brain Res.,* 483: 402–406.

Rossor, M.N., Garrett, N.J., Johnson, A.L., Mountjoy, C.Q., Roth, M. and Iversen, L.L. (1982) A post-mortem study of the cholinergic and GABA systems in senile dementia. *Brain,* 105: 313–330.

Rylett, R.J., Ball, M.J. and Calhoun, E.H. (1983) Evidence for high affinity choline transport in synaptosomes prepared from hippocampus and neocortex of patients with Alzheimer's disease. *Brain Res.,* 289: 169–175.

Schapiro, M.B., Kay, A.D., May, C., Atack, J., Hodes, J.E., Kopp, U., Haxby, J.V., Hanin, I. and Rapoport, S.I. (1989) Cerebrospinal fluid choline in Down syndrome adults at different ages. *Neurobiol. Aging,* (in press).

Schroder, H., Zilles, K., Luiten, P.G.M., Strosberg, A.D. and Aghchi, A.R. (1989) Human cortical neurons contain both nicotinic and muscarinic acetylcholine receptors: an immunocytochemical double-labeling study. *Synapse,* (in press).

Shimohama, S., Taniguichi, T., Fujiwara, M. and Kameyama, M. (1985) Biochemical characterization of the nicotinic cholinergic receptors in human brain: binding of ^{3}H-(−)-nicotine. *J. Neuorchem.,* 45: 604–610.

Sims, N.R., Bowen, D.M., Allen, S.J., Smith, C.C.T., Neary, D., Thomas, D.J. and Davison, A.N. (1983) Presynaptic cholinergic dysfunction in patients with dementia. *J. Neurochem.,* 40(2): 503–509.

Soininen, H.S., Jolkkonen, J.T., Reinikainen, K.J., Halonen, T.O. and Riekkinen, P.J. (1984) Reduced cholinesterase activity and somatostatin-like immunoreactivity in the cerebrospinal fluid of patients with dementia of the Alzheimer type. *J. Neurol. Sci.,* 63: 167–172.

Sugiyama, H. and Yamashita, Y. (1986) Characterization of putative nicotinic acetylcholine receptors solubilized from rat brains. *Brain Res.,* 373: 22–26.

Swanson, L.W., Simmons, D.H., Whiting, P.J. and Lindstrom, J. (1987) Immunohistochemical localization of neuronal nicotinic receptors in rodent central nervous system. *J. Neurosci.,* 7: 3334–3342.

Tucek, S. (1984) Problems in the organization and control of acetylcholine synthesis in brain neurons. *Prog. Biophys. Mol. Biol.,* 44: 1–46.

Vidal, C. and Changeux, J-P. (1989) Pharmacological profile of nicotinic acetylcholine receptors in the rat prefrontal cortex — an electrophysiological study in a slice preparation. *Neuroscience,* 29(2): 261–270.

Whitehouse, P.J. (1987) Neurotransmitter receptor alterations in AD: a review. *Alzheimer Dis. Rel. Disorders* 1: 9–18.

Whitehouse, P.J., Price, D.L., Struble, R.G., Clark, A.W., Coyle, J.T. and DeLong, M.R. (1982) Alzheimer's disease and senile dementia — loss of neurons in the basal forebrain. *Science,* 215: 1237–1239.

Whitehouse, P.J., Martino, A.M., Wagster, M.V., Price, D.L., Mayeux, R., Atack, J.R. and Kellar, K.J. (1988) Reductions in ^{3}H-nicotinic acetylcholine binding in Alzheimer's disease and Parkinson's disease — an autoradiographic study. *Neurology,* 38: 720–723.

Wolf, K.M., Ciarleglio, A. and Chiappinelli, V.A. (1987) κ-Bungarotoxin — binding of a neuronal nicotinic receptor antagonist to chick optic lobe and skeletal muscle. *Brain Res.,* 89: 1–10.

Zweig, R.M., Ross, C.A., Hedreen, J.C., Steele, C., Cardillo, J.E., Whitehouse, P.J., Folstein, M.F. and Price, D.L. (1988) The neuropathology of aminergic nuclei in Alzheimer's disease. *Ann. Neurol.,* 24(2): 233–242.

Zubenko, G.S., Moossy, J., Martinez, A.J., Rao, G.R., Kopp, U. and Hanin, I. (1989) A brain regional analysis of morphologic and cholinergic abnormalities in Alzheimer's disease. *Arch. Neurol.,* 46: 634–638.

S.-M. Aquilonius and P.-G. Gillberg (Eds.)
Progress in Brain Research, Vol. 84
© 1990 Elsevier Science Publishers B.V. (Biomedical Division)

CHAPTER 35

Implications of multiple transmitter system lesions for cholinomimetic therapy in Alzheimer's disease

Vahram Haroutunian, Anthony C. Santucci and Kenneth L. Davis

*Department of Psychiatry, The Mount Sinai School of Medicine, New York, NY 10029,
and The Bronx Veterans Administration Medical Center, Bronx, NY 10468, U.S.A.*

Introduction

Because of the profound cholinergic deficits in Alzheimer's disease (AD) most therapeutic and animal model studies have focused on this system (Santucci et al., 1989). The outcome of treatment studies based on ameliorating the cholinergic deficits in AD has been reviewed many times (Davis and Mohs, 1982; Mohs et al., 1987) and will not be elaborated here. It is important to note, however, that the cholinergic treatment strategy has met with only partial success. Animal model studies, on the other hand, have found cholinergic lesion-induced learning and memory deficits to be readily reversed by cholinomimetic agents. Low doses of physostigmine and other cholinomimetics have repeatedly been shown to reverse n. basalis Meynert (nbM) lesion-induced learning and mem-

ory deficits (Santucci et al., 1989). The experiments described here are based on the hypothesis that the failure of all or some of the other transmitter systems affected in AD contributes to the symptoms of AD and possibly to the efficacy of cholinomimetics in exerting a beneficial effect.

In addition to the cholinergic deficits, the noradrenergic (Bondareff et al., 1982; Arai et al., 1984), serotonergic (Cross, 1987), somatostatinergic (Rossor et al., 1980; Davies et al., 1980; Davies and Terry, 1981), and corticotropin releasing factor (CRF; Powers et al., 1987; DeSouza et al., 1986) systems are among the most severely affected in AD. There are few data regarding the role of CRF in cognition or the interaction of CRF with cholinergic systems. Since pharmacological tools for manipulating CRF systems are not yet available, evaluation of the role of CRF in

TABLE I

Effects of ibotenic acid lesions of the nbM on cortical values of some neurochemical markers

Marker	Sham	nbM	% Depletion
Choline acetyltransferase (nmol ACH/h/mg prot)	19.2 ± 0.3 (12)	14.1 ± 0.7 (14)	26.3 [a]
Acetylcholinesterase (nmol/h/mg prot)	1512 ± 24 (12)	1070 ± 54 (14)	29.1 [a]
Norepinephrine (ng/100 mg tissue)	30.1 ± 0.8 (12)	29.1 ± 0.9 (14)	3.2
Dopamine (ng/100 mg tissue)	6.7 ± 0.2 (12)	6.4 ± 0.3 (14)	5.2
Serotonin (ng/100 mg tissue)	32.2 ± 0.8 (11)	29.0 ± 0.8 (12)	9.9
Somatostatin-LI (pg/mg tissue)	377.8 ± 11 (12)	387 ± 18 (12)	2.6
CRF (pg/mg tissue)	1.9 ± 0.1 (12)	1.8 ± 0.1 (12)	3.1

Values are expressed as means ± SEM (n)
[a] nbM vs. Sham, $p < 0.01$.

AD or with respect to response to cholinomimetics must await future advances in this area. It is clear, however, that in the rat forebrain, CRF is not localized in ACh neurons. Lesions of the cholinergic cells of the basal forebrain do not affect cortical CRF levels (see Table I).

General methods

The general experimental plan in all the studies described was as follows. Male Sprague-Dawley rats (225–250 g) were used in all the experiments described. In those experiments involving lesions of forebrain structures, the animals were allowed to recover from surgery for two weeks before the beginning of behavioral assessment. The rats were trained using a one trial step-through passive avoidance paradigm. Immediately following training each rat received a subcutaneous injection of the drug under study and was returned to its home cage. Retention of passive avoidance was assessed 72 h later. All rats were killed within one week of retention testing: cortices and other areas of interest were dissected on ice and were kept frozen at −80°C until assay.

For ibotenic acid-induced lesions of the nbM, each rat was anesthetized using a combination of ketamine (60 mg/kg i.m.) and pentobarbital (21 mg/kg ip). Following the induction of anesthesia, each rat was positioned in a stereotaxic apparatus with the upper incisor bar set level with the intra-aural line. After a midline incision, burr holes were drilled at coordinates Bregma −0.3, ±2.8 mm lateral to midline. A 33 gauge stainless steel hypodermic cannula was slowly lowered 7.5–8.0 mm ventral to the surface of the skull. One microliter of ibotenic acid (5 μg/μl of phosphate buffer) was infused into the nbM area. The ascending noradrenergic bundle was lesioned by the injection of two microliters of a 4 μg/μl solution of 6-hydroxydopamine (6-OHDA) dissolved in a 0.1% solution of ascorbic acid. The stereotaxic coordinates were Bregma −6.0, 0.8 mm lateral to midline and 6.5 mm ventral to skull. Sham-lesioned rats received identical treatments except for the

infusion of neurotoxins. Rats assigned to combined lesion groups received the nbM and ANB lesions during the same surgical session with the order of structures lesioned randomized. Behavioral testing began two weeks after the surgical procedures. After a 15 min adaptation period to the behavioral testing rooms, rats were placed singly inside the bright, white painted compartment of a two compartment, black/white, shuttle box (28 cm × 14 cm × 15 cm). Sixty seconds later, a guillotine door separating the two compartments was raised. The rat's latency to cross from the bright compartment into the dark, black painted compartment was measured. Upon entry into the dark compartment, the guillotine door was lowered. Each rat then received a 2 s long, 0.6 mA scrambled foot shock delivered through the grid floor of the apparatus. The rat was confined to the dark chamber for an additional 60 s, after which it was removed and injected with the pharmacological agent under study. The drugs administered to the rats were always prepared on the day of the experiment, and were pH adjusted to 7.4. Following the acquisition phase of the passive avoidance protocol and drug administration, each rat was returned to its home cage and was left undisturbed until testing 72 h later. The passive avoidance retention test procedure was identical to that used during training except that the cross-through response into the dark compartment was not punished. The latency to enter the dark, shock-associated compartment was taken as the dependent measure of memory. Within one week of behavioral testing each rat was killed by decapitation. The brain was removed and cortices were dissected and assayed for choline acetyltransferase (Fonnum, 1975), acetylcholinesterase (Johnson et al., 1975) and norepinephrine (Maruyama et al., 1980).

Results and Discussion

Cholinergic / somatostatinergic interactions

The study and manipulation of central somatostatinergic systems, like CRF systems, is hampered by a paucity of pharmacological tools, but central somatostatin levels can be modified by cysteamine (2-mercaptoethylamine). Central somatostatin levels can be depleted by approximately 50% following the systemic administration of cysteamine (Haroutunian et al., 1987). This depletion is rapid, reversible, and under some circumstances leads to impaired performance on tests of learning and memory. Rats received a 150 mg/kg dose of cysteamine immediately following the acquisition of a one-trial passive avoidance response. Each rat was placed in the brightly lit compartment of a two-chambered shuttle box, and after crossing into the dark compartment received a single 0.5–0.8 mA footshock. Different groups of rats then received either an s.c. injection of saline or cysteamine. Retention of the passive avoidance response was assessed 72 h later. The results are shown in Table II, and indicate that retention test performance of cysteamine-treated rats was significantly ($p < 0.01$) worse than saline-injected controls. Cysteamine treated rats crossed into the shock compartment of the shuttle box with latencies comparable to their pre-shock latencies. Saline-treated animals avoided the shock-associated compartment for significant periods. These data suggest that post-acquisition administration of cysteamine leads to significant retention test performance deficits. The mechanism through which cysteamine depletes central somatostatinergic stores and influences performance on

tests of learning and memory is not clear. Whether these mnemonic effects of cysteamine are due to somatostatin depletion per se or to the non-physiological release of somatostatin from central stores remains to be determined (see Haroutunian et al., 1987, for a more complete discussion of these results). These data do demonstrate, however, that perturbation of central somatostatinergic systems does affect performance on tests of learning and memory.

Recent evidence suggests that cysteamine-induced depletion of central somatostatin stores does not significantly affect cholinergic function or response to cholinomimetics (Haroutunian et al., 1989a). The effects of combined nbM and cysteamine-induced somatostatinergic lesions on the retention of a one-trial passive avoidance response are not multiplicative. The superimposition of somatostatinergic lesions upon ibotenic acid-induced lesions of the nbM fails to impair passive avoidance retention test performance beyond the impairment induced by lesions of the nbM alone. There is also clear evidence that cysteamine-induced depletion of central somatostatin stores does not adversely affect the responsivity of "naive" or nbM-lesioned rats to cholinomimetics. In a dose response study of physostigmine, the administration of somatostatin depleting doses of cysteamine failed to prevent physostigmine-induced enhancement of passive avoidance retention test performance in sham-operated or nbM-lesioned rats.

TABLE II

Effects of the administration of different doses of cysteamine to sham-operated and nbM-lesioned rats of the 72-h retention of one-trial passive avoidance using 0.5 mA (replication one) or 0.8 mA (replication two) foot shock

Lesion condition	Cysteamine dose (mg/kg)			
	0.0	25.0	50.0	150.0
Replication one,				
sham-operated	235.3 ± 37	198.4 ± 33	150.7 ± 25 [a]	116.9 ± 23 [a]
nbM-lesioned	44.8 ± 13 [b]	48.7 ± 20 [b]	41.8 ± 12 [b]	37.1 ± 16 [b]
Replication two,				
sham-operated	275.7 ± 24	179.4 ± 39	111.9 ± 27 [a]	138.6 ± 22 [a]
nbM-lesioned	134.9 ± 34 [b]	141.7 ± 18 [b]	144.1 ± 34 [b]	119.0 ± 28 [b]

Values represent mean crossthrough latency (s) at test ± SEM.
[a] vs. sham 0.0 dose, $p < 0.05$; [b] vs same dose sham, $p < 0.05$. Mean crossthrough latency during training did not differ across groups and was 34.8 ± 6.8.

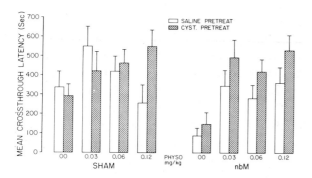

Fig. 1. Effects of various doses of physostigmine on the passive avoidance retention test performance of nbM or sham-lesioned rats with three consecutive days of saline or cysteamine (150 mg/kg) pretreatment. $n = 10-12$.

Different groups of rats received sham operations of ibotenic acid-induced lesions of the nbM. Two weeks following the lesion procedure half of the rats in the lesioned and sham-operated conditions received 3 consecutive daily injections of 150 mg/kg cysteamine. On the fourth day all rats were trained on a one-trial passive avoidance task. Immediately following training, different groups of rats ($n = 10-12$) received a 0.0, 0.03, 0.06, or 0.12 mg/kg s.c. dose of physostigmine. Retention of passive avoidance was assessed 72 h later. The results of this study are summarized in Fig. 1 and indicate that at appropriate doses physostigmine enhanced the retention test performance of sham and nbM-lesioned rats ($p < 0.03$). In addition, cysteamine pretreatment did not adversely affect the efficacy of physostigmine in this paradigm. On the contrary, the pretreatment of rats with cysteamine widened the effective dose range of physostigmine. Neurochemical analysis of cortical ChAT and SLI revealed a 34–37% lesion-induced depletion of ChAT ($p < 0.01$) and an approximately 43% cysteamine-induced depletion of SLI ($p < 0.01$). Thus, currently available data suggest that the depletion of central somatostatin stores does not adversely influence responsivity to cholinomimetics, irrespective of the presence or absence of forebrain cholinergic lesions. It must be kept in mind, however, that somatostatin-specific doses of cysteamine led to only partial depletion of central somatostatin stores. It is possible that different conclusions will be reached when more specific and efficacious anti-somatostatinergic tools become available.

Cholinergic / noradrenergic interactions

It is now apparent that a significant proportion of AD patients suffer considerable cortical noradrenergic depletion, cell loss, and decreased NE turnover (Adolfsson et al., 1979; Bondareff et al., 1982; Arai et al., 1984; Palmer et al., 1987a,b). These results, which have been replicated many times, suggest that noradrenergic deficits contribute to the pathophysiology of AD in at least a significant subpopulation of AD patients. Noradrenergic deficits in AD are not confined to decreased levels of NE and changes in locus coeruleus cell numbers but affect adrenergic receptors as well (Shimohama et al., 1986).

The evidence that noradrenergic dysfunction influences the cognitive deficits of AD is not well established, but significant correlations between brain NE markers and performance on cognitive tests have been reported in AD (Adolfsson et al., 1979; Mann et al., 1980). Animal studies involving lesions of the forebrain noradrenergic system, however, fail to show a strong relationship between noradrenergic function and performance on learning and memory tasks. On the other hand, there is strong and almost unanimous evidence for the involvement of noradrenergic systems in the extinction of learned behaviors (see Haroutunian et al., 1986; Mason, 1979; McNaughton and Mason, 1980 for reviews), and the potentiation of performance on tests of memory (Gold and Zornetzer, 1983). In contrast to the evidence in rodents, lesions of forebrain catecholaminergic systems do result in cognitive impairments in monkeys (Arnsten and Goldman-Rakic, 1985a,b). There also appears to be a strong correlation between age-related forebrain NE depletion and locus coeruleus cell counts and performance on tests of learning and memory in monkeys (Zornetzer, 1985; Arnsten and Goldman-Rakic, 1985b).

Since both cholinergic and noradrenergic systems are involved in AD, the functional interrelationship between these systems must be considered. There are many potential sites, such as the cell bodies, the terminal fields, and common target cells (cf. Andrade and Aghajanian, 1985; Egan and North, 1985; Egan et al., 1983; Engberg and Sevenssen, 1980; Waterhouse et al., 1981, 1986) where interactions between ascending noradrenergic and cholinergic systems can occur. The functional effects of NE and acetylcholine ultimately depend upon the interaction of these transmitters with receptors on post-synaptic target cells. Electrophysiological, neurochemical and behavioral data indicate that these transmitters may interact synergistically. For example, it has recently been shown that in the cerebral cortex norepinephrine and α-adrenergic agonists applied at doses which by themselves have no electrophysiological effects greatly potentiate the responsiveness of somatosensory cortex cells to acetylcholine (Waterhouse et al., 1980, 1981, 1986). Behaviorally, studies of learning and memory employing physostigmine and oxotremorine (Haroutunian et al., 1989b, described below), scopolamine (Decker and Gallager, 1987), oxotremorine following DBH inhibition (Huygens et al., 1980), and a variety of cholinomimetics following noradrenergic lesions (Mason and Fibiger, 1979) provide evidence for

functional interaction between these two systems. These and other studies demonstrate that cholinergic and noradrenergic systems interact at a variety of different sites and suggest that impairment of noradrenergic neurotransmission can significantly modulate the behavioral effects of cholinomimetics.

A combined forebrain cholinergic and noradrenergic lesion preparation has been developed to more closely approximate the neurochemical deficits of AD and to study the functional interaction of these systems. We have examined the consequences of combined forebrain cholinergic and noradrenergic deficits on cognitive performance and responsivity to cholinomimetic agents in the rat.

Several initial studies showed that learning and retention of a passive avoidance response was not impaired by noradrenergic lesions alone. In the first study, groups of 12 rats each received either sham lesions, nbM lesions, ANB lesions or combined nbM + ANB lesions. All rats were trained and tested on the one-trial passive avoidance task two weeks after the lesion. Rats with lesions of the nbM or lesions of the nbM + ANB were severely impaired with respect to the 72 h retention of passive avoidance, whereas ANB lesions by themselves did not impair test performance. Mean cross-through latencies were 306.4 +/− 68, 343.2

TABLE III

Effect of sham, nbM, ANB and nbM + ANB lesions on cortical neurochemical markers

	ChAT (nmol ACH/min prot)	AChE (nmol/min /mg prot)	NE (ng/100 mg tissue)	DA (ng/100 mg/mg tissue)
Sham	1.66 ± 0.06 (12)	2 509 ± 41 (12)	30.1 ± 0.85 (12)	6.7 ± 0.24 (12)
nbM	1.17 ± 0.07 (14)	1 804 ± 83 (14)	29.2 ± 0.92 (14)	6.3 ± 0.28 (14)
% dep	29.5 [a]	28.0 [a]	3.1	5.2
ANB	1.70 ± 0.05 (12)	2 461 ± 77 (12)	1.9 ± 1.22 (12)	6.4 ± 0.34 (12)
% dep	2.4	1.9	93.7 [a]	3.8
nbM + ANB	1.19 ± 0.06 (13)	1 847 ± 65 (13)	3.5 ± 2.21 (13)	5.9 ± 0.36 (13)
% dep	27.7 [a]	26.4 [a]	88.4 [a]	11.2

Results are expressed as means ± SEM (n).
[a] vs. Sham, $p < 0.01$.

+/−71, 113.4 +/−56 and 106.7 +/−48 for sham, ANB, nbM and ANB + nbM lesioned rats, respectively ($F(3/44) = 7.2$, $p < 0.001$). Neurochemically, nbM and nbM + ANB-lesioned rats displayed 26.4% and 28.1% reductions in cortical choline acetyltransferase (ChAT) and acetylcholinesterase (AChE) activity, respectively ($p < 0.01$ vs. sham-operated controls). ANB and nbM + ANB lesioned rats displayed a 95.4% reduction ($p < 0.01$ vs. sham-operated controls) in cortical NE activity (Table III). Lesions of the nbM did not affect cortical NE activity and lesions of the ANB did not alter cortical ChAT, AChE or dopaminergic markers ($p < 0.1$). These results suggest that lesions which deplete cortical cholinergic markers can severely impair performance on a learning and memory task, while noradrenergic lesions alone do not have a similar effect on passive avoidance retention test performance. This pattern of results agrees with earlier studies of cholinergic and adrenergic lesion effects on relatively simple tests of learning and memory in rodents (Mason, 1979; McNaughton and Mason, 1980). Similar results were obtained in another study using a fear potentiation of the acoustic startle response and the measure of learning and memory (Haroutunian et al., 1989b).

In a second study we tested the hypothesis that noradrenergic lesions may block the ability of cholinomimetics to potentiate performance on cognitive tasks. Different groups ($n = 7$) of sham-operated, nbM-lesioned, ANB-lesioned or nbM + ANB-lesioned rats received an s.c. injection of either saline or 0.06 mg/kg physostigmine immediately following the acquisition phase of a one-trial passive avoidance response. When retention for passive avoidance was assessed 72 h later, the nbM-lesioned and nbM + ANB-lesioned rats receiving saline showed poor memory of the passive avoidance response relative to sham-operated controls ($F(3/48) = 9.7$, $p < 0.001$). The administration of physostigmine had a significant retention test performance enhancing effect in the nbM-lesioned rats (Newman-Keuls test, $p < 0.001$), but had no effect on the performance of

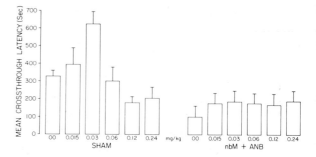

Fig. 2. Effects of different doses of physostigmine on the 72 h retention of one-trial passive avoidance in sham-operated and nbM + ANB-lesioned rats.

the nbM + ANB-lesioned animals ($p > 0.4$). These effects of physostigmine in sham-operated and nbM-lesioned rats directly replicate earlier reports of physostigmine enhancement of retention test performance in nbM-lesioned rats (Haroutunian et al., 1985).

It is possible to argue that the failure of physostigmine to affect retention test performance in nbM + ANB-lesioned rats was due to a shift in physostigmine dose response relationships. To test this possibility, different groups of 11 or 12 rats each with either sham or nbM + ANB lesions were prepared. Two weeks following the lesion procedure the rats were trained in the one-trial passive avoidance paradigm. Immediately following passive avoidance training, 6 doses of physostigmine (0.0, 0.015, 0.03, 0.06, 0.12 and 0.24 mg/kg) were administered to the rats in the two lesion groups. Upon retention testing 72 h later (Fig. 2), the nbM + ANB lesions led to profound memory impairments (ANOVA, $F(1/104) = 12.4$, $p < 0.001$). In addition, there were significant effects of physostigmine ($F(5/104) = 4.5$, $p < 0.002$) and lesion condition by physostigmine interactions ($F(5/104) = 3.5$, $p < 0.01$). The 0.03 mg/kg dose of physostigmine enhanced the retention test performance of sham-operated rats (Newman-Keuls, $p < 0.01$) replicating earlier findings (Haroutunian et al., 1985). The retention test performance of the nbM + ANB-lesioned rats was not improved by any of the doses of physostigmine investigated ($p > 0.10$). Neurochemically, an

88.4% depletion of cortical NE in nbM + ANB-lesioned rats and a 27.7% and 26.4% depletion of frontal cortical ChAT and AChE activity ($p < 0.01$) was observed.

Since a wide dose range of physostigmine was used in this experiment, it is unlikely that the failure of physostigmine to potentiate retention test performance in nbM + ANB-lesioned rats was attributable to lesion-induced shifts in dose response relationships. Thus one reason for the apparent impotency of cholinomimetics in a significant proportion of AD victims may be the presence of noradrenergic and cholinergic deficits.

The α_2 adrenergic agonist clonidine has been reported to enhance the cognitive test performance in aged monkeys suffering forebrain noradrenergic deficits (Arnsten and Goldman-Rakic, 1985a,b), to prevent the amnesia which results from cycloheximide administration to rats (Quartermaine and Botwinick, 1975), and to enhance memory in Korsakoff's psychosis (Mair and McEntee, 1986; McEntee and Mair, 1980). The ability of clonidine, administered alone or in conjunction with physostigmine, to enhance the retention test performance of nbM + ANB-lesioned rats was assessed in the next experiment. Different groups of lesioned and control rats ($n = 11$–12) received one-trial passive avoidance training followed immediately by s.c. injections of either 0.06 mg/kg physostigmine alone, or 0.06 mg/kg physostigmine plus one of several doses (0, 0.01 or 0.5 mg/kg) of the α_2 adrenergic receptor agonist clonidine. Retention of passive avoidance was assessed 72 h later.

The results of this experiment are depicted in Fig. 3. Analyses of variance revealed significant lesion ($F(1/103) = 5.2$, $p < 0.03$), drug ($F(5/103) = 5.4$, $p < 0.001$) and lesion by drug condition interactions ($F(5/103) = 5.9$, $p < 0.001$). Independent group comparisons showed that nbM + ANB lesion induced memory deficits were reversed by either high doses (0.5 mg/kg) of clonidine alone or much smaller doses of clonidine (0.01 mg/kg) administered in conjunction with 0.06 mg/kg physostigmine ($p < 0.01$). In agree-

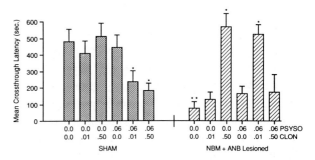

Fig. 3. Effects of post-acquisition administration of clonidine (0, 0.01 and 0.5 mg/kg) and physostigmine (0 and 0.06 mg/kg), either alone or in combination, on the 72 h retention of passive avoidance in nbM + ANB-lesioned rats.

ment with recently published data (Ordy et al., 1988), low doses of clonidine administered alone were without effect. The combination of physostigmine and clonidine had an amnestic effect on the performance of the sham-operated rats ($p < 0.03$).

The generality of these findings was assessed in another experiment using oxotremorine (0.05–0.1 mg/kg) as the cholinomimetic agent. Neither oxotremorine nor clonidine alone were able to reverse nbM + ANB lesion-induced passive avoidance deficits. The combined administration of the two drugs led to significant enhancement of retention test performance ($p < 0.006$). This study also demonstrates that forebrain noradrenergic lesions not only block the activity of physostigmine, but also impede the effects of cholinomimetics with diverse mechanisms of action.

The experiments summarized above suggest that the cognitive deficits of animals refractory to the enhancing effects of cholinomimetics can be reversed by treatments tailored to their specific deficit states. It is also apparent that not only are there behavioral and cognitive deficits which can be associated with cholinergic and noradrenergic systems, but deficits in one system can affect the functioning of the other.

Cholinergic / serotonergic interactions.

Noradrenergic deficits block cholinomimetic enhancement of retention test performance but somatostatinergic deficits do not. These findings demonstrate that not all lesions interfere with cholinomimetic efficacy. It is important, therefore, to evaluate independently the contribution of different system lesions to the responsivity to pharmacological treatments. A substantial literature now shows that serotonergic cells (German et al., 1987; Yamamoto and Hirano, 1985; Curcio and Kemper, 1984;), serotonin levels and metabolites (Palmer et al., 1987ab; Reynolds, et al, 1986; Gottfries et al., 1983), and serotonin S_1 and S_2 receptor numbers (Marcusson et al., 1987; Cross et al., 1986; Middlemiss et al., 1986; Perry et al., 1984) are significantly reduced in AD.

Perturbations of the serotonergic system can significantly affect performance on learning and memory tasks in animal model systems (Quartermain et al., 1988; Flood and Cherkin, 1987; Ogren, 1985, 1986; Altman et al., 1984). The direction of change caused by different manipulations of the serotonergic system appears unpredictable. The inconsistent and often confusing results of studies examining the involvement of the serotonergic system in learning and memory may in part be explained by the neurophysiology of this system. The serotonergic system is generally inhibitory, defuse, highly collateralized, tonically active, has a long duration of action, and has axonal transmitter releasing properties. It is quite possible that this system is involved in the modulation of attentional and arousal states (Fornal and Jacobs, 1987; Waterhouse et al., 1986; Lakoski and Aghajanian, 1985). Suggestive evidence for a primarily "state" modulating role for serotonin can be gleaned from the existing, though meager, results of clinical trials with serotonergic drugs in AD. For example, the administration of the selective serotonin reuptake blockers, alaproclate and zimeldine (Altman et al., 1984), leads to modest positive effects in AD patients, but these improvements are attributable to enhanced emotional function rather than alleviation of memory deficits.

There is little question that serotonergic and cholinergic systems interact in forebrain structures such as the cerebral cortex (Vanderwolf and Stewart, 1986; Lakoski and Aghajanian, 1985; Robinson, 1983), hippocampus (Vanderwolf and Stewart, 1986; Samanin et al., 1978), striatum (Gillet et al., 1985; Ladinsky et al., 1978; Samanin et al., 1978; Euvard, et al, 1977), and the nbM area (Pazos and Palacios, 1985; Pazos et al., 1985; Mitchell et al., 1984). One general conclusion which can be reached from these in vitro studies is that serotonin inhibits cholinergic activity presynaptically and dampens the postsynaptic effects of acetylcholine. Although the in vitro studies of cholinergic/serotonergic interactions have yielded generally consistent results, these results do not lend themselves to simple explanations from a behavioral or Alzheimer's disease perspective. At face value, the in vitro studies suggest that serotonergic hypofunction should result in the release of cholinergic cells from inhibition, leading to the enhancement of cholinergic function. If this hypothesis was correct, a negative correlation between serotonergic and cognitive deficits would be predicted in AD. This is clearly not the case. Furthermore, pharmacological data suggest a synergistic relationship between cholinergic and serotonergic functions. Serotonergic drugs appear to potentiate the effects of muscarinic agonists. Overt behavioral responses attributed to muscarinic receptor stimulation (e.g., purposeless chewing, salivation, tremor) are dependent upon and are enhanced by serotonergic activity (Stewart et al., 1987; Ogren et al., 1985a,b). In view of the conflict between the in vitro and in vivo studies, it must be assumed that the cholinergic and serotonergic systems interact in complex ways which are as yet unpredictable. Extensive pharmacological and neurochemical studies will be required to unravel this puzzle and formulate a hypothesis able to account for some of these data.

To date studies of the 5-HT system have focused on the influence of dl-*p*-chloroamphetamine (PCA) on forebrain neurochemistry, acquisition and retention of passive avoidance in naive rats, reten-

TABLE IV

Effects of pre-acquisition administration of 2.5 mg/kg PCA on short- and long-term passive retention test performance

Treatment	Retetion test interval		
	5 min	1 h	24 h
Saline	658 ± 135	453 ± 120	433 ± 1106
PCA	49 ± 18 [a]	273 ± 69	61 ± 28 [a]

[a] vs. saline-pretreated, $p < 0.01$.

tion of passive avoidance in nbM-lesioned rats, and the effects of single doses of physostigmine in sham-p-chloroamphetamine treated and nbM-lesioned-PCA treated rats. These studies have demonstrated that PCA has a deleterious effect on the acquisition and retention of passive avoidance responses and interferes with the retention test enhancing effects of physostigmine.

The possible effects of PCA on the acquisition of passive avoidance were studied in naive rats. Different groups of rats ($n = 8–10$) received 2.5 mg/kg PCA or saline 30 min before one-trial passive avoidance training. Shock intensity was set to 1.0 mA to minimize the possibility of floor effects. Rats were tested for retention of passive avoidance 5 min, 60 min, or 24 h after the training trial.

The results of this study are shown in Table IV. Saline-pretreated rats showed good retention test performance at all intervals tested. Pretreatment of the rats with PCA led to significant ($p < 0.02$) retention test performance deficits at the 5 min and 24 h intervals, but not at the 1 h retention interval. These data suggest that PCA affects passive avoidance behavior in a complex manner. One explanation of these results is that PCA affects not only mnemonic processes but also emotionality. Thus it is possible that PCA-induced 5-HT release/depletion leads to changes in emotionality, reflected in the 5 min retention test interval performance, and changes in long-term retention, reflected in the 24 h retention test interval deficit. It is also possible, of course, that PCA impairs acquisition directly, but the results of the

one hour retention test interval argue against this possibility.

It is noteworthy that the effects of PCA on performance in the passive avoidance paradigm appear to be restricted to pretraining administration of the drug. When PCA (2.5 mg/kg) was administered to naive rats ($n = 8$) immediately following training on a passive avoidance task, no drug effects could be detected on retention test performance 72 h later.

The effects of pretraining administration of PCA to sham-operated and nbM-lesioned rats were assessed in this experiment. Rats received lesions of the nbM or sham operations. The nbM lesion procedures were identical to those already described except that N-methyl-D-aspartic acid (NMDA-75 nmol) was used as the neurotoxin in this study. Two to three weeks following the operative procedure, lesioned and sham groups were further subdivided into PCA or saline treatment conditions ($n = 7–10$). Each rat received an i.p. injection of either 2.5 mg/kg PCA or saline 30 min before passive avoidance training. Retention of passive avoidance was assessed 72 h later. The training shock intensity was raised to 1.2 mA in this study to allow detection of possible amnesic effects of PCA in the nbM-lesioned rats.

The results of this study were similar to those presented in Table V and showed that (a) rats receiving NMDA lesions of the nbM performed poorly on the retention of passive avoidance relative to sham-operated rats (ANOVA, $p < 0.03$), and (b) that the pretraining administration of PCA to nbM-lesioned rats leads to performance deficits greater than those expected from nbM lesions alone. The infusion of NMDA into the region of the nbM produced consistent and profound depletions of cortical ChAT and AChE. ChAT was depleted by 36.6% ($F(1/23) = 54.4$, $p = 0.00001$) while AChE levels were reduced by 39.7% ($F(1/23) = 47.5$, $p = 0.00001$). There were no differences in the ChAT and AChE deficits between lesioned or sham-operated rats receiving PCA ($F < 1.0$). The results of this study demonstrate that PCA-induced perturbation of central serotonergic systems has profound effects on the retention test performance of rats, even in the presence of significant forebrain cholinergic impairments. It is also possible to argue that serotonergic influences on passive avoidance retention test performance are independent of the forebrain cholinergic system, since forebrain cholinergic lesions fail to block the effects of PCA on passive avoidance behavior.

The failure of forebrain cholinergic lesions to block the effects of PCA does not necessarily imply that cholinergic and serotonergic systems do not interact in the mediation of passive avoidance behavior. The next experiment tested whether perturbation of the serotonergic system would affect the efficacy of physostigmine to potentiate retention test performance.

Forty-three rats received bilateral lesions of the nbM using 50 nmol infusions of NMDA. Forty-seven rats received sham operations. Approximately two weeks later all rats were trained in the standard passive avoidance paradigm using 1 mA shock. Moderate shock (1 mA) was used to ensure that some learning took place in the nbM-lesioned rats allowing for further impairment by PCA. Half the rats in the lesioned and sham-operated conditions received 2.5 mg/kg PCA 30 min before passive avoidance training, the remaining rats received saline injections. Immediately following passive avoidance training each group received either saline or 0.06 mg/kg physostigmine. Retention test performance was assessed 72 h later. Thus four groups of sham-lesioned rats and four groups of nbM-lesioned rats were formed consisting of animals receiving (1) saline before training and saline following training; (2) saline before training and physostigmine following training; (3) PCA before training and saline following training; and PCA before training and physostigmine following training.

Lesions of the nbM led to profound ($p < 0.01$) passive avoidance deficits despite the high intensity of shock employed (Table V). The administration of PCA to sham-operated rats resulted in a significant passive avoidance retention test performance deficit ($p < 0.05$). The administration of

TABLE V

Effects of PCA (2.5 mg/kg) pretreatment on physostigmine-induced enhancement of 72-h retention test performance in sham-operated and nbM-lesioned rats

Condition	SAL/ SAL	SAL/ PHY	PCA/ SAL	PCA/ PHY
Sham nbM-	520 ± 118	351 ± 91	199 ± 67 [a]	111 ± 42 [a]
lesioned	207 ± 87 [a]	375 ± 79 [b]	34 ± 12 [b]	72 ± 29 [b]

[a] vs. Sham SAL/SAL, $p < 0.05$.
[b] vs. nbM-lesioned SAL/SAL, $p < 0.05$.

PCA to nbM-lesioned rats led to an even greater impairment of passive avoidance retention test performance than that produced by the nbM lesion alone ($p < 0.05$). These results constitute a direct replication of our previous findings. Although physostigmine did improve the retention test performance of saline pretreated nbM-lesioned rats ($p < 0.05$), pretreatment with PCA completely blocked responsivity to physostigmine. Furthermore, physostigmine failed to relieve the retention test performance deficit of sham-operated rats pretreated with PCA. Physostigmine dose response studies must still be run in order to determine whether the PCA induced blockade of physostigmine-induced enhancement observed in this study is absolute or represents a shift in the dose response curve. It is evident, however, that serotonergic systems do exert some modulatory influence upon the activity of physostigmine.

The final study in this series examined the neurochemical consequences of PCA treatment. Six groups of six naive male rats (mean weight 270 g) each received an s.c. injection of 2.5 mg/kg PCA. One group of six rats received saline. The PCA treated rats were then killed by decapitation 15 s, 15, 30, 45, 60 and 120 min following the PCA injection. One saline-injected rat was killed at each of these intervals. The results of this study are presented in Table VI, and demonstrate that the systemic administration of PCA to rats leads to significant perturbations of cortical aminergic systems. The administration of PCA led to substantial and significant ($p < 0.05$) decreases in

TABLE VI

Temporal effects of 2.5 mg/kg PCA on cortical neurochemical parameters

	Time (min)					
	0.5	15	30	45	60	120
5-HT	−8	+10	+8	−3	−31 [a]	−52 [a]
5-HIAA	−18 [a]	−22 [a]	−12	−10	−15 [a]	−29 [a]
DA	−37 [a]	−2	+5	+38 [a]	+20	+11
DOPAC	−28	−10	−24	−52 [a]	−55 [a]	−66 [a]
HVA	−39 [a]	−23 [a]	−14	−13	−20 [a]	−37 [a]
NE	−3.5	+7	+16 [a]	+15 [a]	+6	−4

Values represent percent change relative to saline-injected controls.

[a] vs. saline controls, $p < 0.05$.

cortical levels of 5-HT and 5-HIAA 60 and 120 min following drug infusion. It is also apparent that PCA affects not only serotonergic systems, but dopaminergic and noradrenergic systems as well.

The neurochemical analysis of PCA effects allows a more detailed interpretation of the behavioral studies discussed above. Most of the aminergic consequences of PCA administration become evident at least 30 min following its administration. The modulation of memory consolidation processes by drugs is dependent upon a close temporal association between learning and drug effects. It is not surprising, therefore, that post acquisition administration of PCA fails to affect retention test performance. The dopaminergic disturbances observed in this study preclude the attribution of the behavioral and pharmacological effects of PCA to the serotonergic system alone. Although strong evidence implicating the dopaminergic system in the modulation of learning and memory is lacking, its contribution to the present findings cannot be readily dismissed. Our ongoing studies using serotonergic lesions, direct agonists, and antagonists should help clarify these results.

The studies outlined above have demonstrated the necessity for treating Alzheimer's disease as a multitransmitter system disease requiring a multitransmitter approach towards its treatment. Each affected system appears to make a specific contribution to the symptoms of the disease. Some systems, like the forebrain cholinergic system, affect cognitive performance directly. Other transmitter systems, like the noradrenergic system, have a greater influence upon responsivity to cholinomimetics. Still others, like the somatostatinergic system, do not appear to have a dramatic cognitive influence. Our understanding of systems interaction at a central level is not complete enough to allow a priori predictions of the nature and magnitude of these interactions. The currently available animal model systems are at best approximations of the neurochemical deficits in AD. Predictions based on these model systems must be evaluated in extensive clinical trials. Trials to evaluate the ability of adrenergic agents to potentiate the effects of cholinomimetics on cognitive performance are currently under way at our center.

References

Adolfsson, R., Gottfries, C.G., Roos, B.E., and Winblad, B. (1979) Changes in the brain catecholamines in patients with dementia of Alzheimer type. Br. J. Psychiat., 135: 216–223.

Altman, H.J., Nordy, D.A. and Ogren, S.O. (1984) Role of serotonin in memory: Facilitation by alaproclate and zimeldine. Psychopharmacology, 84: 496–501.

Andrade, R.A. and Aghajanian, G.K. (1985) Opiate and α2-adrenoceptor-induced hyperpolarization of locus coeruleus neurons in brain slices: reversal by cyclic-AMP analogues. J. Neurosci., 5: 2359–2364.

Arai, H., Kosaka, K. and Iizuka, R. (1984) Changes of biogenic amines and their metabolites in postmortem brains from patients with Alzheimer's-type dementia. J. Neurochem., 43: 388–393.

Arnsten, A.F.T and Goldman-Rakic, P.S. (1985a) α2-adrenergic mechanisms in prefrontal cortex associated with cognitive decline in aged nonhuman primates. Science, 230: 1273–1279.

Arnsten, A.F.T and Goldman-Rakic, P.S. (1985b) Catecholamines and cognitive decline in aged nonhuman primates. Ann. N.Y. Acad. Sci., 444: 218–234.

Bondareff, W., Mountjoy, C.Q. and Roth, M. (1982) Loss of neurons of origin of the adrenergic projection to cerebral cortex (nucleus locus coeruleus) in senile dementia. Neurology, 32: 164–168.

Cross, A.J. (1987) Serotonin in neurodegenerative disorders. In N.N. Osborn and M. Hamon, (Eds), Neuronal Serotonin, John Wiley, New York, 231–254.

Cross, A.J., Crow, T.J., Ferrier, I.N., and Johnson, J.A. (1986) Selectivity of the reduction of serotonin S2 receptors in Alzheimer-type dementia. *Neurobiol. Aging*, 7: 3–7.

Curcio, C. and Kemper, T. (1984) Nucleus raphe dorsalis in dementia of the Alzheimer's type: Neurofibrillary changes and neuronal packing density. *J. Neuropath. Exp. Neurol.*, 43: 359–368.

Davies, P. and Terry, R.D. (1981) Cortical somatostatin-like immunoreactivity in cases of Alzheimer's disease and senile dementia of Alzheimer's type. *Neurobiol. Aging*, 2: 9–14.

Davies, P., Katzman, R. and Terry, R.D. (1980) Reduced somatostatin-like-immunoreactivity in cerebral cortex from cases of Alzheimer's disease Alzheimer's senile dementia. *Nature*, 288: 279–280.

Davis, K.L. and Mohs, R.C. (1982) Enhancement of memory processes in Alzheimer's disease with multiple dose intravenous physostigmine. *Am. J. Psychiatry*, 139: 1421–1424.

Decker, M.W. and Gallagher, M. (1987) Scopolamine-disruption of radial arm maze performance: Modification by noradrenergic depletion. *Brain Res.*, 417: 59–69.

DeSouza, E.B., Whitehouse, P.J., Kuhar, M.J., Price, D.L. and Vale, W.W. (1986) Reciprocal changes in corticotropin-releasing factor (CRF)-like immunoreactivity and CRF receptors in cerebral cortex of Alzheimer's disease. *Nature*, 319: 593–595.

Egan, T.M. and North, R.A. (1985) Actions of acetylcholine and nicotine on rat locus coeruleus neurons in vitro. *Br. J. Pharmacol.*, 85: 733–738.

Egan, T.M., Henderson, G., North, R.A. and Williams, J.T. (1983) Noradrenaline mediated synaptic inhibition in rat locus coeruleus neurons. *J. Physiol.*, 345: 477–488.

Engberg, G. and Svensson, T.H. (1980) Pharmacological analysis of cholinergic receptor mediated regulation of brain norepinephrine neurons. *J. Neural Trans.*, 49: 137–142.

Euvard, C., Javoy, F., Herbert, A. and Glowinski, J. (1977) Effect of quipazine, a serotonin-like drug, on striatal cholinergic interneurons. *Eur. J. Pharmacol.*, 41: 281–289.

Flood, J.F. and Cherkin, A. (1989) Fluoxetine enhances memory processing in mice. *Psychopharmacology*, 93: 36–43.

Fonnum, F. (1975) A rapid radiochemical method of determination of choline acetyltransferase. *J. Neurochem.*, 24: 407–409.

Fornal, C.A. and Jacobs, B.L. (1987) Physiological and behavioral correlates of serotonergic single-unit activity. In N.N. Osborne and M. Hamon (Eds), *Neuronal Serotonin*, John Wiley, New York, 305–346.

German, D.C., White, C.L. and Sparkman, D.R. (1987) Alzheimer's disease: Neurofibrillary tangles in nuclei that project to the cerebral cortex. *Neuroscience*, 21: 305–312.

Gillet, G., Ammor, S. and Fillon, G. (1985) Serotonin inhibits acetylcholine release from rat striatum slices: Evidence for a pre-synaptic receptor mediated effect. *J. Neurochem.*, 45: 1678–1691.

Gold, P.E. and Zornetzer, S.F. (1983) The mnemon and its juices: Neuromodulation of memory processes. *Behav. Neural Biol.* 38: 151–189.

Gottfries, C.G., Adolfsson, R., Aquilonius, S.-M. Carlsson, A.,

Eckernas, S.-A., Nordberg, L., Oreland, L. Svennerholm, L., Wiberg, A. and Windblad, B. (1983) Biochemical changes in dementia disorders of Alzheimer type (AD/SDAT) *Neurobiol. Aging.* 4: 261–271.

Haroutunian, V., Kanof, P. and Davis, K.L. (1985) Pharmacological alleviation of cholinergic lesions induced memory deficits in rats. *Life Sci.*, 37: 945–952.

Haroutunian, V., Kanof, P.D., Tsuboyama, G.K., Campbell, G.A. and Davis, K.L. (1986) Animal models of Alzheimer's disease: Behavior, pharmacology, transplants. *Can. J. Neurol. Sci.*, 13: 385–393.

Haroutunian, V., Mantin, R., Campbell, G.A., Tsuboyama, G.K. and Davis, K.L. (1987) Cysteamine-induced depletion of central somatostatin-like immunoreactivity: effects on behavior, learning, memory and brain neurochemistry. *Brain Res.* 403: 234–242.

Haroutunian, V., Kanof, P.D. and Davis, K.L. (1989a) Interactions of forebrain cholinergic and somatostatinergic systems in the rat. *Brain Res.*, in press.

Haroutunian, V., Kanof, P.D., Tsuboyama, G. and Davis, K.L. (1989b) Restoration of cholinomimetic activity by clonidine in cholinergic plus noradrenergic lesioned rats. *Brain Res.*, in press.

Huygens, P., Baratti, C.M., Gardella, J.L. and Filinger, E. (1980) Brain catecholamine modifications. The effects on memory facilitation induced by oxotremorine in mice. *Psychopharmacology*, 69: 291–294.

Johnson, C.D. and Russell, R.L. (1975) A rapid, simple radiometric assay for acetylcholinesterase, suitable for multiple determinations. *Anal. Biochem.*, 64: 229–232.

Ladinsky, H., Consolo, S., Peri, G. Crunelli, V. and Samanin, R. (1978) Pharmacological evidence for a serotonergic-cholinergic link in the striatum. In D. Jenden (Ed.), *Advances in Behavioral Biology: Cholinergic Mechanisms and Psychopharmacology*, Plenum Press, New York, 615–627.

Lakoski, J.M. and Aghajanian, G.K. (1985) Effects of ketanserin on neuronal responses to serotonin in the prefrontal cortex, lateral geniculate and dorsal raphe nucleus. *Neuropharmacology*, 24: 265–273.

Mair, R.G. and McEntee, W.J. (1986) Cognitive enhancement in Korsakoff's psychosis by clonidine: A comparison with 1-dopa and ephedrine. *Psychopharmacology*, 88: 374–380.

Mann, D.M., Lincoln, J., Yates, P.O., Stamp, J.E. and Toper, S. (1980) Changes in the monoamine containing neurons of the human CNS in senile dementia. *Br. J. Psychiat.*, 136: 533–541.

Marcusson, J.O., Alafuzoff, I., Backstrom, I.T. Ericson, E., Gottfries, C.G. and Winblad, B. (1987) 5-Hydroxytryptamine-sensitive [3H] imipramine binding of protein nature in the human brain. II: Effect of normal aging and dementia disorders. *Brain Res.*, 425: 137–145.

Maruyama, Y., Oshima, T. and Nakajima, E. III. (1989) Simultaneous determination of catecholamines in rat brain by reversed-phase liquid chromatography with electrochemical detection. *Life Sci.*, 26: 1115–1120.

Mason, S.T. (1979) Noradrenaline: reward or extinction? *Neurosci and Biobehav. Rev.*, 3: 1–10.

Mason, S.T. and Fibiger, H.C. (1979) Possible behavioral function for noradrenaline-acetylcholine interaction in brain. *Nature,* 277: 396–397.

McEntee, W.J. and Mair, R.G. (1980) Memory enhancement in Korsakoff's psychosis by clonidine: Further evidence for a noradrenergic deficit. *Ann. Neurol.* 7: 466–470.

McNaughton, N. and Mason, S.T. (1980) The neuropsychology and neuropharmacology of the dorsal ascending noradrenergic bundle — A review. *Prog. Neurobiol.,* 14: 157–219.

Middlemiss, D.N., Palmer, A.M., Edel, N. and Bowen, D.M. (1986) Binding of the novel serotonin agonist 8-hydroxy-2-(di-*n*-propylamino) tetralin in normal and Alzheimer brain. *J. Neurochem.,* 46: 993–996.

Mitchell, I.J., Stuart, A.M., Slater, P., Unwin, H.P. and Crossman, A.R. (1984) Autoradiographic demonstration of 5HT$_1$ binding sites in the primate basal nucleus of meynert. *Eur. J. Pharmacol.,* 104: 189–190.

Mohs, R.C. and Davis, K.L. (1987) The experimental pharmacology of Alzheimer's disease and related dementias. In H.Y. Meltzer (Ed), *Psychopharmacology: The Third Generation of Progress,* Raven Press, New York, 921–928.

Ogren, S.O. (1985) Evidence for a role of brain serotonergic neurotransmission in avoidance learning. *Acta Physiol. Scand. Suppl.,* 544: 1–71.

Ogren, S.O. (1986) Analysis of the avoidance learning deficit induced by the serotonin releasing compound *p*-chloroamphetamine. *Brain Res. Bull.,* 16: 645–660.

Ogren, S.O., Nordstrom, O., Danielsson, E., Peterson, L.-L. and Bartfai, T. (1985a) In vivo and in vitro studies on the potentiation of muscarinic receptor stimulation by alaproclate, a selective 5-HT uptake blocker. *J. Neural Trans.,* 61: 1–20.

Ogren, S.O., Carlsson, S. and Bartfai, T. (1985b) Serotonergic potentiation of muscarinic agonist evoked tremor and salivation in rat and mouse. *Psychopharmacology,* 86: 258–264.

Ordy, J.M., Thomas, G.J., Volpe, B.T., Dunlap, W.P. and Colombo, P.M. (1988) An animal model of human-type memory loss based on aging, lesions, forebrain ischemia, and drug studies with the rat. *Neurobiol. Aging,* 9: 667–683.

Palmer, A.M., Wilcock, G.K., Esiri, M.M. Francis, P.T. and Bowen, D.M. (1987) Monoaminergic innervation of the frontal and temporal lobes in Alzheimer's disease. *Brain Res.,* 401: 231–238.

Palmer, A.M., Francis, P.T., Benton, J.S., Sims, N.R., Mann, D.M.A., Neary, D., Snowden, J.S. and Bowen, D.M. (1989b) Presynaptic serotonergic dysfunction in patients with Alzheimer's disease. *J. Neurochem.,* 48: 8–15.

Palmer, A.M. Francis, P.T., Bowen, D.M., Neary, J.S., Mann, D.M.A., Snowden, J.S. (1989b) Catecholaminergic neurons assessed antemortem in Alzheimer's disease. *Brain Res.,* 414: 365–375.

Pazos, A. and Palacios, J.M. (1985) Quantitative autoradiographic mapping of serotonin receptors in the rat brain. II: Serotonin-2 receptors. *Brain Res.,* 346: 203–230.

Pazos, A., Cortes, R. and Palacios, J.M. (1985) Quantitative autoradiographic mapping of serotonin receptors in the rat brain. I: Serotonin-1 receptors. *Brain Res.,* 346: 231–249.

Perry, E.K., Perry, R.H., Candy, J.M., Fairbairn, A.F., Blessed,

G., Dick, D.J. and Tomlinson, B.E. (1984) Cortical serotonin-S$_2$ receptor binding abnormalities in patients with Alzheimer's disease: comparisons with Parkinson's disease. *Neurosci. Lett.,* 51: 353–357.

Powers, R.E., Walker, L.C., DeSouza, E.B., Vale, W.W., Struble, R.G., Whitehouse, P.J. and Price, D.L. (1987) Immunohistochemical study of neurons containing corticotropin-releasing factor in Alzheimer's disease. *Synapse,* 1: 405–410.

Quartermaine, D. and Botwinick, C.Y. (1975) Role of biogenic amines in the reversal of cycloheximide-induced amnesia. *J. Comp. Physiol. Psychol.,* 88: 386–401.

Quartermain, D., Judge, M.E. and Leo, P. (1988) Attenuation of forgetting by pharmacological stimulation of aminergic neurotransmitter systems. *Pharmacol. Biochem. Behav.,* 30: 77–81.

Reynolds, G.P., Arnold, L., Rossor, M.N., Iversen, L.L., Mountjoy, C.Q. and Roth, M. (1984) Reduced binding of [^{3}H]ketanserin to cortical 5-HT$_2$ receptors in senile dementia of the Alzheimer's type. *Neurosci. Lett.,* 44: 47–51.

Robinson, S.E. (1983) Effects of serotonergic lesions on cholinergic neurons in the hippocampus, cortex, and striatum. *Life Sci.,* 32: 345–353.

Rossor, M.N., Emson, P.C., Montjoy, C.Q., Roth, M. and Iversen, L.L. (1980) Reduced amounts of immunoreactive somatostatin in the temporal cortex in senile dementia of Alzheimer's type. *Neurosci. Lett.,* 20: 373–377.

Samanin, R., Quattrone, A., Peri, G., Ladinsky, H. and Consolo, S. (1978) Evidence of an interaction between serotonergic and cholinergic neurons in the corpus striatum and hippocampus or the rat brain. *Brain Res.,* 151: 73–82.

Santucci, A.C., Haroutunian, V., Bierer, L.M. and Davis, K.L. (1989) Approaches to the treatment of Alzheimer's disease. In R. Lister and H. Weingartner (Eds.), *Perspectives in Cognitive Neuroscience.* Oxford University Press, in press.

Shimohama, S., Taniguchi, T., Fujiwara, M. and Kameyama, M. (1986) Biochemical characterization of α-adrenergic receptors in human brain and changes in Alzheimer-type dementia. *J. Neurochem.,* 47: 1294–1301.

Stewart, B., Rose, S., Jenner, P. and Marsden, C.D. (1987) Pilocarpine-induced purposeless chewing behaviour in rats is dependent on intact central stores of 5-HT. *Eur. J. Pharmacol.,* 142: 173–176.

Vanderwolf, C.H. and Stewart, D.J. (1986) Joint cholinergic-serotonergic control of neocortical and hippocampal electrical activity in relation to behavior: Effects of scopolamine, ditran, trifluoperazine and amphetamine. *Physiol. Behav.,* 38: 57–65.

Waterhouse, B.D., Moises, H.C. and Woodward, D,J. (1980) Noradrenergic modulation of somatosensory cortical neuronal responses to iontophoretically applied putative neurotransmitters. *Exp. Neurol.,* 69: 30–49.

Waterhouse, B.D., Moises, H.C. and Woodward, D,J. (1981) Alpha-receptor-mediated facilitation of somatosensory cortical neuronal responses to excitatory synaptic inputs and iontophoretically applied acetylcholine. *Neuropharmacology,* 20: 907–920.

Waterhouse, B.D., Moises, H.C. and Woodward, D.J. (1986) Interaction of serotonin with somatosensory cortical neuronal responses to afferent synaptic inputs and putative neurotransmitters. *Brain Res. Bull.,* 17: 507–518.

Yamamoto, T. and Hirano, A. (1985) Nucleus raphe dorsalis in Alzheimer's disease: Neurofibrillary tangles and loss of large neurons. *Ann. Neurol.,* 17: 573–577.

Zornetzer, S. (1985) Catecholamine system involvement in age-related memory dysfunction. *Ann. NY Acad. Sci.,* 444: 242–252.

S.-M. Aquilonius and P.-G. Gillberg (Eds.)
Progress in Brain Research, Vol. 84
© 1990 Elsevier Science Publishers B.V. (Biomedical Division)

CHAPTER 36

Positron emission tomography and cholinergic mechanisms: an overview

M. Mazière, M. Khalili-Varasteh, J. Delforge, M. Janier, D. Leguludec, C. Prenant and A. Syrota

Service Hospitalier Frédéric Joliot, URA CEA-CNRS 1285, 4 Place Gal Leclerc, Commissariat à l'Energie Atomique, 91406 Orsay, France

Introduction

Recent progress in our understanding of the mechanisms involved in neurotransmission is mainly due to technical revolutions that have arisen, in the neuroscience field, in the last decade. Among them, positron emission tomography (PET) has offered new possibilities in clinical research for the in vivo investigation of physiology and pathology of the human brain and heart. It is now possible to measure in an atraumatic manner local tissue functions (glucose and oxygen utilization), pH, cerebral blood flow and neurotransmission systems (receptors-neurotransmitters) using specific radiotracers labeled with positron-emitting isotopes of basic elements and positron-detection systems (positron cameras) for external detection. This paper will deal with the use of PET to study in vivo cholinergic neurotransmission. Some methodological points will be outlined and an overview of the studies carried out to investigate brain and heart physiopathology will be given. An approach of an absolute quantification in vivo of muscarinic receptors (B_{max}, K_d) by using a mathematical model established from PET data will also be presented. The emphasis will be on the work carried out at Service Frederic Joliot, Orsay. To conclude, the applications of the PET methodology will be discussed and future areas of study, in this field of research, will be considered.

Cholinergic radioligands available for PET studies

Among the positron-emitting radioisotopes, carbon 11 is one of the most commonly used for PET studies. In spite of its short half-life of 20.4 min, this externally detectable radioisotope can be used for isotopic labeling of drugs with specific activity high enough to minimize non-specific binding. As shown in Table I, many ligands labeled with carbon 11 have been proposed during the last decade for the in vivo study of nicotinic and muscarinic cholinergic neurotransmission systems. Nicotine, choline and muscarinic receptors have been studied in vivo using PET. However, it is only recently that a great effort has been made in this field. Consequently, we have to wait for its impact on clinical research.

PET studies of nicotinic cholinergic receptors

In Alzheimer's disease, a loss of presynaptic cholinergic markers has been found in the cerebral cortex (Davies and Verth, 1978). However, in contrast to muscarinic receptors, little attention has been paid to possible changes in nicotinic cholinergic receptors. Recently, a consistent and severe loss of nicotinic receptors was found in this disease (Whitehouse et al., 1986). In rats and mice, chronic administration of nicotine increases nico-

348

TABLE I

Cholinergic ligands for PET studies

Nicotinic system
[^{11}C]Nicotine (Mazière et al., 1976)

Muscarinic system
Central nervous system
Antagonist
[^{11}C]Scopolamine (Vora et al., 1983)
                       (Mulholland et al., 1988a)
[^{11}C]Dexetimide, [^{11}C]-
Levetimide (Dannals et al., 1988)
[^{11}C](+)-2α-Tropanyl
benzilate (TRB) (Mulholland et al., 1988b)
[^{11}C]N-Methyl-4-piperidyl
benzilate (NMPB) (Mulholland et al., 1988c)
[^{11}C]Quinuclidinyl benzilate
(QNB) (Prenant et al., 1989)
[^{11}C]Benztropine mesylate
(cogentin) (Dewey et al., 1989)
Agonist
2-Ethyl-8-[^{11}C]methyl
2,8-diazaspiro (4,5)
decane-1,3-dione (RS 86) (Livni and Elmaleh, 1989)
Choline (metabolism,
transport)
[^{11}C]Choline (Bergström et al., 1981)
                  (Gauthier et al., 1985)
[^{11}C]Pyrrolidinocholine (Redies et al., 1988)

Peripheral nervous system
[^{11}C]MQNG (Mazière et al., 1981)
[^{11}C]MTRB (Mulholland et al., 1989)

tinic receptor density in cerebral cortex (Schwartz and Kellar, 1983). To study in vivo by PET the plasticity of nicotinic receptors and nicotine itself, nicotine was labeled with carbon 11. The labeling of the active isomer L-nicotine was performed with high yield and high specific activity (Mazière et al., 1976) by methylation of nor(−)nicotine with [^{11}C]formaldehyde according to Borch's reaction (Borch and Hassid, 1972). After i.v. administration of [^{11}C]nicotine in baboons, PET studies showed that (Mazière et al., 1979) during the first minutes after injection, the radioactivity is quite high in the brain, liver and kidneys. While in the brain the activity decreases sharply with time, in the liver and kidneys the radioactivity decreases less rapidly. In the brain, [^{11}C]nicotine readily penetrates the blood brain barrier and accu-

mulates very rapidly mostly in cortical structures (frontal, temporal, occipital) and less in the cerebellum. In the eyes, the radioactivity remained more stable with time than in the brain. This labeling could correspond to the retina as it has been previously demonstrated with [^{14}C]nicotine (Schmiterlow et al., 1965). Our preliminary results obtained in live baboons using PET were recently confirmed using [^{3}H]nicotine in mice (Broussolle et al., 1989) and [^{11}C]nicotine in man (Nybäck et al., 1989). However, the high non-specific binding of nicotine and its very rapid wash out of the brain makes it difficult to study quantitatively this drug using PET.

PET studies of muscarinic cholinergic receptors

Muscarinic cholinergic receptors are highly distributed throughout the body. In mouse, after labeling by [^{3}H]QNB, it was shown that in the central nervous system, these receptors were mainly concentrated in the cerebral cortex, hippocampus, and colliculi; a moderate concentration was observed in hindbrain nuclei, in the caudate nucleus, putamen and substantia innominata while a low level of binding was observed in thalamic and hypothalamic regions, reticular nuclei and cerebellum (Pauly et al., 1989). In the peripheral nervous system, muscarinic receptor densities were higher in heart, ileum and pancreas. Two different muscarinic receptor subtypes were first characterized: M_1 subtypes which are more dense in the CNS (cerebral cortex, striatum and hippocampus) while M_2 sites predominate in the periphery (heart, ileum, pancreas) as well as in cerebellum and pons-medulla (Hirschowitz et al., 1984). More recently, development of AF-DX 116 a new M_2 antagonist, has led to the suggestion that M_2 receptors may be subdivided into two classes: one with high affinity for AF-DX 116 and one with low affinity (Giachetti et al., 1986). Three subtypes of muscarinic receptor have, now, been mainly proposed: M_1, M_2, M_3 (Dodds et al., 1987). The existence of several subtypes of muscarinic receptors has been confirmed by cloning and sequencing DNA genes which code the receptor proteins (Bonner et al., 1987; Fukuda et al., 1987). Many ligands in vitro appear to show selective properties for M_1 and M_2 subtypes. However, this selectivity is almost relative depending on the degree of the difference in their binding affinities (Hammer et al., 1980). Moreover, pirenzepine (M_1 selective) and AF-DX 116 (M_2 selective) cannot cross the blood–brain barrier and thus cannot be candidates for selective muscarinic receptor ligands for brain studies by PET; but they can be useful to characterize muscarinic receptors on peripheral effector organs. An attempt to study muscarinic receptors by PET was made in our laboratory using [^{11}C]QNB and [^{11}C]MQNB respectively for brain and heart investigations.

Cardiac muscarinic receptors

The neurotransmitters acetylcholine and norepinephrine exert their chronotropic and inotropic effects on the heart by an opposite coupling of the cholinergic and β-adrenergic receptors to adenylate cyclase. While β-adrenoreceptors activate adenylate cyclase, muscarinic receptors inhibit it (Nathanson, 1987). The most commonly used radioligand [^{3}H]QNB (quinuclidinyl benzilate) appears to recognize identical populations of muscarinic receptors. QNB does not differentiate between M_1 and M_2 receptor subtypes. Competition curves for antagonists at the [^{3}H]QNB labeled sites are monophasic. In contrast, the competition curves for muscarinic agonists are biphasic indicating the presence of high and low affinity states of the receptors. However, it has been recently shown that, in the heart, [^{3}H]QNB labels more sites than do two other hydrophilic muscarinic antagonists, [^{3}H]N-methyl scopolamine and [^{3}H]N-methyl QNB ([^{3}H]MQNB), the quarternary derivative of QNB (Brown and Goldstein, 1986). Thus, these findings together with preliminary works on [^{3}H]MQNB (Gibson et al., 1979) strengthen the choice of labeling MQNB with carbon 11 to study the cardiac muscarinic receptor in vivo by PET. MQNB was labeled

TABLE II

[^{11}C]MQNB saturation studies in baboon hearts

[^{11}C]MQNB i.v. injected			[^{11}C]MQNB heart uptake to $+15$ min
mCi	nmol	nmol/kg	
5.04	5.46	0.398	$4.9 \cdot 10^{-2}$
8.91	10.4	0.619	$4.5 \cdot 10^{-2}$
5.9	11.5	0.709	$3.5 \cdot 10^{-2}$
7.45	11.8	0.715	$3.8 \cdot 10^{-2}$
7.84	9.04	0.759	$3.9 \cdot 10^{-2}$
6.04	11.0	0.786	$4.3 \cdot 10^{-2}$
7.86	16.7	1.027	$3.9 \cdot 10^{-2}$
7.87	16.9	1.224	$3.4 \cdot 10^{-2}$
14.3	39.0	2.56	$3.5 \cdot 10^{-2}$
11.4	32.7	2.616	$3.5 \cdot 10^{-2}$
6.65	60.0	4.17	$2.8 \cdot 10^{-2}$
14.2	89.0	5.597	$1.75 \cdot 10^{-2}$
5.37	110.0	7.65	$2.4 \cdot 10^{-2}$
10.2	110.0	9.02	$2.0 \cdot 10^{-2}$
5.66	203.0	14.5	$0.94 \cdot 10^{-3}$

A decrease in the [^{11}C]MQNB heart uptake (% injected dose/cm^3) was observed 15 min after administration of increasing doses of cold MQNB injected together with the radioligand, showing the in vivo saturability of the [^{11}C]MQNB binding in the heart.

semi-automatically with high yield and high specific activity by methylation of QNB with carbon-labeled methyl iodide (Mazière et al., 1983). The first PET study on baboons (Mazière et al., 1981) showed that after i.v. administration of [^{11}C]MQNB, a high and selective concentration of the radioligand was observed in the heart; no accumulation of the radiotracer was seen in the lungs. As shown in Table II, the [^{11}C]MQNB binding in the heart was saturable by administration of increasing doses of cold MQNB. The [^{11}C]MQNB binding was displaceable (Table III) by i.v. injections of either atropine or cold MQNB. In the liver (Fig. 1), a high concentration of radioactivity appears after administration of [^{11}C] MQNB. However, the binding of the radiotracer cannot be displaced by MQNB showing the nonspecific properties of the [^{11}C]MQNB bound in this organ. In contrast, a very high and rapid wash out of the radioactivity was seen in the heart and even in the eyes, indicating the high specificity of the in vivo binding of [^{11}C]MQNB for heart and

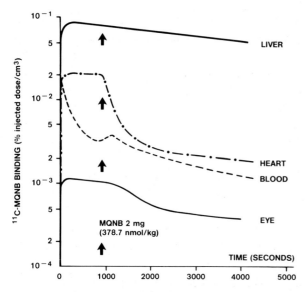

Fig. 1. [¹¹C]MQNB displacement studies in baboon. Displacement of [¹¹C]MQNB by cold MQNB injected 15 min after the radiotracer was observed in the heart and even in the eyes but not in the liver indicating the high specific binding of [¹¹C]MQNB in structures known to be rich in muscarinic receptors.

retina muscarinic receptors. The [¹¹C]MQNB blood radioactivity decreases very rapidly with time. Soon after injection of the cold drug for displacement experiments, a transient increase in the blood activity was observed, indicating a low redistribution of the radiotracer. The stereospecificity of the [¹¹C]MQNB binding was demonstrated; only the pharmacologically active isomer of benzetimide, dexetimide (2 mg), was able to compete with [¹¹C]MQNB, while levetimide injected in the same way and at the same dose was ineffective. Moreover, we were able to demonstrate that the sites labeled with [¹¹C]MQNB were indeed physiologically active receptors and not acceptor sites. During the displacement studies performed either with atropine or cold MQNB, we found a correlation between the increase in [¹¹C]MQNB displaced (indicating the receptor occupancy by the drug) and the simultaneous increase in heart rate resulting from this occupancy (Fig. 2). Thus, all the criteria needed to characterize a receptor (Laduron, 1984) were validated

TABLE III

[¹¹C]MQNB displacement studies in baboon hearts

Cold drug used for displacement	[¹¹C]MQNB i.v. injected			Cold drug i.v. injected		[¹¹C]MQNB displaced from the heart	
	mCi	nmol	nmol/kg	mg	nmol/kg	%	$T_{1/2}$
Atropine	4.5	46.0	2.875	0.05	4.497	26.2	1'56''
	7.86	16.7	10.27	0.25	22.15	56.8	3'07''
	14.2	89.0	5.6	0.5	45.25	69.0	2'37''
	6.9	10.4	0.619	1.0	85.65	78.5	2'45''
	7.45	11.8	0.726	2.0	117.1	87.3	2'57''
	0.81	3.34	0.303	2.0	261.0	92.3	2'40''
MQNB	6.65	60.0	4.17	0.025	4.02	34.5	3'43''
	6.04	11.0	0.786	0.05	8.29	48.7	2'27''
	7.0	10.5	0.812	0.1	16.61	69.3	3'48''
	7.87	16.9	1.224	0.25	41.95	78.0	3'07''
	11.4	32.7	2.616	0.5	92.0	87.8	2'36''
	5.04	5.46	0.396	1.0	168.6	92.3	3'12''
	10.20	110.0	9.02	2.0	378.7	84.6	2'34''

The [¹¹C]MQNB binding in baboon hearts can be displaced by cold atropine or MQNB i.v. administered 20 min after the radioligand. The [¹¹C]MQNB displacement (expressed as a percentage of the radioactivity measured before displacement) is related with the dose of cold drug injected. The radioactivity displaced can be very high and the half-life of the displacement ($T_{1/2}$) very rapid. These data show that more than 90% of the [¹¹C]MQNB can be displaced and thus is specifically bound in the heart.

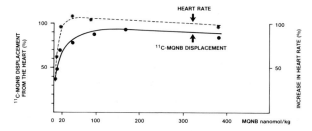

Fig. 2. [¹¹C]MQNB in baboon hearts. A relation between [¹¹C]MQNB labelled receptor occupancy ([¹¹C]MQNB displaced) and simultaneous pharmacological response (increase in heart rate) by increasing doses of cold MQNB can be observed in live primates.

with muscarinic receptors, in an atraumatic manner, by PET, in living baboons. Moreover, displacement studies performed in dogs with PET using various amounts of unlabeled pirenzepine and AF-DX 116 showed that no displacement of bound [¹¹C]MQNB was observed after injection of pirenzepine (1 mg) whereas 25% of the heart radioactivity was displaced after injection of the same dose of AF-DX 116. These in vivo results suggest that M_1 receptors were not detectable by PET in the adult dog heart in these experimental conditions. The results obtained in baboon hearts were confirmed in humans. The ventricular septum and the left ventricle contained high concentrations of [¹¹C]MQNB, the radioactivity in the right ventricle was very low and the atria were never imaged. Saturation experiments showed that the highest concentrations were found in the septum (98 pmol/g of heart) and in the left ventricle (89 pmol/g) (Syrota et al., 1984). In fact, although the receptor concentration could be higher in atria than in ventricules because of their size, ventricles and septum contain more acetylcholine receptors than atria. Saturability of the binding was demonstrated by saturation studies. A few minutes after a bolus injection of [¹¹C]MQNB in a brachial vein in man, the [¹¹C]MQNB blood concentration fell very rapidly to a negligible value. In contrast, the [¹¹C]MQNB radioactive concentration increased rapidly in the myocardium to reach a maximum in 1–5 minutes and then remained constant for 70 minutes. The rapid intravenous injection of un-

labeled atropine led to a rapid decrease in the septal [¹¹C]MQNB. 94% of [¹¹C]MQNB bound in the heart could be displaced. Atropine does not discriminate between heart, brain or glands muscarinic subtypes (Giraldo et al., 1988). Therefore less than 6% of [¹¹C]MQNB bound in the human heart corresponds to non-specific binding. The [¹¹C]MQNB binding is stereospecific since dexetimide but not levetimide can displace [¹¹C]MQNB from its binding sites (Mazière et al., 1981). A correlation between receptor occupancy and a physiological effect has also been demonstrated (Syrota et al., 1985). In a given subject, the MQNB concentration in the ventricular septum was higher when the heart rate was lower. This result seems rather surprising since muscarinic receptor function in the ventricle should be related to inotropic effects rather than to chronotropic ones. However, recent data have shown that the ventricles primarily receive postganglionic cholinergic fibers from ganglion cells localized in the atria. The release of acetylcholine at parasympathetic nerve endings in the ventricles would thus depend on the activity of atrial cells mediating both the atrial chronotropic and the ventricular inotropic effects. The greater [¹¹C]MQNB binding in the septum linked to vagal stimulation could be explained by an increase in either the number or the affinity of antagonist binding sites. In the physiologically active state, acetylcholine is released from the receptor in a low-affinity form (Changeux, 1981) and consequently more sites are available for [¹¹C]MQNB. These findings suggest that PET allows the identification of the physiologically active conformation of the muscarinic receptor under sympathetic and parasympathetic physiological control (Syrota et al., 1985). In patients with hyper and hypothyroidism, myocardial muscarinic receptors were investigated. An increase in the number of high affinity binding sites for acetylcholine was found in hypothyroidism while no significant change was noticed in hyperthyroidism in comparison with normal patients having the same heart rate (Syrota et al., 1988). These results suggest a direct effect of thyroid hormones on heart rate (Heimbach and Crout, 1972; Klein and Levey, 1984; McDevitt, 1968). Changes in myocardial muscarinic receptors were also investigated in patients with tachycardia induced either by exercise stress testing or right ventricular pacing. During exercise, [^{11}C]MQNB radioactivity in the septum increased initially, then decreased significantly during the last six minutes. The mean decrease reached 26% of the value at rest. These data suggest that in the active state, acetylcholine is released from the receptor being in a low affinity form and then leaving more sites for [^{11}C]MQNB. In contrast pacing-induced tachycardia did not influence the [^{11}C]MQNB septal uptake which suggests a lack of change in number or affinity of muscarinic receptor.

Cerebral muscarinic cholinergic receptors

Muscarinic acetylcholine receptors are the major components of the cerebral cholinergic receptors. They are involved in physiological and cognitive processes such as motility, sleep, neuroendocrine functions, memory and attention (Albanus, 1970; Bartus et al., 1987). Moreover, their distribution and characteristics have been shown to be altered in pathological processes affecting the central cholinergic system, such as Alzheimer's disease and Huntington's chorea (Wastek et al., 1976). As shown previously, M_1 receptors are located with a high density in the cerebral cortex, striatum, hippocampus and nucleus accumbens, while M_2 receptors are located with a lower density in the brain stem, cerebellum and hypothalamus. We have explored the feasibility of studying central muscarinic receptors, in an atraumatic manner, in the living baboon, using PET as an external detection system and quinuclidinyl benzilate labeled with carbon 11 ([^{11}C]-QNB) as a specific muscarinic radioligand able to bind to both M_1 and M_2 receptors. QNB has been labeled in our laboratory with the positron emitter carbon 11 (Prenant et al., 1989). The [^{11}C]QNB labeling required two successive steps: formation of [^{11}C]benzilic acid by carbonatation of benzophenone dianion with ^{11}C-CO$_2$—synthesis of

[^{11}C]QNB by esterification of [^{11}C]benzilic acid with 3-quinuclidinol in the presence of carbonyldiimidazole. Preliminary ex vivo assays in rats showed a similar cerebral binding after intravenous administration of either [^{3}H]QNB or [^{11}C]QNB dissolved in saline. Following i.v. administration of [^{11}C]QNB (10 mCi) to baboons, PET studies showed that 40 minutes after injection of the radiotracer, the [^{11}C]QNB total binding reached maximal values in all cerebral structures except in the cerebellum; then, the brain radioactivity seemed to be quite stable till the end of the experiment. Maximal values of regional specific binding of [^{11}C]QNB amounted to 0.64, 0.58, 0.50 and 0.41×10^{-2}% of the injected dose per cm^3 of tissue in the occipital, temporal, frontal cortices and striatum respectively. In contrast to in vitro studies, [^{11}C]QNB specific binding did not appear to be higher in the striatum than in the cerebral cortex. This fact might be due to the small size of the baboon's brain together with the low spatial resolution of the tomograph used in these studies. The radioligand entered more quickly in the cerebellum than in the brain but attained a low maximal level 2 min after injection, then decreased slowly until the end of the experiment. The regional distribution of [^{11}C]QNB in the living baboon's brain for the most part was in agreement with in vitro and ex vivo results reported from the literature (Yamamura et al., 1974a,b; Yamamura and Snyder, 1974). The saturability of the [^{11}C]QNB brain binding was evaluated after a pre-injection of the muscarinic antagonist dexetimide (0.8 mg/kg) performed i.v. 40 min before the radioligand. As seen in Fig. 3 and Table IV the presaturation by dexetimide almost completely inhibited the specific binding of [^{11}C]QNB compared with control experiments. No change in the radiotracer kinetics was noticed in the cerebellum. In order to increase the cerebral [^{11}C]QNB bioavailability, a selective presaturation of the peripheral muscarinic receptors was performed 40 min before the injection of the radiotracer by cold MQNB (0.1 mg/kg). As seen in Fig. 3 and in Table IV, the [^{11}C]QNB specific binding was in-

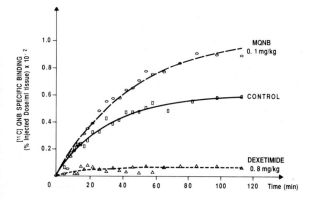

Fig. 3. [^{11}C]QNB saturation experiments in baboon brains. Compared with control studies (without pretreatment), changes in the [^{11}C]QNB specific binding were observed in temporal cortex, after pretreatment with MQNB or dexetimide (i.v. injected 40 min before the radioligand). An increase of the [^{11}C]QNB specific binding was observed after peripheral muscarinic receptor presaturation by MQNB while high inhibition of the [^{11}C]QNB binding was seen after central and peripheral muscarinic receptor presaturation by dexetimide.

TABLE IV

[^{11}C]QNB saturation studies in baboon brains

Cerebral structures	[^{11}C]QNB brain binding (% control)	
	After MQNB (0.1 mg/kg)	After dexetimide (0.8 mg/kg)
Cerebellum	0	0
Frontal cortex	+41.94	−83.33
Temporal cortex	+59.65	−89.47
Occipital cortex	+26.76	−92.31
Striatum	+40.00	−88.88

Compared to control studies (without pretreatment) an increase of the [^{11}C]QNB specific binding (total radioactivity − radioactivity in the cerebellum) is observed in the baboon brains, after peripheral muscarinic receptors are blocked by cold MQNB i.v. injected 40 min before the radiotracer. In contrast, dexetimide injected in the same conditions induced a very significant inhibition of the [^{11}C]QNB brain binding by presaturation of both central and peripheral muscarinic receptors.

creased by this pretreatment particularly in the temporal cortex where it reached 159% of the control values. The [^{11}C]QNB binding was displaceable; when atropine (0.8 mg/kg) or dexetimide (1 mg/kg) were i.v. injected 40 min after the radiotracer, displacements of the [^{11}C]QNB were observed in cerebral cortex and in the striatum, while no significant change in the [^{11}C]QNB bind-

ing was observed in the cerebellum (Table V). Moreover, a higher [^{11}C]QNB displacement by dexetimide could be observed in the cerebral cortex and in the striatum but not in the cerebellum, after peripheral muscarinic receptors pre-saturation by MQNB (Fig. 4 and Table V). During the [^{11}C]QNB displacement experiments, simultaneous effects of dexetimide and atropine were observed in the electroencephalographic activity

TABLE V

[^{11}C]QNB displacement studies in baboon brains

Cerebral structures	[^{11}C]QNB displacement			
	Control		Pretreatment with MQNB (0.1 mg/kg)	
	Atropine (0.8 mg/kg)	Dexetimide (1 mg/kg)	Dexetimide (0.8 mg/kg)	Levetimide (0.8 mg/kg)
Cerebellum	0	0	0	0
Frontal cortex	15.73	24.72	70.79	0
Temporal cortex	12.36	30.34	74.72	0
Occipital cortex	14.89	26.67	74.44	0
Striatum	6.25	12.35	69.15	0

Compared with control values without pretreatment, pretreatment with cold MQNB (i.v. injected 40 min before the radiotracer) increases very significantly the [^{11}C]QNB displaced by dexetimide (expressed as a percentage of the radioactivity measured before displacement) in cerebral structures. No displacement was observed after levetimide injection, showing the stereospecificity of the [^{11}C]QNB binding in the brain.

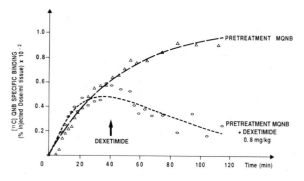

Fig. 4. [¹¹C]QNB displacement in baboon brains. A high displacement of [¹¹C]QNB specific binding induced by dexetimide (i.v. injected 40 min after the radioligand) was observed in temporal cortex after peripheral muscarinic receptors presaturation by MQNB.

acterization of a ligand to a receptor (Laduron, 1988). Using [¹¹C]QNB as in vivo muscarinic radioligand and PET facilities for external detection, most of these criteria (saturability, specificity and stereospecificity of the binding and relation between [¹¹C]QNB labeled receptor occupancy and pharmacological effect) were satisfied in the brain of the living baboon. These studies demonstrated the feasibility of imaging and characterizing the cerebral muscarinic receptors in a living primate, using PET.

Modelization

of the baboons (appearance of slow waves and rapid spikes) which is in agreement with previous studies (Meldrum et al., 1970) suggesting that the sites labelled with [¹¹C]QNB were really receptor sites linked with pharmacological response. For in vivo characterization of receptors, the in vivo binding of a ligand to these receptors should satisfy the same criteria defined in vitro for the char-

Positron emission tomography (PET) coupled with the labeling methods using short-lived positron emitters allows us to determine regional biochemical processes by non-invasive and quantitative methods in any human organ. Using a model and from single-experiment results, it is possible to quantify in vivo the concentration of receptor sites, the ligand affinity for the receptors and all the kinetic parameters corresponding to the

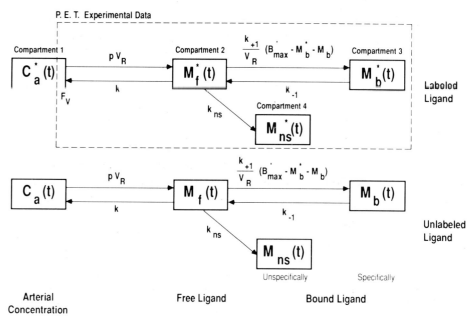

Fig. 5. Compartmental ligand-receptor model.

ligand-receptor interactions. We have used such a model approach (Syrota, 1988) in order to measure in vivo the cardiac muscarinic receptor concentration in dogs using [^{11}C]MQNB as an antagonist ligand (Mazière et al., 1981) and PET for external detection.

The ligand-receptor model

Several models have recently been proposed as a framework for analyzing kinetic data of ligand-receptor interactions (Mintun et al., 1984; Frey et al. 1985; Vera et al., 1985; Perlmutter et al., 1986; Wong et al., 1986, Zeeberg et al., 1988). The model structure may differ depending on the human organ, the molecule or the experimental protocol used. In the model considered in this study and shown in Fig. 5, the free ligand arrived from the capillary lumen with a flux $pV_R C_a^*(t)$ where $C_a^*(t)$ was the radioactive plasma concentration at time t, p an unknown rate constant and V_R the fractional volume of reaction (i.e. the volume of reaction in 1 ml of tissue) expressed without unit. A boundary layer, containing the free ligand at a concentration M_f^*, was formed in the interstitial space close to the cells. This free ligand could bind directly to a free receptor site, bind to a non-specific receptor site or escape with rate constant k. The specific binding probability depended on the rate constant (k_{+1}/V_R) and on the local concentration of free receptors which was equal to $[B_{max}' - M_b^*(t)]$ where B_{max}' was the unknown concentration of receptor sites available for binding and $M_b^*(t)$ the bound ligand concentration. The non-specific binding probability is assumed to be linear (parameter k_{ns}) and irreversible. The rate constant for the dissociation of the bound ligand was denoted by k_{-1}. This model contained six parameters, the two most important of which were the concentration of receptor sites B_{max}' and the ratio of k_{-1} to k_{+1} representing the equilibrium dissociation constant denoted by K_d. This model was nonlinear, which was a big advantage, first, since it could be used whatever the number of occupied receptors or the receptor density B_{max}', and second, because the receptor density B_{max}' and

the association constant k_{+1}/V_R could then be identified separately. We assumed that the unlabeled ligand kinetics was similar to that of the labeled ligand. Since the experimental protocol includes injections of unlabeled ligand, we must incorporate in the model the kinetics of this unlabeled ligand. Indeed, the concentration of the specifically bound unlabeled ligand ($M_b(t)$) has an effect on the local concentration of free receptors and consequently on the binding probability of free labeled ligand. The free unlabeled ligand and the unspecifically bound unlabeled ligand was denoted by $M_f(t)$ and $M_{ns}(t)$ respectively. In this study the model parameters were identified by means of minimization of a weighted least-square cost function defined by (Perlmutter et al., 1986):

$$D(P) = \sum_{i=1}^{m} w_i [y(t_i) - Y(t_i, P)]^2$$

where (t_i) ($i = 1, 2, \ldots, m$) are the data sampling times, (w_i) are the weights associated with the decay corrected measures ($y(t_i)$), $P = [p_1, p_2, \ldots, p_r]^t$ represents the model parameters and $Y(t_i, P)$ are the values predicted by the model from parameter P and from the experimental protocol. This cost function was minimized by using a Marquardt algorithm (Marquardt, 1963) and the weight used was defined by $w_i = (t_i - t_{i-1})/y(t_i)$.

Experimental methods

Five beagle dogs of either sex, weighing 10 to 12 kg and not fed overnight before the experiment, were examined. They were anaesthesized first with a bolus of sodium thiopental (25 mg/kg) followed by a continuous injection at the rate of 5 mg/kg/h. All dogs had undergone an endotracheal intubation. During the experiments, the heart rate was regularly measured but no significant modification was noted. PET studies were performed using the LETI time-of-flight positron camera (Soussaline et al., 1984). Each slice was 13 mm thick and spatial transverse resolution was about 12 mm. One hundred and ten sequential images were obtained. Acquisition times varied from 4 s (during the first 2 min) to 5 min (at the end of the curve) and were chosen as a function of the slope of the curve, taking into account the need to maintain sufficient statistics despite ^{11}C decay. Correction for this decay was automatically obtained during the data acquisition procedure. A region of interest corresponding to an important part of left ventricle was automatically outlined at the 80% isocount contour on an image corresponding to 10 min. Radioactive concentration measured in this region of interest for each image was calculated and expressed in pmol/ml. Identification of model parameters required the knowledge of the plasma time-activity curve $C_a^*(t)$ which was used in the model as input function. Sixty-four arterial blood samples were collected. The time interval between the samples was variable; after an injection of labeled ligand, it was about 5 s for a period of 2 min whereas it was 10 min when the slope of the blood curve was low. In order to avoid too rapid and too high an increase in the plasma concentration, which would be difficult to observe because of the minimum 5-s interval separating two samples, the duration of all injections was about 1 min, the injection flow rate being more or less constant during this time. An estimation of the plasma concentration ($C_a(t)$) of unlabeled ligand was calculated from $C_a^*(t)$ (Delforge, 1990). Studies were performed according to an experimental protocol whose complexity is the consequence of the number of unknown parameters in the model and of our wish to obtain a better justification of the identified parameter values. Indeed, a previous study (Delforge, 1990) on the identifiability of this ligand-receptor model has shown that a single injection of labeled ligand leads to parameter uncertainties so large that most of the parameters must be considered as unidentifiable and when we include a second injection of the cold ligand (displacement experiment) the identification procedure leads to two very different numerical solutions. Consequently, in order to obtain a unique solution, an experimental protocol including a third injection associating both labeled

and unlabeled ligand (co-injection experiment) was used (Delforge, 1990). A bolus of [11C]MQNB (4 nM) was intravenously injected at the beginning of the experiment ($T_0 = 0$ min). At time $T_1 = 30$ min, an additional intravenous injection of unlabeled ligand excess (0.5 mg) was performed (displacement experiment). The injection of cold ligand resulted in an association of free receptors with these molecules and consequently in a competitive inhibition of labeled ligand from its binding sites. This led to an immediate and marked washout of the labeled molecules, the concentration of which fell rapidly. At time $T_2 = 70$ min, a third injection consisted of a simultaneous injection of labeled and unlabeled MQNB (co-injection experiment). The injected labeled and unlabeled ligand quantities were 7 nM and 0.5 mg respectively. Since the concentration of the cold ligand was much larger than the concentration of the labeled ligand, the free receptors were rapidly occupied by the unlabeled ligand and thus the binding probability of the labeled ligand was small. A second displacement was performed at time $T_3 = 120$ min with an injection of unlabeled ligand excess (1 mg) in order to evaluate the nonspecific binding.

Identified parameter values and discussion

Fitting the complete mathematical model to experimental data provided values for kinetic rate constants and receptor densities. The final quality of the fits was very good as can be seen in the example given in Fig. 6. The concentration of receptor sites B_{max}' was found to be 41 ± 12 pmol/g. This value was close to the results obtained in vitro in rat heart homogenates (Syrota et al., 1984) $B_{max} = 228$ pmol/g of protein which corresponds to about 23 pmol/g of tissue and in guinea pig (Gibson et al., 1979) B_{max} about 16.3 pmol/g of tissue. These values could also be compared with those obtained in vitro with QNB since, as pointed out by Gibson (Gibson et al., 1979), the B_{max} values can be considered as similar with both molecules. In particular, a receptor concentration equal to 12 pmol/g was obtained in

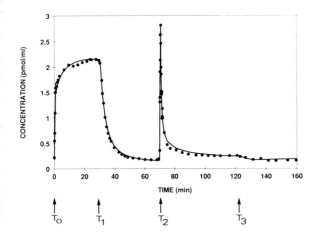

Fig. 6. Validation of the ligand-receptor model. Experimental data (●) resulting from the experiment performed with [^{11}C]MQNB (using the protocol described in the text) correspond to the data predicted by the model (solid line). The corresponding model parameter values are given in the text.

dogs (Wei et al., 1978). Comparison between these results showed that the B_{max} found in vivo by the PET modelling approach was close to those obtained by an in vitro method. However, the $K_d \cdot V_R$ value identified with the model (0.073 ± 0.022 nM) didn't have the same order of magnitude as the K_d values obtained in vitro: $K_d = 0.32$ nM in rat homogenates (Syrota et al., 1984) and $K_d = 0.5$ nM in guinea pig (Gibson et al. 1979). An agreement between these values assumed that the fractional volume of reaction V_R is equal to about 0.23 that is to say that the volume of the boundary layer countaining the free ligand is equal to 23% of the considered tissue volume. The association rate constant (parameter k_{+1}/V_R) is found to be equal to 3.9 ± 0.9 ml pmol^{-1} min^{-1}. The only available in vitro results were obtained in rats: $k_{+1} = 2.7$ ml/(pmol. min) (Syrota et al., 1984). The dissociation rate constant (parameter k_{-1}) was identified to be equal to 0.272 ± 0.030 min^{-1}. This value was close to the dissociation constant found in embryonic chicken heart cell cultures (0.27 min^{-1}) and had the same order of magnitude as the value obtained with rat heart membranes (0.81 min^{-1}) (Syrota et al. 1984). This value meant that, whatever the time, about 27% of

specifically bound ligand was dissociated each minute which was not negligible. The identified values of the other parameters were: $pV_R = 0.65$ ± 0.08 min^{-1}, $k = 4.71 ± 0.94$ min^{-1}, $k_{ns} = 0.047$ ± 0.011 min^{-1}, and $F_v = 0.40 ± 0.10$.

Conclusion

The availability of high affinity cholinergic ligands radiolabeled at high specific activity has made it possible to study the cholinergic system, in a non-invasive way, in the brain and in the heart of animals and humans, using PET. The nicotine cerebral kinetics was studied in the brain of living baboons using [^{11}C]nicotine. The feasibility of investigating heart and brain muscarinic receptors was demonstrated, in humans and baboons, using [^{11}C]MQNB and [^{11}C]QNB respectively. High affinity, saturability, specificity and stereospecificity of the binding of the radiotracers were shown in vivo with PET. Moreover, an increase of muscarinic receptors was found in hypothyroidic patients and transient alterations of muscarinic receptors were seen in subjects with tachycardia induced by exercise but not with tachycardia induced by ventricular pacing. A non-equilibrium non-linear model with identification of 6 parameters was proposed for non-invasive quantification of muscarinic cholinergic receptors in vivo in dog hearts using PET and [^{11}C]MQNB. Although the interest of the data presented in this paper is obvious, an effort to optimize PET methodology to study the cholinergic system is still needed particularly to investigate central muscarinic receptors. More selective and specific radioligands have to be found. Improvements of spatial resolution of positron cameras together with increased sensitivity have to be made. Reliable and quantitative tracer models need to be proposed. Nevertheless, the feasibility of studying the cholinergic system in vivo using PET offers the opportunity to link basic experimental research and clinical applications to investigate alterations of the cholinergic neurotransmission in mental diseases such as Alzheimer's disease and Huntington's chorea.

References

Albanus, L. (1970) Central and peripheral effects of anticholinergic compounds. *Acta Pharmacol. Toxicol.,* 28: 305–326.

Bartus, R.T. Dean, R.L. Flicker, C. (1987) Cholinergic psychopharmacology: an integration of human and animal research on memory; In: *Psychopharmacology: The Third Generation of Progress,* Meltzer H.Y. Ed., Raven Press. pp. 211–218.

Bergström, K. Aquilonius, S.M. Bergson, G. Berggren, B.M. Bergström, M. Brismar, T. Eckernäs, S.A. Ehrin, E. Ericksson, L. Greits, T. Gillberg, P.G. Lagerkranser, M. Litton, J. Lundquist, H. Langström, B. Malmborg, P. Sjöberg, S. Stalnacke, C.G. Widen, L. (1981) Positron emission tomography in cholinergic neuropharmacology. *J. Comput. Assist. Tomogr.,* 5: 938.

Bonner, T.I. Buckley, N.J. Young, A.C. Brann, M.R. (1987) Identification of a family of muscarinic acetylcholine receptor genes. *Science,* 237: 527–532.

Borch, R.F. Hassid, A.I. (1972) A new method for the methylation of amines. *J. Org. Chem.,* 37: 1673–1674.

Broussolle, E.P. Wong, D.F. Fanelli, R.J. London, E.D. (1989) In vivo specific binding of (3H) 1-Nicotine in the mouse brain. *Life Sci.,* 44: 1123–1132.

Brown, J.H. Goldstein, D. (1986) Analysis of cardiac muscarinic receptors recognized selectively by nonquaternary but not by quaternary ligands. *J. Pharmacol. Exp. Therap.,* 238: 580–586.

Changeux, J.P. (1981) The acetylcholine receptor: an "allosteric" membrane protein. Harvey Lect., 75: 85–254.

Dannals, R.F. Langström, B. Ravert, H.T. Wilson, A.A. Wagner, H.N. (1988) Synthesis of radiotracers for studying muscarinic cholinergic receptors in the living human brain using Positron emission tomography: (11C)dexetimide and (11C)levetimide. *Appl. Radiat. Isot.,* 39: 291–295.

Davies, P. Verth, A.H. (1978) Regional distribution of muscarinic acetylcholine receptor in normal and Alzheimer's-type dementia brains. *Brain Res.,* 138: 385–392.

Delforge, J. Syrota, A. Mazoyer, B.M. (1990) Identifiability analysis and parameter identification of an in vivo ligand-receptor model from PET data. *IEEE Trans. Biomed. Eng.* (in press).

Dewey, S.L. Bendriem, B. MacGregor, R. King, P. Fowler, J.S. Christman, D.R. Schlyer, D.J. Wolf, A.P. Volkow, N. Brodie, J.D. (1989) PET studies using (11C) cogentin in baboon brain. *J. Cereb. Blood Flow Metab.,* 9: 1-S13.

Doods, H.N. Mathy, M.J. Davidesko, D. Van Charldorp K.J. De Jonge, A. Van Zwietten P.A. (1987) Selectivity of muscarinic antagonists in radioligand and in vivo experiments for the putative M1, M2 and M3 receptors. *J. Pharmacol. Exp. Ther.,* 242: 257–262.

Frey, K.A. Hichwa, R.D. Ehrenkaufer, R.L.E. Agranoff, B.W. (1985) Quantitative in vivo receptor binding III: Tracer kinetic modeling of muscarinic cholinergic receptor binding. *Proc. Natl. Acad. Sci. USA,* 82: 6711–6715.

Fukuda, K. Kubo, T. Akiba, I. Maeda, A. Mishina, M. Numa, S. (1987) Molecular distinction between muscarinic acetylcholine receptor subtypes. *Nature,* 327: 623–625.

Giachetti, A. Micheletti, R. Montagna, E. (1986) Cardioselective profile of AF-DX 116, a muscarinic M2 receptor antagonist. *Life Sci.,* 38: 1663–1672.

Gauthier, S. Diksic, M. Yamamoto, L. Tyler, J. Feindel, W. (1985) Positron emission tomography with carbon-11 Choline in human subjects. *Can. J. Neurol. Sci.,* 12: 214.

Gibson, R.E. Eckelman, W.C. Vieras, F. Reba, R.C. (1979) The distribution of the muscarinic acetylcholine receptor antagonists, quinuclidinyl benzilate and quinuclidinyl benzilate methiodide (both tritiated) in rat, guinea pig and rabbit. *J. Nucl. Med.,* 20: 865–870.

Giraldo, E. Martos, F. Gomez, A. Garcia, A. Vigano, M.A. Ladinsky, H. Sanchez De La Cuesta, F. (1988) Characterization of muscarinic receptor subtypes in human tissues. *Life Sci.,* 43: 1507–1515.

Hammer, R. Berrie, C.P. Birdsall, N.J.M. Burgen, A.S. Hulme, E.C. (1980) Pirenzepine distinguishes between different subclasses of muscarinic receptors. *Nature,* 283: 90–92.

Heimbach, D.M. Crout, R.J. (1972) Effect of atropine on the tachycardia of hyperthyroidism. *Arch. Int. Med.,* 129: 430–432.

Hirschowitz, B.I. Hammer, R. Giachetti, A. Kevins, J. and Levine, R.R. (1984) Symposium preface. *Trends Pharmacol. Sci.,* 5, Suppl.

Klein, I. Levey, G.S. (1984) New perspectives on thyroid hormone, cathecholamine, and the heart. *Am. J. Med.,* 76: 167–172.

Laduron, P.M. (1984) Criteria for receptor sites in binding studies. *Biochem. Pharmacol.,* 33: 833–839.

Laduron, P.M. (1988) Stereospecificity in binding studies. A useful criterion though insufficient to prove the presence of receptors. *Biochem. Pharmacol.,* 37: 37–40.

Livni, E. Elmaleh, D.R. (1989) Synthesis and biodistribution of 2-ethyl-8-(11C) methyl 2,8-diazaspiro (4,5) decane-1,3-dione (11C-RS 86), a muscarinic acetylcholine receptor agonist. *J. Label Compound Radiopharm.,* 26: 197.

Marquardt, D.W. (1963) An algorithm for least-square estimation of nonlinear parameters. *SIAM Journal,* 11: 431–441.

Mazière, M. Comar, D. Marazano, C. Berger, G. (1976) Nicotine-11C: synthesis and distribution kinetics in animals. *Eur. J. Nucl. Med.,* 1: 255–258.

Mazière, M. Berger, G. Masse, R. Plummer, D. Comar, D. (1979) The in vivo distribution of carbon 11 labeled (−) nicotine in animals a method suitable for use in man. In: Electrophysiological Effects of Nicotine. Remond A. et Izard C. Eds., *Elsevier/North-Holland Biomedical Press.,* pp 31–47.

Mazière, M. Comar, D. Godot, J.M. Collard, Ph.Cepeda, C. Naquet, R. (1981) In vivo characterization of myocardium muscarinic receptors by positron emission tomography. *Life Sci.,* 29: 2391–2397.

Mazière, M. Berger, G. Godot, J.M. Prenant, C. Sastre, J. Comar, D. (1983) 11C- Methiodide quinuclidinyl benzilate, a muscarinic antagonist for in vivo studies of myocardial muscarinic receptors. *J. of Radioanal. Chem.,* 76: 305–309.

McDevitt, D.G. Shanks, R.G. Hadden, D.R. Montgomery, D.A.D. Weaver, J.A. (1968) The role of the thyroid in the control of heart rate. *Lancet,* i: 998–1000.

Meldrum, B.S. Naquet, R. Balzano, E. (1970) Effects of atropine and eserine on the electroencephalogram, on behaviour and on light-induced epilepsy in the adolescent baboon (Papio papio). Electroenceph. *Clin. Neurophysiol.,* 28: 449–458.

Mintun, M.A. Raichle, M.E. Kilbourn, M.R. Wooten, G.F. Welch, M.J. (1984) A quantitative model for the in vivo assessment of drug binding sites with PET. *Ann. Neurol.,* 15: 217–227.

Mulholland, G.K. Jewett, D.M. Toorongian, S.A. (1988a) Routine synthesis of N-(11C-methyl) scopolamine by phosphite mediated reductive methylation with (11C) formaldehyde. *Appl. Radiat. Iso.,* 39: 373–379.

Mulholland, G.K. Otto, C.A. Jewett, D.M. Kilbourn, M.R. Sherman, P.S. Koeppe, R.A. Wieland, D.M. Frey, K.A. Kuhl, D.E. (1988b) Synthesis and preliminary evaluation of (C-11)-(+)-2α-tropanyl benzilate (C-11 TRB) as a ligand for the muscarinic receptor. *J. Nucl. Med.,* 29:932.

Mulholland, G.K. Jewett, D.M. Otto, C.A. Kilbourn, M.R. Sherman, P.S. Kuhl, D.E. (1988c) Synthesis and regional brain distribution of (C-11) N-methyl-4-piperidyl benzilate ((C-11) NMPB) in the rat. *J. Nucl. Med.,* 29: 768.

Mulholland, G.K. Schwaiger, M. Otto, C.A. Sherman, P.S. Jewett, D.M. (1989) Synthesis and animal studies of C-11 tropanyl benzilate methiodide (MTRB). A promising ligand of peripheral muscarinic receptors. *J. Nucl. Med.,* 30: 930.

Nathanson, N.M. (1987) Molecular properties of the muscarinic acetylcholine receptor. *Ann. Rev. Neurosci.,* 10: 195–236.

Nybäck, H. Nordberg, A. Längström, B. Halldin, C. Hartvig, P. Ahlin, A. Swan, C.G. Sedvall, G. (1989) Attempts to visualize nicotinic receptors in the brain of monkey and man by positron emission tomography; In: Progress in Brain Research, Nordberg A., Fuxe K. and Holmstedt B., Eds., Elsevier Science Publishers B.V., pp 313–319.

Pauli, J.R., Stitzel, J.A., Marks, M.J. and Collins, A.C. (1989) An autoradiographic analysis of cholinergic receptors in mouse brain. *Brain Res. Bull.,* 22, 453–459.

Prenant, C. Barre, L. Crouzel, C. (1989) Synthesis of (11C)-3-Quinuclidinylbenzilate (QNB). *J. Label. Compound Radiopharm.* 27, 1257–1265.

Perlmutter, J.S. Larson, K.B. Raichle, M.E. Markham, J. Mintun, M.A. Kilbourn, M.R. Welch, M.J. (1986) Strategies for in vivo measurement of receptor binding using PET. *J. Cereb. Blood Flow Metab.,* 6: 154–169.

Redies, C. Diksic, M. Collier, B. Gjedde, A. Thompson, C.J. Gauthier, S. Feindel, W.H. (1988) Influx of a choline analog to dog brain measured by positron emission tomography. *Synapse,* 2: 406–411.

Schmiterlow, C.G. Hansson, E. Applegren, L.E. and Hoffmann, P.C. (1965) Physiological disposition and biotransformation of 14C-labeled Nicotine. Isotopes in experimental pharmacology. *Roth J. Llyod, Ed., Univ. of Chicago Press.*

Schwartz, R.D. and Kellar, K.J. (1983) Nicotinic cholinergic receptor binding sites in the brain: regulation in vivo, *Science,* 220: 214–216.

Soussaline, F. Campagnolo, R. Verrey, B. Bendriem, B. Bouvier, A. Lecomte, J.L. Comar, D. (1984) Physical characterization of a time-of-flight positron emission tomograph system for whole-body quantitative studies. *J. Nucl. Med.,* 25: 46.

Syrota, A. (1988) Receptor binding studies of the living heart. *New Concepts Cardiac Imag.,* 4: 141–166.

Syrota, A. Paillotin, G. Davy, J.M. and Aumont, M.C. (1984) Kinetic of in vivo binding of antagonist to muscarinic cholinergic receptor in the human heart studied by positron emission tomography. *Life Sci.,* 35: 937–945.

Syrota, A. Comar, D. Paillotin, G. Davy, J.M. Aumont, M.C. Stulzaft, O. Mazière, B. (1985) Muscarinic cholinergic receptor in the human heart evidenced under physiological conditions by positron emission tomography. *Proc. Natl. Acad. Sci. USA,* 82: 584–588.

Syrota, A. Le Guludec, D. Prenant, C. Fournier, D. Crouzel, M. Aumont, M.C. Crouzel, C. (1988) PET investigation of myocardial muscarinic acetylcholine receptor in patients with hyper and hypothyroidism. *J. Nucl. Med.,* 29: 808.

Vera, D.R. Krohn, K.A. Scheibe, P.O. and Stadalnik, R.C. (1985) Identifiability analysis of an in vivo receptor-binding radiopharmacokinetic system. *IEEE Trans. Biomed. Eng.,* 32: 312–322.

Vora, M.M. Finn, R.D. and Boothe, T.E. (1983) Ethyl-11C-Scopolamine: Synthesis and distribution in rat brain. *J. Label. Compound Radiopharm.,* 20: 1229–1236.

Wastek, G.J. Stern, L.Z. Johnson, P.C. and Yamamura, H.I. (1976) Huntington's disease: regional alteration in muscarinic cholinergic receptor binding in human brain. *Life Sci.,* 19: 1033–1040.

Wei, J.W. and Sulakhe, P.V. (1978) Regional and subcellular distribution of myocardial muscarinic cholinergic receptors. *Eur. J. Pharmacol.,* 52: 235–238.

Whitehouse, P.J. Martino, A.M. Antuono, P.G. Lowenstein, P.R. Coyle, J.T. Price, D.L. Kellar, K.J. (1986) Nicotinic acetylcholine binding sites in Alzheimer's disease. *Brain Res.,* 371: 146–151.

Wong, D.K. Gjedde, A. and Wagner, H.N. (1986) Quantification of neuroreceptors in the living human brain. *J. Cereb. Blood Flow Metab.,* 6: 137–146.

Yamamura, H.I. and Snyder, S.H. (1974) Muscarinic cholinergic binding in rat brain. *Proc. Nat. Acad. Sci. USA,* 71: 1725–1729.

Yamamura, H.I. Kuhar, M.J. Greenberg, D. and Snyder, S.H. (1974a) Muscarinic cholinergic receptor binding: regional distribution in monkey brain. *Brain Res.,* 171: 473–480.

Yamamura, H.I. Kuhar, M.J. and Snyder, S.H. (1974b) In vivo identification of muscarinic cholinergic receptor binding in rat brain. *Brain Res.,* 80: 170–176.

Zeeberg, B.R. Gibson, R.E. and Reba, R.C. (1988) Accuracy of in vivo neuroreceptor quantification by PET and review of steady-state, transient, double injection and equilibrium models. *IEEE Trans. Med. Imag.,* 7: 203–212.

S.-M. Aquilonius and P.-G. Gillberg (Eds.)
Progress in Brain Research, Vol. 84
© 1990 Elsevier Science Publishers B.V. (Biomedical Division)

CHAPTER 37

Spinal cholinergic mechanisms

Per-Göran Gillberg, Håkan Askmark and Sten-Magnus Aquilonius

Department of Neurology, University Hospital, S-751 85 Uppsala, Sweden

Cholinergic structures within the spinal cord

Ventral horn

Several decades ago the presence (Macintosh, 1941) and synthesis (Feldberg and Vogt, 1948) of acetylcholine (ACh) in the spinal cord was demonstrated in animal experiments and the first applications of acetylcholinesterase (AChE) histochemistry (Giacobini and Holmstedt, 1958) depicted intense staining of the motor neurons. The highest activity of choline acetyltransferase (ChAT) is found in the ventrolateral part of the ventral horn (Aquilonius at al., 1981; Gillberg et al., 1982) which corresponds closely to the distribution pattern of AChE (Ishii and Friede, 1967; Silver and Wolstacroft, 1971). The main part of this high ChAT activity is probably located in the motor neurons, as it can be traced into the human ventral root region (Aquilonius et al., 1981; Gillberg et al., 1981). In immunohistochemical studies using monoclonal antibody to ChAT, staining is found in the ventral horn of large motor neurons (Kimura et al., 1981; Houser et al., 1983; Satoh et al., 1983; Barber et al., 1984; Borges and Iversen, 1986). In addition, large ChAT immunoreactive boutons (5 μm) have been observed on the soma and proximal dendrites of large and medium sized somatic motor neurons (Fig. 1, cell 1). These large morphologically distinct terminals may be the cholinergic boutons of recurrent axon collaterals (Cullheim et al., 1977; Cullheim and Kellerth, 1978) since Ia fibers and descending projections to motor neurons have smaller boutons (Borges and

Iversen, 1988). A number of small dense ChAT-positive neurons have also been found in the motor neuronal pools (Barber et al., 1984; Borges and Iversen, 1986; Houser et al., 1983). Small motor neuronal somatas have rarely been associated closely with ChAT-positive terminal-like elements. It is likely that many of them are gamma motor neurons, since combined physiological and anatomical studies have demonstrated that gamma motor neurons are generally smaller in size than α motor neurons and that the two types of cell are intermingled in the motor nuclei (Bryan et al., 1972) (Fig. 1, cell 2). The finding of ChAT-posi-

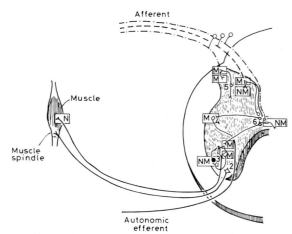

Fig. 1. Schematic diagram of some cholinergic structures in the spinal cord. M = muscarinic receptors. N = nicotinic receptors. 1. Alpha motor neuron. 2. Gamma motor neuron. 3. Renshaw cell (cholinoceptive and inhibitory to motor neuron). 4. Intermediolateral cell column. 5. Interneuron in lamina III. 6. Lamina X neuron.

tive terminals within the neurophil and around the cell bodies of unstained neurons in lamina VII (Houser et al., 1983; Barber et al., 1984; Borges and Iversen, 1986) is consistent with the results of previous morphological studies indicating that the axon collaterals of motor neurons terminate on Renshaw cells in these locations (Lagerbäck et al., 1981). The Renshaw cell is inhibitory to the motor neuron (Renshaw, 1941; Eccles et al., 1954; Curtis et al., 1957; Wilson et al., 1960) (Fig. 1, cell 3).

Dorsal horn

Heavy staining of AChE has been found in the dorsal horn, especially corresponding to laminae III and IV of Rexed (1954). Also a relatively high activity of ChAT activity has been demonstrated in the spinal cords of the cat (Gwyn et al., 1972), the cow (Aquilonius et al., 1981) and man (Aquilonius et al., 1981; Gillberg et al., 1982). Subcellular studies performed on spinal cord from the cow have revealed that the major proportion of dorsal horn ChAT is present in a particulate form, indicating a main location in nerve terminals (Aquilonius et al., 1981). With immunohistochemical techniques using monoclonal antibody to ChAT, numerous small punctate structures have been found in lamina III and some fewer in lamina I (Kimura et al., 1981; Houser et al., 1983; Barber et al., 1984; Borges and Iversen, 1986). Electron microscopy has revealed that many of these punctate structures are terminals containing synaptic vesicles and abundant ChAT-positive reaction products (Barber et al., 1984). ChAT-positive cell bodies are also present in the dorsal horn, those located in laminae III–V extending dendrites dorsally into lamina III (Houser et al., 1983; Barber et al., 1984; Borges and Iversen, 1986) (Fig. 1, cell 5). The autonomic neurons in the thoraco-lumbar (sympathetic) and lumbosacral (parasympathetic) levels of the spinal cord are ChAT-positive (Fig. 1, cell 4). Partition neurons are characterized as intensely ChAT-positive cells whose somal axes average 24×36 μm (Barber et al., 1984). Partition neurons form a ChAT-positive network across the intermediate spinal region of non-autonomic levels

extending from the central canal to the lateral edge of the grey matter, thereby delineating the dorsal from the ventral horn.

Small ChAT-positive neurons have been observed throughout the spinal cord (Barber et al., 1984; Borges and Iversen, 1986). These cells, which are more numerous in the upper lumbar than in the thoracic level of the cord, are grouped together in the central grey matter encircling the central canal within lamina X (Fig. 1, cell 6).

In the central intermediate grey–lamina X there are neurons which project to dorsal, intermediate and ventral grey matter and appear to provide integration between the sensory, motor and autonomic segments of the spinal cord (Borges and Iversen, 1986) (Fig. 1, cell 6).

Cholinergic receptors within the spinal cord

In vitro receptor autoradiography is an adequate technique to localize and quantitate neuroreceptors within sections of spinal cord. To map muscarinic antagonistic receptors [^{3}H]quinuclidinylbenzilate (QNB) (Gillberg et al., 1984; Seybold and Elde, 1984; Scatton et al., 1984; Gillberg and Aquilonius, 1985: Seybold, 1985; Villiger and Faull, 1985; Gillberg and Wiksten, 1986; Manaker et al., 1988; Gillberg and Askmark, 1989), [^{3}H]methylscopolamine (Wamsley et al., 1981; Whitehouse et al., 1983; Wamsley et al., 1984) or [^{3}H]pirenzepine (Yamamura et al., 1983; Villiger and Faull, 1985) have been used. α-[^{3}H]Bungarotoxin (α-Btx) has been used for mapping nicotinic receptors in the spinal cord (Arimats et al., 1981; Ninkovic and Hunt, 1983; Gillberg and Aquilonius, 1985; Gillberg and Wiksten, 1986; Gillberg and Askmark, 1989) but the use of this ligand is of doubtful significance because in most neurophysiological studies α-Btx has not been able to inhibit the response of nicotinic drugs within the central nervous system (CNS). The receptor distribution visualized in the spinal cord by the use of this ligand, however, is in close agreement with that obtained by means of ^{3}H-ACh

(Gillberg et al., 1988), which might imply a functional significance for the binding sites.

Muscarinic receptors

The highest densities of both agonistic and antagonistic muscarinic binding sites are found in lamina IX and in the substantia gelatinosa (laminae II–III). In lamina IX, motor neuron area, the muscarinic receptors are mainly of the high-affinity agonist type (Whitehouse et al., 1983; Wamsley et al., 1984), while in the substantia gelatinosa they are mostly of the low-affinity agonist type (Whitehouse et al., 1983; Wamsley et al., 1984). When pirenzepine, a selective M_1 antagonist, has been used as a ligand, a 20–30% higher density of labelling has been found in lamina II compared with lamina IX (Yamamura et al., 1983; Villiger and Faul, 1985). Taken together, these results conclusively show that M_2 receptors predominate in lamina IX of the ventral horn, while M_1 receptors occur in a higher proportion than M_2 receptors in the posterior horn. Muscarinic receptors have also been reported to be located in the intermediolateral cell column (IML). On the basis of in vitro autoradiographic grain counting in the IML, Seybold and Elde (1984) have suggested that these receptors are located postsynaptically on neuronal perikarya and dendrites. There is also an accumulation of binding sites around the central canal (lamina X) (Seybold, 1985; Gillberg et al., 1988). The antagonistic muscarinic binding sites in the posterior horn are reduced by 30% after dorsal root ligation (Gillberg and Askmark, 1989) and after dorsal rhizotomies the number of binding sites are already reduced after 12 h and continue to decrease for up to 20 days of survival time (Gillberg and Wiksten, 1986). These two studies indicate that at least 30% of the binding sites are located presynaptically on the primary afferents in the posterior horn (Fig. 1). After ventral root rhizotomies the number of muscarinic antagonistic binding sites is reduced in the motor neuron area ipsilateral to the lesion (Gillberg and Wiksten, 1986; Gillberg and Askmark, 1989). The number of α motor neurons is reduced after ventral rhizotomy (Kellerth, personal communication) and it is plausible that muscarinic receptors are located on these neurons. The view that muscarinic ACh receptors are located on α motor neurons is supported by the results of an iontophoretic study in the cat by Ziegelgänsberger and Reiter (1974) and a study by Gillberg and Wiksten (1986). In the latter study, small areas within lamina IX with low grain density, the size of which roughly corresponded to a motor neuron, were observed on the ipsilateral side of a ventral rhizotomy. The number of binding sites for the antagonist QNB are considerably higher than in the number for the agonist ACh. This difference might be due to binding to different subtypes of muscarinic receptors in the spinal cord. Agonist binding sites seem to be less sensitive to axonal damage than antagonist binding sites as there is no significant decrease of muscarinic ACh binding in the motor neuron area after ventral rhizotomy while there is a clearcut decrease of QNB binding (Gillberg and Askmark, 1989) (Fig. 1).

Nicotinic receptors

The largest number of nicotinic ACh binding sites is found in the apical part of the dorsal horn and in lamina X around the central canal (human and cat) (Gillberg et al., 1988). With our incubation technique, nicotinic binding sites have not been detected within the ventral horn in man and cat. There are two types of excitatory response for ACh on Renshaw cells (Curtis and Ryall, 1966). The neurophysiologically defined muscarinic receptors are similar to the muscarinic receptors in peripheral effector organs. The nicotinic receptors, on the other hand, seem to be intermediate between those of peripheral nicotinic and muscarinic receptors (King and Ryall, 1981). These nicotinic recognition sites could have been displaced from the Renshaw cells by the co-incubation with 1.5 μM atropine in our experiments. In the dorsal horn of the rat spinal cord, α-Btx binding sites are concentrated in lamina I, in the marginal cell layer, and in lamina III, the nucleus propius, with low levels of binding sites in lamina II, the substantia gelatinosa. High concentration of binding sites have also been detected in lamina X around the central canal (Ninkovic and Hunt, 1983; Gillberg and Wiksten, 1986). The lack of reduction of nicotinic, ACh and α-Btx binding ipsilateral to ventral rhizotomy means that it is less likely that nicotinic receptors are located on the α motor neurons. There is much evidence that nicotinic receptors are instead located on the Renshaw cells in the ventral horn (Ninkovic and Hunt, 1983) which are not reduced after ventral rhizotomy (Kellerth, personal communication).

Studies on the terminations of primary afferent fibres within the spinal cord generally suggest that the large and intermediate diameter myelinated fibres project mainly into layers III and IV of the dorsal horn, while the majority of A δ and C fibres terminate more superficially within layers I and II (Light and Perl, 1979). Ninkovic and Hunt (1983) have found a reduction of the grains generated from α-Btx in lamina III with little loss in other laminae after dorsal root section (Fig. 1). This might indicate that α-Btx binding sites are located on myelinated afferent fibres. In two other studies the authors have not been able to detect significant reduction of binding sites in the posterior horn after dorsal rhizotomy (Gillberg and Wiksten, 1986) or ligation (Gillberg and Askmark, 1989).

Ascending and descending cholinergic fibres in the spinal cord?

Receptors frequently react rapidly, with an increase or decrease in their number, to environmental changes such as drug treatment (Taylor et al., 1982; Churchill et al., 1984) or deafferentation (Rotter et al., 1979; Kayaalp and Neff, 1980; Charlton et al., 1981; Jerusalinsky et al., 1983; Gillberg and Wiksten, 1986). The location of receptors can be both post- and presynaptic and also non-synaptic (Hamel and Beaudet, 1984). When a lesion is produced in a fibre tract and a reduction in the number of receptors is detected

relatively soon afterwards in the termination area, these receptors are probably located presynaptically or non-synaptically. A second response may then appear, namely an increase to the normal level or above, and this response occurs from postsynaptic receptors. In yet another situation no receptor response at all can be detected. One possible reason for this is that neurons completely inside the CNS may not be able to react by changing the number of receptors (Rotter et al., 1979). To determine whether there are ascending and/or descending cholinergic fibres in the spinal cord the most comonly used technique has been to perform spinal cord lesions (hemisections) above the segment under study. The observation that ChAT activity in the ventral horn is reduced ipsilateral to and below a spinal cord lesion suggests — although there is no change in cholinergic receptors — that cholinergic mechanisms may be influenced from higher levels (Gillberg and Wiksten, 1986). This is not in agreement with a report from an earlier ChAT study (Kanazawa et al., 1979), but is in accordance with results of Gwyn et al. (1966, 1972), who found evidence of ascending and descending cholinergic fibres in the spinal cord by AChE accumulation distal and proximal to a lesion in the spinal cord white matter. It is possible that the AChE staining observed within the funiculi may have been in monoaminergic axons. Borges and Iversen (1986) could not with immunohistochemical techniques involving monoclonal antibody to ChAT observe any evidence of cholinergic fibers within the dorsolateral or dorsal funiculus that would support a descending cholinergic projection to the dorsal horn. However, they observed fine ChAT immunoreactive fibres entering the midlateral funiculus from the ventral grey matter. These fibres appeared to represent cholinergic propriospinal neurons (neurons which are intraspinal), perhaps from recurrent axon collaterals of motor neurons.

Cholinergic receptor studies give evidence both in favour of (Charlton et al., 1981) and against (Kayaalp and Neff, 1980) the existence of descending and ascending cholinergic tracts in the spinal cord. In vitro receptor autoradiography cannot detect cholinergic connections in the spinal cord after spinal lesions (Gillberg and Wiksten, 1986). There are several possible explanations for this negative finding. (1) The cholinergic projection from supraspinal areas is too small and too widely spread in the spinal cord sections to be detected by in vitro autoradiographic techniques. It is known that the propriospinal neurons are numerically predominant (97% of the total neurons of the spinal cord) and that the long tract neurons make up approximately 1% and motor neurons 1–2% of the total neurons of the spinal cord (Chung et al., 1984). (2) The change in properties of receptor binding could have been undetected by these studies. (3) The phenomenon of supersensitivity may not occur in the spinal system.

Functional aspects of the cholinergic system within the spinal cord

The best-known cholinergic neurons are the spinal motor neurons which project from the ventral horn to skeletal muscle. These neurons are responsible for the muscle contraction directly as well as indirectly by influencing neighboring anterior horn neurons via recurrent axon collaterals. The spinal cholinergic cells within laminae I–III in the posterior horn and around the central canal lamina X are capable of affecting nociception. Receptors in the region surrounding the central canal may modulate sensory input to the reticular formation (Nahin et al., 1983).

Nociception

More than fifty years have now elapsed since the first observation was made that the cholinesterase inhibitor physostigmine increased the pain threshold in man (Pellandra, 1933). The spinal antinociception action of morphine in the rat is potentiated by physostigmine when they are intrathecally co-administered (Dirksen and Nijhuis, 1983). Physostigmine is an AChE inhibitor, which increases the endogenous level of acetylcholine acting on both muscarinic and nicotinic cholinergic receptors (Taylor, 1986). A dose-related effect has been shown for physostigmine in the nociceptive tail immersion test (Gordh et al., 1989).

The effects of physostigmine after spinal administration last about 30 min, probably due to rapid systemic uptake and elimination of this lipophilic AChE inhibitor (Hartvig et al., 1986). Spinal administration of neostigmine also gives increased tail immersion latency in the nociceptive test but the effect is of considerably longer duration. This longer effect is due to its quarternary ammonium ion which passes only poorly from the cerebrospinal fluid to the blood. The antinociceptive effects of both physostigmine and neostigmine are promptly reversed by atropine. This response indicates that a selective muscarinic receptor-mediated action produces the antinociceptive effect (Gordh et al., 1989). The tail immersion test involves a spinal motor reflex and this effect is mediated locally in the spinal cord. The hot plate latency times are controlled from the brain. Contrary to the effect in the tail immersion test, physostigmine does not affect the hot plate latency times. This indicates that the drug, given by intrathecal (IT) injection, mainly produces an effect on the spinal cord with less pronounced supraspinal actions.

Clinically, an analogue effect has been demonstrated after intravenous administration of physostigmine to patients with postoperative pain (Peterson et al., 1986). A potent spinally mediated antinociception by the ACh receptor agonist carbachol has been demonstrated in the rat (Yaksh et al., 1985; Gillberg et al., 1989). These effects have been postulated to be due to muscarinic receptor agonism, since the antinociception can be completely antagonized by atropine. Both the selective M_1 antagonist pirenzepine and the M_2 selective antagonist AFDX 116 are capable of blocking the antinociceptive effects produced by IT carbachol. Thus, the carbachol effects are probably mediated by both M_1 and M_2 receptor activation (Gillberg et al., 1989a).

It has been postulated from experiments in anaesthetized rats that subarachnoid nicotine has an antinociceptive effect (Aceto et al., 1986). However, the antinociceptive action of IT administered nicotine receptor agonists, such as cytisine and nicotine, in rats is not convincing (Gillberg et al., 1989b). Yaksh and collaborators (1985) were also unable to obtain antinociception response from IT nicotine. Antinociception induced by nicotine after systemic and intracerebroventricular administration points to a selective central action of the drug (Phan et al., 1973; Mattila et al., 1968; Sahley and Berntson, 1979; Tripathi et al., 1982; Aceto et al., 1986; Molinero and Del Rio, 1987). The effect was blocked by the centrally acting nicotine receptor blocker mecamylamine but not by selective antagonists unable to pass the blood brain barrier.

It can be concluded that the main analgesic effect of nicotine is of supraspinal origin, since nicotine gives no obvious antinociception after subarachnoid administration.

IT injections of nicotine, cytisine and 9-amino-1,2,3,4-tetrahydroacridine (THA) cause spontaneous behavioral symptoms such as gnawing on the test cage, vocalization and hyperactivity (Gillberg et al., 1989). These effects can be antagonized with mecamylamine, which indicates that they are mediated by cholinergic nicotinic receptors (Gillberg et al., 1989). Thus, nicotinic receptors may have a role in spinal sensory transmission, but not in antinociception.

The cholinergic system interacts with other transmitter systems in spinal antinociception

To test the hypothesis that spinal α_2-adrenoceptor-mediated antinociception may be influenced by cholinergic receptor agonism, both clonidine and physostigmine have been administered simultaneously. When combining 10 μg of clonidine, which in itself has a moderate effect on latency times in the tail immersion test, with 15 μg of physostigmine, an additive antinociception occurs in the duration and the degree of the peak effect (Gordh et al., 1989). The clonidine (15 μg

IT) produced increase of latency times is attenuated by administration of atropine (15 μg, IT) (Gordh et al., 1989). This indicates that a part of the clonidine effects might be cholinergic in nature, although clonidine is generally regarded as a selective α_2-adrenoceptor agonistic drug (Yaksh, 1985; Werner, 1986).

Buccafusco and Aronstam (1986) have shown that clonidine may interact with cholinergic mechanisms in the central nervous system in at least three different ways. In the first place, clonidine may be agonistic at presynaptic α_2-adrenoceptors located on cholinergic neurons, resulting in an inhibition of ACh release from cholinergic nerve terminals. This effect would decrease a cholinergic agonistic effect in antinociception. Secondly, clonidine interacts directly with muscarinic receptors, blocking the effects of ACh. Thirdly, clonidine inhibits the activity of AChE. This action would therefore increase the concentration of endogenously released ACh in the synaptic cleft, and would promote cholinergic antinociception.

Selective chemical destruction of spinal noradrenergic nerve terminals with 6-hydroxydopamine abolishes the antinociceptive effect of physostigmine, and pharmacological α-receptor blockade causes a significant attenuation of the action of physostigmine (Gordh et al., 1989). In rats pretreated with a systemic dose of N-2-chloroethyl-N-ethyl-2-bromobenzylamine (DSP4), which is a selective CNS noradrenaline neurotoxin, carbachol still gives increased latency times as compared to control rats. However, the effect is significantly attenuated 30 and 60 min after administration in comparison to non-lesioned animals (Gillberg et al., 1989a). Taken together, these findings indicate that the spinal noradrenergic system is necessary for the optimal function of the spinal cholinergic system and vice versa: unimpaired cholinergic mechanisms are required for optimal function of the α_2-adrenoceptor-mediated effects.

One possibility that must be considered in order to explain the interaction between spinal noradrenergic and cholinergic neuronal structures is the existence of a cholinergic interneuron in lamina III (see structure section), terminating on the primary afferent or on the secondary sensory neuron in the dorsal horn. This cholinergic interneuron could, hypothetically, receive noradrenergic tracts which are involved in the modulation of the transmission of nociceptive input. If muscarinic receptors, located in the dorsal horn on the sensory primary afferent or the secondary sensory neuron, are blocked with atropine, descending bulbospinal noradrenergic excitatory input to this cholinergic interneuron may produce release of ACh. In this situation, ACh would not be able to stimulate the postsynaptic muscarinic receptors in the presence of atropine. This would lead to attenuation of the antinociceptive effect of clonidine by blockade of its cholinergic link of action.

Destruction of the spinal noradrenergic nerve terminals extinguishes the antinociceptive effect of physostigmine (Gordh et al., 1989) but not that of carbachol (Gillberg et al., 1989a). To explain this interaction, the postulated cholinergic interneuron located in the dorsal horn may be of importance. Hypothetically, if the spinal noradrenergic nerve endings are destroyed, this would lead to the disappearance of noradrenergic excitatory input, normally activating the cholinergic interneuron. When this activation is absent, ACh will not be released, leaving the postsynaptic muscarinic receptors located on the primary afferent without input. The main effect of physostigmine, as an AChE inhibitor, is to increase the amount of endogenously available ACh in the synaptic gap. If this speculation is correct, it explains why physostigmine antinociception is blocked by destruction of spinal noradrenergic nerve terminals. Carbachol analgesia in rats is unaffected by α-adrenoceptor blockade with phentolamine (Yaksh et al., 1985). Carbachol, however, is a much stronger muscarinic agonist than physostigmine. This difference may explain why carbachol gives rise to antinociception in spite of α-adrenoceptor blockade or DSP4 lesion of noradrenergic terminals.

There is also interaction between the enkephalin and cholinergic systems since morphine and physostigmine are additive when co-administered and IT morphine antinociception in rats has been shown to be attenuated by atropine (Dirksen and Nijhuis, 1983). However, the carbachol antinociception is not reversed by naloxon (Yaksh et al., 1985).

Spontaneous motor activity

The spontaneous motor activity of rats has been studied after IT injection of cholinergic drugs using computerized test boxes. Physostigmine and THA significantly decrease total activity, locomotion and rearing as compared to control animals. The motor effects of physostigmine are attenuated with IT atropine more markedly than are those of THA. Mecamylamine, however, cannot antagonise effects (Gillberg et al., 1989b). This indicates that these effects are mediated mainly via cholinergic muscarinic receptors. These findings are in agreement with a study by Ryall and Haas (1975) who have suggested that the muscarinic receptors on Renshaw cells are the physiologically active ones.

Physostigmine and THA increase the level of ACh within the spinal cord by inhibition of ChAT (Enz, 1988). Microiontophoretically applied ACh onto the motor neuron gives a depolarization of the cells, whereas Renshaw cells respond with both a rapid depolarization and an increase of firing rate (Zieglgänsberger and Reiter, 1974). Renshaw cells have both nicotinic and muscarinic receptors on the perikarya (Curtis and Ryall, 1966; King and Ryall, 1981) and are inhibitory to the motor neuron (Renshaw, 1941; Eccles et al., 1954; Curtis et al., 1957; Wilson et al., 1960). The decrease of spontaneous activity of the motor neuron caused by physostigmine and THA, might be explained by both a direct depolarization of the motor neuron and an inhibition mediated via Renshaw cells. The Renshaw cells are not an integral part of the spinal central pattern generator for locomotion, nor do they control the timing of the motor neuron or Ia interneuron bursts of firing during fictive locomotion. The Renshaw cells instead limit the firing rates of motor neurons and Ia interneurons during each burst (Noga et al., 1987).

According to one study (Gillberg et al., 1989b) spinal cholinergic nicotinic receptors have no significant effect on total activity, locomotion and rearing. When cytisine, another nicotinic agonist, has been used, a significant decrease of total activity and locomotion has been observed. These effects are mediated via nicotinic cholinergic receptors as indicated by antagonism with mecamylamine. Thus, cytisine may activate Renshaw cells thus causing inhibition of the motor neuron and hence a reduced spontaneous motor activity. AChE inhibitors increase the level of ACh and thereby stimulate muscarinic receptors on the motor neuron whereas cytisine only activates the nicotinic receptors on Renshaw cells.

Acknowledgement

Studies in the laboratory of the authors were supported by the Swedish Medical Research Council (grant No 4373). The authors are indebted to Mrs Gun Kärrlander for secretarial help.

References

Aceto, M.D., Bagley, R.S., Dewey, W.L., Fu, T.C. and Martin, B.R. (1986) The spinal cord as a major site for the antinociceptive action of nicotin in the rat. *Neuropharmacology,* 25: 1031–1036.

Aquilonius, S.-M., Eckernäs, S.-Å. and Gillberg, P.-G. (1981) Topographical localization of choline acetyltransferase within the human spinal cord and a comparison with some other species. *Brain Res.,* 211: 329–340.

Arimatsu, Y., Seto, A. and Amano, T. (1981) An atlas of α-bungarotoxin binding sites and structures containing acetylcholinesterase in the mouse central nervous system. *J. Comp. Neurol.,* 198: 603–631.

Barber, R.P., Phelps, P.E., Houser, C.R., Crawford, G.D., Salvaterra, P.M. and Vaughn, J.E. (1984) The morphology and distribution of neurons containing choline acetyltransferase in the adult rat spinal cord: An immunocytochemical study. *J. Comp. Neurol.,* 229: 329–346.

Borges, L. and Iversen, S.D. (1986) Topography of choline acetyltransferase immunoreactive neurons and fibers in the rat spinal cord. *Brain Res.,* 362: 140–148.

Buccafusco, J.J. and Aronstam, R.S. (1986) Clonidine protection from the toxicity of soman, an organophosphate acetylcholinesterase inhibitor in the mouse. *J. Pharmacol. Exp. Ther.,* 239: 43–47.

Bryan, R.N., Trevino, D.L. and Willis, W.D. (1972) Evidence for a common location of α and gamma motoneurons. *Brain Res.,* 38: 193–196.

Charlton, G., Brennan, M.J.W. and Ford, D.M. (1981) Alterations in neurotransmitter receptor binding sites in the spinal cord after transection. *Brain Res.,* 218: 372–375.

Chung, K., Kevetter, G.A., Willis, W.D. and Coggeshall, R.F. (1984) An estimate of the ratio or propriospinal to long tract neurons in the sacral spinal cord of the rat. *Neurosci. Lett.,* 44: 173–177.

Churchill, L., Pazdernik, T.L., Samson, F. and Nelson, S.R. (1984) Topographical distribution of down-regulated muscarinic receptors in rat brains after repeated exposure to diisopropyl phosphorofluoridate. *Neuroscience,* 11: 463–473.

Cullheim, S., Kellerth, J.O. and Conradi, S. (1977) Evidence for direct synaptic interconnections between cat spinal and motoneurones via recurrent axon collaterals: a morphological study using intracellular injection of horseradish peroxidase. *Brain Res.,* 132: 1–10.

Cullheim, S. and Kellerth, J.O. (1978) A morphological study of the axons and recurrent axon intracellular staining with horseradish peroxidase. *J. Comp. Neurol.,* 178: 537–538.

Curtis, D.R. and Ryall, R.W. (1966) The excitation of Renshaw cells by cholinomimetics. *Exp. Brain Res.,* 2: 49–65.

Curtis, D.R., Eccles, J.C. and Eccles, R.M. (1957) Pharmacological studies of spinal reflexes. *J. Physiol.,* 136: 420–434.

Dirksen, R.N. and Nijhuis, G.M.M. (1983) The relevance of cholinergic transmission at the spinal level to opiate effectiveness. *Eur. J. Pharmacol.,* 91: 215–221.

Eccles, J.C., Fatt, P. and Koketsu, K. (1954) Cholinergic and inhibitory synapses on a pathway from motor axon collaterals to motoneurons. *J. Physiol.,* 126: 524–562.

Enz, A. (1988) Accumulation and turn-over of acetylcholine after administration of acetylcholinesterase inhibitors in rat brain. In E. Giacobini and R. Becker (Eds.), *Current Research in Alzheimer Therapy,* Taylor and Francis, London, pp. 43–51.

Feldberg, W. and Vogt, M. (1948) Acetylcholine synthesis in different regions of the central nervous system. *J. Physiol.,* 107: 372–381.

Giacobini, E. and Holmstedt, B. (1958) Cholinesterase content of certain regions of the spinal cord as judged by histochemical and cartesian diver technique. *Acta Physiol. Scand.,* 42: 12–27.

Gillberg, P.-G. and Askmark, H. (1989) Changes of cholinergic and opioid receptor in the rat spinal cord, dorsal root and sciatic nerve after ventral and dorsal root lesion. Submitted.

Gillberg, P.-G. and Wiksten, B. (1986) Effects of spinal cord lesions and rhizotomies on cholinergic and opiate receptor binding sites in rat spinal cord. *Acta Physiol. Scand.,* 126: 575–582.

Gillberg, P.-G., Aquilonius, S.-M., Eckernäs, S.-Å., Lundqvist, G. and Winblad, B. (1982) Choline acetyltransferase and substance P-like immunoreactivity in the human spinal cord: changes in amyotrophic lateral sclerosis. *Brain Res.,* 250: 394–397.

Gillberg, P.-G., Nordberg, A. and Aquilonius, S.-M. (1984) Muscarinic binding sites in small homogenates and in autoradiographic sections from rat and human spinal cord. *Brain Res.,* 300: 327–333.

Gillberg, P.-G. and Aquilonius, S.-M. (1985) Cholinergic, opioid and glycine receptor binding sites localized in human spinal cord by in vitro autoradiography: changes in amyotrophic lateral sclerosis. *Acta Neurol. Scand.,* 72: 299–306.

Gillberg, P.G., d'Argy, R. and Aquilonius, S.-M. (1988) Autoradiographic distribution of ^{3}H-acetylcholine binding sites in the cervical spinal cord of man and some other species. *Neurosci. Lett.,* 90: 197–202.

Gillberg, P.-G., Gordh, T., Hartvig, P., Jansson, I., Pettersson, J. and Post, C. (1989a) Characterization of antinociception induced by intrathecally administered carbachol. *Pharmacol. Toxicol.,* 64: 340–343.

Gillberg, P.-G., Hartvig, P., Gordh, T., Sottile, A., Jansson, I., Archer, T. and Post, C. (1989b) Behavioral effects after intrathecal administration of cholinergic receptor agonists in the rat. Submitted.

Gordh, T., Jansson, I., Hartvig, P., Gillberg, P.-G. and Post, P. (1989) Interactions between noradrenergic and cholinergic mechanisms involved in spinal nociceptive processing. *Acta Anaesthesiol. Scand.,* 33: 39–47.

Gwyn, D.G. and Wolstencroft, J.H. (1966) Ascending and descending cholinergic fibers in cat spinal cord: histochemical evidence. *Science,* 153: 1543–1544.

Gwyn, D.G., Wolstencroft, J.H. and Silver, A. (1972) The effect of a hemisection on the distribution of acetylcholinesterase and choline acetyltransferase in the spinal cord of cat. *Brain Res.,* 47: 289–301.

Hamel, E. and Beaudet, A. (1984) Electron microscopic autoradiographic localization of opioid receptors in rat neostriatum. *Nature,* 312-155-157.

Hartvig, P., Wiklund, L. and Lindström, B. (1986) Pharmacokinetics of physostigmine after intravenous, intramuscular and subcutaneous administration to surgical patients. *Acta Anaesthesiol. Scand.,* 30: 177–182.

Houser, C.R., Crawford, G.D., Barber, R.P., Salvaterra, P.M. and Vaughn, J.E. (1983) Organization and morphological characteristics of cholinergic neurons: an immunocytochemical study with a monoclonal antibody to choline acetyltransferase. *Brain Res.,* 266: 97–119.

Ishii, T. and Friede, R.L. (1967) A comparative histochemical mapping of the distribution of acetylcholinesterase and nicotinamide adenine dinucleotide-diaphorase activities in the human brain. In Pfeiffer and Smythies (Eds.), *International Review of Neurobiology,* Academic Press, New York, pp. 231–275.

Jerusalinsky, D., Medina, J.H. and Robertis, D. (1983) Lesion of forebrain nuclei reveals possible presynaptic cholinergic muscarinic receptors in rat cerebral cortex. *Neuropharmacology,* 22: 835–838.

Kanazawa, I., Sutoo, D., Oshima, I. and Saito, S. (1979) Effect of transection on choline acetyltransferase, thyrotropin releasing hormone and substance P in the cervical spinal cord. *Neurosci. Lett.,* 13: 325–330.

Kayaalp, S.O. and Neff, N.H. (1980) Region distribution of cholinergic muscarinic receptors in spinal cord. *Brain Res.,* 196: 429–436.

Kimura, H., Mcgeer, P.L., Peng, J.H. and Mcgeer, F.G. (1981) The central cholinergic system studied by choline acetyltransferase immunohistochemistry in the cat. *J. Comp. Neurol.,* 200: 151–200.

King, K.T. and Ryall, R.W. (1981) A re-evaluation of acetylcholine receptors on feline Renshaw cells. *Br. J. Pharmacol.,* 73: 455–460.

Lagerbäck, P.-Å., Ronnevi, L.-O., Cullheim, S. and Kellerth, J.-O. (1981) An ultrastructural study of the synaptic contacts of α-motoneurone axon collaterals. I. Contacts in lamina IX and with identified α-motoneurone dendrites in lamina VII. *Brain Res.,* 207: 247–266.

Light, A.R. and Perl, E.R. (1979) Spinal termination of functionally identified primary afferent neurons with slowly conducting myelinated fibers. *J. Comp. Neurol.,* 186: 133–150.

Macintosh, F.C. (1941) The distribution of acetylcholine in the peripheral and the central nervous system. *J. Physiol.,* 99: 436–442.

Manaker, S., Caine, S.B. and Winokur, A. (1988) Alterations in receptors for thyrotropin-releasing hormone, serotonin, and acetylcholine in amyotrophic lateral sclerosis. *Neurology,* 38: 1464–1474.

Mattila, M.J., Ahtee, L. and Saarnivaara, L. (1968) The analgesic and sedative effects of nicotine in white mice, rabbits and golden hamsters. *Ann. Med. Exp. Fenn.,* 46: 78–84.

Molinero, M.T. and Del Rio, J. (1987) Substance P, nicotinic acetylcholine receptors and antinociception in the rat. *Neuropharmacology,* 26: 1715–1720.

Nahin, R.L., Madsen, A.M. and Giesler, G.R., Jr. (1983) Anatomical and physiological studies of the gray matter surrounding the spinal cord central canal. *J. Comp. Neurol.,* 220: 321–335.

Ninkovic, M. and Hunt, S.P. (1983) Alpha-bungarotoxin binding sites on sensory neurones and their axonal transport in sensory afferents. *Brain Res.,* 272: 57–69.

Noga, B.R., Shefchyk, S.J. Jamal, J. and Jordan, L.M. (1987) The role of Renshaw cells in locomotion: antagonism of their excitation from motor axon collaterals with intravenous mecamylamine. *Exp. Brain Res.,* 66: 99–105.

Pellandra, C.L. (1933) La geneserine-morphine adjuvant de l'anesthesia generale. *Lyon. Med.,* 151: 653.

Petersson, J., Gordh, T.E., Hartvig, P. and Wiklund, L. (1986) A double-blind trial of the analgesic properties of physostigmine in postoperative patients. *Acta Anaesthesiol. Scand.,* 30: 283–288.

Phan, D.V., Doda, M., Bite, A. and György, I. (1973) Antinociceptive activity of nicotine. *Acta Physiol. Acad. Sci. Hung.,* 1: 85–93.

Renshaw, B. (1941) Influence of discharge of motoneurons upon excitation of neighboring motoneurons. *J. Neurophysiol.,* 4: 167–183.

Rexed, B. (1954) A cytoarchitectonic atlas of the spinal cord in the cat. *J. Comp. Neurol.,* 100: 297–379.

Rotter, A., Birdsall, N.J.M., Burgen, A.S.V., Field, P.M., Smolen, A. and Raisman, G. (1979) Muscarinic receptors in the central nervous system of the rat. IV. A comparison of the effects of axotomy and deafferentation on the binding of ³H-propylbenzilycholine mustard and associated synaptic changes in the hypoglossal and pontine nuclei. *Brain Res. Rev.*, 1: 207–224.

Ryall, R.W. and Haas, H.L. (1975) On the physiological significance of muscarinic receptors on Renshaw cells: a hypothesis. In P.G. Waser (Ed.), *Cholinergic Mechanisms,* Raven Press, New York, pp. 335–341.

Sahley, T. and Berntson, G.G. (1979) Antinociceptive effects of central and systemic administration of nicotine in the rat. *Psychopharmacology,* 65: 279–283.

Satoh, H., Armstrong, D.M. and Fibiger, H.C. (1983) A comparison of the distribution of central cholinergic neurons as demonstrated by acetylcholinesterase pharmacohistochemistry and choline acetyltransferase immunohistochemistry. *Brain Res. Bull.,* 11: 693–720.

Scatton, B., Dubois, A., Javoy-Agid, F. and Camus, A. (1984) Autoradiographic localization of muscarinic cholinergic receptors at various segmental levels of the human spinal cord. *Neurosci. Lett.,* 49: 239–245.

Seybold, V.S. (1985) Distribution of histaminergic, muscarinic and serotonergic binding sites in cat spinal cord with emphasis on the region surrounding the central canal. *Brain Res.,* 342: 291–296.

Seybold, V.S. and Elde, R. (1984) Receptor autoradiography in thoracic spinal cord: correlation of neurotransmitter binding sites with sympathoadrenal neurons. *J. Neurosci.,* 4: 2533–2542.

Silver, A. and Wolstencroft, J.H. (1971) The distribution of cholinesterases in relation to the structure of the spinal cord in the cat. *Brain Res.,* 34: 205–227.

Taylor, P. (1986) Anticholinesterase agents. In A. Goodman Gilman, L.S. Goodman, T.W. Rall and F. Murad (Eds.), *The Pharmacological Basis of Therapeutics,* MacMillan Publishing Co, New York, pp 110–129.

Taylor, J.E., Yaksh, T.L. and Richelson, E. (1982) Agonist regulation of muscarinic acetylcholine receptors in spinal cord. *J. Neurochem.,* 39: 521–524.

Tripathi, H.L., Martin, B.R. and Aceto, M.D. (1982) Nicotine-induced antinociception in rats and mice: Correlation with nicotine brain levels. *J. Pharmacol. Exp. Ther.,* 221: 91–96

Wamsley, J.K., Lewis, M.S., Scott Young III, W. and Kuhar, M.J. (1981) Autoradiographic localization of muscarinic cholinergic receptors in rat brainstem. *J. Neurosci.,* 1: 176–191.

Wamsley, J.K., Zarbin, M.A. and Kuhar, M.J. (1984) Distribution of muscarinic cholinergic high and low affinity agonist binding sites: A light miscoscopic autoradiographic study. *Brain Res. Bull.,* 12: 233–243.

Werner, N. (1986) Drugs that inhibit adrenergic nerves and block adrenergic receptors. In A. Goodman Gilman, L.S. Goodman, T.W. Rall and F. Murad (Eds.), *The Pharmacological Basis of Therapeutics,* MacMillan Publishing Co, New York, pp 181–214.

Whitehouse, P.J., Wamsley, J.K., Zarbin, M.A., Price,. D.L., Tourtellotte, W.W. and Kuhar, M.J. (1983) Amyotrophic lateral sclerosis alterations in neurotransmitter receptors. *Ann. Neurol.,* 14: 8–16.

Villiger, J.W. and Faull, R.L.M. (1985) Muscarinic cholinergic receptors in the human spinal cord: differential localization of ³H-pirenzepine and ³H-quinuclidinylbenzilate binding sites. *Brain Res.,* 345: 196–199.

Wilson, V.J., Talbot, W.H. and Diecke, F.P.J. (1960) Distribution of recurrent facilitation and inhibition in cat spinal cord. *J. Neurophysiol.,* 23: 144–153.

Yamamura, H.I., Wamsley, J.K., Deshmukh, P. and Roeske, W.R. (1983) Differential light microscopic autoradiographic localization of muscarinic cholinergic receptors in the brainstem and spinal cord of the rat using ³H-pirenzepine. *Eur. J. Pharmacol.,* 91: 147–149.

Yaksh, T.L., Dirksen, R. and Harty, G.J. (1985) Antinociceptive effects of intrathecal cholinomimetic drugs in the rat and cat. *Eur. J. Pharmacol.,* 117: 81–88.

Zieglgänsberger, W. and Reiter, Ch. (1974) A cholinergic mechanism in the spinal cord of cats. *Neuropharmacology,* 13: 519–527.

S.-M. Aquilonius and P.-G. Gillberg (Eds.)
Progress in Brain Research, Vol. 84
© 1990 Elsevier Science Publishers B.V. (Biomedical Division)

CHAPTER 38

Neuropharmacology of amyotrophic lateral sclerosis

H. Askmark, S.-M. Aquilonius and P.-G. Gillberg

Department of Neurology, University Hospital, S-751 85 Uppsala, Sweden

Introduction

In spite of extensive research, attractive hypotheses and new treatment strategies, amyotrophic lateral sclerosis (ALS) remains an enigmatic and incurable disease. ALS and other degenerative disorders such as Parkinson's disease and dementia of the Alzheimer type are neuropathologically characterized by preferential vulnerability of some neuronal systems and relative resistance of other neuronal systems. Irrespective of the aetiology, the progressive neuronal degenerations should be accompanied by transmitter dysfunction at the synapses of the fibre tracts involved. Insight into such mechanisms might lead to the development of symptomatic pharmacological therapy. L-DOPA treatment in Parkinson's disease and clinical trials of cholinergic agents in Alzheimer's disease have been based on this principle. Knowledge of the transmitter mechanisms involved could also provide clues to the aetiology of the disorder.

In ALS the degenerative changes are mainly restricted to the cortical spinal tracts and to the lower motor neurons in the brainstem and spinal cord, although the involvement of non-motor pathways has been increasingly recognised (see Tandan and Bradley, 1985 for review). The aim of the present chapter is to overview the neuropharmacology of ALS, as expressed in studies on transmitter-related enzymes and receptors in the CNS and skeletal muscle, with emphasis on cholinergic mechanisms. Closely allied therapeutic trials and the search for neurotrophic disturbances and neurotoxic factors in ALS are included.

Abnormalities of neuronal receptors and transmitters

In the human spinal cord the highest activity of choline acetyltransferase (ChAT) is found in the ventrolateral part of the ventral horn (Aquilonius et al., 1981). This activity is probably mainly located in the motor neurons, cells of an undoubtedly cholinergic nature. Another area with high ChAT activity can be demarcated in the apical part of the dorsal horn. Not unexpectedly, profound reductions in ChAT activity within the motor neuron areas are found in ALS (Kanazawa, 1977; Gillberg et al., 1982; Nagata et al., 1982). In this disease the ChAT activity is also considerably decreased in the area in the dorsal horn, which normally shows high activity (Gillberg et al., 1982). The morphological counterparts of the latter reductions are at present unknown, but a relationship to degeneration of large afferent neurons (Kawamura et al., 1981) seems probable.

Until recently little was known about the location of other markers of classical neurotransmitters and peptides in the spinal cord of ALS patients and controls. When substance P-like immunoreactivity (SPLI) was measured in tissue parts dissected from human spinal cord, the highest value was found in the dorsal horn at all segment levels (Gillberg et al., 1982). This result is in agreement with the findings in a previous detailed immunohistochemical study (Cuello et al., 1976). No clearcut changes in SPLI were found in spinal cords from ALS cases, which is in accordance with the observations in a recent study by Dietl et al. (1989). However, in two other investigations (Patten and Croft, 1984; Schoenen et al., 1985), severe loss of spinal SP-containing fibres in ALS was demonstrated by immunohistochemical methods. Schoenen et al. (1985) also studied 5-HT, met- and leu-enkephalin and cholecystokinin (CCK) fibers and found them unchanged in ALS. Since the loss of SP-fibres was restricted to the motor neuron areas (lamina IX) and seemed to precede motor neuron degeneration, they proposed that SP-fibres descending from supraspinal regions might normally exert trophic influence on the lower motor neurons.

Another peptide, thyrotropin-releasing hormone (TRH), has received considerable interest in relation to ALS. The highest TRH immunoreactivity within the human spinal cord is found in the anterior horn. Some investigators have noted reduced TRH levels in the anterior horn of ALS cases (Mitsuma et al., 1984), whereas others have not found any change in spinal TRH levels in ALS (Jackson et al., 1986). The latter investigators found increased concentrations of the putative TRH metabolite histidyl proline diketopiperazine and concluded that TRH neurons are probably not primarily affected in ALS. In other studies the effects of TRH on cultured motor neurons have indicated that TRH plays a role as a neurotrophic factor (Banda et al., 1985; Schmidt-Achert et al., 1984).

With the use of specific radioactive ligands it has been possible to identify and measure neurotransmitter receptors in the central nervous tissues. Hayashi and colleagues (1981) in studies of homogenates of spinal cords, found reduced glycinergic receptor binding in the anterior grey matter in ALS cases, but no change in muscarinic, cholinergic, dopaminergic, gamma-aminobutyric acid (GABA)-ergic or beta-adrenergic receptor binding.

Today in vitro receptor autoradiography is the most adequate technique for localizing and quantitating neuroreceptors within sections of human spinal cord (Whitehouse et al., 1983; Whitehouse, 1985; Gillberg et al., 1984; Gillberg and Aquilonius, 1985; Scatton et al., 1984; Manaker et al., 1985, 1988). In these studies, [^{3}H]quinuclidinylbenzilate or [^{3}H]methylscopolamine has been used as a radioactive ligand for muscarinic and α-[^{3}H]bungarotoxin (α-BuTx) for nicotinic binding sites. The receptor distribution visualized in the human spinal cord with use of these ligands is in close accordance with that observed by means of [^{3}H]ACh (Gillberg et al., 1988), which might suggest that the binding sites have functional significance. The highest densities of muscarinic binding sites are found in lamina IX and in the substantia gelatinosa (laminae II–III) (Whitehouse et al., 1983; Gillberg et al., 1984; Scatton et al., 1984). In ALS the muscarinic binding sites are markedly reduced in lamina IX and slightly reduced in laminae II–III (Whitehouse et al., 1983; Gillberg et al., 1985; Manaker et al., 1988). The pronounced reduction in such binding sites in lamina IX seems to parallel the degeneration of motor neurons. It is not known to what extent these binding sites are located on motor neuron somata, on collaterals and on Renshaw cells. The muscarinic subtype mainly reduced in lamina IX corresponds to the "high-affinity agonist site" (Whitehouse et al., 1983).

TRH binding sites are also mainly distributed within laminae IX and II–III, the highest density being seen in the latter areas (Manaker et al., 1985). Interestingly, in ALS the changes in spinal TRH binding sites are similar to those in muscarinic sites, discussed earlier. Thus, TRH receptors in lamina IX are reduced by almost 90% and the corresponding reduction in lamina II is about 50% (Manaker et al., 1988). Substance P binding has also recently been found to be reduced in spinal cords from ALS cases, especially in the ventral horn (Dietl et al., 1986). In contrast to the reductions of the above-mentioned binding sites, increases of up to 140% in the densities of serotonin type IA receptors have been observed in lamina IX from ALS cases (Manaker et al., 1988).

Autoradiographic studies of other spinal receptor binding sites, namely [^{3}H]α-BuTx, opioid, benzodiazepines, glycine (Whitehouse et al., 1983; Gillberg et al., 1985), beta-adrenergic and norepinephrine (Manaker, 1988), have shown relatively unchanged or slightly reduced densities in ALS.

The findings in the above-mentioned autoradiographic studies point to the usefulness of this receptor mapping technique in understanding the changes in neuronal populations that occur in the neurodegenerative diseases. It may be concluded (Table I) from the relatively limited number of post-mortem studies that the most consistent changes in transmitter-related markers in spinal cords from ALS cases are pronounced reductions in the activity of ChAT, in muscarinic binding sites and in TRH receptors. Treatment strategies intended to restore spinal cholinergic and TRH mechanisms in ALS will be discussed below.

Increasing interest has been devoted to glutamate and aspartate, potentially neuroexcitotoxic compounds, which are considered to be the transmitters of the corticospinal pathways (Young et al., 1981; Potachner et al., 1986) which are markedly involved in ALS. Decreased contents of these amino acids in the brain and spinal cord

(Robinson et al., 1968; Perry et al., 1987) and abnormality of their metabolism (Plaitakis and Caroscio, 1987) have been observed. A partial deficiency of glutamate dehydrogenase (GDH) and abnormal glutamate metabolism have also been identified in late-onset multi-system atrophic disorders which can present as atypical ALS (Plaitakis et al., 1984). Serum aspartate has been reported to correlate inversely with the severity of the disease (Patten et al., 1978). A glutamate analogue, β-N-methylamino-L-alanine, isolated from *Cycas circinalis* (false sago palm) is toxic to the motor system in animal experiments and has been proposed to be the cardinal aetiological factor underlying the high incidence of ALS and Parkinson-dementia complex in Guam (Spencer, 1987).

The contents of GABA have been found to be reduced in some brain regions (Perry et al., 1987) and in the CSF (Ziegler et al., 1980) from patients with ALS. The content of taurine, an amino acid with possible inhibitory effects on neuronal firing (Curtis and Johnston, 1974), has been reported to be increased in the motor cortex of ALS cases (Yoshino et al., 1979; Perry et al., 1987). Abnormal concentrations of other amino acids in CSF and plasma from ALS patients have also been observed (Patten et al., 1978), including elevated CSF concentrations of lycine and leucine.

The finding of increased levels of norepineph-

TABLE I

Neurotransmitter-related spinal changes in ALS

Markers of transmitters and peptides

Region	ChAT	5-HT	SP	TRH	Enkephalin	CCK
Anterior horn	↓↓↓	–	↓–	↓–	–	–
Posterior horn	↓↓	–	–	–	–	–

Binding sites

Region	Muscarinic	α-BuTx	Opioid	Glycine	SP	TRH	Benzo-diazepine	5-HT	β-adreno-ceptor	Norepinephrine
Anterior horn	↓↓↓	–	–	↓–	↓↓	↓↓↓	↓	↑↑↑	–	–
Posterior horn	↓	–	–	–	–	↓↓	–	–	–	–

For abbreviations see text.

rine in the plasma and CSF from ALS patients (Ziegler et al., 1980) is surprising, since bedridden controls have been found to have decreased plasma norepinephrine levels and this suggests that the autonomic nervous system might be affected in ALS. Belendiuk and colleagues (1981) have reported a slightly increased concentration of serotonin and significantly increased monoaminoxidase activity in the platelets, and decreased plasma levels of free and bound tryptophan, all correlating with the severity of the disease. They concluded that the increased platelet monoaminoxidase activity might be related to the elevated levels of plasma epinephrine and that the increased platelet serotonin and low plasma tryptophan levels could be an attempt to compensate either for dysfunction of the monoaminergic neurons which normally facilitate motor function (White and Neuman, 1983) or for motor neuron degeneration. Decreased activity of central dopaminergic neurons in ALS has been suggested by Szulc-Kuberska et al. (1988) on the basis of their finding of an exaggerated prolactin response to metoclopramide in ALS patients.

The reactions of skeletal muscle to denervation involve the widespread appearance of extrajunctional ACh receptors, a process which seems to be unimpaired in ALS. Thus, increased extrajunctional binding of $[^{125}I]\alpha$-BuTx has been demonstrated in muscle biopsy specimens taken from the motor point zone in cases of ALS (Drachman and Famebrough, 1976). In vitro autoradiography of a whole biceps brachii muscle from an ALS patient revealed pronounced $[^{3}H]\alpha$-BuTx binding distributed over the entire muscle (Askmark et al., 1985).

Search for neurotrophic disturbances in ALS

It has been suggested that neurotoxic factors or limitation or a reduction or blockade of trophic factors necessary for the survival of motor neurons are involved in the aetiology of ALS. Conradi and Ronnevi (1982, 1985) observed that a cytotoxic factor in plasma from ALS patients provoked haemolysis of normal erythrocytes. Studies on effects of ALS sera on ciliary neurons in culture failed to establish that the sera had any clear influence on the survival of these cells or on the choline acetyltransferase levels (Touzeau and Kato, 1983). On the other hand, sera from ALS patients have been reported to contain antibodies against a 56,000 mol. wt. protein which enhances terminal sprouting and muscle reinnervation (Gurney, 1984; Gurney et al., 1984). Later studies of this antigen by Gurney et al. (1986) led to the isolation and cloning of neuroleukin, a factor suggested to address sensory and motor neurons as well as lymphocytes. Recent sequence comparisons, however, have shown neuroleukin to be glucose-6-phosphate isomerase, a ubiquitous cytoplasmic enzyme (Gurney et al., 1986; Chaput et al., 1988). Cytotoxic effects of ALS sera on cultured neonatal mouse motor neurons from the ventral horn have also been reported (Roisen et al., 1982), as has enhanced binding of serum immunoglobulins from ALS patients to rat spinal cord neurons (Digby et al., 1985). Doherty et al. (1986) reported that ALS serum decreased the concentration of neurophilament proteins in cultured chick spinal neurons. These authors, however, found no neurotoxic activity in immunoglobulin fractions of ALS serum and there was no evidence of circulating antibodies that could have neutralized muscle-derived neurotrophic factors or induced lysis of spinal neurons. Touzeau and Kato (1986) reported that ALS sera had no effects on cultured human spinal cord neurons.

In a recent study Ebendal et al. (1989) observed that extracts of spinal cord and muscle from ALS cases and controls stimulated the survival of chicken ciliary neurons in a similar way. Ventral horn extracts were about five times as effective as muscle extracts in promoting the survival of ciliary neurons with no differences between control and ALS samples. Sera from ALS patients, as well as normal sera if present in a proportion of above 5% in the medium, suppressed fibre outgrowth from chicken sympathetic ganglia induced by added nerve growth factor (NGF). The presence of sera (also from healthy volunteers) substantially reduced the survival of ciliary neurons supported by trophic activity in choroid extract. The most pronounced inhibitory effects were observed in sera from some ALS patients, but the ALS sera as a group did not appear to differ significantly from the controls. This could indicate the presence of neurotoxic activity in the sera of some of the ALS patients, a hypothesis supported by the apparent relationship between the clinical severity of the disease and the inhibition of neuron survival. Whether a toxic effect is a cause or a consequence of the disease remains to be determined.

Therapeutic trials

The different hypotheses concerning the aetiology of ALS are reflected by the large number of treatment strategies which have been tried (Table II). The results of controlled studies have in general been disappointing and no drug has proved to have symptomatic effects of clinical usefulness or to halt the progression of the disorder. One has to bear in mind that long-term controlled trials are difficult in ALS for the reasons that a high rate of patient loss (both from death and discontinuation of treatment) and variations in the natural history of the disease complicate the analysis and interpretion of the results. Another difficulty is that generally accepted standardized instructions for the conductance of therapeutic trials in ALS are still lacking. To perform a placebo-controlled trial is also an ethical dilemma in such a desolate disease as ALS. The whole spectrum of clinical trials has been summarized elsewhere (Tandan and Bradley, 1985; Mitsumoto et al., 1988) and in the following only some studies with direct relations to the aforementioned neurotransmitter mechanisms will be discussed.

On the basis of the assumption that TRH has excitatory or trophic effects on motorneurons, large doses of the hormone have been administered in therapeutic trials in ALS. In contrast to the reported acute or subacute effects observed in the initial trials of intravenous or subcutaneous

TABLE II

Hypothetical causes and treatment trials in ALS

Findings/hypothetical cause	Trials
Heavy metal exposure	penicillamine
Viral cause	guanidine, amantadine, idoxuridine, isoprinosine, tilerone, transfer factor, snake venom, interferon, thymic hormone
Immunological changes	corticosteroids, azathioprine, cyclophosphamide, cyclosporin, methotrexate, cytosine-arabinoside, plasmapheresis, total lymphoid irradiation
Defective androgen receptors	testosterone
Cholinergic hypofunction	guanidine hydrochloride, edrophonium, neostigmine, physostigmine, tetrahydroaminoacridine
Abnormal thyrotropin-releasing hormone (TRH)	TRH
Increased neuronal catabolism	growth hormone
Decreased trophic factor	growth hormone
Decreased collateral sprouting and axonal regeneration	bovine gangliosides
Neuroexcitotoxic amino acids	branched-chain amino acids, dextromethorphan

TRH therapy in ALS (Engel et al., 1984, 1985; Gracco et al., 1984; Sufit et al., 1984; Conrad et al., 1985; Guiloff et al., 1986; Serratrice et al., 1986), and in one trial of intrathecal treatment with this hormone (Munsat et al., 1984), all controlled studies (Imoto et al., 1985; Brooke et al., 1986; Caroscio et al., 1986; Mitsumoto et al., 1986) except for one (Brooks et al., 1987) have given negative results. Most authors also agree that the clinical course of ALS is not altered with TRH treatment.

Assuming the presence of cholinergic hypofunction of clinical significance in ALS, it has seemed reasonable to administer cholinergic agents in an attempt to restore spinal cholinergic transmission. Earlier trials with guanidine-hydrochloride (Norris et al., 1974), which increases the acetylcholine output, and with the "cholinergic precursor" lecithin (Keleman et al., 1982) have, however, had negative results. Mulder et al. (1959) reported improvement of muscle strength after injection of edrophonium and neostigmine in four patients with ALS with myasthenia-like fatiguability. However, neither of these cholinesterase inhibitors penetrates into the CNS. The results of post-mortem studies indicating that cholinergic structures at different locations within the spinal cord are profoundly, although not selectively involved in ALS, prompted us to examine the effect of physostigmine, a tertiary ACh esterase inhibitor that penetrates into the CNS (Aquilonius et al., 1986). Seven patients with ALS participated in a double-blind cross-over trial of oral physostigmine versus neostigmine (10 and 45 mg/day, respectively, for 3 days). Six of the patients were also given intravenous injections (1 and 1.5 mg, respectively) of the drugs in an open trial. A myometric technique was used to measure muscle strength before and 5, 10, 30 and 60 min after intravenous injection of the drugs and on the third day of oral medication. A test battery of neurophysiological variables (decremental response, H-reflex, tonic vibration reflex, flexion reflex and somatosensory evoked potentials) that might reflect changes in neuromuscular and spinal transmission was applied before medication, 10–30 min after injection and on the third day of oral medication. With this design it seemed probable that any direct pharmacological effects on cholinergic hypofunction would be detectable. Plasma concentrations of the ACh-esterase inhibitors were not determined, but cholinergic side-effects indicated a clinically significant bioavailability. However, the results of the trial were negative throughout, as no increase in muscle strength or changes in the neurophysiological variables were observed. It was concluded that the logical basis of using an ACh-esterase inhibitor in ALS might be wrong or that the lack of effect may have been due to the presence of such a degree of degeneration in synaptic structures that functional restoration was impossible.

The reports of a beneficial effect of the cholinesterase inhibitor tetrahydroaminoacridine (THA) in Alzheimer's disease (Summers et al., 1986; Nybäck et al., 1988; Gauthier et al., 1988) prompted us to try this drug in ALS in spite of the negative results of the physostigmine trial (Askmark et al., to be published). Alzheimer's disease is a disorder which is often attributed in part to a deficit in cholinergic activity (Bartus et al., 1982). Apart from its inhibition of cholinesterase, THA interacts with subtypes of muscarinic and nicotinic receptors and induces ACh release in Alzheimer brain tissue (Nordberg et al., 1988). Moreover, in the neuromuscular junction THA has been shown to be more effective than physostigmine and 4-aminopyridine in reversing cholinergic block (Bradley et al., 1988). In addition, THA has recently been reported to be an NMDA-receptor antagonist (Davenport et al., 1988), which is of special interest, as it has been suggested that neuroexcitotoxic amino acids may be implicated in the pathophysiology of ALS (Spencer, 1987). Seven patients with amyotrophic lateral sclerosis were treated with 100–200 mg of THA together with 11 g lecithin daily for up to 7 weeks. In a separate experiment the patients were given 30 mg THA intravenously. After injection of THA increased muscle strength was observed in two of the patients. No beneficial effect was seen, however, during oral medication and side-effects were frequent. No conclusive changes in the studied neurophysiological variables were observed after drug administration. The plasma clearance of THA was high and the oral bioavailability low, with large interindividual differences (6–36%).

The increase in muscle strength after injection of THA cannot have been due to an effect on the transmission in the neuromuscular junction, as no change in the decremental response was observed. THA might in some way exert its action on cerebral or spinal neurotransmission. Muscarinic ACh receptors seem to be present both on the pyramidal cells (Krnjevic and Phillis, 1963; Crawford and Curtis, 1966; Stone, 1972) and on the motor neurons (Gillberg and Wiksten, 1986) and it is conceivable that the effect of THA is mediated by some of these receptors. Glutamate and aspartate are considered to be the transmitters in the cortical spinal pathway (Young et al., 1981; Potachner et al., 1986), but there are data suggesting that ACh may play a role as an excitatory modulator of motor neuron activity (Zieglgänsberger and Reiter, 1974). One possibility is that THA increases the activity of the Renshaw cells, which have nicotinic as well as muscarinic receptors (King and Ryall, 1981). Stimulation of the Renshaw cells causes inhibition of the motor neuron. THA might then protect the motor neurons from overstimulation by excitatory amino acids, a mechanism which could be of importance in the pathophysiology of ALS. A discrepancy between the effects of physostigmine and THA may be due to differences both in the pharmacokinetic and pharmacodynamic properties of the drugs. THA has higher affinity than physostigmine for both muscarinic and nicotinic receptors in human brain tissue (Nordberg et al., 1988). It has also been shown to be more potent than physostigmine in antagonizing central and cholinergic effects (Gershon and Olariu, 1960) and also effects of morphine (Shaw and Shulman, 1985). THA might also influence other transmitter systems (Drukarch et al., 1988).

Even if THA may have an acute effect of theoretical interest on the muscle strength in some ALS patients, we must conclude that the drug probably has no place in the treatment of the disease. At present it does not seem reasonable to try other cholinergic agents in ALS.

On the basis of the hypothesis that a defect in glutamatergic transmission mechanisms are of importance in ALS, the branched chain amino acids L-leucine and L-isoleucine, which can activate GDH, have recently been administered in a pilot trial (Plaitakis et al., 1988). The patients in the treatment group were reported to show less progression of the disease. The results must be interpreted with caution, however, because of the small sample size and in view of the substantial variation in the natural history of the disease. Based on a similar assumption that excitatory amino acids may be involved in the pathogenesis of ALS, we have recently started a double-blind placebo-controlled trial with dextromethorphan, an NMDA receptor antagonist (Wong et al., 1987; Aryanpur et al., 1988).

The ideas of treatment with branched chain amino acids and NMDA-receptor antagonists are attractive, but it must be kept in mind that many treatments that initially have been reported to be beneficial have later proved to be of no value. It is possible that specific treatment of ALS will become available only after the pathogenesis has been discovered, but therapeutic trials could also provide clues to the aetiology of the disease. It is at the same time depressing and demanding to further research that the aetiology of ALS is the same enigma today as it was when the disorder was first described more than 100 years ago.

Acknowledgements

The authors are indebted to Mrs Gun Kärrlander for secretarial help. Our studies were supported by the Swedish Medical Research Council (No 4303), and by the Pharmacia and NHR foundations, Sweden.

References

Aquilonius, S.-M., Eckernäs, S.-Å. and Gillberg, P.-G. (1981) Topographical localization of choline acetyltransferase within the human spinal cord and a comparison with some other species. *Brain Res.*, 211: 329–340.

Aquilonius, S.-M., Askmark, H., Eckernäs, S.-Å., Gillberg, P.-G., Hilton-Brown, P., Rydin, E. and Stålberg, E. (1986) Cholinesterase inhibitors lack therapeutic effect in amyotrophic lateral sclerosis. A controlled study of physostigmine versus neostigmine. *Acta Neurol. Scand.*, 73: 628–632.

Aryanpur, J.J., Eccles, C., Cole, A.E. and Fisher, R.S. (1988) Dextromethorphan and dextrorphan selectively block depolarization by NMDA in rat hippocampal slice. *Neurology*, 38: (Suppl 1): 301.

Askmark, H., Gillberg, P.-G. and Aquilonius, S.-M. (1985) Autoradiographic visualization of extrajunctional

378

acetylcholine receptors in whole human biceps brachii muscle. (1985) *Acta Neurol. Scand.,* 72: 344–347.

Banda, R., Means, E. and Samaha, F.J. (1985) Trophic effect of thyrotropin-releasing hormone on murine ventral horn neurons in culture. *Neurology,* 35 (Suppl 1): 93.

Bartus, R.T., Dean, R.I., Beer, B. and Lipa, A.S. (1982) The cholinergic hypothesis of geriatric memory dysfunction. *Science,* 217: 408–417.

Belendiuk, K., Belendiuk, G.W., Freedman, D.X. and Antel, J.P. (1981) Neurotransmitter abnormalities in patients with motor neuron disease. *Arch. Neurol.,* 38: 415–417.

Bradley, R.J., Edge, M.T., Moran, S.G. and Freeman, A.M. (1988) Effects of cholinergic drugs used in Alzheimer therapy at the mammalian neuromuscular junction. In E. Giacobini and R. Becker (Eds.), *Current Research in Alzheimer Therapy,* Taylor and Francis, New York, pp. 199–209.

Brooke, M.H., Florence, J.M., Heller, S.L. Kaiser, K.K., Phillips, D., Gruber, A., Babcock, D. and Miller J.P. (1986) Controlled trial of thyrotropin releasing hormone in amyotrophic lateral sclerosis. *Neurology,* 36: 146–151.

Brooks, B.R., Sufit, R.L., Montgomery, G.K., Beaulieu, D.A. and Erickson, L.M. (1987) Intravenous thyrotropin-releasing hormone in patients with amyotrophic laterals sclerosis. Dose-response and randomized concurrent placebo-controlled pilot studies. *Neurol. Clin.,* 5: 143–157.

Caroscio, J.T., Cohen, J.A., Zawodniak, J., Takai, V., Shapiro, A., Blaustein, S., Mulvihill, M.N., Loucas, S.P., Gudesblatt, M., Rube, D. and Yahr, M.D. (1986) A double-blind, placebo-controlled trial of TRH in amyotrophic lateral sclerosis. *Neurology,* 36: 141–145.

Chaput, M., Claes, V., Portetelle, D., Cludts, I., Cravador, A., Burny, A., Gras, H. and Tartar, A. (1988) The neurotrophic neuroleukin factor is 90% homologous with phosphohexose isomerase. *Nature,* 332: 454–456.

Conrad, J., Clough, J., Sufit, R.L. and Brooks, B.R. (1985) Isokinetic assessment of muscle torque in amyotrophic lateral sclerosis (ALS) patients after administration of saline and thyrotropin-releasing hormone (TRH). *Neurology,* 35: (Suppl)· 73

Conradi, S. and Ronnevi, L.-O. (1982) Cytotoxic factor in plasma from ALS patients provokes haemolysis of normal erythrocytes. *Acta Neurol. Scand.,* 65 (Suppl. 90): 246–247.

Conradi, S. and Ronnevi, L.-O. (1985) Cytotoxic activity in the plasma of amyotrophic lateral sclerosis (ALS) patients against normal erythrocytes. Quantitative determinations. *J. Neurol. Sci.,* 68: 135–145.

Crawford, J.M. and Curtis, D.R. (1966) Pharmacological studies on feline Betz cells. *J. Physiol. (Lond.),* 1986: 121–138.

Cuello, A.C., Polak, J.M. and Pearse, A.G.E. (1976) Substance P: Naturally occurring transmitter in human spinal cord. *Lancet,* ii: 1054–1056.

Curtis, D.R. and Johnston, G.A.T. (1974) Amino acid transmitters in the mammalian nervous system. *Ergeb. Physiol. Biol. Chem. Exp. Pharmacol.,* 69: 97–188.

Davenport, C.J., Monyer, H. and Choi, D.W. (1988) Tetrahydroaminoacridine selectively attenuates NMDA receptor-mediated neurotoxicity. *Eur. J. Pharmacol.,* 154: 73–78.

Digby, J., Warrison, R., Jehanli, A., Lunt, G.G. and Clifford-Rose, F. (1985) Cultured rat spinal cord neurons: interaction with motor neuron disease immunoglobulins. *Muscle Nerve,* 8: 595–605.

Dietl, M.M., Sanchez, M., Probst, A. and Palacios, J.M. (1989) Substance P receptors in the human spinal cord: decrease in amyotrophic lateral sclerosis. *Brain Res.,* 483: 39–49.

Doherty, P., Dickson, J.G., Flanigan, T.P., Kennedy, P.G. and Walsh, F.S. (1986) Effects of amyotrophic lateral sclerosis serum on cultured chick spinal neurons. *Neurology,* 36: 1330–1334.

Drachman, D.B. and Fambrough, D.M. (1976) Are muscle fibers denervated in myotonic dystrophy? *Arch. Neurol.,* 33: 485–488.

Drukarch, B., Leysen, J.E. and Stoof, J.C. (1988) Further analysis of the neuropharmacological profile of 9-amino-1,2,3,4-tetrahydroacridine (THA), an alleged drug for the treatment of Alzheimer's disease. *Life Sci.,* 42: 1011–1017.

Ebendal, T., Askmark, H. and Aquilonius, S.-M. (1989) Screening for neurotrophic disturbances in amyotrophic lateral sclerosis. *Acta Neurol. Scand.,* 79: 188–193.

Engel, W.K., Van den Bergh, P. and Askanas, V. (1984) Subcutaneous thyrotropin-releasing hormone seems ready for wider trials in treating lower motor neuron-produced weakness and spasticity. *Ann. Neurol.,* 16: 109–110.

Engel, W.K., Siddique, T. and Nicoloff, J.T. (1985) Effect on weakness and spasticity in amyotrophic lateral sclerosis of thyrotropin-releasing hormone. *Lancet,* ii: 73–75.

Gauthier, S., Masson, H., Gauthier, L., Bouchard, R., Collier, B., Bacher, Y., Bailey, R., Becker, R., Bergman, H., Charbonneau, R., Dastor, D., Gayton, D., Kennedy, J., Kissel, C., Krieger, M., Kushnir, S., Lamontagne, A., St-Martin, M., Morin, J., Nair, N.V.P., Neirinck, L., Ratner, J., Suissa, S., Tesfaye, Y. and Vida, S. (1988) Tetrahydroaminoacridine and lecithin in Alzheimers disease. In E. Giacobini and R. Becker (Eds.), *Current Research in Alzheimer Therapy,* Taylor & Francis, New York, pp. 237–245.

Gershon, S. and Olariu, J. (1960) JB 329 — A new psychotomimetic. Its antagonism by tetrahydroaminactin and its comparison with LSD, mescaline and sernyl. *J. Neuropsychiat.,* 1: 283–292.

Gillberg, P.-G. and Aquilonius, S.-M. (1985) Cholinergic, opioid and glycine receptor binding sites localized in human spinal cord by in vitro autoradiography. *Acta Neurol. Scand.,* 72: 299–306.

Gillberg, P.-G. and Wiksten, B. (1986) Effects of spinal cord lesions and rhizotomies on cholinergic and opiate receptor binding sites in rat spinal cord. *Acta Physiol. Scand.,* 126: 575–582.

Gillberg, P.-G., Aquilonius, S.-M., Eckernäs, S.-Å., Lundqvist, G. and Winblad, B. (1982) Choline acetyltransferase and substance P-like immuno-reactivity in the human spinal cord: changes in amyotrophic lateral sclerosis. *Brain Res.,* 250: 394–397.

Gillberg, P.-G., Nordberg, A. and Aquilonius, S.-M. (1984) Muscarinic binding sites in small homogenates and in autoradiographic sections from spinal cord of rat and man. *Brain Res.,* 300: 327–333.

Gillberg, P.-G., D'Argy, R. and Aquilonius, S.-M. (1988) Auto-radiographic distribution of ^{3}H-acetylcholine binding sites in the cervical spinal cord of man and some other species. *Neurosci. Lett.,* 90: 197–202.

Gracco, V.L., Caligiuri, M., Abbs, J.H., Sufit, R.L. and Brooks, B.R. (1984) Placebo controlled computerized dynametric measurements of bulbar and somatic muscle strength increase in patients with amyotrophic lateral sclerosis following intravenous infusion of 10 mg/kg thyrotropin-releasing hormone. *Ann. Neurol.,* 16: 110.

Guiloff, R.J., Demain, D., Eckland, D. and Lightman, S. (1986) Acute neurological effects of a TRH analogue (RX 77368) in patients with motorneurone disease. A controlled study. *Muscle Nerve,* 9(suppl): 100.

Gurney, M.E. (1984) Suppression of sprouting at the neuro-muscular junction by immune sera. *Nature,* 307: 546–548.

Gurney, M.E., Belton, A.C., Cashman, N. and Antel, J.P. (1984) Inhibition of terminal axonal sprouting by serum from patients with amyotrophic lateral sclerosis. *N. Engl. J. Med.,* 311: 933–939.

Gurney, M.E., Heinrich, S.P., Lee, M.R. and Yin, H.-S. (1986) Molecular cloning and expression of neuroleukin, a neuro-trophic factor for spinal and sensory neurons. *Science,* 234: 566–574.

Hayashi, H., Suga, M., Satake, M., and Tsubaki, T. (1981) Reduced glycine receptor in the spinal cord in amyotrophic lateral sclerosis. *Ann. Neurol.,* 9: 292–294.

Imoto, K., Saida, K., Iwanmura, K., Saida, T. and Nishitani, H. (1985) Amyotrophic lateral sclerosis: a double-blind crossover trial of thyrotropin-releasing hormone. *J. Neurol. Neurosurg. Psychiat.,* 47: 1332–1334.

Jackson, II., Adelman, L.S., Munsat, T.L., Forte, S. and Lechan, R.M. (1986) Amyotrophic lateral sclerosis: Thyrotropin-re-leasing hormone and histidyl proline diketopiperazine in the spinal cord and cerebrospinal fluid. *Neurology,* 36: 1218–1223.

Kanazawa, I. (1977) Neurotransmitters and motor neuron disease. *Jpn. J. Clin. Med.,* 35: 4025–4029.

Kawamura, Y., Dyck, P.J., Shimono, M., Okazaki, H., Tateishi, J. and Doi, H. (1981) Morphometric comparison of the vulnerability of peripheral motor and sensory neurons in amyotrophic lateral sclerosis. *J. Neuropathol. Exp. Neurol.,* 40: 667–675.

Keleman, J., Hedlund, W., Murray-Douglas, P. and Munsat, T. (1982) Lecithin is not effective in amyotrophic lateral sclerosis. *Neurology,* 32: 315–316.

King, K.T. and Ryall, R.W. (1981) A re-evaluation of acetylcholine receptors on feline Renshaw cells. *Br. J. Pharmacolol.,* 73: 455–460.

Krnjevic, K. and Phillis, J.W. (1963) Acetylcholine sensitive cells in the cerebral cortex. *J. Physiol. (Lond.),* 166: 296–327.

Manaker, S., Winokur, A., Thodes, C.H. and Rainbow, T.C. (1985) Autoradiographic localization of thyrotropin-releas-ing hormone (TRH) receptors in human spinal cord. *Neurology,* 35: 328–332.

Manaker, S., Caine, S.B. and Winokur, A. (1988) Alterations in receptors for thyrotropin-releasing hormone, serotonin, and

acetylcholine in amyotrophic lateral sclerosis. *Neurology,* 38: 1464–1474.

Mitsuma, T., Nogimori, T., Adachi, K., Mukoyama, M. and Ando, K. (1984) Concentrations of immunoreactive thyrotropin-releasing hormone in spinal cord of patients with amyotrophic lateral sclerosis. *Am. J. Med. Sci.,* 287: 34–36.

Mitsumoto, H., Salgado, E.D., Negroski, D., Hanson, M.R., Salanga, V.D., Wilber, J.F., Wilbourn, A.J., Breuer, A.C. and Leatherman, J. (1986) Amyotrophic lateral sclerosis: effects of acute intravenous and chronic subcutaneous ad-ministration of thyrotropin-releasing hormone in controlled trials. *Nerurology,* 36: 152–159.

Mitsumoto, H., Hanson, M.R. and Chad, D.A. (1988) Amyotrophic lateral sclerosis. Recent advances in patho-genesis and therapeutic trials. *Arch. Neurol.,* 45: 189–202.

Mulder, D.W., Lambert, E.H. and Eaton, L.M. (1959) Myasthenic syndrome in patients with amyotrophic lateral sclerosis. *Neurology,* 9: 627–631.

Munsat, T.L., Mora, J.S., Robinton, J.E., Lechan, R., Hedlund, W., Taft, J., Reichlin, S. and Scheife, R. (1984) Intrathecal TRH in amyotrophic lateral sclerosis: preliminary observa-tions. *Neurology,* 34: (Suppl): 239.

Nagata, Y., Okuya, M., Watanabe, T. and Honda, M. (1982) Regional distribution of cholinergic neurons in human spi-nal cord transection in the patients with and without motor neuron disease. *Brain Res.,* 224: 223–229.

Nordberg, A., Nilsson, L., Adem, A., Hardy, J. and Winblad, B. (1988) Effect of THA on acetylcholine release and cholinergic receptors in Alzheimer brains. In E. Giacobini and R. Becker (Eds.), *Current Research in Alzheimer Ther-apy,* Taylor & Francis, New York, pp. 247–257.

Norris, F.H., Calanchini, P.R., Fallat, R.J., Panchart, R.P.T. and Jewett, B. (1974) The administration of guanidine in amyotrophic lateral sclerosis. *Neurology,* 24: 721–728.

Nybäck, H., Nyman, H., Ohman, G., Nordgren, I. and Lin-dström, B. (1988) Preliminary experiences and results with THA for the amelioration of symptoms of Alzheimer's disease. In E. Giacobini and R. Becker (Eds.), *Current Research in Alzheimer Therapy,* Taylor & Francis, New York, pp. 231–236.

Patten, B.M. and Croft, S. (1984) Spinal cord substance P in amyotrophic lateral sclerosis. In F. Clifford Rose (Ed.) *Research Progress in Motor Neuron Disease,* Pitman Press, Bath, pp. 283–289.

Patten, B.M., Harati, Y., Acosta, L., Jung, S.-S. and Felmus, M.T. (1978) Free amino acid levels in amyotrophic lateral sclerosis. *Ann. Neurol.,* 3: 305–309.

Perry, T.L., Hansen, S. and Jones, K. (1987) Brain glutamate deficiency in amyotrophic lateral sclerosis. *Neurology,* 37: 1845–1848.

Plaitakis, A. and Caroscio J.T. (1987) Abnormal glutamate metabolism in amyotrophic lateral sclerosis. *Ann. Neurol.,* 22: 575–579.

Plaitakis, A., Berl, S. and Yahr, M.D. (1984) Neurological disorders associated with deficiency of glutamate dehydro-genase. *Ann. Neurol.* 15: 144–153.

Plaitakis, A., Mandeli, J., Smith, J. and Yahr, M.D. (1988) Pilot trial of branced-chain aminoacids in amyotrophic lateral sclerosis. *Lancet,* 1015–1018.

Potachner, S.J. and Dymczyk, L. (1986) Amino acid levels in the Guinea pig spinal gray matter after axotomy of primary sensory and descending tracts. *J. Neurochem.,* 47: 412–422.

Robinson, N. (1968) Chemical changes in the spinal cord in Friedreich ataxia and motor neuron disease. *J. Neurol. Neurosurg. Psychiat.,* 3: 330–333.

Roisen, F.J., Bartfeld, H., Donnenfeld, H. and Baxter, J. (1982) Neuron specific in vitro cytotoxicity of sera from patients with amyotrophic lateral sclerosis. *Muscle Nerve,* 5: 48–53.

Scatton, B., Dubois, A., Javoy-Agid, F. and Camus, A. (1984) Autoradiographic localization of muscarinic cholinergic receptors at various segmental levels of the human spinal cord. *Neurosci. Lett.* 49: 239–245.

Schmidt-Achert, K.M., Askanas, V. and Engel, W.K. (1984) Thyrotropin-releasing hormone enhances choline acetyltransferase and creatine kinase in cultured spinal ventral horn neurons. *J. Neurochem.,* 43: 586–589.

Schoenen, J., Reznik, M., Delwaide, P.J. and Vanderhaeghen, J.-J. (1985) Étude immmunocytohimique de la distribution spinale de substance P, des enképhalines, de cholécystokinine et de sérotonine dans la sclérose latérale amyotrophique. *C.R. Soc. Biol. (Paris),* 179: 528–534.

Serratrice, G., Desnuelle, C., Crevat, A., Guelton, C. and Meyer-Dutour, A. (1986) Traitement de la sclerose laterale amyotrophique par le facteur de liberation de l'hormone thyreotrope (TRH). *Rev. Neurol.,* 142: 133–139.

Shaw, F.H. and Shulman, A. (1955) Treatment of intractable pain with large doses of morphine and diamino-phenylthiazole. *Br. Med. J.,* 4: 1367–1369.

Spencer, P.S. (1987) Guam ALS-/parkinsonism-dementia: A long-latency neurotoxic disorder caused by "slow toxin(s)" in food? *Can. J. Neurol. Sci.,* 14: 347–357.

Stone, T.W. (1972) Cholinergic mechanisms in the rat somatosensory cerebral cortex. *J. Physiol. (Lond.),* 225: 485–499.

Sufit, R., Beaulieu D, Sanguq, M., Paulson, D., Reddan, W., Erickson, L., Montgomery, G., Braun, S., Peters, H. and Brooks, B.R. (1984) Placebo controlled quantitative measurements of neuromuscular function following intravenous infusion of 10 mg/kg thyrotropin-releasing hormone in 16 male patients with amyotrophic lateral sclerosis. *Ann. Neurol.,* 16: 110–11.

Summers, W.K., Majovski, L.V., Marsh, G.M., Tachiki, K. and Kling, A. (1986) Oral tetrahydroaminoacridine in long-term treatment of senile dementia, Alzheimer type. *N. Engl. J. Med.,* 315: 1241–1245.

Szulc-Kuberska, J., Stepien, H., Klimek, A. and Cieslak, D. (1988) Effect of bromocriptine and metoclopramide on serum prolactin levels in patients with amyotrophic lateral sclerosis. *J. Neurol. Neurosurg. Psychiat.,* 51: 643–645.

Tandan, R. and Bradley, W.G. (1985) Amyotrophic lateral sclerosis: Part 1. Clinical features, pathology, and ethical issues in management. *Ann. Neurol.,* 18: 271–280.

Touzeau, G. and Kato, A. (1983) Effects of amyotrophic lateral sclerosis sera on cultured cholinergic neurons. *Neurology,* 33: 317–322.

Touzeau, G. and Kato, A. (1986) ALS serum has no effect on three enzymatic activities in cultured human spinal cord neurons. *Neurology,* 36: 573–576.

White, S.R. and Neuman, R.S. (1983) Pharmacological antagonism of facilitatory but not inhibitory effects of serotonin and norepinephrine on excitability of spinal motoneurons. *Neuropharmacology,* 22: 489–494, 1983.

Whitehouse, P.J. (1985) Receptor autoradiography: application in neuropathology. *Trends Neurosci.,* 8: 434–437.

Whitehouse, P.J., Wamsley, J.K., Zarbin, M.A., Price, D.L., Tourtellotte, W.W. and Kuhar, M.J. (1983) Amyotrophic lateral sclerosis: Alterations in neurotransmitter receptors. *Ann. Neurol.,* 14: 8–16.

Wong, B., Coulter, D., Choi, D. and Priner, D. (1987) Dextrorphan and dextromethorphan common antitissives are antiepileptic and antagonze NMDA in brain slices. *Soc. Neurosci. Abstr.,* 13: 1560.

Young, A.B., Bromberg, M.B. and Penny, J.B. Jr. (1981) Decreased glutamate uptake in subcortical areas deafferented by sensorimotor cortical ablation. *J. Neurosci.* 1: 241–249.

Yoshino, Y., Koike, H. and Akai, K. (1979) Free amino acids in motor cortex of amyotrophic lateral sclerosis. *Experientia,* 35: 219–220.

Ziegler, M.G., Brooks, B.R., Lake, C.R., Wood, J.H.. and Enna, S.J. (1980) Norepinephrine and gamma-aminobutyric acid in amyotrophic lateral sclerosis. *Neurology (NY),* 30: 98–101.

Zieglgänsberger, W. and Reiter, W. (1974) A cholinergic mechanism in the spinal cord of cats. *Neuropharmacol.,* 13: 519–527.

S.-M. Aquilonius and P.-G. Gillberg (Eds.)
Progress in Brain Research, Vol. 84
© 1990 Elsevier Science Publishers B.V. (Biomedical Division)

CHAPTER 39

An animal model of motor neuron disease in guinea pigs

Stanley H. Appel, Jozsef I. Engelhardt and Katalin Jakob

Department of Neurology, Baylor College of Medicine, Houston, TX, U.S.A

Introduction

The etiology and pathogenesis of amyotrophic lateral sclerosis are unknown, as are the etiology and pathogenesis of syndromes confined to lower motor neurons. Clearly some cases are of genetic origin, but the genes or gene products for neither lower motor neuron syndromes such as the spinal muscular atrophies, upper and lower motor neuron syndromes of amyotrophic lateral sclerosis, nor bulbospinal forms have been isolated and characterized. Furthermore, the vast majority of motor neuron disease cases are sporadic, and viral, toxic and endocrine approaches have provided limited insight. Recent circumstantial evidence supports the role of autoimmune factors in the pathogenesis of ALS due to increased incidence of associated autoimmune disorders (Appel, 1986) and increased incidence of paraproteinemias (Shy, 1986).

Prior to the last several decades our understanding of myasthenia gravis was similarly limited, and it was not until the discovery of a specific acetylcholine receptor antagonist, alpha-bungarotoxin (Lee, 1972), and the fortuitous development of an animal model of myasthenia gravis (Patrick, 1973), that an unraveling of the autoimmune pathogenesis of MG was made possible.

In order to provide evidence for the autoimmune basis of motor neuron disease, our own efforts have concentrated on development of an appropriate animal model. Guinea pigs injected with bovine motor neurons develop symptoms of neuromuscular degeneration marked by weakness, evidence of denervation by electromyographic and morphological criteria, and the loss of motor neurons within the spinal cord (Engelhardt, 1989). These guinea pigs develop high serum titers of IgG-class antibodies to motor neuron constituents. Immunohistochemistry demonstrates the presence of IgG within spinal cord motor neurons and at the end plates of immunized animals. This experimental model offers a relatively specific immune-mediated destruction of motor neurons which should permit detailed investigation of the mechanism of motoneuron loss and of therapeutic agents which may ameliorate the process.

Methods and Results

Motor neuron isolation and inoculation

Bovine spinal cord motor neurons were isolated by a modification of the method for isolation of swine motor neurons (Engelhardt, 1985). By light microscopy, motor neurons appear to be the only cellular constituent present. The purity of the preparation was greater than 95% and only capillary fragments are present as contaminants. Choline acetyltransferase (ChAT) activity was 14.2 ± 1.2 nmol/mg protein per h (mean $\pm$ S.D.). Muscarinic receptive binding sites were present at a concentration of 25.3 ± 3.6 fmol/mg protein. All cells stained with the anti-ChAT antibody (Fig. 1A,B).

The isolated bovine motor neurons were homogenized in complete Freund's adjuvant and in-

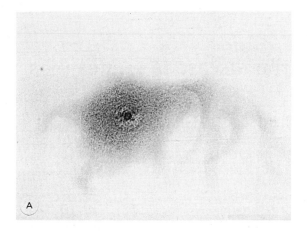
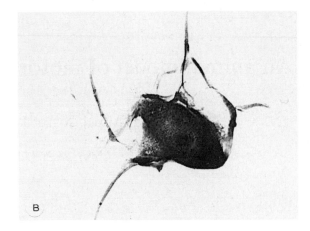

Fig. 1. Isolated bovine spinal motor neurons. A. Without stain. B. Stained with peroxidase-labeled anti-choline acetyltransferase monoclonal antibody. ×800.

jected into male and female albino Hartley guinea pigs. Subsequent injections of motor neurons suspended in incomplete Freund's adjuvant were administered four times at 4-weekly intervals. Control guinea pigs were similarly inoculated with complete Freund's adjuvant followed by monthly injections of incomplete Freund's adjuvant in carrier solution without motor neurons.

Clinical syndrome

After the fourth antigen injection, four of nine female guinea pigs and four of five male guinea pigs developed the gradual onset of disease symptoms with slow but continuous worsening. The animals demonstrated decreased muscle tone in the extremities, especially in the hind legs (Fig. 2). The animals moved sluggishly and had difficulty assuming a normal posture and supporting their body weight. When held upright, they exhibited bilateral foot-drop. There were no detectable sensory changes, skin trophic changes, or signs of bulbar or sphincter disturbances. By EMG examination with concentric needle electrodes in the immunized symptomatic animals, there was a patchy moderate reduction of motor unit activity in most muscles sampled with areas of discrete motor unit firing activity compatible with chronic partial denervation. The immunized asymptomatic

animals had no abnormalities noted on EMG, and five control pairs were also normal. Repeat studies of affected animals over several weeks showed similar findings as on the original examination.

Pathology

Histological examination of the hind leg muscles showed scattered and small group muscle fiber atrophy of both type I and type II fibers, by ATPase reaction and reinnervation as evidenced by small and large groups of type I and type II

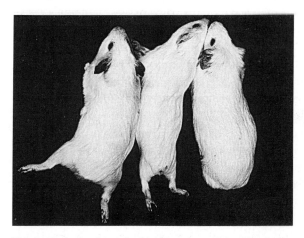

Fig. 2. Control guinea pig (right), and two immunized guinea pigs with hind limb weakness (left).

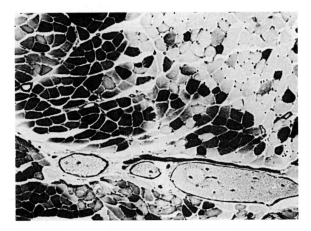

Fig. 3. Grouping of type I (light) and type II (dark) fibers in skeletal muscle of animal with experimental autoimmune motor neuron disease (ATPase reaction ×100).

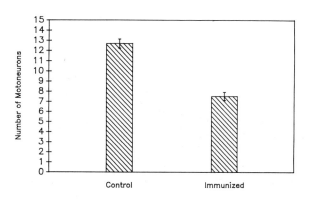

Fig. 5. The numbers of motor neurons in sections of the lateral motor columns of lumbar enlargement in the spinal cord of 6 control guinea pigs and 7 animals with experimental autoimmune motor neuron disease (mean ± S.D.).

fibers (Fig. 3). This evidence of denervation was present in 30–50% of the specimens examined.

Within the central nervous system, the sole pathological findings were limited to lower motor neurons in the spinal cord and brainstem. Loss of Nissl substance, shrinkage, and cell death with consequent satellitosis and neuronophagia were commonly seen (Fig. 4). There was no pathology of cortical neurons or descending pyramidal tracts, nor were there any pathological changes in parenchymal organs. To estimate the extent of

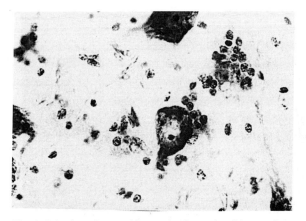

Fig. 4. Spinal cord ventral horn of guinea pig with experimental autoimmune motor neuron disease demonstrating motor neuron undergoing degeneration and phagocytosis. (Cresyl violet stain; ×350).

motor neuron loss, the lumbar enlargement was dissected, and horizontal sections prepared and stained with cresyl violet. Animals with clinical symptomatology had approximately 30–40% fewer motor neurons and an increased number of degenerating motor neurons compared to control or immunized asymptomatic animals (Fig. 5). There were no inflammatory foci in the meninges, cortical gray matter, cortical, subcortical or spinal cord white matter, or spinal cord gray matter. Furthermore, there was no evidence of perivascular inflammation.

Immunological studies

IgG reactivity to bovine motor neurons in the sera of guinea pigs immunized with motor neurons reached a titer of 1 : 102,400 after the second antigen injection and remained at this level. There were no detectable IgG antibodies to bovine myelin basic protein, ganglioside, or cerebroside. The IgG class antibodies reacted strongly with the membrane fraction of guinea pig spinal cord gray matter homogenate, and less extensively with cerebellar membrane fractions, cerebral cortical membrane fractions, and minimally with sciatic nerve, liver, and muscle homogenate membrane fractions. The sera did not react with bovine liver or torpedo electric organ membrane fractions. None of the control animals demonstrated reactivity of IgG with motor neurons or with any other antigen preparation. Titers of IgM reactivity with motor neurons reached a maximal level of 1 : 3200 in most animals whether they were immunized with motor neurons or only with Freund's adjuvant without motor neurons.

In an effort to define the potential role of anti-motor neuron antibodies and the loss of the motor unit, direct immunohistochemical evaluation of the guinea pigs spinal cord, brainstem, and cerebrum was carried out. In all motor neuron immunized animals including those which were asymptomatic, intensive staining for IgG was ob-

served in the motor neurons of the spinal cord and brainstem (Figs. 6A,B). The cytoplasm was stained in a characteristic course granular and patchy pattern and the nuclei were spared (Figs. 6C,D).

By electron microscopy, IgG could be localized to elements of the cytoskeletal apparatus, primarily microtubules, to the rough endoplasmic reticulum, and to lysosomes (Figs. 7A,B). No ferritin-labelled anti-guinea pig IgG antibody was found in association with the Golgi apparatus. Occasionally large cells in the posterior horn of the spinal cord were stained for IgG, but such staining was also present in control animals. In

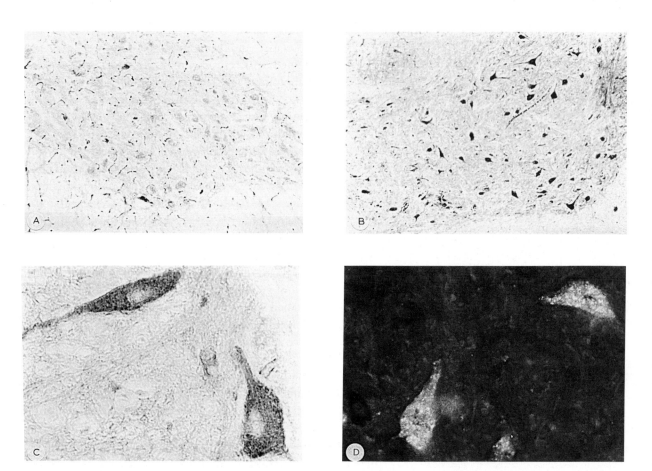

Fig. 6. Immunohistochemical reactivity of ventral horn cells. A. No IgG reactivity in motor neurons of control guinea pig. B. Positive IgG reactivity in guinea pig with experimental autoimmune motor neuron disease (Peroxidase-conjugated goat anti-guinea pig IgG ×50). C . Higher magnification of two positive motor neurons from immunized guinea pig (peroxidase reaction ×400). D. Motor neurons from immunized guinea pig reacted with fluorescein isothiocyanate conjugated goat anti-guinea pig IgG antibody.

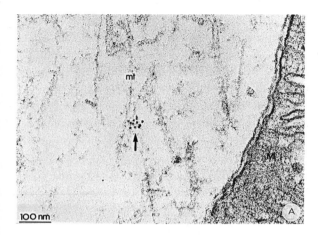 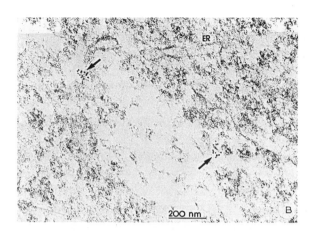

Fig. 7A. Longitudinal section of axon of ventral horn motor neuron from guinea pig with experimental autoimmune motor neuron disease. IgG cluster in the vicinity of a microtubule. Detected with 1 : 200 dilution of biotin-conjugated goat anti-guinea pig IgG and ferritin conjugated avidin. B. Detail of endoplasmic reticulum in ventral horn motor neuron from same animal. The localization of ferritin-labeled IgG is indicated by arrows.

control animals no reactivity for IgG could be detected in any anterior horn constituents with the same detecting antibody dilutions.

Immunoglobulin could also be detected at the end plate of immunized animals employing either peroxidase-labeled goat anti-guinea pig IgG antibody or fluorescein isothiocyanate-labeled anti-guinea pig IgG antibody. After staining sections with the fluorescein-labelled anti-guinea pig IgG antibody followed by incubation with rhodamine labeled alpha bungarotoxin, approximately one-third of the end plates defined by bungarotoxin staining were also positive for guinea pig IgG. The intensity of the stain and the shape of the neuro-muscular junction as defined by rhodamine-bungarotoxin differed slightly from the intensity and morphology noted with fluorescein anti-guinea pig IgG suggesting a presynaptic localization. In control animals, end plates prepared with rhodamine-bungarotoxin demonstrated only nonspecific FITC localization, but no co-localization of bungarotoxin and guinea pig IgG.

Studies were also carried out to determine the ability of IgG from guinea pigs immunized with motor neurons to stain normal guinea pig spinal cord, brainstem, and cerebrum. Using indirect immunohistochemical techniques, similar intense staining for IgG was observed in the motor neurons of the spinal cord and brainstem when the serum of any of the motor neuron immunized animals was employed. The staining pattern was similar to that observed with direct studies in that the cytoplasm of motoneurons was stained in a patchy distribution, and no nuclear staining was noted. No such staining was observed with any of the control guinea pig sera. In addition, occasional cortical cells as well as cerebellar Purkinje cells were also slightly more reactive when motor neuron immunized animal sera were employed than the control animals' sera.

Discussion

Our results document the development of an animal model with relatively specific compromise of lower motor neurons accompanied by electrical and morphological evidence of denervation and elevated titers of motor neuron antibodies. Only lower motor neurons were lost and other constituents of the central and peripheral nervous system appeared unaffected. This syndrome of experimental autoimmune motor neuron disease is distinct from experimental allergic encephalomyelitis produced by the inoculation of myelin basic protein as well as other myelin constituents (Van den Bark, 1984), and also distinct from experimental allergic neuritis which compromises peripheral nerve function (Waksman, 1956). When whole spinal cord is used to induce experimental allergic encephalomyelitis, dysfunction of proximal motor root has been described; but no evidence for degeneration and loss of spinal cord motor neurons was presented (Pender, 1988). In our studies the purity of the isolated bovine motor neurons was critical because even small contamination with myelin gave rise to a different clinical syndrome, which was associated with inflammatory foci throughout the neuraxis. Our model of experimental motor neuron disease manifested clinical weakness only after several months of inoculations, whereas EAE was more acute in onset, spared the motor unit, compromised myelinated structures within the CNS and gave rise to ataxia, weakness, and sphincter disturbances.

At a light microscopic level, it was not possible to determine the exact localization of endogenous IgG in motoneurons. Plant lectins that bind tightly to membrane glycoproteins have been shown to appear in the Golgi apparatus (Trojanowski, 1981); and our IgG staining resembles that for agrin localization within the Golgi apparatus of torpedo, frog, and chick motoneurons (Magill-Dolc, 1988). Nevertheless our electron microscopic studies localize the IgG to the endoplasmic reticulum and microtubules with no reactivity with the Golgi apparatus. These results suggest that the IgG reactivity in the motoneuron may relate to an antigenic moiety which is being synthesized and transported.

The high titer of serum antibodies against motor neurons as well as the presence of IgG, both at the neuromuscular junction and within anterior horn cells, suggest the potential pathogenic role for such immunoglobulin in experimental autoimmune motor neuron disease. Immunoglobulin can definitely be taken up at the axon terminal and may reach the cell body by retrograde axoplasmic transport (Fabian, 1986; Yamamoto, 1987; Fa-

bian, 1988). The presence of IgG at the neuromuscular junction and within motor neuron somas of animals immunized with motor neurons, and its absence in animals inoculated with myelin basic protein suggest the relevance of the IgG, but in no sense can such localization define a causal role. Only the passive transfer of motor neuron dysfunction with serum derived from guinea pigs with experimental autoimmune motor neuron disease will shed light on the pathogenesis of the disorder. Such studies are currently in progress in our laboratories.

Acknowledgements

These studies were supported by grants from the Muscular Dystrophy Association, as well as the Jack Wagner Foundation and the Robert C. and Helen Kleberg Foundation.

References

Appel, S.H., Appel, V., Stewart, S.S. and Kerman, R.H. (1986) Amyotrophic lateral sclerosis: Associated clinical disorders and immunologic evaluations. *Arch Neurol.*, 43: 234–238.

Engelhardt, J.I., Appel, S.H. and Killian, J.M. (1989) Experimental autoimmune motor neuron disease. *Ann. Neurol.*, in press.

Engelhardt, J. and Joo, F. (1986) An immune-mediated guinea pig model for lower motor neuron disease. *J. Neurol. Immunol.*, 12: 279–290.

Engelhardt, J., Joo, F., Pakski, M. and Kasa, P. (1985) An improved method for the bulk isolation of spinal motor neurons. *J. Neurol. Sci.*, 15: 219–227.

Fabian, R.H. and Ritchie, T.C. (1986) Intraneuronal IgG in the central nervous system. *J. Neurol. Sci.*, 73: 257–267.

Fabian, R.H. (1988) Uptake of plasma IgG by CNS motor neurons. Comparison of anti-neuronal and normal IgG. *Neurology*, 38: 1775–1780.

Latov, N., Hayes, A.P., Donofrio, P.D., et al. (1988) Monoclonal IgM with unique specificity to gangliosides GM1 and GD1B and to lacto-*N*-tetrose associated with human motor neuron disease. *Neurology*, 38: 763–768.

Lee, C.Y. (1972) Chemistry and pharmacology of polypeptide toxins in snake venoms. *Annu. Rev. Pharmacol.*, 12: 265–286.

Magill-Dolc, C. and McMahon, U.J. (1988) Motor neurons contain again-like molecules. *J. Cell Biol.*, 107: 1825–1833.

Patrick, J. and Lindstrom, J. (1973) Autoimmune response to acetylcholine receptor. *Science*, 180: 871–872.

Pender, M.P. (1988) The pathophysiology of acute experimental allergic encephalomyelitis induced by whole spinal cord in the Lewis rat. *J. Neurol. Sci.,* 84: 209–222.

Shy, M.E., Rowland, L.P., Smith, T., et al. (1986) Motor neuron disease and plasma cell dyscrasia. *Neurology,* 36: 1429–1436.

Trojanowski, J.Q., Gonatas, J.O. and Gonatas, N.K. (1981) A light and electron microscopic study of the intraneuronal transport of horse radish peroxidase and wheat germ agglutinin-peroxidase conjugates in the rat visual system. *J. Neurocytol.,* 10: 441–456.

Van den Bark, A.A. and Raus, J.C.M. (1984) Experimental autoimmune encephalomyelitis: Pathogenesis and prevention. In A. Van den Bark and J.C.M. Raus (Eds.), *Immunoregulatory Processes and Experimental Allergic Encephalomyelitis and Multiple Sclerosis.* Elsevier, Amsterdam, 99–125.

Waksman, B.H. and Adams, R.D. (1956) Comparative study of experimental allergic neuritis in the rabbit, guinea pig and mouse. *J. Neuropathol. Exp. Neurol.,* 15: 293–314.

Yamamoto, T., Iwasaki, Y., Konno, H., et al. (1987) Retrograde transport in differential accumulation of serum proteins in motor neurons: Implications for motor neuron diseases. *Neurology,* 37: 843–846.

S.-M. Aquilonius and P.-G. Gillberg (Eds.)
Progress in Brain Research, Vol. 84
© 1990 Elsevier Science Publishers B.V. (Biomedical Division)

CHAPTER 40

Antimuscarinic drugs in the treatment of movement disorders

Stanley Fahn, Robert Burke and Yaakov Stern

*Department of Neurology, Columbia University College of Physicians and Surgeons, and The Neurological Institute of New York,
Columbia-Presbyterian Medical Center, New York, NY 10032-3784, U.S.A.*

Introduction and historical aspects

Movement disorders are a group of neurological dysfunctions in which there is either (1) a paucity of voluntary movement in the absence of weakness or spasticity (and is referred to as akinesia, bradykinesia or hypokinesia) or (2) an excess of movement referred to as abnormal involuntary movements (also known as dyskinesias or hyperkinesias). The hypokinetic syndromes are basically parkinsonian states.

The various movement disorders are listed in Table I. In addition to the classical parkinsonian states, other disorders presenting solely as shuffling gait — not due to weakness, spasticity, or to another hypokinetic or hyperkinetic disorder — are also listed in this table as gait disorders. Gait disorders comprise a heterogeneous group of conditions including the senile gait disorder, fear of falling syndrome, and psychogenic gait disorders.

The localization of the brain's highest activities of the synthesizing and degrading enzymes of acetylcholine to the neostriatum (Fahn and Cote, 1968; Fahn, 1976) would make it almost predictable that acetylcholine plays a role in at least some movement disorders, since these conditions are related to dysfunction of the basal ganglia. There-

fore, drugs which influence acetylcholine function could be expected to influence the symptomatology of some of the movement disorders. The development of the use of drugs which block cholinergic muscarinic receptors in brain, so-called antimuscarinic drugs, has a long history, beginning before the turn of the century.

TABLE I

List of movement disorders

A. Hypokinesias
 1. Parkinson's disease
 2. Symptomatic parkinsonism
 3. Parkinsonism plus syndromes
 4. Other gait disorders

B. Hyperkinesias
 1. Akathitic movements
 2. Asynergia/ataxia
 3. Athetosis
 4. Ballism
 5. Chorea
 6. Dysmetria
 7. Dystonia
 8. Hyperekplexias
 9. Myoclonus
10. Neuroleptic malignant syndrome
11. Painful legs, moving toes
12. Paroxysmal dyskinesias
13. Restless legs
14. Stereotypy
15. Stiff-man syndrome
16. Tics
17. Tremor

Correspondence to: Dr. Stanley Fahn, Neurological Institute, 710 West 168th Street, New York, NY 10032, U.S.A.

Other than through the ingestion of alcohol, which suppresses essential tremor, antimuscarinics were probably the first effective therapeutic agents to ameliorate a movement disorder, namely parkinsonism. The belladonna alkaloids, atropine and scopolamine, were introduced by Charcot (1879) and Erb (1909), respectively, at the turn of the century. Since that time, a mild amount of symptomatic relief for parkinsonism has been achieved with the use of these and other anticholinergic agents. Because of fewer systemic side effects, the synthetic centrally acting anticholinergic drugs, introduced in the late 1940s and early 1950s, largely replaced the belladonna alkaloids in the management of parkinsonian symptoms and signs (Doshay and Constable, 1949; Corbin, 1949). The first synthetic anticholinergic, trihexyphenidyl (Artane), was soon joined by a host of others, such as benztropine (Cogentin), biperidine (Akineton), cycrimine (Pagitane), ethopropazine (Parsidol), and procyclidine (Kemadrin).

Since the development of dopamine replacement therapy, the anticholinergics today play a minor role in the treatment of Parkinson's disease. However, they still remain the treatment of choice for drug-induced parkinsonism (Simpson and May, 1985). In fact, the anticholinergics are commonly used with the introduction of neuroleptics in the treatment of psychosis in order to prevent drug-induced parkinsonism and acute dystonic reactions (Simpson and May, 1985).

Moreover, the anticholinergics have since been found useful in the treatment of some of the hyperkinetic movement disorders. The first of these disorders found to be benefited by these agents was the acute dystonic reaction from dopamine receptor blocking agents (DBRA) which consists mainly of antipsychotic drugs and anti-nausea and anti-vomiting agents (such as metoclopramide) (Casteels et al., 1970; Gatrad, 1976; Pinder et al., 1976). These reactions usually occur in the early stages of treatment with DRBA, more often in children, adolescents and young adults, and consist of acutely developed sustained,

forceful contractions in any part of the body that are extremely uncomfortable, are often painful, and can even be fatal (Reasbeck and Hossenbocus, 1979). These acute dystonic reactions gradually fade over several days if the offending drug is discontinued. The discovery in 1960 that anticholinergics can dramatically relieve them was a major advance (Paulson, 1960; Waugh and Metts, 1960). Although today acute dystonic reactions are usually treated by parenteral injections of antihistamines (Smith and Miller, 1961), their effect is probably due to their anticholinergic properties, which, although weaker than standard anticholinergics, are adequate to control the acute dystonia.

Because of such anticholinergic properties, the antihistamines are also often used in the treatment of parkinsonism in patients unable to tolerate standard anticholinergics due to adverse effects. Commonly used antihistamines for parkinsonism include diphenhydramine (Benadryl) and orphenadrine (Disipal, Norflex).

Based partly on the dramatic benefit of anticholinergics on acute dystonic reactions, these agents were evaluated, beginning in 1969, for their possible benefit in idiopathic torsion dystonia (Fahn, 1979). By slowly increasing the dosage to avoid adverse effects, Fahn (1983) reached an average dose of 40 mg/day in children and found benefit in 60%. Because of poorer tolerance by adults, only lower doses could be reached, and benefit was observed in only 40%. Today, high-dosage anticholinergics remain the most often used class of medications for the dystonic syndromes, and they result in a greater percentage of patients being improved than any other oral medication studied (Greene et al., 1988).

Following the introduction of high-dosage anticholinergics for idiopathic torsion dystonia, a similar approach was then attempted with other types of movement disorders, with success being reported for cerebellar intention tremor (Jabbari et al., 1983), tardive dystonia (Kang et al., 1986), essential myoclonus (Chokroverty et al., 1987), symptomatic myoclonus (Sasaki et al., 1987), and palatal myoclonus and pendular nystagmus (Jabbari et al., 1987). This chapter covers the clinical aspects of anticholinergic therapy for all these disorders, and the clinical pharmacokinetics and behavioral adverse effects of high-dosage anticholinergics in the treatment of dystonia.

Parkinsonism

Over a century ago, naturally occurring belladonna alkaloids were used to treat parkinsonism, and subsequently a number of synthetic antimuscarinics, developed in the 1940s, were the mainstay of treatment until the advent of levodopa. The current explanation for the beneficial response with anticholinergics is that with the loss of the nigrostriatal dopaminergic neurons, the normal inhibitory influence of these neurons on the postsynaptic cholinergic cells is lost in this disorder. This results in an excessive cholinergic state in the striatum. By reducing cholinergic activity with antimuscarinic drugs, symptoms lessen.

Since the introduction of levodopa in 1967 by Cotzias et al (1967), dopamine replacement therapy has been recognized as the most effective form of symptomatic therapy for Parkinson's disease. The ergoline dopamine agonists, bromocriptine, pergolide and lisuride (Calne et al., 1974; Lieberman and Goldstein, 1982), are also much more effective than the anticholinergics in this disorder. Therefore at present the anticholinergics are relegated (1) to treatment predominantly in the early, mild stage of Parkinson's disease, (2) as adjunctive treatment for intractable symptoms, and (3) in drug-induced parkinsonism and in Parkinsonism-Plus syndromes (Jankovic, 1989) in which dopamine replacement therapy is ineffective. Parkinsonian tremor-at-rest is often relatively intractable to levodopa, and anticholinergics can be quite effective in suppressing this symptom for many patients when used in combination with levodopa. Anticholinergics are not effective for the action tremor of parkinsonism, are mildly effective for bradykinesia and rigidity, and are rarely effective for postural instability. They are particu-

larly good for sialorrhea, which is a common complaint in parkinsonism.

Typical doses in Parkinson's disease are trihexyphenidyl 6 to 10 mg/day, ethopropazine up to 200 mg/day, and benztropine 6 mg/day. Adverse effects can be divided into central nervous system (CNS) and peripheral adverse effects. The former consist of memory loss and toxic psychosis, while the latter comprise difficulty with micturition, dry mouth, and mydriasis with blurred vision. The peripheral side effects can usually be overcome with a peripherally acting acetylcholinesterase inhibitor, such as pyridostigmine at a dosage of 30 to 60 mg four times daily. But the central side effects can only be overcome by reducing the dosage of the anticholinergic agent or using a milder anticholinergic. Because anticholinergics are particularly likely to produce central adverse effects in older individuals, these drugs should be avoided in the elderly parkinsonian patient. Our rule of thumb is not to use these agents in patients older than 70 years of age. If anticholinergics are deemed worthy of a trial in parkinsonian patients who otherwise are prone to CNS side effects, the antihistamines with their milder anticholinergic property can be utilized instead. Diphenhydramine 50 mg t.i.d. or orphenadrine 50–100 mg t.i.d. can be utilized safely and with some mild anti-tremor effect.

Amantadine appears to have anticholinergic properties in addition to its role in releasing dopamine from or blocking reuptake at the dopamine terminals. This drug is often used in the early stages of Parkinson's disease or in advanced stages in which the dopaminergics are no longer active enough. The usual dosage of amantadine is 200–300 mg/day.

Dystonia

Acute dystonic reaction

Acute dystonic reactions occur in the first few days following the introduction of medications that block dopamine receptors. Those most susceptible to develop this reaction are children and juveniles; boys are more often affected than girls. The reactions can affect all parts of the body, but cranial structures are more frequently involved. The jaw can remained pulled down or up, the tongue grotesquely protruded, the neck twisted, bent or hyperextended, the eyes deviated, the face distorted, the arm pulled behind the back or up, the trunk twisted, flexed or extended. These are descriptions of just some of the sustained postures that represent the acute dystonic reaction that can develop after oral or systemic administration of DRBAs.

These grotesque, distorted, painful postures fortunately respond dramatically to parenteral administration of anticholinergics or antihistaminics (Paulson, 1960; Waugh and Metts, 1960, Smith and Miller, 1961). An intramuscular injection of benztropine mesylate, 2 mg, is usually effective. More commonly a slow intravenous injection of the antihistaminic diphenhydramine, 50 mg, is given. The dose can be repeated if necessary.

Torsion dystonia, idiopathic and symptomatic

The abnormal movements making up dystonia are diverse, with a wide range in speed, amplitude, rhythmicity, torsion, forcefulness, distribution in the body, and relationship to rest or voluntary activity (Fahn, 1988). The common type of involuntary movement in all the dystonias is that the movements consist of sustained muscle contractions, frequently causing twisting and repetitive movements, or abnormal postures. Before their recent use in high dosage for the treatment of the dystonias (Fahn, 1983), antimuscarinics had been used occasionally with benefit. In fact, one of the first patients described with dystonia (Schwalbe, 1908; translation by Truong and Fahn, 1988) was successfully treated with scopolamine (Regensburg, 1930). Based originally on open-label trials (Fahn, 1983), the efficacy of anticholinergic drugs given in high dosages has been substantiated by double-blind investigations (Burke et al., 1986) and by other open-label trials on large numbers of patients (Fahn and Marsden, 1987). In general, all these studies show that approximately 50% of

children and 40% of adults with idiopathic dystonia obtain moderate to dramatic benefit from this class of drugs.

A subgroup of idiopathic torsion dystonia, known as dopa-responsive dystonia because the signs and symptoms completely disappear with low-dosage levodopa, also responds to anticholinergics, usually at low dosage (Fahn and Marsden, 1988). Secondary dystonia can often respond to anticholinergics also, but less often than does idiopathic dystonia (Greene et al., 1988). Two forms of symptomatic dystonia that respond particularly well to antimuscarinics are that associated with perinatal injury and the chronic form of dystonia known as tardive dystonia (Burke et al., 1982) due to dopamine receptor blocking agents. About 40% of patients with tardive dystonia have a beneficial response to antimuscarinics (Kang et al., 1988). Athetosis associated with cerebral palsy can be considered a variant of dystonia, and can partially respond to high-dosage anticholinergics.

A significant problem with high-dosage anticholinergic therapy of dystonia is that the dose is limited in most patients because of adverse effects, both peripheral (dry mouth, blurred vision, micturition difficulty, weight loss) and central (memory impairment, and even confusion, hallucinations and psychosis). To evaluate the effect of high doses on memory and attention, we carried out a prospective evaluation, which is discussed below.

Myoclonus

Jabbari and his colleagues (1987) have found that anticholinergics can ameliorate palatal myoclonus and other rhythmical movements, including pendular nystagmus. No other reports attempting to duplicate this finding have been published so far. There are also reports that some patients with nonrhythmic myoclonus, both essential myoclonus and symptomatic myoclonus, respond to anticholinergics (Chokroverty et al., 1987; Sasaki et al., 1987).

Cerebellar intention tremor

Jabbari and his colleagues (1983) also found that high-dosage antimuscarinics can ameliorate cerebellar intention tremor. The basis as to why this type of tremor and some of the myoclonias respond to anticholinergics is not understood.

Worsening of other movement disorders

Classical tardive dyskinesia with rhythmical choreic movements tends to worsen in the presence of antimuscarinics (Fahn, 1984). This is in contrast to the beneficial response seen in tardive dystonia. Regular chorea (random, not rhythmical movements) may also be aggravated or even induced by anticholinergics (Fahn and David, 1972). Another disorder reported to worsen with the administration of anticholinergic drugs is Gilles de la Tourette syndrome. Patients who have both tics and dystonia have been observed to have a worsening of tics when the dystonia is treated with anticholinergics (personal observations).

Evaluation of memory and attentional functions with anticholinergics

Since the treatment of choice for many patients with dystonia is anticholinergic medication and since several studies have shown that acute administration of high doses of anticholinergic compounds can produce memory and attentional deficits (Drachman and Leavitte, 1974), we are assessing the long-tern effects of exposure to anticholinergics. We designed a study of memory and attentional performance in patients with dystonia who were initiating anticholinergic therapy.

Subjects: Subjects were recruited from the Dystonia Clinical Research Center at The Neurological Institute, Columbia-Presbyterian Medical Center. All subjects received medication for treatment of their dystonia; all decisions regarding drug titration and dosage were made by the treating neurologist with the aim of optimizing treatment of dystonia symptoms.

While in the course of their treatment most patients were evaluated several times, scores from only two evaluations are included in the final analysis: the evaluation before initiation of anticholinergic medication (baseline), and the evaluation when the patient was on the highest dose of anticholinergics for the longest period of time. The time between the first and the second evaluation therefore varied from patient to patient. In 2 cases, the study began with patients already receiving medications, in this case the "baseline" testing occurred when treatment was terminated.

Twenty-six patients (18 females and 8 males) were selected from a larger cohort that gave informed consent for the final analysis in this study. All of them were treated with anticholinergic medications on a long-term basis: 18 of them (13 females and 5 males) with ethopropazine hydrochloride (Parsidol) and 8 (5 females, 3 males) with trihexyphenidyl hydrochloride (Artane). Eighteen patients had idiopathic dystonia; the rest were symptomatic and ranged from stroke and tardive to unknown but suspected symptomatic causes.

Neuropsychological assessment: Memory was assessed with the Selective Reminding Test (SRT) (Buschke and Fuld, 1974). This is a list-learning task in which the subject is given 12 trials to learn a list of 12 words. After each recall attempt, the subject is reminded of the words not recalled and asked to again attempt to recall the entire list.

Several summary scores were calculated. They included (1) total recall — the total of all words recalled on all trials (maximum score = 144, 12 words × 12 trials); (2) long-term storage — words recalled on two successive trials without an intervening reminder are considered to be in long-term storage in all subsequent trials; (3) long-term retrieval — words actually retrieved from long-term storage; (4) consistent long-term retrieval — words recalled on all successive trials without intervening reminders; (5) intrusions — words reported by the subject that are not actually on the list; (6) delayed recall — a recall trial administered approximately 15 minutes after the original testing.

Attention was assessed by a Continuous Performance Task (CPT) (Stern et al., 1984). Ten different letters flash in random order on a computer screen. Letters remain on the screen for 100 ms, and the interstimulus interval ranged in random steps between 400 and 500 ms. The task lasted 15 min. The letter X was the critical stimulus and was responded to with a press of a space bar on a standard computer key board. It occurred with a probability of 20%. Performance measures for the CPT included omission errors (not pressing for an X); percent hits (percent of correct responses to the critical stimulus); incorrect responses (to letters other than X); and reaction time (to the critical stimulus).

Results: Demographic characteristics of the patients are described in Table II. Patients taking ethopropazine were significantly older than those taking trihexyphenidyl.

Performance of patients on the SRT and CPT at baseline and highest dose are summarized in Table III. Paired *t*-tests were used to compare performance under these two conditions and there was a significant difference for variables on almost all aspects of the SRT. On the CPT, there were more errors of omission, but incorrect responses and reaction time did not change between the two conditions.

The drug effect did not relate to age of the patients, type of drug (trihexyphenidyl vs. ethopropazine), dose, or the amount of time the patient was taking the drug. The only exception to this was for delayed recall on the SRT, where

TABLE II

Patient demographics for memory and attention testing

	Mean	SD
Age	43.7	16.4
Education	14.2	4.0
Age at onset	38.5	16.6
Duration of illness	6.9	7.3
Follow-up time (yrs)	0.46	0.43
Drug dosage:		
Trihexyphenidyl (*n* = 7)	26.9	20.3
Ethopropazine (*n* = 19)	31.9	14.3

TABLE III

Test scores for memory and attention testing at baseline and highest dose

	Baseline		Highest dose		*p* <
	Mean	SD	Mean	SD	
SRT					
Total recall	116.9	12.5	109.7	8.4	0.05
Long-term storage	115.5	17.6	104.4	26.8	0.01
Long-term retrieval	107.3	19.9	96.2	28.3	0.05
Consistent LTR	87.5	29.7	74.9	35.5	0.05
Intrusions	1.7	1.9	3.3	3.1	0.01
Delayed recall	10.5	1.9	9.1	2.8	0.05
CPT					
Omission errors	29.9	31.2	39.2	26.4	0.05
Percent hits	73.8	19.9	69.6	21.5	NS
Incorrect responses	10.6	12.6	24.0	30.8	NS
Reaction time (s)	0.43	0.02	0.38	0.15	NS

p values are for repeated-measures *t*-tests.

older patients showed a smaller decrement in performance on drug than the younger patients.

While there was a significant drug effect on memory and attention test performance, this appeared to be reversible. In two cases patients were tested while taking medication for a long period of time and then again after medication was discontinued. In both cases, there was an increase in test scores after drug cessation. In addition, several patients undergoing rapid changes in dose while hospitalized showed dose-dependent changes, with return to baseline either when receiving placebo or when drug was discontinued.

Discussion: These findings suggest that chronic administration of anticholinergic medications can affect patients' performance on a memory task. Only one measure on the attention task was affected, suggesting that attention is relatively less affected by the anticholinergic medications. Both the memory and the attentional changes appear to be reversible. We are currently assessing patients with more in depth batteries of tests in order to more fully delineate the nature of the drug effects. In addition, we are now assessing potential interactions of other variables, including the patient's mood at time of testing.

Pharmacokinetics of trihexyphenidyl

In spite of their long use and their efficacy, little is known about the pharmacokinetics or clinical pharmacology of the antimuscarinics. In part, this lack of information has been due to the lack of sensitive physico-chemical methods to detect these compounds in body fluids. More recently, there have been developed sensitive radioreceptor assays for the measurement of small quantities of compounds which interact with biological receptors (Enna, 1978), and such an assay has been developed for the detection of antimuscarinic drugs (Tune and Coyle, 1980). We have used this assay to study the pharmacokinetics and clinical pharmacology of trihexyphenidyl (THP) in dystonic patients treated with high dosage.

The radioreceptor assay for THP measures the ability of a specimen, in this case serum, to displace a known amount of a potent muscarinic ligand, [^{3}H]QNB, from a standard preparation of rat brain membranes, which contain the muscarinic receptor. Using a standard curve of per cent [^{3}H]QNB bound in the presence of known quantities of THP, serum THP is determined. Although this assay is sensitive, it is not specific for THP; any compound which antagonizes muscarinic binding is measured. Thus, not only THP but also any pharmacologically active metabolites are measured. For that reason, results are expressed as THP equivalents.

We initially studied the absorption and serum half-life of THP in dystonic patients by administering oral THP (5–10 mg) and assaying serum THP levels over time. $T_{1/2}$ was determined from the terminal portion of a log [THP] vs time curve, as illustrated in Fig. 1. Among 17 dystonic patients we found that peak serum level was achieved 1.3 ± 0.2 h after an oral dose (Burke and Fahn, 1985a). Among these patients the half-life was 3.7 ± 0.4 h. We found no relationship between the duration of therapy and the $T_{1/2}$; thus, there was no evidence for an induction of THP metabolism with prolonged exposure to the drug. We had previously noted during treatment of some pa-

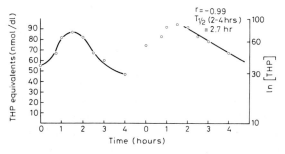

Fig. 1. Serum concentration–time curve following a single 10 mg oral dose of trihexyphenidyl in a patient treated chronically. Data are plotted linearly on the left and semilogarithmically on the right. The four terminal points of the semilogarithmic plot closely conform to the best-fit line determined by linear regression analysis ($r = -0.99$), indicating first-order kinetics of elimination. The slope of this line indicates that the rate constant of elimination is $= 0.26$ h^{-1} and half-life ($T_{1/2}$) is 2.7 h. Peak serum level occurs at 1.5 h. Reproduced from Burke and Fahn (1985a) with permission from the publisher.

tients that efficacy was lost; this would suggest that this loss was not, in general, attributable to more rapid metabolism of the drug. Our study showed that there was a correspondence in time between when patients suffered acute antimuscarinic side effects (dry mouth, visual blurring, confusion, forgetfulness) and the occurrence of peak serum levels. However, there was no similar correspondence between serum levels and response of dystonia to therapy. Dystonia did not fluctuate in its response to therapy with fluctuations in the serum level. We observed that many patients did not show their maximum benefit from a fixed dose until after they had been on that dose for several months, long after a steady state in serum trough levels would have been achieved (Burke and Fahn, 1985a). Furthermore, we observed that some patients who were weaned off therapy did not show deterioration until it had been discontinued for weeks, long after the drug would have been eliminated. Thus, response of dystonia to antimuscarinic treatment is not tightly coupled to serum levels.

We also studied relationships between total daily dose, serum levels, side effects, and efficacy in dystonic patients treated chronically with high dosage (Burke and Fahn, 1985b). We found that daily trough levels (those obtained in the morning before the day's first dose) correlated with the total daily dose, as anticipated ($r = 0.67$, $p < 0.01$). Thus, serum levels were useful in monitoring patient compliance. However, trough serum levels were not predictive of response to therapy. There was no correlation between level and response to therapy as measured by a standardized clinical rating scale (Burke et al., 1985). Even when we examined this relationship within a single diagnostic type of primary dystonia (e.g., the non-Jewish, autosomal dominant torsion dystonia group), a relationship did not emerge.

Although we observed a relationship between peak serum levels and the occurrence of cerebral side effects in particular individuals, we did not observe such a relationship at the population level. For example, in a group of children (< 18 years) with dystonia, the few who had cerebral side effects had them at THP levels which were well tolerated by other children. The most important factor related to the likelihood of these side effects was age. While most children tolerated doses of THP up to 120 mg/day, and serum levels up to 180 nmol/dl, adults frequently had cerebral side effects at lower levels. This greater susceptibility of adults to anticholinergic side effects had previously been observed (Fahn, 1983), and these results indicate that the explanation for this sensitivity does not lie in peripheral serum levels or rate of metabolism. The explanation probably lies in alterations in central cholinergic systems with aging (Burke and Fahn, 1985b).

What do these studies of THP pharmacokinetics and serum levels tell us about the mechanism of action of THP in the treatment of dystonia? First, we think it is likely that THP mediates benefit by its antimuscarinic properties. Although it has other pharmacological effects, such as an ability to block dopamine re-uptake (Coyle and Snyder, 1969), it shares antimuscarinic properties with structurally distinct compounds, such as ethopropazine, which also mediate benefit in dystonia (Greene et al., 1988). On the other hand, other drugs which also possess dopamine re-up-

take blocking properties, including diphenhydramine and some tricyclics (Coyle and Snyder, 1969), have not emerged as efficacious in the treatment of dystonia. THP and other antimuscarinic drugs do not, however, appear to alleviate dystonia directly by simple competitive antagonism at the muscarinic receptor. As pointed out, there is not a close relationship in time between achievement of THP serum levels and the relief of dystonia, nor is there a simple direct relationship between levels and degree of improvement. This lack of a clear relationship is most compatible with the concept that THP (and other anticholinergics) act centrally, rather than peripherally, to alleviate dystonia. This concept is also supported by our anecdotal observations that peripherally-acting quarternary ammonium anticholinergics are not effective. While the central site of action of anticholinergics to modify dystonia is unknown, one major possibility is the striatum, which plays a major role in motor control; it is frequently implicated on pathological grounds in the dystonias; and it is the locus of an important group of cholinergic neurons.

References

Burke, R.E. and Fahn, S. (1985a) Pharmacokinetics of trihexyphenidyl after short-term and long-term administration to dystonic patients. *Ann. Neurol.*, 18: 35–40.

Burke, R.E. and Fahn, S. (1985b) Serum trihexyphenidyl levels in the treatment of torsion dystonia. *Neurology*, 35: 1066–1069.

Burke, R.E., Fahn, S., Jankovic, J., Marsden, C.D., Lang, A.E., Gollomp, S. and Ilson, J. (1982) Tardive dystonia: Late-onset and persistent dystonia caused by antipsychotic drugs. *Neurology*, 32: 1335–1346.

Burke, R.E., Fahn, S., Marsden, C.D., Bressman, S.B., Moskowitz, C. and Friedman, J. (1985) Validity and reliability of a rating scale for the primary torsion dystonias. *Neurology*, 35: 73–77.

Burke, R.E., Fahn, S. and Marsden, C,D. (1986) Torsion dystonia: a double-blind, prospective trial of high-dosage trihexyphenidyl. *Neurology*, 36: 160–164.

Buschke, H. and Fuld, P.A. (1974) Evaluating storage, retention and retrieval in disordered memory and learning. *Neurology*, 24: 1019–1025.

Calne, D.B., Teychenne, P.F., Claveria, L.E., Eastman, R., Greenacre, J.K. and Petrie, A. (1974) Bromocriptine in parkinsonism. *Br. Med. J.*, 4: 442–444.

Casteels-Van Daele, M., Jaeken, J., Van Der Schueren, P., Zimmerman, A., and Van Der Bon, P. (1970) Dystonic reactions in children caused by metoclopramide. *Arch. Dis. Child.*, 45: 130–133.

Charcot, J. M. (1879) *Clinical Lectures on Diseases of the Nervous System, vol. I*, 2nd edn., translated by Sigerson, G., Philadelphia, Henry C. Lea

Chokroverty, S, Manoch, M.K. and Duvoisin, R.C. (1987) A physiologic and pharmacologic study in anticholinergic-responsive essential myoclonus. *Neurology*, 37: 608–615.

Corbin, K.B. (1949) Trihexyphenidyl. Evaluation of the new agent in the treatment of parkinsonism. *JAMA*, 141: 377–382.

Cotzias, G. C., Van Woert, M.H., and Schiffer, L. M. (1967). Aromatic amino acids and modification of parkinsonism. *N. Engl. J. Med.*, 276, 374–379

Coyle, J.T. and Snyder, S.H. (1969) Antiparkinsonian drugs: Inhibition of dopamine uptake in the corpus striatum as a possible mechanism of action. *Science*, 166: 899–901.

Doshay, L.J. and Constable, K (1949) Artane therapy for parkinsonism. *JAMA*, 140: 1317–1322.

Drachman, D.A. and Leavitte, J. (1974) Human memory and the cholinergic system. *Arch. Neurol.*, 30: 113–121.

Enna, S.J. (1978) Radioreceptor assay techniques for neurotransmitters and drugs. In Yamamura, H.I., Enna, S.J. and Kuhar, M.J. (Eds.), *Neurotransmitter Receptor Binding.* Raven Press, New York: pp. 127–137.

Erb, W. (1909). Paralysis agitans (Parkinson's disease). In Church, A. (ed.), *Diseases of the Nervous System*, D. Appleton, New York, pp. 801–898.

Fahn, S. (1976) Regional distribution studies of GABA and other putative neurotransmitters and their enzymes. In E. Roberts, T.N. Chase, and D.B. Tower (Eds.), *GABA in Nervous System Function*. Raven Press, New York, pp. 169–186.

Fahn, S. (1979) Treatment of dystonia with high-dosage anticholinergic medication. *Neurology*, 29:605.

Fahn, S. (1983) High dosage anticholinergic therapy in dystonia. *Neurology*, 33: 1255–1261.

Fahn, S. (1984) The tardive dyskinesias. In Matthews, W.B., Glaser, G.H., (Eds) *Recent Advances in Clinical Neurology, Vol 4.*, Churchill Livingstone, Edinburgh pp 229–260.

Fahn, S. (1988) Concept and classification of dystonia. *Adv. Neurol.*, 50:1–8.

Fahn, S. and Cote, L.J. (1968) Regional distribution of choline acetylase in the brain of the Rhesus monkey. *Brain Res.*, 7: 323–325.

Fahn, S. and David, E. (1972) Oral-facial-lingual dyskinesia due to anticholinergic medication. *Trans. Am. Neurol. Assoc.*, 97: 277–299.

Fahn, S. and Marsden, C.D. (1987) The treatment of dystonia. In Marsden, C.D. and Fahn, S. (Eds), *Movement Disorders 2* Butterworths, London. pp. 359–382.

Gatrad, A.R. (1976) Dystonic reactions to metoclopramide. *Dev. Med. Child Neurol.*, 18: 767–769.

Greene, P., Shale, H., and Fahn, S. (1988) Analysis of open-label trials in torsion dystonia using high dosages of anticholinergics and other drugs. *Movement Disord.*, 3: 46–60.

Jabbari, B., Gunderson, C.H. and McBurney, J.W. (1983) Improvement of ataxic hemiparesis with trihexyphenidyl. *Neurology*, 33: 1627–1628.

Jabbari, B., Rosenberg, M., Scherokman, B., Gunderson, C.H., McBurney, J.W. and McClintock, W. (1987) Effectiveness of trihexyphenidyl against pendular nystagmus and palatal myoclonus: evidence of cholinergic dysfunction. *Movement Disord.*, 2: 93–98.

Jankovic, J. (1989) Parkinsonism-plus syndromes. *Movement Disord.*, 4: S95–S119.

Kang, U.J., Burke, R.E, and Fahn, S. (1986) Natural history and treatment of tardive dystonia. *Movement Disord.*, 1: 193–208.

Lieberman, A.N. and Goldstein, M. (1982) Treatment of advanced Parkinson's disease with dopamine agonists. In Marsden, C.D. and Fahn, S. (Eds.), *Movement Disorders,* Butterworth Scientific, London, 146–165.

Paulson, G. (1960) Procyclidine for dystonia caused by phenothiazine derivatives. *Dis. Nerv. Syst.*, 21: 447–448.

Pinder, R.M, Brogden, R.N., Sawyer, P.R., Speight, T.M. and Avery, G.S. (1976) Metoclopramide: a review of its pharmacological properties and clinical use. *Drugs* 12: 81–131.

Reasbeck, P. G. and Hossenbocus, A. (1979) Death following dystonic reaction to oral metoclopramide. *Br. J. Clin. Pract.*, 33: 31–33.

Regensburg, J. (1930) Zur Klinik des hereditaren torsiondystonischen Symptomenkomplexes. *Msch. Psychiat. Neurol.*, 75: 323–345.

Sasaki, H., Sudoh, K., Hamada, K., Hamada, T. and Tashiro, K. (1987) Skeletal myoclonus in olivopontocerebellar atrophy: treatment with trihexyphenidyl. *Neurology*, 37: 1258–1262.

Schwalbe, W. (1908) Eine eigentumliche tonische Krampfform mit hysterischen Symptomen. *Inaug. Diss.*, G. Schade, Berlin.

Simpson, G.M. and May, P.R.A. (1985) Schizophrenia: somatic treatment. In H.I. Kaplan and B.J. Sadock, (Eds.), *Comprehensive Textbook of Psychiatry*, 4th edition. Williams & Wilkins, Baltimore, pp. 713–724.

Smith, M.J. and Miller, M.M. (1961) Severe extrapyramidal reaction to perphenazine treated with diphenhydramine. *N. Engl. J. Med.*, 264: 396–397.

Stern, Y., Mayeux, R. and Cote, L. (1984) Reaction time and vigilance in Parkinson's disease: Possible role of altered norepinephrine metabolism. *Arch. Neurol.*, 41: 1086–1089.

Truong, D.D. and Fahn, S. (1988) An early description of dystonia: Translation of Schwalbe's thesis and information on his life. *Adv. Neurol.*, 50: 651–664.

Tune, L. and Coyle, J.T. (1980) Serum levels of anticholinergic drugs in treatment of acute extrapyramidal side effects. *Arch. Gen. Psychiatry*, 37: 293–297.

Waugh, W.H. and Metts, J.C. Jr. (1960) Severe extrapyramidal motor activity induced by prochloprperzine. *N. Engl. J. Med.*, 262: 353–354.

S.-M. Aquilonius and P.-G. Gillberg (Eds.)
Progress in Brain Research, Vol. 84
© 1990 Elsevier Science Publishers B.V. (Biomedical Division)

CHAPTER 41

Cholinergic agents in clinical anaesthesiology

Lars Wiklund and Per Hartvig

Department of Anaesthesiology and The Hospital Pharmacy, University Hospital of Uppsala, S-751 85 Uppsala, Sweden

Introduction

While anticholinergics such as atropine and scopolamine have been used in clinical anaesthesia for many years, the use of cholinomimetics as pharmaceutic agents in this area has a relatively short history. Only choline esterase inhibitors have been in general use as antidotes to neuromuscular blockade of the curare type. Thus, neostigmine has been and continues to be the classic drug for this purpose although the more rapidly acting edrophoneum is sometimes used instead. These pharmaceutical agents have consequently been extensively investigated and documented as part of a routine method for reversal of neuromuscular block. The following report concentrates on the central nervous effects of cholinomimetics.

Effects of systemic administration on postoperative somnolence and analgesia

Although it is a predecessor of the choline esterase inhibitors and has been known about for many years, physostigmine was not considered suitable for use in clinical anaesthesia when muscular relaxants were adopted in clinical anaesthesia in the 1950s (Burke et al., 1948). It was not until the late 1960s and the 1970s that a number of anaesthesiologists (Duvoisin and Katz, 1968; Rupreht and Dworacek, 1976; Thompson, 1976; Hill et al., 1977) discovered the usefulness of the central nervous effects that followed the administration of

physostigmine. By then Longo (1966) had defined the so-called central anticholinergic syndrome, which consists of dizziness, impairment of thought and recent memory, drowsiness up to the point of unconsciousness, excitement, and hallucinations combined with ataxia, and which is possible to reverse by the use of physostigmine. In typical cases the central anticholinergic syndrome was seen after (Tune et al., 1981) the administration of atropine-like pharmaceutics in sufficiently large doses. The most pronounced syndrome is often seen in elderly patients who have been premedicated by scopolamine (Holzgrafe et al., 1973), with the result that in spite of adequate doses of neostigmine and naloxone, the patient does not breathe at all and remains unconscious postoperatively. Usually these individuals have to be put back on the ventilator again until the anticholinergic has been eliminated. During the past ten years, however, these patients have usually been treated successfully by the administration of physostigmine (Thompson, 1976; Hill et al., 1977).

The effects of physostigmine in reversing neuromuscular block of the curare-type have been compared with those of neostigmine (Burke et al., 1948; Baraka, 1978; Salmenperä and Nilsson, 1981), and it has been shown that physostigmine is not as suitable as neostigmine. The physicochemical difference between the two substances is mainly due to the fact that neostigmine contains an ammonium ion, which gives a positive charge to the molecule so that as a consequence the molecule is hydrophilic and does not pass the blood-brain barrier easily. Physostigmine, on the other hand, with its tertiary amino function, is a non-charged molecule which is lipophilic instead, which explains its unreliable effects on the neuromuscular block and its quick passage through the blood-brain barrier.

After the central anticholinergic syndrome was described, it was soon demonstrated that physostigmine also effectively antagonized drugs other than the anticholinergics. It was shown that physostigmine successfully counteracted oversedation after large doses of fenothiazines or neuroleptics (Bernhards, 1973). It was similarly shown that although its duration of action was short, physostigmine could be used as an antidote to the tricyclic antidepressants (Aquilonius and Hedstrand, 1978). In addition, it was soon demonstrated that physostigmine antagonized sedation by the benzodiazepines (DiLiberti et al., 1975), and that ventilation was often stimulated by physostigmine after the administration of opioids (Weinstock et al., 1980, 1982; Snir-Mor et al., 1983). In fact, physostigmine seemed to be a rather omnipotent antidote to most pharmaceuticals with hypnotic or sedative actions, which led some investigators to the opinion that the drug was an analeptic (Havasi et al., 1982).

It has long been known that anticholinergic drugs also possess an anti-analgesic effect, and adrenergics (Tulunuy ct al., 1976) as well as cholinergics cause analgesia when administered parenterally (Flodmark and Wramner, 1945; Saxena, 1958; Harris et al., 1969; Ireson, 1970). These rather old findings caused Dirksen and Nijhuiis (1983) to investigate the significance of cholinergic neurotransmission at the spinal level in the effectiveness of opioids. In particular, the interaction between atropine or physostigmine and the opioids was evaluated. It was found that atropine reduced the antinociceptive effects while physostigmine markedly potentiated morphine analgesia. They proposed that this difference is related to a specific cholinergic mechanism involved in antinociception at the spinal level, and

that cholinergic mechanisms are relevant to opioid effectiveness. These findings encouraged our group to intensify our efforts to use physostigmine both clinically and for experimental research. For quite some time we had been using physostigmine postoperatively for the reversal of oversedation. Thus a clinical study where physostigmine was given in 2 mg bolus doses i.v. in the early postoperative phase demonstrated an analgesic effect of physostigmine which was of the same magnitude as that produced by 50 mg of pethidine (Pettersson et al., 1986). Unfortunately, the duration of analgesia produced by physostigmine was very short. Our findings soon became important to many neurosurgical patients at our hospital. We found that 0.5–2.0 mg of physostigmine i.v. given immediately post-operatively in combination with very small doses of naloxone (1–2 μg/kg) very effectively abolished the remaining sedation present at the end of surgery without producing increased postoperative pain (Wiklund, 1986). Thus, the combination of these two pharmaceutical agents resulted in such a rapid return of consciousness to anaesthetized patients who had just undergone surgery that we were almost immediately able to speak to them and examine their neurological signs and symptoms. However, many patients became resedated after 45–60 min. This clinical finding was explained when the pharmacokinetics of physostigmine were revealed (Hartvig et al., 1986). Subcutaneous and intramuscular forms of administration were investigated in order to circumvent these difficulties but were found to have little effect on the duration. However, the combination of an i.v. bolus and a subcutaneous injection resulted in an approximately 50% increase in duration. From a clinical point of view greater duration is desirable, and therefore we instituted an investigation of the possibilities of achieving good clinical effects with a constant two-rate infusion of physostigmine (Hartvig et al., 1989). In a previous study we had postulated that in order to get a sufficient clinical effect the plasma concentration should ideally be between 3 and 5 ng/ml (Hartvig et al., 1986).

During the course of this investigation, however, we found that different patients seemed to need very different amounts of physostigmine, i.e. a sufficient effect was sometimes not achieved until the plasma concentration was twice or three times the one we previously considered adequate. The explanation for these different demands may possibly be due to the patient himself, as well as to the kind of anaesthetic he had received. It was pointed out that the findings of this investigation were in line with the view that patients are subject to quite different levels of anticholinergic effects right after undergoing anaesthesia, which results in totally different requirements for physostigmine. An individual approach for determining suitable doses is therefore necessary. In addition, it should be mentioned that the analgesic effect in conjunction with the two-rate infusion was considered not better or less than that seen after intravenous bolus injections.

At this stage we had to consider alternatives to physostigmine. The first pharmaceutic agent that appeared suitable to us was tetrahydroaminoacridine (THA), which was used in clinical anaesthesia as early as the 1950s and '60s (Hunter, 1965) and has been registered in Australia ever since. It has been used primarily as a ventilatory stimulant after the administration of opioids, but has also been utilized to increase the duration of succinylcholine-induced neuromuscular block by a partial inhibition of the plasma acetylcholinesterase (Hunter, 1965). We have given a series of 10 patients 30 mg THA i.v. during the immediate postoperative period in the same way as we previously used physostigmine (Hartvig et al., 1989). The results showed that THA caused a prompt recovery of consciousness, similar to that of physostigmine, with an effect of the same magnitude. The duration of effect of THA, however, was clearly longer than that produced by physostigmine, although still not in proportion to its slow elimination from the plasma. The doses used did not result in any significant analgesic effect. The cholinergic side effects were also of less magnitude than those encountered after the administration of

1–2 mg of physostigmine (Hartvig et al., 1989). Unfortunately, THA is known to be hepatotoxic, especially when administered orally (Ames et al., 1988). Although this hepatotoxicity is probably less important after i.v. administration than after oral administration, alternatives which are less toxic than THA should be considered. So far we have not had any trials of galentamine.

Spinal analgesic effects

Another line of research that has been followed in our institution (T. Gordh Jr and coworkers) is one pursued in order to elucidate the analgesic effects after spinal administration of the cholinergic agents. So far these investigations have been almost purely experimental. They were carried out because it was known that both oral and parenteral administration of physostigmine and THA in selected clinical cases rendered good analgesia and potentiated the effect of the opioids (Tinel et al., 1933; Stone and Moon, 1961; Spillane et al., 1971; Schott and Loh, 1984). Similarly, T. Gordh Jr et al. also found that the α_2-adrenergic agent clonidine proved to have significant analgesic properties both experimentally and clinically (Tamsen and Gordh, 1984; Post et al., 1987), especially when administered spinally along with opioids. Thus the subarachnoidal administration of physostigmine was found to significantly increase the tail immersion response latency in rats, and this effect was attenuated if atropine was given simultaneously. In addition, it was possible to show that the combination of clonidine and physostigmine given intrathecally to the rats resulted in a potentiation of effect and that this effect was dependent upon a spinal cord containing noradrenergic functioning neurons. It was also demonstrated that phentolamine and atropine attenuated the tail immersion response latency caused by physostigmine. In addition, intrathecally administered neostigmine caused a very pronounced increase in the duration of tail immersion response latencies which also was attenuated by atropine (Gordh et al., 1988). The whole experimental series (Gillberg et al., 1989; Gordh, 1989) is believed to demonstrate that the cholinergic and adrenergic nervous systems in the spinal cord interact, and that both systems are necessary for the analgesic effects of adrenergic (e.g. clonidine) and cholinergic drugs (e.g. physostigmine, neostigmine and carbachol). It is still not possible to investigate the cholinomimetics after intrathecal or epidural administration in the clinical setting, as proper toxicological data are not yet available. Toxicological investigations are under way, however, and clinical trials will be performed in the near future if the results are found to be satisfactory. So far, however, we have been able to confirm that the use of oral physostigmine in selected patients with intractable pain has proved to be successful.

Postoperative fatigue

Excessive sedation and fatigue have proved to be a problem not only immediately postoperatively but for a rather long time during convalescence. Clinical experience indicating that 4–6 weeks are necessary for full recovery, even after minor surgery under regional or general anaesthesia, has also proved to be valid by scientific standards (Christensen et al., 1982; Christensen and Kehlet, 1984; Hjortsö et al., 1985; Schultze et al., 1988). Furthermore, increased demands for a quicker recovery after surgery have been advanced by society and industry so that surgical patients can return to health and production, thereby reducing hospital costs and insurance benefits during sick-leave. It seems to us that the goals for future research should conform to these expectations and consequently aim at developing different pharmacological principles which can make such a future possible.

In order to judge whether there is any probability of influencing the rate of reversal from general anaesthesia, a short review of current theories regarding the mechanisms of general anaesthesia would seem appropriate (cf. Ueda and Kamaya,

1984). Although general anaesthesia often causes decreased oxygen consumption, it seems that suggested chemical mechanisms, such as uncoupling, inhibited electron transport via the electron transport chain, and inhibited use of ATP through block of its hydrolysis, now seem less probable owing to the fact that no changes in the turnover of intracellular energy metabolites have been found. In contrast to this, the finding that virtually all known general anaesthetic agents inhibit the luminescence of luciferin, which consumes ATP and molecular oxygen and is catalysed by the firefly light-emitting enzyme (luciferase), seems to show that volatile anaesthetic agents may also influence a complicated protein (Franks and Lieb, 1984; Firestone, 1988). A vivid debate concerning the effect of general anaesthetics has taken place between those who have claimed that general anaesthetics unspecifically influence the physical-chemical properties in macromolecules of central nervous system neurons, and those who instead have claimed that the effect is probably mediated through specific receptors (Ueda and Kamaya, 1984; Franks and Lieb, 1987). The first of these two main mechanisms has been supported by the fact that the potency of different anaesthetics is directly correlated to their lipophilicity (cf. Ueda and Kamaya, 1984), and that the inert gas xenon (Cullen and Gross, 1957), which cannot be a part of ionic formation, hydrogen or covalent binding with other atoms, is also a very potent general anaesthetic. Another finding which has supported the unspecific mode of action of the anaesthetics is the fact that anaesthesia induced by all known general anaesthetics is wholly reversed if the animal is exposed to high ambient pressure (Miller et al., 1973). Other unspecific theories must also be added here, such as those which take into account the influence of general anaesthetics on the intracellular water phase forming microcrystals (Pauling, 1961; Miller, 1961), and, perhaps most importantly, the effect of general anaesthetics on lipoprotein cell membrane elements, called fluidization (for review see Ueda and Kamaya, 1984). Recently, however, experiments using nuclear magnetic resonance (Evers et al., 1987) have resulted in data suggesting the existence of a saturable anaesthetic site for halothane in the brain, thus not supporting the concept of anaesthetic action by non-specific membrane perturbation. In addition, Buch et al. (1989) have published experimental evidence which seems to prove that the fluidization of membranes does not appear to be a realistic alternative. After noting these and other results indicating involvement of specific receptors (Artru et al., 1980; Ori et al., 1989) Cheng and Brunner (1987) modified their previous GABA theory somewhat, so as to take new facts into consideration, by suggesting that general anaesthetics have a site of action immediately adjacent to the protein part of the cell membrane in the neurons, i.e. the specific receptor itself. Thus, it is suggested that the GABA-receptor complex immediately adjacent to lipid-protein interface is influenced by general anaesthetics in the same way that the chloride channel is shut off by GABA. As late as the year before last further interesting experiments were published to elucidate these phenomena (Moody et al., 1988). It was found that volatile anaesthetic agents have the characteristic of modifying the benzodiazepin/GABA/chloride channel complex in a way which is similar to what has been found for barbiturates and alcohols. These results show that general, gaseous as well as volatile, anaesthesics in clinical concentrations stimulate chloride uptake in a concentration-dependent, picrotoxin-sensitive way, which also modulates muscimol and pentobarbital-stimulated chloride uptake.

In conclusion, the most recent findings and theories within the area of general anaesthesia seem to indicate that both the volatile and the i.v. agents act on the benzodiazepine/GABA/chloride channel complex by direct and indirect mechanisms. Interestingly, Geller et al. (1988) and Roald et al. (1988) recently reported that a partial reversal of the central nervous effects of isoflurane and halothane takes place after the administration of the benzodiazepine antagonist flumazenil. It has also been claimed that this agent possesses analgesic properties (Davidovich et al., 1988; Schwartz et al., 1989). However, our own experimental data (unpublished observations) do not support the idea of a spinal mechanism involved in flumazenil analgesia. These most recent findings thus make it likely that we must again consider the receptor theories in our search for the explanation of mechanisms involved in general anaesthesis.

Do the cholinergic mechanisms and receptors appear to be involved in the mechanisms of general anaesthesia? Since Braswell and Kitz (1977) have found that dog brain and human erythrocyte acetylcholinesterase were reversibly inhibited in a dose-dependent manner by a number of general anaesthetics, admittedly in superclinical concentrations, plus the knowledge that general anaesthetics influence the nicotinic acetylcholine receptor-rich membranes from the *Torpedo* (Blanchard et al., 1979; Firestone et al., 1986), it seems that this is still an open issue (Ueda and Kamaya, 1984). In contrast, it seems that opioid administration significantly influences the turnover of acetylcholine in the brain (Dayton and Garrett, 1973; Domino and Wilson, 1973; Zsilla et al., 1976; Moroni et al., 1977; Schmidt and Buxbaum, 1978; Romano and Shih, 1983). Thus there is only scanty evidence indicating that cholinergic receptors are primarily involved in the molecular mechanism of general anaesthesia, and we must point out that facts rather seem to favor the opinion that cholinergic neurotransmission is merely secondarily involved. It is possible, for instance, to reverse benzodiazepine-induced sedation by physostigmine.

During the next few years the highest priority in our lab will be to elucidate the connection between the different kinds of receptors known to be involved in the process of general anaesthesia, and the interactions between these different mechanisms in the central nervous system, in order to obtain a powerful pharmacological means not only for the reversal of anaesthesia, but also for a possibly more rapid full recovery and earlier return to work after anaesthesia and surgery.

References

Ames, D.J., Bhathal, P.S., Davies, B.M. and Fraser, J.R.E. (1988) Hepatotoxicity of tetrahydroacridine. *Lancet,* 1: 887.

Aquilonius, S.-M. and Hedstrand, U. (1978) The use of physostigmine as an antidote in tricyclic anti-depressant intoxication. *Acta Anaesthesiol. Scand.,* 22: 40–45.

Artru, A.A., Steen, P.A. and Michenfelder, J.D. (1980) Cerebral metabolic effects of naloxone administered with anesthetic and subanesthetic concentrations of halothane in the dog. *Anesthesiology,* 52: 217–220.

Baraka, A. (1978) Antagonism of neuromuscular block by physostigmine in man. *Br. J. Anaesth.,* 50: 1075–1077.

Bernards, W. (1973) Case history 74: Reversal of phenothiazine-induced coma with physostigmine. *Anesth. Analg.,* 52: 938–941.

Braswell, L.M. and Kitz, R.J. (1977) The effect in vitro of volatile anesthetics on the activity of cholinesterases. *J. Neurochem.,* 29: 665–671.

Buck, K.J., Allan, A.M. and Harris, R.A. (1989) Fluidization of brain membranes by A2C does not produce anesthesia and does not augment muscimol-stimulated 36Cl-influx. *Eur. J. Pharmacol.,* 160: 359–367.

Burke, J.C., Linegar, C.R., Frank, M. and McIntyre, A. (1948) Eserine and neostigmine antagonism to d-tubocurarine. *Anesthesiology,* 9: 251–257.

Cheng, S.-C. and Brunner, E.A. (1987) A hypothetical model on the mechanism of anesthesia. *Med. Hypotheses,* 23: 1–9.

Christensen, T. and Kehlet, H. (1984) Postoperative fatigue and changes in nutritional status. *Br. J. Surg.,* 71: 473–476.

Christensen, T., Bendix, T. and Kehlet, H. (1982) Fatigue and cardiorespiratory function following abdominal surgery. *Br. J. Surg.,* 69: 417–419.

Cullen, S. and Gross, E. (1951) The anesthetic properties of xenon in animals and human beings, with additional observations on krypton. *Science,* 113: 580–582.

Davidovich, S., Niv, D., Geller, E. and Urca, G. (1988) RO 15-1788 produces naloxone-reversible analgesia in the rat. *Eur. J. Pharmacol.,* 146: 175–179.

Dayton, H.E. and Garrett, R.L. (1973) Production of analgesia by cholinergic drugs. *Proc. Soc. Exp. Biol. Med.,* 142: 1011–1013.

DiLiberti, J., Brebner, J., Galloon, S. and Young, P.S. (1975) The use of physostigmine as an antidote in accidental diazepam intoxication. *J. Pediat.,* 86: 106–107.

Dirksen, R. and Nijhuis, G.M.M. (1983) The relevance of cholinergic transmission at the spinal level to opiate effectiveness. *Eur. J. Pharmacol.,* 91: 215–221.

Domino, E.F. and Wilson, A. (1973) Effects of narcotic analgesic agonists and antagonists on rat brain acetylcholine. *J. Pharmacol. Exp. Ther.,* 184: 18–32.

Duvosin, R. and Katz, R. (1968) Reversal of central anticholinergic syndrome in man by physostigmine. *JAMA,* 206: 1963–1965.

Evers, A.S., Berkowitz, B.A. and d'Avignon, A. (1987) Correlation between the anaesthetic effect of halothane and saturable binding in brain. *Nature,* 328: 157–160.

Firestone, L.L. (1988) General anesthetics. *Int. Anesthesiol. Clin.,* 26: 248–253.

Firestone, L.L., Sauter, F., Braswell, L.M. and Miller, K.W. (1986) Actions of general anesthetics on acetylcholine receptor-rich membranes from Torpedo californica. *Anesthesiology,* 64: 694–702.

Flodmark, S. and Wramner, T. (1945) The analgesic action of morphine, eserine and prostigmine studied by a modified Hardy-Wolff-Goodell method. *Acta Physiol. Scand.,* 9: 88–96.

Frank, M. and McIntyre, A. (1948) Eserine and neostigmine antagonism to d-tubocurarine. *Anesthesiology,* 9: 251.

Franks, N.P. and Lieb, W.R. (1984) Do general anaesthetics act by competitive binding to specific receptors? *Nature,* 310: 599–601.

Franks, N.P. and Lieb, W.R. (1987) What is the molecular nature of general anaesthetic target sites? *Trends. Pharmacol. Sci.,* 8: 169–174.

Geller, A., Weinbrum, A., Schiff, B., Speiser, Z., Nevo, Y., Halpern, P. and Cohen, S. (1988) The effects of flumazenil on the process of recovery from halothane anaesthesia, *Eur. J. Anaesthesiol.,* Suppl 2: 151–153.

Gillberg, P.G., Gordh, T Jr., Hartvig, P., Jansson, I., Petterson, J. and Post, C. (1989) Characterization of the antinociception induced by intrathecally administered carbachol. *Pharmacol. Toxicol.,* 64: 340–343.

Gordh, T Jr., Jansson, I., Hartvig, P., Gillberg, P.G. and Post, C. (1989) Interactions between noradrenergic and cholinergic mechanisms involved in spinal nociceptive processing. *Acta Anaesthesiol. Scand.,* 33: 39–47.

Harris, L.S., Dewey, W.L., Howes, J.F., Kennedy, J.S. and Pars, H. (1969) Narcotic-antagonist analgesics. Interactions with cholinergic systems. *J. Pharmacol. Exp. Ther.,* 169: 17–22.

Hartvig, P., Pettersson, E., Wiklund, L. and Lindström, B. Pharmacokinetics and effects of 9-amino-1,2,3,4-tetrahydroacridine, Tacrine, in the immediate postoperative period in neurosurgical patients. *In manus.*

Hartvig, P., Askmark, H., Aquilonius, S.-M., Wiklund, L. and Lindström, B. Clinical pharmacokinetics of intravenous and oral 9-amino-1,2,3,4-tetrahydroacridine. *Eur. J. Clin. Pharmacol.,* Submitted.

Hartvig, P., Wiklund, L. and Lindström, B. (1986) Pharmacokinetics of physostigmine after intravenous, intramuscular and subcutaneous administration in surgical patients. *Acta Anaesthesiol. Scand.,* 30: 177–182.

Hartvig, P., Lindström, B., Petterson, E. and Wiklund, L. (1989) Reversal of postoperative somnolence using a two rate infusion of physostigmine. *Acta Anaesthesiol. Scand.,* In press.

Havasi, G., Havasi, I., Gintautas, J. and Kraynack, B.J. (1982) Is physostigmine a pure analeptic agent? A clinical evaluation. *Proc. West. Pharmacol. Soc.,* 25: 35–37.

Hill, G.E., Stanley, T.H. and Sentker, C.R. (1977) Physostigmine reversal of postoperative somnolence. *Can. Anaesth. Soc. J.,* 24: 707–711.

Hjortsø, N.C., Neuman, P., Frøsig, F., Andersen, T., Lindhard, A., Rogon, E. and Kehlet, H. (1985) A controlled study on the effect of epidural analgesia with local anaesthetics and morphine on morbidity after abdominal surgery. *Acta Anaesthesiol. Scand.,* 29: 790–796.

Holzgrafe, R., Vondell, J.J. and Mintz, S.M. (1973) Reversal of postoperative reactions to scopolamine with physostigmine. *Anesth. Analg* (Cleve.), 52: 921–928.

Hunter, A.R. (1965) Tetrahydroaminacrine in anaesthesia. *Br. J. Anaesth.,* 37: 505–513.

Ireson, J.D. (1970) A comparison of the antinociceptive actions of cholinomimetic and morphine-like drugs. *Br. J. Pharmacol.,* 40: 92–101.

Longo, V.G. (1966) Behavioral and electroencephalographic effects of atropine and related compounds. *Pharmacol. Rev.,* 18: 965–996.

Miller, S.L. (1961) A theory of gaseous anesthetics. *Proc. Natl. Acad. Sci. USA,* 47: 1515–1524.

Moody, E.J., Suzdak, P.D., Paul, S.M. and Skolnick, P. (1988) Modulation of the benzodiazepine/γ-aminobutyric acid receptor chloride channel complex by inhalational anesthetics. *J. Neurochem.,* 51: 1386–1393.

Moroni, F., Cheney, D.L. and Costa, E. (1977) b-endorphin inhibits ACh turnover in nuclei of the rat brain. *Nature,* 267: 267–268.

Ori, C., Ford-Rice, F. and London, E.D. (1989) Effects of nitrous oxide and halothane on μ and k opioid receptors in guinea-pig brain. *Anesthesiology,* 70: 541–544.

Pauling, P. (1961) A molecular theory of gaseous anesthesia. *Science,* 134: 15–21.

Pettersson, J., Gordh, T.E., Hartvig, P. and Wiklund, L. (1986) A double-blind trial of the analgesic properties of physostigmine in postoperative patients. *Acta Anaesthesiol. Scand.,* 30: 283–288.

Post, C., Gordh, T Jr., Minor, B., Archer, T. and Freedman, J. (1987) Antinociceptive effects and spinal cord tissue concentrations after intrathecal injection of guanfacine or clonidine into rats. *Anesth. Analg.,* 66: 317–324.

Roald, O.K., Forsman, M. and Steen, P.A. (1988) Partial reversal of the cerebral effects of isoflurane in the dog by the benzodiazepine antagonist flumazenil. *Acta Anaesthesiol. Scand.,* 32: 209–212.

Romano, J.A. and Shih, T.-M. (1983) Cholinergic mechanisms of analgesia produced by physostigmine, morphine and cold water swimming. *Neuropharmacology,* 22: 827–833.

Rupreht, J. and Dworacek, B. (1976) Central anticholinergic syndrome in anesthetic practice. *Acta Anaesth. Bel.,* 27: 45–60.

Salemenperä, M. and Nilsson, E. (1981) Comparison of physostigmine and neostigmine for antagonism of neuromuscular block. *Acta Anaesthesiol. Scand.,* 25: 387–390.

Saxena, P.N. (1958) Mechanism of cholinergic potentiation of morphine analgesia. *Ind. J. Med. Res.,* 46: 653–658.

Schmidt, D.E. and Buxbaum, D.M. (1978) Effect of acute morphine administration of regional acetylcholine turnover in the rat. *Brain Res.,* 147: 194–200.

Schott, G.D. and Loh, L. (1984) Anticholinesterase drugs in the treatment of chronic pain. *Pain.* 20: 201–206.

Schulze, S., Roikjaer, O., Hasselstrøm, L., Jensen, N.H. and Kehlet, H. (1988) Epidural bupivacaine and morphine plus systemic indomethacine eliminates pain but not systemic response and convalescence after cholecystectomy. *Surgery,* 103: 321–327.

Schwartz, A.E., Maneksha, F.R., Kanchuger, M.S., Sidhu, U.S. and Poppers, P.J. (1989) Flumazenil decreases the minimum alveolar concentration of isoflurane in dogs. *Anesthesiology,* 70: 764–766.

Snir-Mor, I., Weinstock, M., Davidson, J.T. and Bahar, M. (1983) Physostigmine antagonizes morphine-induced respiratory depression in human subjects. *Anesthesiology,* 59: 6–9.

Spillane, J.D., Nathan, P.W., Kelly, R.E. and Marsden, C.D. (1971) Painful legs and moving toes. *Brain,* 94: 541–556.

Stone, V. and Moon, W. (1961) Treatment of intractable pain with morphine and tetrahydroaminacredine. *Br. Med. J.,* 471–473.

Tamsen, A. and Gordh, T. (1984) Epidural clonidine gives analgesia. *Lancet,* ii: 876–877.

Thompson, D.E.A. (1976) Physostigmine as an adjunct to neurolept anesthesia in neurosurgical procedures. *Can. Anesth. Soc. J.,* 23: 582–586.

Tinel, J., Eck, M. and Stewart, W. (1933) Causalgie de la main guérie par l'acétylcholine. *Rev. Neurol.,* 2: 38–43.

Tulunay, F.C., Yano, I. and Takemori, A.E. (1976) The effect of biogenic amine modifiers on morphine analgesia and its antagonism by naloxone. *Eur. J. Pharmacol.,* 35: 285–292.

Tune, L., Holland, A., Folstein, M.F., Damluji, N.F., Gardner, T.J. and Coyle, J.T. (1981) Association of postoperative delirium with raised serum levels of anticholinergic drugs. *Lancet,* ii: 651–652.

Ueda, I. and Kamaya, H. (1984) Molecular mechanisms of anesthesia. *Anesth. Analg.,* 63: 929–945.

Weinstock, M., Davidson, J.T., Rosin, A.J. and Schnieden, H. (1982) Effect of physostigmine on morphine-induced postoperative pain and somnolence. *Br. J. Anaesth.,* 54: 429–434.

Wiklund, L. (1986) Reversal of sedation and respiratory depression after anaesthesia by the combined use of physostigmine and naloxone in neurosurgical patients. *Acta Anaesthesiol. Scand.,* 30: 374–377.

Zsilla, G., Cheney, D.L., Racagni, G. and Costa, E. (1976) Correlation between analgesia and the decrease of acetylcholine turnover rate in cortex and hippocampus elicited by morphine, meperidine, viminol R2 and azidomorphine. *J. Pharmacol. Exp. Ther.,* 199: 662–668.

S.-M. Aquilonius and P.-G. Gillberg (Eds.)
Progress in Brain Research, Vol. 84
© 1990 Elsevier Science Publishers B.V. (Biomedical Division)

CHAPTER 42

Acetylcholine and acetylcholine receptor subtypes in REM sleep generation

Javier Velazquez-Moctezuma [2], Priyattam J. Shiromani [1] and J. Christian Gillin [1]

[1] Department of Psychiatry, San Diego VA Medical Center, University of California San Diego, La Jolla, CA, U.S.A., and [2] Universidad Autonoma Metropolitana-Iztapalapa, Mexico City, Mexico

Introduction

The neuronal mechanisms underlying the generation and maintenance of sleep stages are still poorly understood. Several theories have proposed complex interactions between different neurotransmitter systems but no fully accepted theory has yet emerged which attempts to explain the three states of consciousness: wakefulness, REM sleep (also called paradoxical or D sleep) and non-REM sleep (or slow-wave sleep). Nevertheless, a great deal of information has been accumulated in the last three decades implicating the cholinergic system in the regulation of REM sleep.

REM sleep was discovered by Aserinsky and Kleitman in 1953. Nowadays, it is well known that REM sleep is characterized by the simultaneous presence of tonic components, such as cortical desynchronization, atonia of antigravitory muscles and hippocampal theta rhythm, as well as phasic components, such as rapid eye movements and ponto-geniculo occipital spikes. Cholinergic stimulation of the brainstem is capable of eliciting a state that is behaviorally and polygraphically indistinguishable from naturally occurring REM sleep, and specific sites within the brainstem are capable of inducing a selective increase of one of the components as well.

Cholinomimetic agents and REM sleep

Since Hernandez-Peon's pioneering work (1963), it has been well known that cholinergic stimulation of a number of brain regions can increase either slow-wave sleep or REM sleep. From these studies a cholinergic hypnogenic pathway was proposed. This pathway included the hypothalamus, amygdala, hippocampus, the medial anterior pre-optic area, temporal and cingulate cortex, as well as some areas of the brainstem where the medial pontine reticular formation is specially relevant. In the same year, Cordeau et al. (1963) induced REM sleep by the administration of a solution of acetylcholine bromide in the caudal mesencephalon and in the medulla of freely moving cats.

The main pharmacological tool in the analysis of cholinergic control of REM sleep has been carbachol, a mixed cholinergic receptor agonist. In 1964, George et al. reported increased REM sleep following the administration of smaller doses of carbachol (0.2–5 μg) directly in the giganto-cellular tegmental field (FTG), an area located in the medial pontine reticular formation. Hernandez-Peon (1963) reported success in eliciting REM sleep when carbachol crystals were applied directly in the medial forebrain, midbrain, pons and medulla of freely moving cats. Six years later,

Baxter (1969) reproduced these results by applying carbachol crystals in the central grey and in the fourth ventricle.

During the 1970s and 1980s the number of papers reporting the effects of carbachol on REM sleep increased markedly (for review see Shiromani et al., 1987). It is now clear that carbachol readily triggers REM sleep when applied to the FTG, but it can also selectively increase one of the components of REM sleep or even induce the suppression of REM signs (Amatruda et al., 1975; Baghdoyan et al., 1984b). This indicates that carbachol has a site-specific effect within the brainstem (Baghdoyan et al., 1987b; Hobson et al., 1986). Moreover, Shiromani and McGinty (1986b) reported that a great percentage of medial pontine reticular cells are not activated or are even inactivated in the presence of carbachol. These results have been interpreted as evidence that only a subpopulation of medial pontine cells are necessary and sufficient for the generation of naturally occurring REM sleep.

In contrast to carbachol, oxotremorine is a selective muscarinic agonist and, when infused in the FTG, it elicits an increase in REM sleep in freely moving cats, with doses as small as those used for carbachol (George et al., 1964). Bethanechol (Hobson et al., 1983), another selective muscarinic agonist, is also capable of increasing REM sleep when infused within the medial pontine reticular formation. Appropriate systemic administration of muscarinic agonists such as arecoline (Sitaram et al., 1980) or RS 86 (Spiegel, 1984) shortens REM latency in humans.

The above data indicate that the cholinergic control of REM sleep is mediated exclusively by muscarinic receptors. Nevertheless, the lack of nicotinic participation is not completely clear. George et al. (1964) reported that nicotine had no behavioral and polygraphic effects when it was administered in the FTG. Moreover, nicotine failed to change the food-induced cataplexy test in narcoleptic dogs (Delashaw et al., 1979). On the other hand, however, Domino and Yamamoto in 1965 reported that small doses of nicotine given intravenously in freely behaving cats significantly increased REM sleep. This effect could be blocked by administering mecamylamine (a nicotine blocker), which crosses the blood brain barrier, and was not blocked with trimethidinium, which does not enter the brain readily. The results were reproduced by Jewett et al. (1986) with subcutaneous administration of nicotine. In the same study, Jewett reported that doses higher than 100 μg/kg increased the wake time as well.

The hypothesis that the physiological liberation of acetylcholine facilitates REM sleep is further supported by studies using anticholinesterases, which prevent the breakdown of acetylcholine. The intravenous administration of eserine (physostigmine) in cats and rats increases the amount of REM sleep and of its phasic and tonic components (Domino et al., 1968; Jouvet, 1977; Karczmar, 1970). Eserine is also capable of eliciting PGO bursts in cats (Magherini et al., 1971) and when infused in humans shortens REM latency in normal volunteers (Sitaram et al., 1976). Another potent anticholinesterase drug, neostigmine, increases REM sleep, particularly PGO waves, when administered in the mPRF (Baghdoyan et al., 1984a, 1987a).

Cholinolytic agents and REM sleep

If acetylcholine is involved in the onset of REM sleep, then the blockade of cholinergic transmission should decrease REM sleep. This prediction has been successfully tested either with the inhibition of the synthesis of acetylcholine or with the blockade of the cholinergic receptor.

In 1970, Hazra reported that low doses of hemicholinum (an acetylcholine synthesis blocker), applied in the fourth ventricle of the cat, totally suppressed REM sleep; in addition, it increased slow-wave sleep in a dose-dependent manner. These results were replicated by Domino and Stawinski (1970), who administered hemicholinum in the lateral ventricle of cats.

At the receptor level, atropine and scopolamine (muscarinic receptor blockers) have been able to block the induction of REM sleep by cholino-mimetics. Velluti and Hernandez-Peon (1963) reported that local application of atropine blocked the REM sleep increase otherwise produced by cholinergic stimulation in the same atropinized point or in other sites of the hypnogenic circuit distant from the atropinized area.

Atropine potently inhibits REM sleep as well as REM components. Jouvet (1977) administered atropine to reserpine-pretreated cats and blocked the enhancement of PGO waves that characterize this preparation. These results were similar to those obtained with the administration of atropine in PCPA-pretreated cats (Jacobs et al., 1972). Baghdoyan et al. (1989) reported that atropine blocks the increase of REM sleep induced either with neostigmine or with carbachol. Shiromani and Fishbein (1986a) reported that the chronic administration of scopolamine into the pons significantly reduced naturally occurring REM sleep in the rat.

Furthermore, during the withdrawal period after the chronic administration of scopolamine there is an increase of REM sleep which coincides with the increase in muscarinic receptor binding in the hippocampus and caudate (Sutin et al., 1986). In addition, in the canine model of narcolepsy there is an increase in muscarinic receptors in the medial pontine reticular formation (Killduff et al., 1986), a region involved in REM sleep generation.

The Flinders Sensitive Line of rats, a proposed animal model of depression, also have significantly higher amounts of REM sleep as well as increased binding of muscarinic receptors in several brain regions (Shiromani et al., 1988b).

Cholinergic receptor subtypes and REM sleep

The above studies support the hypothesis that the cholinergic system is triggering REM sleep by acting through muscarinic receptors. Recently, muscarinic receptors have been divided into several subtypes. The most widely accepted subclassification of muscarinic receptors is that proposed by Hammer and Gianchetti (1982) and this is based on the affinity of the muscarinic receptor for the antagonist pirenzepine. M_1 receptors have high affinity for pirenzepine, while the M_2 receptors have low affinity for pirenzepine. Spencer et al. (1986), using autoradiographic techniques, have reported that the distribution of muscarinic receptor subtypes in the brain follows different patterns. The M_1 receptors are located preferentially in forebrain areas, while the M_2 subtype predominates in posterior areas, where the medial pontine reticular formation is included.

In order to elucidate the role of the different muscarinic receptor subtypes in the generation of REM sleep, we have administered drugs with high selectivity either for M_1 or for the M_2 receptor subtype. When infused in the medial pontine reticular formation of freely moving cats, the selective M_2 agonists cismethyldioxolane and oxotremorine-M increased REM sleep to the same extent as carbachol but with a 4-fold lower dose compared to carbachol. This increase in REM sleep closely corresponded with a decrease in slow-wave sleep, while wake percentage remained unaltered. On the other hand, McN 343-A, a selective M_1 agonist, did not show any change in REM sleep, slow-wave sleep or wake percentage when compared to Ringer's control (Velazquez-Moctezuma et al., 1989).

Recent data obtained from experiments using atropine and pirenzepine support our hypothesis that the enhancement of REM sleep induced by cholinergic stimulation is mediated selectively by the M_2 muscarinic receptors subtype.

Cholinergic neuronal pathways involved in REM sleep generation

Even though considerable evidence from pharmacological drug infusion studies had accumulated which linked the cholinergic system with REM sleep generation, until recently there was no clear map of the distribution of cholinergic pathways in the brain. With the development of antibodies against choline acetyltransferase, the acetylcholine synthesizing enzyme, cholinergic neuroanatomy has become more clear. In the brainstem, there are two major collections of cholinergic cell bodies located in the lateral dorsal tegmental (LDT) and pedunculopontine pontine tegmental (PPT) nuclei. We have shown that some cholinergic neurons from these two groups project to the area in the medial pontine from where REM sleep can be readily induced by cholinergic stimulation (Shiromani et al. 1988a). Thus, we hypothesize that physiological REM sleep may occur as a result of an interaction between cholinergic LDT/PPT neurons and cholinoceptive medial pontine. Of course, as hypothesized by Hobson and McCarley (1975), these neurons in turn interact with catecholamine and serotonin neurons.

Clinical implications

Short REM latency (the elapse time from the onset of sleep until the first REM period) is characteristic of some clinical syndromes, particularly depression and narcolepsy. A better understanding of the physiological mechanisms of sleep would contribute to the elucidation of the pathophysiology of these disorders

In 1972, Janowsky et al. proposed the cholinergic-aminergic imbalance hypothesis of affective disorders, which suggested that depression is associated with a predominance of central cholinergic to aminergic neurotransmission, while mania was associated with a predominance of aminergic to cholinergic neurotransmission. The data originally cited in support of the hypothesis were derived mostly from inferences about the mechanisms of action of drugs known to treat or induce affective disorders (Dilsaver et al., 1984; Dilsaver, 1988; Janowsky et al., 1988). Consistent with this hypothesis, cholinesterase inhibitors have been reported to induce anergy, lethargy and dysphoria in man and to antagonize manic symptoms (Bowers et al., 1964; Carroll et al., 1973; Davis et al., 1978; Gershon et al., 1961; Janowsky et al., 1973; Risch et al., 1981). In addition, choline, a biosynthetic precursor of acetylcholine, has been reported to

induce depression in schizophrenic patients when administered for the treatment of tardive dyskinesia (Davis et al., 1979; Tamminga et al., 1976). Choline or lecithin may also have antimanic effects (Cohen et al., 1982). Deanol, which is also a precursor to acetylcholine, has been reported to exacerbate depression symptoms in schizophrenic patients with a history of depressive symptoms (Casey, 1979). Arecoline has also been reported to induce depressive-like symptoms in some volunteers or patients (Risch et al., 1983).

The objective sleep changes associated with depression may also be consistent with the cholinergic-aminergic imbalance hypothesis (Gillin et al., 1979b). EEG sleep patterns in depression are characterized by short REM latency, increased REM density (a measure of ocular activity during REM sleep), increased duration of the first REM period, and reduced total sleep time, sleep efficiency (the proportion of time in bed spent asleep) and Delta (stage 3 and 4) sleep (Gillin et al., 1979a, 1984; Reynolds et al., 1987).

We have earlier suggested that the sleep disturbances of depression might be associated with muscarinic supersensitivity (Gillin et al., 1979b). This hypothesis was based on a study in normal volunteers in which scopolamine withdrawal induced muscarinic supersensitivity produced short REM latency, increased REM density, increased sleep latency, and reduced total sleep time and sleep efficiency (Gillin, 1979b; Sitaram et al., 1979). Using a discriminate function analysis which we had previously shown to separate sleep records of depressed, normal and insomniac patients (Gillin et al., 1979a), we identified the records of the normal subjects as "normal" before scopolamine treatment and as predominately "depressed" afterwards (Gillin et al., 1979b).

In order to test the hypothesis that functional muscarinic supersensitivity resulted from daily administration of scopolamine in normal volunteers, we developed the cholinergic REM induction test (CRIT) with arecoline (Sitaram et al., 1979). In this test, the elapsed time from the infusion of arecoline during the second NREM period to the onset of the second REM period is measured. In the original studies, which were conducted primarily in patients with bipolar disorders, patients enter REM sleep significantly more quickly in a dose response fashion compared with normal controls (Sitaram et al., 1980, 1982). Since then, this finding has been replicated (Dube et al., 1987; Jones et al., 1985; Nurberger et al., 1989; Sitaram et al., 1987). These six studies represent two separate studies at the Intramural Program of the National Institute of Menthal Health in Bethesda, Maryland (Nurberger et al., 1989; Sitaram et al., 1980, 1982), three reports apparently based on overlapping data bases from the Lafayette Clinic in Detroit, Michigan (Dube et al., 1987; Jones et al., 1985; Sitaram et al., 1987), and our current unpublished report from the San Diego Veterans Administration Center in San Diego, California. In all six reports, patients with affective disorder showed a statistically faster response than normal controls at at least one dose; in addition, in the Dube et al. (1987) and Jones et al. (1985) studies, patients with major depressive disorder, endogenous type, showed a significantly shorter response than nonendogenous depressed patients, patients with primary anxiety disorder with or without secondary depression, and from nonaffective patients. It should be noted that the contrast in the Sitaram et al. (1987) paper was between "ill" and "well" first-degree relatives of probands with both affective disorder and short response to the CRIT. That study, as well as the twin study of Nurnberger et al. (1983), suggests that a short response on the CRIT may be modulated by genetic factors and could be a weak genetic marker for affective disorder (see also Nurberger et al., 1989). In addition, Wager et al. (1988) have presented preliminary data supporting the CRIT with arecoline in atypical depressed patients.

Further evidence also supports a more sensitive sleep response to cholinergic agonists in depression than controls: the greater awakening response to physostigmine reported by Berger et al. (1989) and the faster induction of REM sleep following oral administration of RS 86, an orally active M_1 agonist (Berger et al., 1983; Berger et al., 1985; Riemann et al., 1988).

Acknowledgements

Funded by NIH-NS25212 (PJS), American Narcolepsy Association (PJS), NIMH-38738 (JCG) and VA Research Service.

References

Amatruda, T., Black, D., McKena, T., McCarley, R.W. and Hobson, J.A. (1975) Sleep cycle control and cholinergic mechanisms: differential effects of carbachol injections at pontine brainstem sites. *Brain Res.*, 98: 501–515.

Aserinsky, E. and Kleitman, N. (1953) Regularly occurring periods of eye motility and concomitant phenomena during sleep. *Science*, 118: 273–274.

Baghdoyan, H.A., Monaco, A.P., Rodrigo-Angulo, M.L., Assens, F., McCarley, R.W. and Hobson, J.A. (1984a) Microinjection of neostigmine into the pontine reticular formation of cats enhances the desynchronized sleep signs. *J. Pharmacol. Exp. Ther.*, 231: 173–180.

Baghdoyan, H.A., Rodrigo-Angulo, M.L., McCarley, R.W. and Hobson, J.A. (1984b) Site-specific enhancement and supression of desynchronized sleep signs following cholinergic stimulation of three brainstem regions. *Brain Res.*, 306: 39–52.

Baghdoyan, H.A., Lydic, R., Callaway, C.W. and Hobson, J.A. (1987a) Increased pontogeniculo-occipital wave frequency following central administration of neostigmine. *Neurosci. Lett.*, 82: 278–284.

Baghdoyan, H.A., Rodrigo-Angulo, M.L., McCarley, R.W. and Hobson, J.A. (1987b) A neuroanatomical gradient in the pontine tegmentum for the cholinoceptive induction of desynchronizcd sleep signs. *Brain Res.*, 414: 245–261.

Baghdoyan, H.A., Lydic, R., Callaway, C.W. and Hobson, J.A. (1989) The carbachol-induced enhancement of desynchronized sleep signs is dose dependent and antagonized by centrally administered atropine. *Neuropsychopharmacology*, 2: 67–79.

Baxter, B.L. (1969) Induction of both emotional behavior and a novel form of REM sleep by chemical stimulation applied to cat mesencephalon. *Exp. Neurol.*, 23: 220–230.

Berger, M., Lund, R., Bronisch, T. and Zerssen, D.von (1983) REM latency in neurotic and endogenous depression and the cholinergic REM induction test. *Psychiat. Res.*, 10: 113–123.

Berger, M., Hochli, D. and Zulley, J. (1985) Cholinomimetic drug RS 86, REM sleep and depression. *Lancet*, ii: 1385–1386.

Berger, M., Riemann, D., Hochli, D. and Spiegel, R. (1989) The cholinergic REM sleep induction test with RS 86. State or trait-marker of depression? *Arch. Gen Psychol.*, 46: 421–428.

412

Bowers, M.D., Goodman, E. and Sim, V.M. (1964) Some behavioral changes in man following anticholinesterase administration. *J. Nerv. Ment. Dis.*, 138: 383–389.

Casey, D.E (1979) Mood alteration during deanol therapy. *Psychopharmacology*, 62: 187–191.

Carroll, B.J., Frazer, A., Schless, A. and Mendels J. (1973) Cholinergic reversal of manic symptoms. *Lancet*, i: 427.

Cohen, B.M., Lipinsky, J.F. and Altesmar, R.F. (1982) Lecithin in the treatment of mania. *Am. J. Psychiat.*, 138: 1162–1164.

Cordeau, J.P., Moreau, A., Beaulnes, A. and Laurin C. (1963) EEG and behavioral changes following microinjections of acetylcholine and adrenaline in the brain stem of cats. *Arch. Ital. Biol.*, 101: 30–47.

Davis, K.L., Berger, P.A., Hollister, L.E. and Defraites E. (1978) Physostigmine in man. *Arch. Gen. Psychiat.*, 136: 1581–1584.

Davis, K.L., Hollister, L.E. and Berger, P.A. (1979) Choline chloride and schizophrenia. *Am. J. Psychiat.*, 136: 1581–1584.

Delashaw, J.B., Foutz, A.S., Guilleminuault, C. and Dement, W.C. (1979) Cholinergic mechanisms and narcolepsy in dogs. *Exp. Neurol.*, 66: 745–757.

Dilsaver, S.C. (1988) Pharmacological perturbation of cholinergic systems. Applications to the study of pathophysiological mechanisms in affective disorders. *Hillside J. Clin. Psychiat.*, 10: 38–54.

Dilsaver, S.C. and Greden, J.F. (1984) Antidepressant withdrawal phenomena. *Biol. Psychiat.*, 19: 237–255.

Domino, E.F. and Stawinski, M. (1970) Effect of cholinergic antisynthesis agent HC-3 on the awake-sleep cycle in the cat. *Psychophysiology*, 7: 315–316.1970.

Domino, E. and Yamamoto, K. (1965) Nicotine: effect on the sleep cycle of the cat. *Science*, 150: 637–638.

Domino, E.F., Yamamoto, K. and Dren, A.T. (1968) Role of cholinergic mechanisms in states of wakefulness and sleep. *Prog. Brain. Res.*, 28: 113–133.

Dube, S., Kumar, N., Ettedgul, E., Pohl, R., Jones, D. and Sitaram, N. (1987) Cholinergic REM induction response. separation of anxiety and depression. *Biol. Psychiat.*, 20: 408–418.

George, R., Haslett, E.L. and Jenden, D.J. (1964) A cholinergic mechanism in the brainstem reticular formation: induction of paradoxical sleep. *Int. J. Neuropharmacol.*, 3: 541–552.

Gershon, S and Shaw, F.H. (1961) Psychiatric sequelae of chronic exposure to organophosphorous insecticides. *Lancet*, i: 1371–1374.

Gillin, J.C., Duncan, W.C., Pettigrew, K., Frankel, B.L. and Synder, F. (1979a) Successful separation of depressed, normal and insomniac subjects by EEG sleep data. *Arch. Gen. Psychiat.*, 36: 85–90.

Gillin, J.C., Sitaram, N. and Duncan, W.C. (1979b) Muscarinic supersensitivity. A possible model for the sleep disturbance of primary depression? *Psychiat. Res.*, 1: 17–22.

Gillin, J.C., Sitaram, N., Wehr, T., Duncan, W., Poot, R.M., Murphy, D.L., Mendelson, W.B., Wyatt, R.J. and Bunney, W.E. Jr. (1984) Sleep and affective illness. In: R.M. Post and J.C. Ballenger (Eds.), *Neurobiology of Mood Disorders.*

Vol. 1. Frontiers of Clinical Neuroscience. Baltimore, Williams and Wilkins, Baltimore, pp. 157–189.

Hazra, J. (1970) Effect of hemicholinum-3 on slow wave and paradoxical sleep of cat. *Eur. J. Pharmacol.*, 11: 395–397.

Hammer, R. and Gianchetti, A. (1982) Muscarinic receptor subtypes: M_1 and M_2 biochemical and functional characterization. *Life Sci.*, 31: 2991–2998.

Hernandez-Peon, R., Chavez-Ibarra, G., Morgane, P.J. and Timo-Iaria, C. (1963) Limbic cholinergic pathways involved in sleep and emotional behavior. *Exp. Neurol.*, 8: 93–111.

Hobson, J.A., McCarley, R.W. and Wyzinski, P.W. (1975) Sleep cycle oscillation: reciprocal discharge by two brainstem neuronal group. *Science*, 189: 55–58.

Hobson, J.A., Goldberg, M., Vivaldi, E. and Riew D. (1983) Enhancement of desynchronized sleep signs after pontine microinjection of the muscarinic agonist bethanechol. *Brain Res.*, 275: 127–136.

Hobson, J.A., Lydic, R. and Baghdoyan, H.A. (1986) Evolving concepts of sleep cycle generation: from brain centers to neuronal population. *Behav. Brain Sci.*, 9: 371–348.

Jacobs, B.L., Henriksen, S.J. and Dement, W.C. (1972) Neurochemical base of the PGO wave. *Brain Res.*, 48: 406–411.

Janowsky, D.S., Davis, J.M., El-Yousef, M.K. and Sekerke, H.J. (1972) A cholinergic-adrenergic hypoothesis of mania and depression. *Lancet* ii: 632.

Janowsky, D.S., El-Yousef, M.K., Davis, J.M. and Sekerke, H.J. (1973) Parasympathetic suppression of manic symptoms of physostigmine. *Arch. Gen. Psychiat.*, 28: 542–547.

Janowsky, D.S., Golden, R.N., Rapaport, M., Cain, J.J. and Gillin, J.C. (1988) Neurochemistry of depression and mania. In: A. Georgotas and R. Cancro (Eds.), *Depression and Mania*, Elsevier, New York, pp. 244–264.

Jewett, R.E. and Norton, S. (1986) Effect of some stimulant and depressant drugs on sleep cycles of cats. *Exp. Neurol.*, 15: 463–474.

Jones, B., Kewala, S., Bell, S., Dube, S., Jackson, E. and Sitaram, N. (1985) Cholinergic REM induction response correlation with endogenous major depressive subtype. *Psychiat. Res.*, 14: 99–110.

Jouvet, M. (1977) Neuropharmacology of the sleep-waking cycle. In: L.L. Iversen and S.H. Snyder (Eds.), *Handbook of Psychopharmacology.*, Plenum Press, New York.

Karczmar, A.G., Longo, V.G. and DeCarolis, A.S. (1970) A pharmacological model of paradoxical sleep: the role of cholinergic and monoamine systems. *Physiol. Behav.*, 5: 175–182.

Kilduff, T., Bowersox, S., Kaitin, K., Baker, T.L., Ciaranerlo, R.D. and Dement W.C. (1986) Muscarinic cholinergic receptors and the canine model of narcolepsy. *Sleep*, 9: 102–106.

Magherini, P., Pompeiano, O. and Thoden, U. (1971) The neurochemical basis of REM sleep: a cholinergic mechanism responsible for rhytmic activation of the vestibulo-oculomotor system. *Brain Res.*, 35: 565–569.

Nurberger, J. Jr., Sitaram, N., Gershon, E.S. and Gillin, J.C. (1983) A twin study of cholinergic REM induction. *Biol. Psychiat.*, 18: 10.

413

Nurberger, J. Jr., Berretini, W., Mendelson, W.B., Sack, D. and Gershon, E.S. (1989) Measuring cholinergic sensitivity. I. Arecoline effects in bipolar patients. *Biol. Psychiat.*, 25: 610–617.

Reynolds, C.F. and Kupfer, D.J. (1987) Sleep research in affective illness: State of the art circa 1987. *Sleep*, 10: 199–215.

Riemann, D., Joy, D., Hochll, D., Lauer, C., Zulley, J. and Berger, M. (1988) The influence of the cholinergic agonist RS 86 on sleep with regard to gender and age. *Psychiat. Res.*, 24: 137–147.

Risch, S.C., Cohen, R.M., Janowsky, D.S., Kalin, N.H., Sitaram, N., Gillin, J.C. and Murphy, D.J. (1981) Physostigmine induction of depressive symptomatology in normal subjects. *Psychiat. Res.*, 4: 89–94.

Risch, S.C., Siever, L.J., Gillin, J.C., et al. (1983) Differential mood effects of arecoline in depressed patients and normal volunteers. *Psychiat. Bull.*, 19: 696–698.

Shiromani, P.J. and Fishbein, W. (1986a) Continuous pontine cholinergic microinfusion via mini-pump induces sustained alterations in rapid eye movement (REM) sleep. *Pharmacol. Biochem. Behav.*, 25: 1253–1261.

Shiromani, P.J. and McGinty, D. (1986a) Pontine neuronal response to local cholinergic infusion: relation to REM sleep. *Brain Res.*, 386: 20–31.

Shiromani, P.J., Gillin, J.C. and Henriksen, S.J. (1987) Acetylcholine and the regulation of REM sleep: basic mechanisms and clinical implications for affective illness and narcolepsy. *Annu. Rev. Pharmacol. Toxicol.*, 27: 137–156.

Shiromani, P.J., Armstrong, D.M., and Gillin, J.C. (1988a) Cholinergic neurons from the dorsolateral pons project to the medial pons: a WGA-HRP and choline acetyltransferase immunohistochemical study. *Neurosci. Lett.*, 95: 19–23.

Shiromani, P.J., Overstreet, D., Levy, D., Goodrich, C.A., Campbell, S.S. and Gillin, J.C. (1988b) Increased REM sleep in rats selectively bred for cholinergic hyperactivity. *Neuropsychopharmacology*, 1: 127–133.

Sitaram, N., Wyatt, R.J., Dawson, S. and Gillin, J.C. (1976) REM sleep induction by physostigmine infusion during sleep. *Science*, 191: 1281–1283.

Sitaram, N., Moore, A.J. and Gillin, J.C. (1979) Scopolamine induced muscarinic supersensitivity in man: changes in sleep. *Psychiat. Res.*, 1: 9–16.

Sitaram, N., Nurberger, J.I., Gershon, E.S. and Gillin, J.C. (1980) Faster cholinergic REM induction in euthymic patients with primary affective illness. *Science*, 208: 200–202.

Sitaram, N., Nurberger, J.I., Gershon, E.S. and Gillin, J.C. (1982) Cholinergic regulation of mood and REM sleep: Potential model and marker of vulnerability to affective disorder. *Am. J. Psychiat.*, 139: 571–576.

Sitaram, N., Dube, S., Keshavan, M., Davies, A. and Reynal, P. (1987) The association of supersensitive cholinergic REM-induction and affective illness within pedigrees. *J. Psychiat Res.*, 21: 487–497.

Spencer, D.G., Horvath, E. and Traber, J. (1986) Direct autoradiographic determination of M_1 and M_2 muscarinic acetylcholine receptor distribution in the rat brain: relation to cholinergic nuclei and projections. *Brain Res.*, 380: 59–68.

Spiegel, R. (1984) Effects of RS 86, an orally active cholinergic agonist on sleep in man. *Psychiat. Res.*, 11: 1–13.

Sutin, E.L., Shiromani, P.J., Kelsoe, J.R., Storch, F.I. and Gillin, J.C. (1986) Rapid eye movement sleep and muscarinic receptor binding in rats are augmented during withdrawal from chronic scopolamine treatment. *Life Sci.*, 39: 2419–2427.

Tamminga, C., Smith, R.C., Change, S., Harasztl, J.S. and Davis, J.M. (1976) Depression associated with oral choline. *Lancet*, ii: 905.

Velazquez-Moctezuma, J., Gillin, J.C. and Shiromani, P.J. (1989) The effect of M_1 and M_2 receptor agonists on REM sleep generation. *Brain Res.*, 503: 128–131.

Velluti, R. and Hernandez-Peon, R. (1963) Atropine blockade within a cholinergic hypnogenic circuit. *Exp. Neurol.*, 8: 20–29.

Wager, S. Robinson, D., Goetz, R., Nunes, E., Gulley, R. and Quitkin, F. (1988) The arecoline-REM induction test in atypical depression – a pilot study. *Sleep Res.*, 17: 133.

S.-M. Aquilonius and P.-G. Gillberg (Eds.)
Progress in Brain Research, Vol. 84
© 1990 Elsevier Science Publishers B.V. (Biomedical Division)

CHAPTER 43

Future prospects of research on central cholinergic mechanisms

Agneta Nordberg [1], Stanley H. Appel [2], C. G. Gottfries [3] and Marsel M. Mesulam [4]

[1] *Department of Pharmacology, University of Uppsala, Uppsala, Sweden,* [2] *Department of Neurology, Baylor College of Medicine, Houston, U.S.A.,* [3] *Department of Psychiatry and Neurochemistry, St Jörgen's Hospital, Hisings Backa, Sweden, and* [4] *Department of Neurology, Beth Israel Hospital, Boston, U.S.A.*

The research frontier concerning central cholinergic mechanisms has moved quickly during the last 20 years. From early studies dealing with measurement of levels of endogenous acetylcholine (ACh), turnover of ACh in brain and the influence of various drugs, the research frontier has moved towards receptor characterizations and linkage of cholinergic mechanisms to second messenger systems. The recent rapid development of molecular biology techniques has revealed a whole family of receptor genes for the muscarinic as well as for the nicotinic receptors in brain. Together with results obtained from receptor binding experiments performed in tissue homogenates and thin tissue slices (autoradiography) valuable information about the existence of multiple binding sites and their distribution in brain has been obtained. Techniques for functional studies such as transmittor release are available both in vitro and in vivo. The in vitro methods have given valuable information concerning the role of the presynaptic muscarinic and nicotinic receptors for regulation of the ACh release. From studying in vivo release of ACh by cortical cups in the past, new techniques (microdialysis) now allow measurement of

ACh release in deeper structures of the brain. During recent years the research on cholinergic mechanisms in brain has become more clinically oriented. Great attention has been paid especially to the involvement of cholinergic mechanisms in the pathophysiology of neurodegenerative diseases such as Alzheimer's disease. For the future, several questions concerning the cholinergic system have to be solved. The aim of this chapter is to focus on some of the crucial questions for future basic and clinical research on central cholinergic mechanisms.

Our knowledge about the cholinergic system in brain is mainly based on animal studies. One important question is to what extent animal data can be extrapolated to man. Another question is whether we can compare data obtained in vitro and in vivo. What is the correlation between receptor binding data and functional studies? It is well known that in functional transmittor studies a much higher concentration of a drug is needed to observe a pharmacological effect than is revealed in ligand binding studies. For the muscarinic receptors five distinct receptor genes (m1, m2, m3, m4, m5) have been isolated but pharmacological tools to characterize the corresponding receptor subtypes are still lacking. The M_1 and M_2 receptors have been well characterized in rodent and human brain and the regional distribution is well known from autoradiographical

Correspondence to: Agneta Nordberg MD, PhD, Department of Pharmacology, Box 591, S-751 24 Uppsala, Sweden.

studies. Whether these receptors are solely or partly presynaptically or postsynaptically located has to be solved. Another important question is whether the muscarinic agonist and antagonist binding sites are equivalent sites or different conformational states of the same receptor or binding sites on quite distinct receptor molecules.

Progress in unraveling the organization of cortical cholinergic innervation has been substantial. However, additional advances need to be made in a number of areas. It would be desirable to understand even more closely the normal neuroanatomy of central cholinergic pathways. Do the cholinergic cells of the basal forebrain communicate with each other, are there collateral projections from one neuron to several cortical regions? Do the more recently described muscarinic receptor subtypes (M_3, M_4, M_5, etc.) display regional variations similar to those described for the M_1 and M_2 subtypes?

Another important issue is the extent of interindividual variations in central cholinergic innervation. It has been known for some time, for example, that maze-bright and maze-dull rats may have different levels of choline acetyltransferase in the brain. How are these differences reflected at the level of neuroanatomical organization? Are there anatomical variations of cholinergic pathways in primates? If such variations exist, do they reflect some aspects of individual cognitive skills?

Species differences need to be taken seriously. The rodent neocortex contains intrinsic choline acetyltransferase-containing neurons. Such neurons may appear in the fetal monkey brain but are apparently absent in adult non-rodent brains. Furthermore, acetylcholinesterase-rich cortical pyramidal neurons in layers III and V are numerous in the adult human brain but rare in the adult monkey brain. These differences are interesting in themselves and also introduce some limitations to the applicability of cross-species models.

During recent years it has become evident that the nicotinic receptors are widely distributed in the brain and play a role for example in the regulation of the release of other transmitters. It has finally been established that the effects of smoking are mediated by activation of central nicotinic receptors. Further studies concerning the functional role of the nicotinic receptors in brain are needed for the understanding of the underlying mechanisms for dependence and tolerance.

Although receptor binding techniques and even functional release studies have been applicable to human post-mortem brain tissue it is still an open question whether the second messenger systems can be explored in human brain. The agonal state of the brain tissue might be an important limiting factor especially for molecular biology studies. It is to be hoped that cell culture techniques and in vivo imaging techniques (positron emission tomography) will provide further valuable information.

A great deal needs to be discovered about the relationship of central cholinergic innervation to human behaviour and disease states. Many observations indicate that cortical cholinergic deficiency may be an important component in Alzheimer's disease. However, it is highly unlikely that this deficiency constitutes the prime mover of the complex neuropathology which characterizes this disease. It is conceivable that there are conditions of truly primary central cholinergic deficiency in the human brain (i.e. the CNS equivalent of myesthenia gravis or of the Eaton-Lambert syndrome). One of the greatest challenges for the future will be to figure out how to recognize such putative cholinergic deficiency states and their impact on mental state.

With the availability of molecular biology approaches, research in Alzheimer's disease is accelerating at a rapid rate. It is clear that both degeneration and regeneration are going on at a tissue level. Although previous hypotheses implicated alterations in nerve growth factors (NGF) as responsible for the lack of compensatory trophic effects, current data suggest that there may be minimal alterations in most growth factors, including NGF, and no direct evidence that they are produced in abnormal amounts associated with abnormal sprouting. Instead, more recent data might suggest that the precursor for the beta amyloid peptide may induce growth and toxic actions. The compensatory release of growth factors, possibly including components of the amyloid precursor protein itself, would encourage neuritic in-growth and increase the availability of more amyloid precursors. The new growth would be more than offset by the enhanced proteolysis resulting in increased amyloid deposition and increased disconnection of networks.

With respect to future prospects, the ideal therapeutic effort would be to interfere with the initiating event. Since the etiology is currently unknown for Alzheimer's disease, we need to direct our attention towards those events in the pathogenesis the interruption of which would prevent deterioration and presumably enhance function. The primary goal at present should be to curtail the overall catabolic state. It will also be important to attempt to enhance regeneration, and thereby return the participating neuron to a net regenerative rather than degenerative mode. Agents which interfere with proteolysis may be of significant benefit. Clearly, neurotrophic factors may also be of a positive value in reversing the net imbalance of degeneration and regeneration. NGF alone is probably not the solution. Interestingly NGF seems to have some connection with the cholinergic system. Other factors also exist currently which may play an important restorative role. Some, such as insulin growth factor, may also have a neuromodulatory role (increase acetylcholine release). The prospects are currently quite exciting for understanding both those processes of enhanced catabolism as well as those of enhanced regeneration. Therapeutic intervention with respect to both facets of the process are likely to yield important new avenues for therapy.

It is well documented that there is a deficiency of the cholinergic system in dementia of Alzheimer type (AD/SDAT). It is, however, also well established that not only the cholinergic system but also other neurotransmitter systems are disturbed in AD/SDAT, such as the monoaminergic systems, the neuropeptides and amino acids. Of

interest is that changes are recorded not only in neurotransmitter systems but also in the metabolism of gangliosides and white matter components. At the present level of knowledge it is not possible to single out one of these changes and give it special importance for AD/SDAT. Either it must be assumed that there is a more fundamental disturbance in the brains of Alzheimer-afflicted patients which can explain the multiple disturbances recorded, or that AD/SDAT is a heterogenous disorder from an etiopathogenetic point of view. Disturbance of the cholinergic system, however, has evidently pathogenetic importance. Behavioural disturbances assumed to be related to disturbances in the cholinergic system are impairment of memory, confusion and neuroendocrine disturbances. Based on these findings pharmacological treatment stategies have been formulated. Efforts to stimulate the cholinergic system on a presynaptic, synaptic and/or postsynaptic level have been made. These trials include investigations with precursors, enzyme inhibitors and to some extent also receptor agonists. In total these pharmacological investigations have been almost negative. An important question to answer is why the cholinergic hypotheses in AD/SDAT cannot be applied in the same way as the dopaminergic one in Parkinson's disease. One reason for the negative effect of therapeutic intervention in AD/SDAT may be that we still do not have an effective drug on the effector site. It is obvious that not only is the synthesis of acetylcholine (ACh) of importance but also the release and receptor interaction. In order to definitely answer the question whether cholinergic drugs are of use in AD/SDAT effective and clinically usable muscarinic and/or nicotinic receptor agonists are needed. One limiting factor might be that the Alzheimer brains can no longer respond to feed back activation or perhaps to pharmacological challenges in the way we expect them to.

One factor that may also be of importance for the absence of positive effect with cholinergic drugs is that the neurotransmitter systems in the brain are to a great extent integrated. It is probably not sufficient to only substitute one system at a time. Combined treatment with, for instance, cholinergic and monoaminergic drugs may be of value.

Another factor of importance when interpreting results of pharmacological drug interventions is that the capacity to diagnose dementia syndromes is still on a primitive level. AD/SDAT is an exclusion diagnosis and in principle all primary degenerative dementias are brought to the group of AD/SDAT, when no other obvious explanation for the dementia can be found. There is a great need for ante mortem biological markers, especially as the post mortem neuropathological markers, senile plaques and fibrillary tangles, are rather unspecific. Brain imaging techniques have advanced much during recent years. It is hoped that this technique will provide the clinicians with a diagnostic tool made ante mortem and based on the localization of the brain disorder. There is a great need for future research in clinical diagnoses of dementia disorders. This research has to go hand in hand with neuropathological and neurochemical research if a treatment progress is to be achieved. At present, promising avenues for studying central cholinergic function in the living individual include the examination of CSF metabolites, Single Photon Emission Computer Tomography (SPECT) and PET studies with suitable markers, quantitation of the P300 response (which may be sensitive to cholinergic transmission) and possibly also dose-response studies while challenging patients with cholinoactive agents during specific cognitive tasks.

SECTION IV

Achievements in Cholinergic Research 1969–1989

S.-M. Aquilonius and P.-G. Gillberg (Eds.)
Progress in Brain Research, Vol. 84
© 1990 Elsevier Science Publishers B.V. (Biomedical Division)

CHAPTER 44

The cell and molecular biology of the cholinergic synapse: twenty years of progress

V.P. Whittaker

Arbeitsgruppe Neurochemie, Max-Planck-Institut für biophysikalische Chemie, Postfach 2841, D-3400 Göttingen, F.R.G.

Introduction

A series of publications summarizing the results of eight conferences on cholinergic mechanisms which took place between 1970 and 1986 (Table I), together with the recent appearance of a 750-page monograph (Whittaker 1988a) on the cholinergic synapse, show how much our knowledge of the cell and molecular biology of this synapse has advanced during the past two decades. Until the early 1960s, our knowledge of cholinergic synaptic transmission was based almost entirely on electrophysiological techniques which led, in the hands of Katz and coworkers (review, 1966), to the discovery of the quantized release of transmitter. With the development of electron microscopy and

TABLE I

Conferences on cholinergic mechanisms, 1970–1989

Date	Location	Conference book
1970	Skokloster, Sweden	Heilbronn and Winter (1970)
1974	Boldern, Switzerland	Waser (1975)
1977	La Jolla, CA, USA	Jenden (1978)
1980	Florence, Italy	Pepeu and Ladinsky (1981)
1983	Oglebay Park, WV, USA	Hanin (1986)
1986	Buxton, UK	Dowdall and Hawthorne (1987)
1989	Lidingö, Sweden	Present volume

In addition, a conference on the cholinergic synapse, not in this series, was held in Žinkovy, ČSSR, in 1978 (Tuček, 1979).

the discovery of synaptic vesicles, there was a clear presumption that the latter provided the morphological basis for such release. The next step, well under way by 1969, was to apply subcellular fractionation techniques to isolate from mammalian brain, first, complete functional nerve terminals (synaptosomes) and then all the other component parts of the terminal, including synaptic vesicles, which were found to contain transmitter in the requisite amount. Further progress was however hampered by the fact that, in mammalian brain, cholinergic terminals are outnumbered 20:1 by non-cholinergic, and tissues with a purely cholinergic innervation have too low a synaptic content. This led to the intensive use of the electromotor innervation of *Torpedo* as a model cholinergic system; the electric organ has 500–1000-times more cholinergic synapses than muscle, and the electric lobes are rich sources of cholinergic cell bodies. The subsequent identification on the electromotor terminals of a cholinergic-specific surface antigen conserved between *Torpedo* and mammals made possible the immunoisolation of purely cholinergic synaptosomes from mammalian brain.

The most important results from work with *Torpedo* have been (a) the complete sequencing of the acetylcholine receptor, (b) the discovery that synaptic vesicles exist in two different stimulus-regulated functional states (reserve and recycling), and (c) the implication, in the mechanism of vesicular transmitter uptake, of a V-type proton-translocating ATPase. The main gap in our present knowledge is an understanding of the molecular mechanism of the stimulus-evoked exocytosis of vesicles with its attendant quantized transmitter release.

Acetylcholine is stored in and released from synaptic vesicles

The recognition of vesicular metabolic heterogeneity resolves a paradox of transmitter release

With the discovery of synaptic vesicles in the mid '50s, there was a clear presumption that these provided the morphological basis for transmitter release and it became apparent that chemical transmission, like so many other functions of nerve cells, utilized, in modified, even hypertrophied form, a general cellular property — in this case secretion by exocytosis of storage vesicles — rather than a totally new mechanism unique to nerve cells. Transmitter release was seen as a miniaturized version of cell secretion, in which the basic cellular mechanism had been modified by the exigencies imposed by the geometry of the neurone, in which the release site in the axon terminal is often far distant from the site of vesicle generation and repair in the perikaryon and in which transmitter release must be maintained at a rate far surpassing that of axonal transport. Direct evidence for the participation of synaptic vesicles in tissue storage and release only came, however, with the application of the then novel techniques of cell biology — subcellular fractionation followed by biochemical and electron microscopical characterization of fractions — and with the isolation from mammalian brain, first, of detached, sealed nerve terminals (synaptosomes) (Gray and Whittaker, 1960, 1962) and then, from these, morphologically pure fractions of synaptic vesicles (Whittaker et al., 1964). The latter were demonstrated to contain transmitter in amounts in satisfactory agreement with the size of a quantum (Whittaker and Sheridan, 1965; Whittaker, 1988b). The story has been told more than once (Whittaker, 1965; Gray and Whittaker, 1984; Whit-

taker, 1988c,d). The results were quickly confirmed in several laboratories, but there followed a period of difficulty when it was observed that the acetylcholine released from terminals in which the acetylcholine stores had been labelled with a radioactive precursor far exceeded in specific radioactivity the main fraction of isolated, mono-disperse synaptic vesicles (Barker et al., 1972; Chakrin et al., 1972) and were closest to that of the cytosolic fraction of transmitter. This paradox was resolved when it was realised that a second fraction of synaptic vesicles associated with and carried down a sucrose density gradient by presynaptic plasma membranes contained acetylcholine of specific radioactivity comparable to that of released transmitter. Such vesicles were identified as a fraction of recycling vesicles which filled with radioactive acetylcholine synthesized in the cytoplasm after previous release of "cold" acetylcholine from vesicles recruited from the reserve pool. Thus the concept of the metabolic heterogeneity of cholinergic vesicles was arrived at. Preferential release of transmitter from recycling vesicles could explain the high specific radioactivity of transmitter release by stimulation without abandoning a vesicular origin for the released transmitter. The work of von Schwarzenfeld (1979) (see also von Schwarzenfeld et al., 1979) confirmed this conclusion and, in addition, ruled out a cytoplasmic origin. She succeeded in labelling the recycling vesicular and cytoplasmic pools in mammalian cerebral cholinergic nerve terminals differentially by making use of "false transmitters" — analogues of acetylcholine which are formed in the cytoplasm from appropriate precursors and, along with acetylcholine, taken up into vesicles and released on stimulation. This is a technique first used successfully in the adrenergic system (reviewed by Smith, 1972). By selecting false transmitter precursors which are good substrates for cytoplasmic choline acetyltransferase but whose acetylated products are poor substrates for the vesicular acetylcholine transporter, marked differences can be induced between the acetylcholine:false transmitter ratio in cytoplasm and that in recycling vesicles. Indeed, some choline analogues can themselves act as false transmitters by gaining access to recycling vesicles without prior acetylation (Luqmani et al., 1980; Welner and Collier, 1984, 1985). To generate a pool of recycling vesicles loaded with false transmitter a "loading stimulus" is required. This is followed by a "release stimulus", and the ratio in which true and false transmitters are released is compared with that in the cytoplasm and recycling vesicles. The result of such experiments is unequivocal: the ratio in which transmitters are released on stimulation always matches that in which they are present in recycling vesicles whatever the ratio may be in the cytosol. This result has been repeated in a number of cholinergic synapses, including the electromotor terminals of *Torpedo* (Luqmani et al., 1980), rat brain synaptosomes (Welner and Collier, 1984) and the superior cervical ganglion (Welner and Collier, 1985).

The concept of vesicle metabolic heterogeneity has been strongly reinforced in work with *Torpedo* electromotor synapses and guinea-pig myenteric plexus. In both preparations, vesicles can be isolated directly from the tissue after perfusion with labelled precursors; reserve and recycling vesicles are found to differ sufficiently in biophysical properties (density and size) to be separable by high-resolution centrifugal density-gradient separation in a continuous sucrose gradient (Zimmermann and Whittaker, 1977; Zimmermann and Denston, 1977b; Agoston et al., 1985) or by particle-exclusion chromatography (Giompres et al., 1981a). The differences in biophysical properties between reserve and recycling vesicles are reversible: during a period of rest after stimulation, the recycling pool, identified by its content of isotopically labelled transmitter, reacquires the biophysical properties of the reserve pool from which it was originally derived (Zimmermann and Denston, 1977a; Agoston et al., 1986). This reversibility has been shown to be a consequence of changes in vesicular water space osmotically induced by variable loading with transmitter and ATP (Giompres et al., 1981b; Giompres and Whittaker,

1984, 1986); partial loading during recycling and the attendant reduced osmotic load leads to osmotic dehydration, a decrease in vesicle diameter and an increase in vesicle density, while complete reloading during a relatively prolonged period of rest is accompanied by rehydration, swelling, a reduction in density and a reincorporation of the recycling population into the reserve population. Reserve electromotor vesicles contain about 250 000 molecules of acetylcholine per vesicle, actively recycling perhaps a tenth of that amount. These concentrations are higher than those estimated for mammalian cholinergic vesicles; this is a consequence of the greater size of the electromotor vesicle (diameter 90 nm versus 50–60 nm for mammalian synaptic vesicles) and the higher osmotic pressure of *Torpedo* body fluids, which permits a higher level of osmotic loading without excessive shrinking or swelling.

In addition to the heterogeneity imposed on the vesicle population by the exigencies of quantal release and stimulus-enhanced recycling, another type of vesicle heterogeneity has recently been recognized in electromotor terminals: the presence in the nerve terminal of a small population of largely empty vesicles newly arrived from the cell body by axonal transport (Kiene and Stadler, 1987; Agoston et al., 1989; see also review by Whittaker, 1986). These vesicles can be isolated from electromotor axons: they have the same diameter but much less (less than one-thousandth) of the acetylcholine (and ATP) content of reserve synaptic vesicles; they are also less dense, perhaps because lighter inorganic ions have taken the place of denser organic ions. Pulse-chase experiments (Stadler and Kiene, 1987) using vesicular proteoglycan covalently labelled with ^{35}S have shown that on entering the terminal, such vesicles fill with acetylcholine and ATP and then join the reserve population. The label ultimately works its way through into the recycling population and eventually disappears, perhaps as a result of the elimination, by retrograde flow, of the membranous component of exhausted recycled vesicles.

Although stimulation greatly increases the proportion of recycling vesicles in the total vesicle population, all three classes of vesicle — reserve, recycling and newly arrived — are also present, to varying extents, in unstimulated, "resting" terminals. This has been particularly clearly shown in recent work (Whittaker, 1990) in which the acetylcholine and vesicle content of each fraction in a density gradient after centrifugal fractionation of a cytoplasmic extract of nerve terminals has been compared. In Fig. 1 the number of molecules of acetylcholine per vesicle (the "molecular acetylcholine content", MAC) has been calculated for each fraction in two experiments, one (a) in which a block of electric tissue was processed immediately after removal from an anaesthetized fish, another (b) in which a block was perfused with [^{3}H]acetate for 1 h before being processed.

It will be seen that the distribution of acetylcholine in the gradient takes the form of a single, smooth, more or less symmetrical peak. By contrast there is considerable variation in the MAC, some of which is due to random counting errors. Nevertheless, the vesicles can be classified into three subpopulations: a main one with a mean MAC of about 250 000, close to that previously determined (Ohsawa et al., 1979) for the peak acetylcholine fractions, and two others flanking it, respectively less dense and more dense than the main population and each with considerably lower mean MACs. The differences between the mean MACs of the flanking and peak populations are significant ($p < 0.01$). The denser fraction corresponds to the recycling fraction of vesicles isolated from stimulated tissue since it acquires radioactive (i.e. newly synthesized) acetylcholine (Fig. 1b) when a radioactive precursor is perfused through the tissue before vesicle isolation. The less dense fraction corresponds to the vesicles isolated from electromotor axons (Kiene and Stadler, 1987; Agoston et al., 1989). That these vesicles, too, are not artifacts of the isolation procedure is shown by their ability to acquire newly synthesized acetylcholine while still in situ in the perfused block.

The proportion of the total number of synaptic vesicles present in the recycling vesicle fraction is

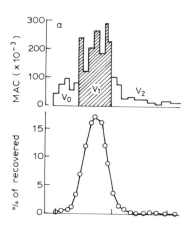

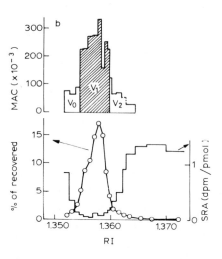

Fig. 1. Distribution in zonal density gradients of vesicular acetylcholine (circles) after extraction of synaptic vesicles from blocks (a) frozen immediately after dissection or (b) after perfusion with radioactive acetate for 1 h. The upper histograms in a and b show the number of acetylcholine molecules per vesicle (molecular acetylcholine content, MAC) of the vesicles in each fraction, the lower one (in b only) the specific radioactivity of each fraction. Vesicle numbers were evaluated from the number of profiles in vesicle pellets (Ohsawa et al., 1979). In spite of some fraction-to-fraction variance, the main population (V_1) of vesicles is seen to have an MAC of about 250 000 (upper histograms, hatched area) and this is flanked by populations of newly arrived (V_0) and recycling (V_2) vesicles with lower MACs. Stimulation greatly increases the $V_2 : V_1$ ratio. That both V_0 and V_2 populations were present in the blocks and are not artifacts of vesicle isolation is shown by their ability (b, lower histogram) to incorporate radioactive acetylcholine generated from [^{3}H]acetate during perfusion (Whittaker, 1990).

quite variable, probably because it is difficult to dissect out electric tissue without adventitiously stimulating it — as anyone who has done the dissection with bare hands can testify — but the mean ($\pm$SEM) of four experiments is $34 \pm 6\%$. The proportion in the "immature" or "newly arrived" vesicles is much smaller and shows less variance — $13 \pm 1\%$.

Cytoplasmic release of acetylcholine

Since the site of synthesis of acetylcholine is the terminal cytoplasm and acetylcholinesterase is an exo-enzyme, a cytoplasmic pool of acetylcholine undoubtedly exists. In electromotor terminals, a non-invasive technique (Weiler et al., 1982) has estimated this as about 20% of the total.

Acetylcholine is continuously leaking out from cholinergic terminals at a low rate in a non-quantized fashion: this is shown by the inability of quantal release in resting terminals (spontaneous miniature end-plate frequency multiplied by any reasonable estimate of the size of the quantum) to account for the amount of bioassayable acetylcholine released and the lack of effect on the latter of changes in ionic composition of the extracellular medium which greatly modify quantal frequency (Mitchell and Silver, 1963; Katz and Miledi, 1977). Cytoplasmic release is also detectable by false transmitters; the composition of the transmitters released at rest corresponds to that of the cytoplasmic compartment (Luqmani et al., 1980). The released acetylcholine is rapidly destroyed in the absence of an anticholinesterase by the acetylcholinesterase in the cleft and the products of hydrolysis — choline and acetate — are salvaged by carrier-mediated uptake into the presynaptic nerve terminal. In electromotor terminals, at least, acetate is a good substrate for acetylcholine synthesis. What is the significance of this apparently futile recycling which costs the terminal metabolic energy? The background release of acetylcholine may have a regulatory effect on the receptor and/or in the kinetics of acetylcholine synthesis and storage. For the experimenter, the futile recycling of the cytoplasmic compartment

enables it to be labelled readily. Since recycling vesicles draw upon cytoplasmic acetylcholine for refilling, high rates of stimulated release would be expected to lower cytoplasmic acetylcholine while leaving vesicular acetylcholine levels more or less unchanged. There is evidence that this happens (Dunant et al., 1972). Although several alternative explanations are possible (Zimmermann and Whittaker, 1974) these authors interpret their results to mean that the evoked (i.e. quantal) release of acetylcholine is also primarily from the cytoplasmic compartment. The balance of evidence is strongly against this. It is possible to perturb the level of cytoplasmic acetylcholine widely, but this has no effect on the size or time course of miniature end-plate potentials (Dunant et al., 1977; van der Kloot, 1978). What type of gated channel or carrier in the presynaptic plasma membrane would be able to deliver batches of acetylcholine comprising some 6000 molecules from the cytoplasmic compartment at a rate independent of cytoplasmic concentration and non-electrogenically, with, moreover, the same specificity for acetylcholine analogues as synaptic vesicles? A functional membrane component with these to some extent contradictory properties would be unprecedented.

The structure and function of cholinergic synaptic vesicles

Pure cholinergic synaptic vesicles from electromotor nerve terminals have about 6 μmol of acetylcholine and 1.2 μmol of ATP per mg of protein. Such vesicles can be readily prepared from cytoplasmic extracts of frozen and crushed electric organ by high-resolution centrifugal density-gradient separation in a zonal (dynamically loaded and unloaded) rotor, either preceded by a step-gradient centrifugation to remove soluble cytoplasmic protein (Tashiro and Stadler, 1978) or followed by particle exclusion chromatography (Ohsawa et al., 1979). The lipid and protein analyses by Ohsawa et al. (1979), the analysis of water spaces by Giompres et al. (1981c), the biophysical studies of Giompres and Whittaker (1986) and the nuclear magnetic resonance measurements of Stadler and

Füldner (1981) and Füldner and Stadler (1982) are all consistent with a model of the vesicle in which a predominantly aqueous core of diameter 82 nm and pH of 5.5 contains free acetylcholine and ATP and is surrounded by a 4-nm-thick semipermeable lipoprotein membrane with a fairly high degree of hydration (~ 30%) and a 2 : 1 lipid : protein ratio.

The pioneer work of Tashiro and Stadler (1978) and Stadler and Tashiro (1979) (reviewed by Whittaker and Stadler, 1980) showed that such vesicles have a relatively simple protein composition which differs from that of presynaptic plasma membrane; components of molecular mass 220, 200, 160, 147, 115, 76, 52, 42, 37, 34 and 25 kDa are the most abundant. Such vesicles also contain a heparan sulphate-type proteoglycan (Stadler and Dowe, 1982; Agoston et al., 1989), synaptophysin (Agoston et al., 1989), synapsin I (Volknandt et al., 1987), Mg^{2+} and Ca^{2+}-activated ATPase (Breer et al., 1977) and carriers for ATP (Stadler and Fenwick, 1983; Lee and Witzemann, 1983) and acetylcholine (Giompres and Luqmani, 1980), all of which appear to be intrinsic membrane proteins (for review see Zimmermann, 1988). However, it is not yet possible to state with certainty how many intrinsic vesicle proteins there are in how many copies per vesicle and what their function is. This is an important task for the next 2–5 years.

It is now accepted that the driving force for acetylcholine and probably also ATP uptake is the acidification of the vesicle core by a proton-translocating ATPase. This generates a pH gradient and a membrane potential. Acetylcholine cations move in exchange for H^+ whereas permeant anions move in to neutralize the pH gradient. The acetylcholine carrier has so far resisted identification; it migrates as a smear in gel electrophoresis (Parsons et al., 1989), suggesting that it may be highly glycosylated.

Recent work (Yamagata and Parsons, 1989) has also shown that there are two ATPases in electromotor synaptic vesicle preparations: a vanadate-sensitive enzyme which accounts for 50–85% of the total ATPase activity of the preparation and a vanadate-insensitive enzyme; both are inhibited by N-ethylmaleimide (NEM). The vanadate-sensitive enzyme consists of several subunits of molecular mass 98–110 kDa and one of molecular mass about 60 kDa. Its properties identify it as a so-called P-type enzyme, similar to the Na^+,K^+-activated ATPase of plasma membranes. The vanadate-insensitive ATPase consists of subunits of molecular mass 72, 54 and 38 kDa; it conforms in properties to the proton-translocating vacuolar or V-type ATPase and closely resembles the corresponding enzyme of chromaffin granules. Since acetylcholine uptake is also vanadate-insensitive and NEM-sensitive, it is thought that this enzyme is the one that provides the energy for acetylcholine uptake.

Sequenced synaptic vesicle proteins

Recently, considerable progress has been made using the recombinant DNA technique in the sequencing of synaptic vesicle proteins. Such proteins are of two types, those whose functions are related to the particular transmitter being stored and those common to all synaptic vesicles and perhaps to storage particles in general. As examples of the former, the vesicular acetylcholine and ATP transporters of cholinergic vesicles already mentioned may be cited. Those of the latter "universal" type may be involved in the interaction of the vesicle with elements of the cytoplasm and the plasma membrane and with such processes as vesicular movement, exocytosis and retrieval. Interestingly, proton-translocating ATPases seem to be widespread in storage organelles; those in vesicles storing organic cations (acetylcholine, catecholamines, amino acids) create a proton-motive gradient which, in conjunction with specific transporters, drives the uptake of the cations in question; those in particles storing propeptides may activate cathepsins which carry out post-translational modification during axonal transport, a good example of evolutionary adaptation.

Two of the vesicle proteins that have recently been cloned and sequenced, synaptophysin or p38

(Jahn et al., 1985; Wiedenmann and Franke, 1985) and synapsin I (Ueda and Greengard, 1977), belong to the "universal" class. Synaptophysin (molecular mass 38 kDa) possesses four hydrophobic regions which are believed to represent transmembrane segments (Johnston et al., 1989). Both the amino- and carboxy-terminal domains are thought to be cytoplasmic; the latter has an unusual structure comprising 10 copies of a tyrosine- and proline-rich repeat which may become phosphorylated on the tyrosine residues. The cytoplasmic and transmembrane regions are highly conserved among mammals (ox, rat, human) but the connecting loops in the lumen of the synaptic vesicle are much less highly conserved. This suggests that synaptophysin may act as a docking protein in exocytosis or be essential to the interaction of the vesicle with elements of the surrounding cytoplasm.

Synapsin I, a protein of molecular mass 80 kDa, is an extrinsic vesicle protein with three protein kinase phosphorylation sites: one of these is both Ca^+-calmodulin- and cAMP-dependent; the other two are Ca^{2+}-calmodulin-dependent only. Synapsin I has recently been sequenced by the cloning method. According to one report (McCaffery and DeGennaro, 1986) the carboxy-terminal "tail" domain is collagen-like and contains the Ca^{2+}-calmodulin-dependent phosphorylation sites; these are flanked by three regions of repeating amino acid sequences which are thought to be vesicle-binding domains and have some homology with the actin-binding proteins profilin and villin. Phosphorylation in this part of the molecule is known to regulate the binding of synapsin I to vesicles. A central region of about 270 amino acid residues may exist as a globular core. The remaining 439 residues define the N-terminal region of the protein and contain the cAMP-dependent phosphorylation site; this domain is collagenase-insensitive. The molecule has some immunoreactive sites in common with the erythrocyte spectrin-binding protein 4.1 (Baines and Bennett, 1985) but is not identical with it. Further work with synapsin I fragments and lipid vesicles of varying composition containing a photoactivatable analogue of phosphatidylcholine (Benfenati et al., 1989a,b) has indicated that synapsin I first interacts electrostatically with acidic phospholipids and then inserts its collagenase-insensitive head domain into the hydrophobic core of the bilayer. The collagen-like tail region interacts strongly with synaptic vesicles or synaptic vesicle proteins reconstituted into a lipid bilayer but not with phospholipids. The central region has F-actin binding and bundling activity (Bähler et al., 1989). Such observations strengthen the notion that synapsin I is involved in coupling vesicles to the cytoskeleton, though the precise way in which this is done and its implications for vesicle mobilization remain uncertain. One possibility is that the role of non-phosphorylated synapsin I is to provide an inhibitory constraint to vesicle mobilization by cross-linking the vesicle to the terminal F-actin meshwork; phosphorylation, by reducing the attachment of synapsin I to the vesicle, would mobilize the latter and make it available for recycling. Inflow of Ca^{2+} might be the trigger.

A third synaptic vesicle protein that has been recently sequenced is VAMP-1, a protein of molecular mass 13 kDa first detected immunochemically in electromotor synaptic vesicles from *T. californica*. It has a hydrophobic, putatively transmembrane region and a cytoplasmic portion which resembles the collagen tail of synapsin I (Trimble et al., 1988).

Modern techniques such as these should enable the structure of synaptic vesicles to be understood rather completely in the coming decade, but success will depend on the production of vesicle preparations in bulk of high purity and homogeneity.

Cholinergic terminals often contain neuropeptides which are differently packaged from acetylcholine

Classical notions of chemical transmission have had to undergo considerable modification in recent years with the discovery, initially by immunocytochemical techniques, that terminals using classical transmitters often also contain neuropeptides. This has sometimes been referred to as a violation of Dale's Law but this is totally unjustified historically (Whittaker, 1984). The peptide vasoactive intestinal polypeptide (VIP) is one of the best-established cholinergic co-transmitters. Here, the immunocytochemical evidence has been supplemented by co-purification with cholinergic synaptosomes separated by immunoadsorption (Agoston et al., 1988a).

Like other neuropeptides, VIP is not stored in synaptic vesicles but in larger, dense-cored vesicles (Lundberg, 1981) which are unable to recycle in the terminal and, at any rate in the myenteric plexus, are preferentially released by an exocytotic mechanism activated through L-type voltage-sensitive calcium channels: these, in contrast to the N-type channels involved in synaptic vesicle exocytosis and acetylcholine release, are preferentially activated by relatively high frequencies (50 Hz) of stimulation; there are thus marked differences in the frequency-dependency of release of the two co-transmitters, acetylcholine release being favoured by low, that of VIP by high frequencies of stimulation (Agoston et al., 1988b; Agoston and Lisziewicz, 1989). Hemicholinium-3, a drug that blocks vesicle recycling by inhibiting the uptake of choline and the resynthesis of acetylcholine, rapidly reduces the stimulus-induced release of acetylcholine from the ileum without affecting VIP release; by contrast, colchicine, a drug which blocks axonal transport, has little effect on acetylcholine release, at least over the time-scale of 1–2 h, but speedily blocks VIP release. This shows that VIP cannot be recycled at the terminal and that its supply is determined by its rate of axonal transport.

The presynaptic plasma membrane also has an important role in synaptic transmission

General functions

The presynaptic plasma membrane (PSPM) has so far been less intensively studied than synaptic vesicles but it has many important general functions. These include: (i) the uptake of energy-yielding metabolites and released transmitters or their precursors; (ii) the mediation of ion fluxes via channels which sustain the invasion of the terminal by axon potentials and permit the ingress of Ca^{2+} needed to activate vesicle exocytosis; (iii) participation in vesicle exocytosis; (iv) the maintenance of the ionic composition of the resting terminal; (v) the detection of trophic factors; (vi) the display, on its external surface, of molecular components important in cell-cell recognition, synaptogenesis, adhesion and synaptic consolidation. The regulation of such components could be important in synaptic plasticity and thus in learning and memory.

Some of these functions are common to all PSPMs but others may well be more or less transmitter-specific.

The following section of the review will cover work done so far on the function of the PSPM in cholinergic synapses.

Uptake of precursors of vesicle constituents

Choline. Acetylcholine released from cholinergic terminals is rapidly hydrolysed by the relatively high concentration of acetylcholinesterase in the synaptic cleft to choline and acetate. Vesicular ATP is similarly hydrolysed to adenosine by an exo-ATPase. Choline is salvaged for acetylcholine resynthesis by a high-affinity ($K_T \sim 2 \mu M$) choline uptake system in the cholinergic PSPM. Electromotor PSPMs are a rich source of a rather stable high-affinity choline transporter. The specificity and characteristics of the *Torpedo* system are indeed now quite well understood; it has been reconstituted in an artificial membrane (Ducis and Whittaker, 1985) and something is now known about its molecular constitution.

Briefly, while not completely specific for choline, the deviations from the choline structure the carrier can tolerate are relatively small (Dowdall, 1977; Whittaker and Luqmani, 1980). It can accommodate one-carbon additions either to the *N*-methyl groups or as an extension of the 2-hydroxyethyl groups but not as a substituent or bridge involving the carbon atom of the latter carrying the OH group. Compounds in which the N-methyls are bridged, either to form a tricyclic ring, or by ethylene to form a pyrrolidine ring, are effective substrates. The former of these, known as choline mustard aziridinium, acts as a site-directed alkylating agent and has been useful in identifying the part of the carrier that contains the choline recognition site. This has a molecular mass of about 42 kDa (Rylett, 1989). The complete system seems to have a molecular mass of 100 kDa, comprising a subunit of molecular mass 58 kDa and the 42 kDa subunit. By contrast, the transporter of cholinergic insect neurones appears to consist of a single molecule of molecular mass 80 kDa; a monoclonal antibody raised to it which blocks choline uptake into insect-derived synaptosomes (Knipper et al., 1989a,b) failed to cross-react with any protein of the *Torpedo* PSPM (V.P. Whittaker, unpublished observations with antibody kindly provided by Dr H. Breer).

Vesiculated fragments of electromotor PSPMs energized by an inwardly directed Na^+ and outwardly directed K^+ gradient, or corresponding artificial lipid vesicles containing membrane proteins derived from PSPMs, have proved useful for determining the ionic requirements of the carrier (Ducis and Whittaker, 1985). There is an absolute dependence for Na^+; Cl^- is required but can be partially replaced by Br^- but not by other anions, and K^+ is partly replaceable by Rb^+, NH_4^+, Cs^+ and Li^+ with decreasing effectiveness in that order.

Acetate. The kinetics of acetate uptake by *Torpedo* electromotor synaptosomes also indicate the existence of a transporter system for this transmitter precursor (O'Regan, 1983); however, its affinity for acetate is not particularly high ($K_T \sim 17 \, \mu M$). Little is known of its specificity or other characteristics beyond the fact that propionate is a poor substrate. The claim (O'Regan, 1983) that incoming propionate is synthesized to propionylcholine has not stood up to critical reinvestigation (Kosh and Whittaker, 1985).

Radiolabelling experiments have shown that in mammalian brain, acetate is poorly utilized as a source of acetyl coenzyme A for acetylcholine synthesis, the preferred source being pyruvate; in electromotor terminals, however, it is quite an effective source (reviewed by Tuček, 1988).

Adenosine. Besides being an essential energy metabolite in the nerve terminal, ATP is a constituent of cholinergic vesicles in electromotor and other cholinergic terminals (Dowdall et al., 1974). Vesicular ATP is recycled in a manner quite comparable to that of vesicular acetylcholine (Zimmermann, 1978). This involves its breakdown by ATPase and 5'-nucleosidase to adenosine. The last-named is transported into electromotor synaptosomes by a saturable, high-affinity ($K_T \sim 2.2 \, \mu M$) uptake system (Zimmermann et al., 1979; Meunier and Morel, 1978). Adenine and 2-deoxyadenosine are poor substrates for this relatively specific transporter.

Participation in vesicle exocytosis

Immunocytochemical and cryosubstitution studies have demonstrated vesicle recycling in cholinergic nerve terminals. Jones et al. (1982a,b), using an antiserum directed against the core proteoglycan of vesicles, demonstrated exteriorization of the antigen during stimulation of electromotor nerve terminals and its reinternalization after a period of rest following stimulation. Valtorta et al. (1988) demonstrated incorporation of synaptophysin into the PSPM in motor terminals immunocytochemically under conditions of vesicle depletion, and its subsequent reinternalization. The cryosubstitution studies of Torri-Tarelli et al. (1985) established a temporal coincidence between synaptic vesicle fusion events and quantal acetylcholine secretion in a cholinergic terminal (motor innervation of frog cutaneous pectoris muscle).

Cholinergic-specific surface groups

In the Göttingen group it was argued that if there were cholinergic-specific surface groups, *Torpedo* electromotor nerve terminals should be rich in them and such groups should show a considerable degree of evolutionary conservation. Antisera to electromotor PSPM were therefore raised and their capacity to recognize cholinergic nerve terminals was tested by determining their ability selectively to induce the complement-mediated lysis of the cholinergic subpopulation of mammalian brain synaptosomes (Jones et al., 1981; Richardson et al., 1982). Such selective lysis was indeed found to occur. The antigens recognized by the antielectromotor PSPM antiserum in mammalian brain are two gangliosides (Ferretti and Borroni, 1986), designated Chol-1 α and β; the α behaves like a tetrasialo- and the β like a trisialo-ganglioside, but both migrate a little more slowly than the main tetra- and triganglioside fractions (GQ and GT1b). Chol-1 β has been tentatively identified as Cer-Glc-Gal(S_1 S_2)-GalN-Ac(S_3)-Gal (Giuliani et al., 1990).

The function of Chol-1 is not known. In the developing mammalian brain it is expressed at about the same time as the classical cholinergic marker choline acetyltransferase, and is not present in growth cones (Derrington and Borroni, 1989). In electric organ it is also expressed concomitantly with choline acetyltransferase and is not present in electromotor growth cones (Fiedler et al., 1986). It may therefore be concerned with synaptic consolidation or perhaps with the expression of cholinergic function, e.g. as a receptor for a cholinotrophic factor (discussed in a later section) which "turns on" cholinergic function.

Axonal transport: the link between cell body and terminal

Axonal transport is a general property of neurones and thus it is unlikely that cholinergic neurones would display transmitter-specific features in this function. There is ample evidence that cholinergic synaptic vesicles and other components of the cholinergic terminal are synthesized in the cell body and conveyed to the terminal at different rates by axonal transport. Choline acetyltransferase moves at the "slow" rate (Davies et al., 1977), synaptic vesicles at the "fast" rate. The latter process is difficult to follow by measurements of acetylcholine movement alone since much of the transmitter in the axon is not vesicle-

bound, but may be followed immunochemically by measuring the accumulation of putative vesicle-specific membrane-bound antigens above a ligature (Jones et al., 1982ab; Dahlström et al., 1985) or radiochemically by labelling a stable vesicle component in vivo (Kiene and Stadler, 1987). It has recently been shown (Agoston et al., 1989) that electromotor axonal synaptic vesicles have a lower Mg^{2+}-ATPase and a much lower acetylcholine and ATP content than terminal vesicles; they are also less dense, which enables them to be separated from the terminal as a subpopulation distinct from the reserve and recycling vesicles. As previously mentioned, they constitute just over 10% of the population in resting terminals. As we have seen, pulse-chase experiments with ^{35}S-labelled vesicular proteoglycan have shown that these light, almost empty newly arrived vesicles fill up with acetylcholine and ATP and soon join the main pool of fully charged vesicles (Kiene and Stadler, 1987). Possibly the newly arrived vesicles' proton-translocating ATPase is switched on when the vesicle reaches the terminal and this causes the denser organic ions ATP and acetylcholine to exchange with lighter inorganic ions, forming a replete, significantly denser terminal vesicle.

As mentioned in a previous section, many cholinergic nerve terminals, including electromotor nerve terminals, store and release VIP as well as acetylcholine. The intracellular dynamics of the storage organelles storing the two neuroactive substances are quite different. Recent comparisons of axonal and terminal storage particles in *Torpedo* have shown that in contrast to synaptic vesicles, the large, dense VIP-containing storage particles are fully preformed with identical densities, Mg^{2+}-ATPase activities and transmitter content in axon and terminal (Agoston et al., 1989).

Trophic factors

An important area of interest in contemporary neurobiology is that of trophic factors (for recent reviews see Whittlemore and Sieger, 1987, and

Barde, 1989). These are substances released by target or supporting cells (glia) which maintain neurones and regulate their function. Such factors may be of great importance in guiding development. Neurones are often overproduced in the early stages of differentiation and many are subsequently eliminated in a process — known as programmed or naturally occurring cell death — which adjusts the size of the neuronal pool to the size of the area to be innervated. If target cells produce trophic factors essential for neuronal survival, only those neurites reaching the target area may get enough trophic factor to survive. A dearth of trophic factors in old age or, prematurely, in certain disease states, might explain "natural" or pathological regressions in the number of healthy neurones of a particular type possessed by an individual. If only certain types of neurone (e.g. cholinergic) were primarily affected, this would point to an involvement of transmitter-specific trophic factors.

As an example of how trophic factors can be detected some experiments of the Göttingen group on embryonic electromotor neurones may be cited (Richardson et al., 1985). In 50-mm-long *Torpedo* embryos electromotor neurones express only a low level of choline acetyltransferase activity and a wave of cell death affects the population of these neurones in the electric lobes at this stage of development. Explants taken at this time have a low choline acetyltransferase and do not survive 7 days in unsupplemented culture medium. If, however, the medium is supplemented with extracts of electric organ (the target tissue) from 80-mm embryos or longer, cells survive 7 days or more and express choline acetyltransferase. That at least two trophic factors are involved, one of which is concerned with cell survival and another with the expression of choline acetyltransferase activity, is shown by the observation that heat treatment of extracts greatly reduces the ability of the cells to express the enzyme without affecting their survival. Experiments with extracts from embryos of different ages show that the two trophic factors begin to be expressed at about 60 mm embryo length, just at a time when the wave of naturally occurring cell death in the electric lobes is coming to an end and their choline acetyltransferase activity rapidly rises. Presumably the release of the trophic factors by the target tissue stabilizes the surviving lobe population and brings about the rapid rise in choline acetyltransferase seen in the lobe cells after 60 mm.

Several factors are known which promote the survival and growth of cholinergic neurones or which induce or enhance the expression of the cholinergic phenotype (for review see Richardson, 1988). Some of these have been purified and their molecular masses (also in some cases isoelectric points and sedimentation coefficients) have been

TABLE II

Cholinergic factors

Factor	Molecular mass (kDa)	Source	Effect on target	References
Ciliary neuronotrophic factor	20	Eye of 15-day-old chick embryo; chick and ox heart	Promotes survival and growth of ciliary ganglion cells	Barbin et al. (1984)
Cholinergic specifying factor	21	Rat heart; C6 glioma cells	Induces or enhances expression of cholinergic phenotype in sympathetic ganglia and spinal cord	Weber (1981), Fukada (1985)
Nerve growth factor	26	Male mouse submaxillary glands	Increases choline acetyltransferase in some central cholinergic neurones	Gnahn et al. (1983)

determined (Table II). In the periphery, two factors have been fairly well characterized, a trophic factor necessary for the development of embryonic cholinergic chick ciliary ganglion cells and a "cholinergic specifying factor" which induces the expression of cholinergic features in embryonic sympathetic ganglia and enhances the choline acetyltransferase activity of spinal cord explants. Interestingly, extracts of late-stage (66 mm onwards) embryonic electric organ were active in the chick ciliary ganglion system with about 2.5% of the activity per unit weight of the embryonic chick eye (Richardson et al., 1985).

The best-characterized of the trophic factors active on cholinergic neurones is nerve growth factor (NGF), albeit only on a limited class of such neurones. NGF is present in high concentration in male mouse submaxillary glands; extracts of these glands were found to stimulate neurite outgrowth in explants of embryonic mouse sympathetic ganglia (for a historical review see Levi-Montalcini, 1987). Antibodies to NGF injected into neonatal mice immunochemically sympathectomize them; this demonstrates that NGF is needed for normal development. Recent evidence indicates that NGF is taken up by neurones dependent on it and after retrograde axonal transport to the cell body regulates gene expression in the nucleus (reviewed by Barde, 1989). A similar mechanism may apply to other trophic factors.

NGF is without action on central adrenergic neurones but does act on cholinergic neurones of the basal forebrain that project to the hippocampus and cortex (Schwab et al., 1979). This has been shown by the ability of such neurones to take up ^{125}I-NGF by retrograde transport — as do adrenergic neurones of sympathetic ganglia — and by the rise in choline acetyltransferase which occurs in the hippocampus, cortex and septum following injection of NGF (Gnahn et al., 1983). NGF is also able to "rescue" axotomized cholinergic septal neurones after they have undergone retrograde degeneration (Hefti, 1986). Such observations hold out the promise of eventually being able to stimulate the regeneration of central nervous system neurones injured by trauma or disease.

The cholinoceptive cell

The two main types of acetylcholine receptor

No account of the progress made over the last twenty years in our understanding of the cell and molecular biology of the cholinergic synapse would be complete without mentioning the cholinoceptive target cells of cholinergic neurones and the way in which acetylcholine interacts with them. Pharmacologists discovered early in the history of chemical transmission that the responses that the natural transmitter evoked in its target cell could be mimicked by chemical analogues of the transmitter. In the case of acetylcholine, the structural requirements for such analogues were quite different from those of substrates for acetyl- or butyrylcholinesterase, proteins recognizing acetylcholine and present in high concentration at the cholinergic synapse. Thus, to give a rather striking example, the carbon analogue of acetylcholine, 3,3-dimethylbutylacetate, is an effective substrate for acetylcholinesterase (it is hydrolysed at about 30% of the rate of acetylcholine) but it is an extremely poor cholinergic agonist, having less than 0.01% of the potency of acetylcholine, less than that of choline (Banister and Whittaker, 1951). Such observations led to the concept of pharmacological receptors. They were assumed to be proteins, like enzymes, but with their own unique specificity and embedded in the membrane, able to mediate ion fluxes or second messenger activity in response to activation by the agonist. In the case of the acetylcholine receptor two main classes of receptor could be defined pharmacologically, the muscarinic and nicotinic receptors, and this classification still retains its usefulness today. In spite of some pioneer attempts, receptors eluded identification and molecular characterization, and remained for many years purely theoretical concepts.

The nicotinic acetylcholine receptor

The discovery of a rich source — the electric organ of *Torpedo* — of the nicotinic acetylcholine receptor and of powerful ligands for it in the form of certain snake venoms, especially those of the banded krait (*Bungarus multicinctus*) and the cobra (*Naja naja*) (Lee, 1972), provided the prerequisites for progress. The relevant toxins were conjugated to columns of Sepharose and used to pick out proteins of cholinergic postsynaptic membranes prepared by subcellular factionation of electric tissue. *Naja naja* toxin proved to be the most satisfactory since its affinity for the receptor is high enough to be effective but not so high as to prevent the elution of the receptor-protein complex from the column (Karlsson et al., 1972). All the techniques — subcellular fractionation, improved methods of solubilizing membrane proteins and the use of affinity chromatography — were comparatively new at the time and came together to contribute to a spectacular advance in biochemical pharmacology: the isolation, for the first time, of a transmitter receptor.

The *Torpedo* electric organ nicotinic acetylcholine receptor (nAChR) is now known to consist of 4 similar peptides (α, β, γ and δ, of molecular masses 40, 50, 60 and 65) which form a pentameric molecule in which the α peptide is represented twice. All four peptides have been sequenced (Noda et al., 1983); they each have four hydrophobic domains and thus are thought to cross the membrane four times (for a dissenting view see Maelicke, 1988) and the funnel-shaped hole at the centre of the cluster of 20 transmembrane domains forms the channel of the ionophore (Brisson and Unwin, 1985, and references therein). Attachment of two molecules of acetylcholine to the two α subunits causes an allosteric modification (not yet fully understood) which opens the ion channel, thus permitting the rapid exchange of Na^+ and K^+ which gives rise to the electrical signal known as the postsynaptic potential.

The muscarinic acetylcholine receptor

The primary structure of the second type of acetylcholine receptor, the muscarinic (mAChR), has been elucidated by Kubo et al. (1986). It is composed of a single 70 kDa, 460-amino acid peptide. The sequence suggests that the N-terminal portion of the molecule faces the extracellular space and is followed by seven hydrophobic domains which may represent transmembrane regions. If the molecule traverses the membrane seven times this would put the C-terminal region on the cytoplasmic side of the membrane. This transmembrane organization strongly resembles those proposed for the β-adrenergic receptor and rhodopsin.

The purified receptor retains the binding sites for ligands and the guanine nucleotide binding protein (known as G_i or N_i), the first in a chain of membrane proteins which are responsible for catalysing the metabolic effects induced by muscarinic agonists — a fall in cAMP, a rise in cGMP and an increased phosphatidyl inositol turnover which in turn mobilizes Ca^{2+}. Both cAMP and Ca^{2+} have regulatory roles through their ability to control protein phosphorylation and are thus known as "second messengers", in contrast to the transmitter itself (the "first messenger"). The muscarinic action of acetylcholine has thus been described as a metabo(lo)tropic action, in contrast to its nicotinic action, described as ionotropic (see Eccles and McGeer, 1979, and comment on etymology by Whittaker, 1979).

Molecular biological investigations have shown that there are regional variations in mAChRs undetectable by currently available agonists and antagonists. If these variations could be exploited, drugs could be much more effectively directed than at present.

Experimental autoimmune myasthenia gravis

Work on the nAChR had an initially unexpected byproduct of considerable medical significance. When the purified receptor was injected into rabbits, a hind-limb paralysis developed (Patrick and Lindstrom, 1973; Heilbronn and Mattsson, 1974). Electrophysiological analysis of the affected animals showed a strong resemblance of the condition to the human disease myasthenia gravis. This led to the concept that the latter begins with an inflammation of the postsynaptic muscle membrane which causes it to shed receptor molecules. These, being highly antigenic, induce the formation of antibodies which combine with membrane-bound receptor to block muscular transmission, thus generating the myasthenia (muscle weakness). Other mechanisms can also be envisaged, e.g. induction of a complement-mediated lysis of cholinoceptive postsynaptic membranes (Toyka, 1988). This autoimmune theory of myasthenia gravis is not without difficulties owing to the frequent occurrence of "atypical" cases; even in patients with demonstrable circulating anti-nAChR antibodies it is often difficult to establish a correlation, especially between patients, between the anti-nAChR titre and the severity of the disease. Nevertheless, the interaction between basic research on the receptor and the application of the knowledge so gained to a human disease provides us with an example which one hopes will in future extend to many other areas of progress in cholinergic neurobiology in the course of the *next* two decades.

References

Agoston, D.V. and Lisziewicz, J. (1989) Calcium uptake and protein phosphorylation in myenteric neurones, like the release of vasoactive intestinal polypeptide and acetylcholine, are frequency-dependent. *J. Neurochem.*, 52: 1637–1640.

Agoston, D.V., Kosh, J.W., Lisziewicz, J. and Whittaker, V.P. (1985) Separation of recycling and reserve synaptic vesicles from cholinergic nerve terminals of the myenteric plexus of guinea pig ileum. *J. Neurochem.*, 44: 299–305.

Agoston, D.V., Dowe, G.H.C., Fiedler, W., Giompres, P.E., Roed, I.S., Walker, J.H., Whittaker, V.P. and Yamaguchi, T. (1986) A kinetic study of stimulus-induced vesicle recycling in electromotor nerve terminals using labile and stable vesicle markers. *J. Neurochem.*, 47: 1584–1592.

Agoston, D.V., Borroni, E. and Richardson, P.J. (1988a) Cholinergic surface antigen Chol-1 is present in a subclass of VIP-containing rat cortical synaptosomes. *J. Neurochem.*, 50: 1659–1662.

Agoston, D.V., Conlon, J.M. and Whittaker, V.P. (1988b) Selective depletion of the acetylcholine and vasoactive intestinal polypeptide of the guinea-pig myenteric plexus by differential mobilization of distinct transmitter pools. *Exp. Brain Res.*, 72: 535–542.

Agoston, D.V., Dowe, G.H.C. and Whittaker, V.P. (1989) Isolation and characterization of secretory granules storing a vasoactive intestinal polypeptide-like peptide in *Torpedo* cholinergic electromotor neurones. *J. Neurochem.*, 52: 1729–1740.

Bähler, M., Benfenati, F., Valtorta, F., Czernik, A.J. and Greengard, P. (1989) Characterization of synapsin I fragments produced by cysteine-specific cleavage: a study of their interactions with F-actin. *J. Cell Biol.*, 108: 1841–1849.

Baines, A.J. and Bennett, V. (1985) Synapsin I is a spectrin-binding protein immunologically related to erythrocyte protein 4.1. *Nature (Lond.)*, 315: 410–413.

Banister, J. and Whittaker, V.P. (1951) Pharmacological activity of the carbon analogue of acetylcholine. *Nature (Lond.)*, 167: 605.

Barbin, G., Manthorpe, M. and Varon, S. (1984) Purification of the chick eye ciliary neuronotrophic factor. *J. Neurochem.*, 43: 1468–1478.

Barde, Y.-A. (1989) Trophic factors and neuronal survival. *Neuron*, 2: 1525–1534.

Barker, L.A., Dowdall, M.J. and Whittaker, V.P. (1972) Choline metabolism in the cerebral cortex of guinea pig. *Biochem. J.*, 130: 1063–1075.

Benfenati, F., Greengard, P., Brunner, J. and Bähler, M. (1989a) Electrostatic and hydrophobic interactions of synapsin I and synapsin I fragments with phospholipid bilayers. *J. Cell Biol.*, 108: 1851–1862.

Benfenati, F., Bähler, M., Jahr, R. and Greengard, P. (1989b) Interaction of synapsin I with small synaptic vesicles: distinct sites in synapsin I bind to vesicle phospholipids and vesicle proteins. *J. Cell Biol.*, 108: 1863–1872.

Breer, H., Morris, S.J. and Whittaker, V.P. (1977) Adenosine triphosphatase activity associated with purified cholinergic synaptic vesicles of *Torpedo marmorata*. *Eur. J. Biochem.*, 80: 313–318.

Brisson, A. and Unwin, P.N.T. (1985) Quaternary structure of the acetylcholine receptor. *Nature (Lond.)*, 315: 474–477.

Chakrin, L.W., Marchbanks, R.M., Mitchell, J.F. and Whittaker, V.P. (1972) The origin of the acetylcholine released from the surface of the cortex. *J. Neurochem.*, 19: 2727–2736.

Dahlström, A., Larsson, P.-A., Carlson, S.S. and Bööj, S. (1985) Localization and axonal transport of immunoreactive cholinergic organelles in rat motor neurons — an immunofluorescent study. *Neuroscience*, 14: 607–625.

Davies, L.P., Whittaker, V.P. and Zimmermann, H. (1977) Axonal transport in the electromotor nerves of *Torpedo marmorata*. *Exp. Brain Res.*, 30: 493–510.

Derrington, E. and Borroni, E. (1990) The developmental expression of the cholinergic-specific gangliosidic antigen Chol-1 in the central and peripheral nervous system of the rat. *Dev. Brain Res.*, 52: 131–140.

Dowdall, M.J. (1977) The biochemistry of *Torpedo*, cholinergic neurons. In: Osborne, N.N. (Ed.), *Biochemistry of Characterised Neurons*, Pergamon Press, Oxford and New York, pp. 177–216.

Dowdall, M.J. and Hawthorne, J.N. (Eds.) (1987) *Cellular and Molecular Basis of Cholinergic Function.* Ellis Horwood, Chichester, xviii + 941 pp.

Dowdall, M.J., Boyne, A.F. and Whittaker, V.P. (1974) Adenosine triphosphate, a constituent of cholinergic synaptic vesicles. *Biochem. J.,* 140: 1–12.

Ducis, I. and Whittaker, V.P. (1985) High-affinity sodium-gradient-dependent transport of choline into vesiculated presynaptic plasma membrane fragments from the electric organ of *Torpedo marmorata* and reconstitution of the solubilized transporter into liposomes. *Biochim. Biophys. Acta,* 815: 109–127.

Dunant, Y., Gautron, J., Israël, M., Lesbats, B. and Manaranche, R. (1972) Les compartiments d'acétylcholine de l'organe électrique de la torpille et leurs modifications par la stimulation. *J. Neurochem.,* 19: 1989–2002.

Dunant, Y., Israël, M., Lesbats, B. and Manaranche, R. (1977) Oscillation of acetylcholine during nerve activity in the *Torpedo* electric organ. *Brain Res.,* 125: 123–140.

Eccles, J.C. and McGeer, P.L. (1979) Ionotropic and metabotropic neurotransmission. *Trends Neurosci.,* 2: 39–40.

Ferretti, P. and Borroni, E. (1986) Putative cholinergic-specific gangliosides in guinea pig forebrain. *J. Neurochem.,* 46: 1888–1894.

Fiedler, W., Borroni, E. and Ferretti, P. (1986) An immunohistochemical study of synaptogenesis in the electric organ of *Torpedo marmorata* by use of antisera to vesicular and presynaptic plasma membrane components. *Cell Tiss. Res.,* 246: 439–446.

Fukada, K. (1985) Purification and partial characterization of a cholinergic neuronal differentiation factor. *Proc. Natl. Acad. Sci. USA,* 82: 8795–8799.

Füldner, H.H. and Stadler, H. (1982) ^{31}P-NMR analysis of synaptic vesicles: status of ATP and internal pH. *Eur. J. Biochem.,* 121: 519–524.

Giompres, P.E. and Luqmani, Y.A. (1980) Cholinergic synaptic vesicles isolated from *Torpedo marmorata*: demonstration of acetylcholine and choline uptake in an in vitro system. *Neuroscience,* 5: 1041–1052.

Giompres, P.E. and Whittaker, V.P. (1984) Differences in the osmotic fragility of recycling and reserve synaptic vesicles from the cholinergic electromotor nerve terminals of *Torpedo* and their possible significance for vesicle recycling. *Biochim. Biophys. Acta,* 770: 166–170.

Giompres, P.E. and Whittaker, V.P. (1986) The density and free water of cholinergic synaptic vesicles as a function of osmotic pressure. *Biochim. Biophys. Acta,* 882: 398–409.

Giompres, P.E., Zimmermann, H. and Whittaker, V.P. (1981a) Purification of small dense vesicles from stimulated *Torpedo* electric tissue by glass bead column chromatography. *Neuroscience,* 6: 765–774.

Giompres, P.E., Zimmermann, H. and Whittaker, V.P. (1981b) Changes in the biochemical and biophysical parameters of cholinergic synaptic vesicles on transmitter release and during a subsequent period of rest. *Neuroscience,* 6: 775–785.

Giompres, P.E., Morris, S.J. and Whittaker, V.P. (1981c) The water spaces in cholinergic synaptic vesicles from *Torpedo*

measured by changes in density induced by permeating substances. *Neuroscience,* 6: 757–763.

Giuliani, A., Calappi, E., Borroni, E., Whittaker, V.P., Sonnino, S. and Tettamanti, G. (1990) Purification and partial characterization of a ganglioside recognized by a cholinergic-specific antigen. *Arch. Biochem. Biophys.* (in press).

Gnahn, H., Hefti, F., Heumann, R., Schwab, M.E. and Thoenen, H. (1983) NGF-mediated increase of choline acetyltransferase (ChAT) in the neonatal rat forebrain: evidence for a physiological role of NGF in the brain? *Dev. Brain Res.,* 9, 45–52.

Gray, E.G. and Whittaker, V.P. (1960) The isolation of synaptic vesicles from the central nervous system. *J. Physiol.,* 153, 35–37P.

Gray, E.G. and Whittaker, V.P. (1962) The isolation of nerve endings from brain: an electron-microscopic study of cell fragments derived by homogenization and centrifugation. *J. Anat.,* 96, 79–88.

Gray, E.G. and Whittaker, V.P. (1981) This week's citation classic. *Current Contents,* 24, 16.

Hanin, I. (Ed.) (1986) *Dynamics of Cholinergic Function.* Plenum Press, New York, xvii + 1273 pp [*Advances in Behavioral Biology Vol. 30*].

Hefti, F. (1986) Nerve growth factor (NGF) promotes survival of septal cholinergic neurons after fimbrial transection. *J. Neurosci.,* 6, 2155–2162.

Heilbronn, E. and Mattsson, C. (1974) The nicotinic cholinergic receptor protein: improved purification method, preliminary aminoacid composition, and observed autoimmune response. *J. Neurochem.,* 22, 315–317.

Heilbronn, E. and Winter, A. (Eds) (1970) *Drugs and Cholinergic Mechanisms in the CNS.* Försvarets Forskningsanstalt, Stockholm, xxiv + 577 pp.

Jahn, R., Schiebler, W., Ouimet, C. and Greengard, P. (1985) A 38,000-dalton membrane protein (p38) present in synaptic vesicles. *Proc. Natl. Acad. Sci. USA,* 82, 4137–4141.

Jenden, D.J. (Ed.) (1978) *Cholinergic Mechanisms and Psychopharmacology.* Plenum Press, New York, xiv + 885 pp. [*Advances in Behavioral Biology Vol. 24*]

Johnston, P.A., Jahn, R. and Südhof, T.C. (1989) Transmembrane topography and evolutionary conservation of synaptophysin. *J. Biol. Chem.,* 264, 1268–1272.

Jones, R.T., Walker, J.H., Richardson, P.J., Fox, G.Q. and Whittaker, V.P. (1981) Immunohistochemical localization of cholinergic nerve terminals. *Cell Tiss. Res.,* 218, 355–373.

Jones, R.T., Walker, J.H., Stadler, H. and Whittaker, V.P. (1982a) Immunohistochemical localization of a synaptic vesicle antigen in a cholinergic neuron under conditions of stimulation and rest. *Cell Tiss. Res.,* 223, 117–126.

Jones, R.T., Walker, J.H., Stadler, H. and Whittaker, V.P. (1982b) Further evidence that glycosaminoglycan specific to cholinergic synaptic vesicles recycles during electrical stimulation of the electric organ of *Torpedo marmarata.* *Cell Tiss. Res.,* 224, 685–688.

Karlsson, E., Heilbronn, E. and Widlund, L. (1972) Isolation of the nicotinic acetylcholine receptor by biospecific chromatography and insolubilized *Naja naja* neurotoxin. *FEBS Lett.,* 28, 107–111.

434

Katz, B. (1966) *Nerve, Muscle and Synapse*. McGraw Hill, New York

Katz, B. and Miledi, R. (1977) Transmitter leakage from motor nerve endings. *Proc. R. Soc. Lond.,* B196, 59–72.

Kiene, M.-L. and Stadler, H. (1987) Synaptic vesicles in electromotoneurones. I. Axonal transport, site of transmitter uptake and processing of a core proteoglycan during maturation. *EMBO J.,* 6, 2209–2215.

Knipper, M., Krieger, J. and Breer, H. (1989a) Hemicholinium-3 binding sites in the nervous tissue of insects. *Neurochem. Int.,* 14, 211–215.

Knipper, M., Strotmann, J., Mädler, U., Kahle, C. and Breer, H. (1989b) Monoclonal antibodies against the high affinity choline transport system. *Neurochem. Int.,* 14, 217–222.

Kosh, J.W. and Whittaker, V.P. (1985) Is propionylcholine present in or synthesized by electric organ? *J. Neurochem.,* 45, 1148–1153.

Kubo, T., Fukada, K., Mikami, A., Maeda, A., Takahashi, M., Mishina, M., Haga, T., Haga, K., Ichiyama, A., Kangawa, K., Kojimo, M., Matsuo, H., Hirose, T. and Numa, S. (1986) Cloning, sequencing and expression of complementary DNA encoding the muscarinic acetylcholine receptor. *Nature (Lond.),* 323, 411–416.

Lee, C.Y. (1972) Chemistry and pharmacology of polypeptide toxins in snake venoms. *Annu. Rev. Pharmacol.,* 12, 265–286.

Lee, D.A. and Witzemann, V. (1983) Photoaffinity labeling of a synaptic vesicle specific nucleotide transport system from *Torpedo marmorata. Biochemistry,* 22, 6123–6130.

Levi-Montalcini, R. (1987) The nerve growth factor: thirty-five years later. *EMBO J.,* 6, 534–569.

Lundberg, J.M. (1981) Evidence for coexistence of vasoactive intestinal polypeptide and acetylcholine in neurons of cat exocrine glands: Morphological, biochemical and functional studies. *Acta Physiol. Scand. Suppl.,* 496, 1–57.

Luqmani, Y.A., Sudlow, G. and Whittaker, V.P. (1980) Homocholine and acetylcholine: false transmitters in the cholinergic electromotor system of *Torpedo. Neuroscience,* 5, 153–160.

Maelicke, A. (1988) Structure and function of the nicotinic acetylcholine receptor. *Handb. Exp. Pharmacol.,* 86, 267–313.

McCaffery, C.A. and DeGennaro, L.J. (1986) Determination and analysis of the primary structure of the nerve terminal specific phosphoprotein, synapsin I. *EMBO J.,* 5, 3167–3173.

Meunier, F. and Morel, N. (1978) Adenosine uptake by cholinergic synaptosomes from *Torpedo* electric organ. *J. Neurochem.,* 31, 845–851.

Mitchell, J.F. and Silver, A. (1963) The sponteneous release of acetylcholine from the denervated hemidiaphragm of the rat. *J. Physiol. (Lond.),* 165, 117–129.

Noda, M., Takahashi, H., Tanabe, T., Toyosato, M., Kikyotani, S., Furutani, Y., Hirose, T., Takashima, H., Inayama, S., Miyata, T. and Numa S. (1983) Structural homology of *Torpedo californica* acetylcholine receptor subunits. *Nature (Lond.),* 302, 528–532.

Ohsawa, K., Dowe, G.H.C., Morris, S.J. and Whittaker, V.P.

(1979) The lipid and protein content of cholinergic synaptic vesicles from the electric organ of *Torpedo marmorata*, purified to constant composition: implications for vesicle structure. *Brain Res.,* 161, 447–457.

O'Regan, S. (1983) The uptake of acetate and propionate by isolated nerve endings from the electric organ of *Torpedo marmorata* and their incorporation into choline esters. *J. Neurochem.,* 41, 1596–1601.

Parsons, S.M., Yamagata, S.K., Rogers, G.A., Noremberg, K. and Bahr, B.A. (1989) Newly identified proteins of the cholinergic synaptic vesicle. *Abstr. Conf. Cell Biol. of the Presynapse,* Estoril, April 1989 (unpaginated).

Patrick, J. and Lindstrom, J.M. (1973) Autoimmune response to acetylcholine receptor. *Science,* 180, 871–872.

Pepeu, G. and Ladinsky H. (Eds) (1981) *Cholinergic Mechanisms: Phylogenetic Aspects, Central and Peripheral Synapses, and Clinical Significance.* Plenum Press, New York, xx + 989 pp. [*Advances in Behavioral Biology Vol. 25*]

Richardson, G.P. (1988) Development of the cholinergic synapse: role of trophic factors. *Handb. Exp. Pharmacol.,* 86, 81–100.

Richardson, G.P., Rinschen, B. and Fox, G.Q. (1985) *Torpedo* electromotor system development: developmentally regulated neuronotrophic activities of electric organ tissue. *J. Comp. Neurol.,* 231, 339–352.

Richardson, P.J., Walker, J.H., Jones, R.T. and Whittaker, V.P. (1982) Identification of a cholinergic-specific antigen Chol-1 as a ganglioside. *J. Neurochem.,* 38, 1605–1614.

Rylett, R.J. (1989) Affinity labelling and identification of the high-affinity choline carrier from synaptic membranes of *Torpedo* electromotor nerve terminals with [³H]choline mustard. *J. Neurochem.,* 51, 1942–1945.

Schwab, M.E., Olten, U., Agid, Y. and Thoenen, H. (1979) Nerve growth factor (NGF) in the rat CNS: absence of specific retrograde axonal transport and tyrosine hydroxylase induction in locus coeruleus and substantia nigra. *Brain Res.,* 168, 473–483.

Schwarzenfeld, I. von (1979) Origin of transmitters released by electrical stimulation from a small, metabolically very active vesicular pool of cholinergic synapses in guinea-pig cerebral cortex. *Neuroscience,* 4, 477–493.

Schwarzenfeld, I. von, Sudlow, G. and Whittaker, V.P. (1979) Vesicular storage and release of cholinergic false transmitters. *Prog. Brain Res.,* 49, 163–174.

Smith, A.D. (1972) Cellular control of the uptake, storage and release of noradrenaline in sympathetic nerves. *Biochem. Soc. Symp.,* 36, 103–131.

Stadler, H. and Dowe, G.H.C. (1982) Identification of a heparan sulphate-containing proteoglycan as a specific core component of cholinergic synaptic vesicles from *Torpedo marmorata. EMBO J.,* 1, 1381–1384.

Stadler, H. and Fenwick, E.M. (1983) Cholinergic synaptic vesicles from *Torpedo marmorata* contain an atractyloside binding protein related to the mitochondrial ADP/ATP carrier. *Eur. J. Biochem.,* 136, 377–382.

Stadler, H. and Füldner, H.H. (1981) ³¹P-NMR analysis of ATP in synaptic vesicles and its relationship to in vivo conditions. *Biomed. Res.,* 2, 673–676.

Stadler, H. and Tashiro, T. (1979) Isolation of synaptosomal plasma membranes from cholinergic nerve terminals and a comparison of their proteins with those of synaptic vesicles. *Eur. J. Biochem.*, 101, 171–178.

Tashiro, T. and Stadler, H. (1978) Chemical composition of cholinergic synaptic vesicles from *Torpedo marmorata* based on improved purification. *Eur. J. Biochem.*, 90, 479–487.

Torri-Tarelli, F., Grohovaz, F., Fesce, R. and Ceccarelli, B. (1985) Temporal coincidence between synaptic vesicle fusion and quantal secretion of acetylcholine. *J. Cell Biol.*, 101, 1386–1399.

Toyka, K.V. (1988) Disorders of cholinergic synapses in the peripheral nervous system. *Handb. Exp. Pharmacol.*, 86, 697–724.

Trimble, W.S., Cowan, D.M. and Scheller, R.H. (1988) VAMP-1: a synaptic vesicle-associated integral membrane protein. *Proc. Natl. Acad. Sci. USA*, 85, 4538–4542.

Tuček, S. (Ed.) (1979) *The Cholinergic Synapse*. Elsevier, Amsterdam, xx + 511 pp [*Progress in Brain Research, Vol. 49*].

Tuček, S. (1988) Choline acetyltransferase and the synthesis of acetylcholine. *Handb. Exp. Pharmacol.*, 86, 125–165.

Ueda, T. and Greengard, P. (1977) Adenosine 3′:5′-monophosphate-regulated phosphoprotein system of neuronal membranes. *J. Biol. Chem.*, 252, 5155–5163.

Valtorta, R., Jahn, R., Fesce, R., Greengard, P. and Ceccarelli, B. (1988) Synaptophysin (p38) at the frog neuromuscular junction: its incorporation into the plasma membrane and recycling after intense quantal secretion. *J. Cell Biol.*, 107, 2719–2730.

Van der Kloot, W. (1978) Quantal size is not altered by abrupt changes in nerve terminal volume. *Nature (Lond.)*, 271, 561–562.

Volknandt, W., Naito, S., Ueda, T. and Zimmermann, H. (1987) Synapsin I is associated with cholinergic nerve terminals in the electric organs of *Torpedo, Electrophorus* and *Malapterurus* and copurifies with *Torpedo* synaptic vesicles. *J. Neurochem.*, 49, 342–347.

Waser, P.G. (Ed.) (1975) *Cholinergic Mechanisms*. Raven Press, New York, xviii + 555 pp.

Weber, M. (1981) A diffusible factor responsible for the determination of cholinergic functions in cultured sympathetic neurons. *J. Biol. Chem.*, 256, 3447–3453.

Weiler, M., Roed, I.S. and Whittaker, V.P. (1982) The kinetics of acetylcholine turnover in a resting cholinergic nerve terminal and the magnitude of the cytoplasmic compartment. *J. Neurochem.*, 38, 1187–1191.

Welner, S.A. and Collier, B. (1984) Uptake, metabolism, and releasability of ethyl analogues of homocholine by rat brain. *J. Neurochem.*, 43, 1143–1151.

Welner, S.A. and Collier, B. (1985) Accumulation, acetylation and releasability of diethylhomocholine from a sympathetic ganglion. *J. Neurochem.*, 45, 210–218.

Whittaker, V.P. (1965) The application of subcellular fractionation techniques to the study of brain function. *Prog. Biophys. Mol. Biol.*, 15, 39–96.

Whittaker, V.P. (1979) Re: metabotropic neurotransmission. *Trends Neurosci.*, 2, VII.

Whittaker, V.P. (1984) What is Dale's Principle? In: V. Chan-Palay and S.L. Palay (Eds.), *Coexistence of Neuroactive Substances*, John Wiley and Sons, New York, pp. 137–140.

Whittaker, V.P. (1987) Cholinergic synaptic vesicles from the electromotor nerve terminals of *Torpedo*: composition and life cycle. *Ann. N.Y. Acad. Sci.*, 493, 77–91.

Whittaker, V.P. (Ed.) (1988a) *The Cholinergic Synapse*. Springer-Verlag, Berlin, Heidelberg, xxvi + 762 pp [*Handbook of Experimental Pharmacology, Vol. 86*].

Whittaker, V.P. (1988b) Model cholinergic systems: an overview. *Handb. Exp. Pharmacol.*, 86, 3–22.

Whittaker, V.P. (1988c) The cellular basis of synaptic transmission: an overview. In: H. Zimmermann (Ed.), *Cellular and Molecular Basis of Synaptic Transmission, NATO ASI Series Vol. H21*. Springer-Verlag, Berlin, Heidelberg, pp. 1–23.

Whittaker, V.P. (1988d) This week's citation classic. *Current Contents*, 31, 15.

Whittaker, V.P. (1990) Cholinergic synaptic vesicles are metabolically and biophysically heterogeneous even in resting terminals. *Brain Res.*, 511, 113–121.

Whittaker, V.P. and Luqmani, Y.A. (1980) False transmitters in the cholinergic system: implications for the vesicle theory of transmitter storage and release. *Gen. Pharmacol.*, 11, 7–14.

Whittaker, V.P. and Sheridan, M.N. (1965) The morphology and acetylcholine content of isolated cerebral cortical synaptic vesicles. *J. Neurochem.*, 12, 363–372.

Whittaker, V.P. and Stadler, H. (1980) The structure and function of cholinergic synaptic vesicles. In: R.A. Bradshaw and D.M. Schneider (Eds.), *Proteins of the Nervous System*, 2nd edn. Raven Press, New York, pp. 231–255.

Whittaker, V.P., Michaelson, I.A. and Kirkland, R.J.A. (1964) The separation of synaptic vesicles from nerve ending particles ('synaptosomes'). *Biochem. J.*, 90, 293–303.

Whittlemore, S.R. and Seiger, Å. (1987) The expression, localization and functional significance of β-nerve growth factor in the central nervous system. *Brain Res.*, 434 (Brain Res. Rev. 12) 439–464.

Wiedenmann, B. and Franke, W.W. (1985) Identification and localization of an integral membrane glycoprotein of M_r 38 000 (synaptophysin) characteristic of presynaptic vesicles. *Cell*, 41, 1017–1028.

Yamagata, S.K. and Parsons, S.M. (1989) Cholinergic synaptic vesicles contain a V-type and a P-type ATPase. *J. Neurochem.*, 53, 1354–1362.

Zimmermann, H. (1978) Turnover of adenine nucleotides in cholinergic synaptic vesicles of the *Torpedo* electric organ. *Neuroscience*, 3, 827–836.

Zimmermann, H. (1988) Cholinergic synaptic vesicles. *Handb. Exp. Pharmacol.*, 86, 349–382.

Zimmermann, H. and Denston, C.R. (1977a) Recycling of synaptic vesicles in the cholinergic synapses of the *Torpedo* electric organ during induced transmitter release. *Neuroscience*, 2, 695–714.

Zimmermann, H. and Denston, C.R. (1977b) Separation of synaptic vesicles of different functional states from the cholinergic synapses of the *Torpedo* electric organ. *Neuroscience*, 2, 715–730.

Zimmermann, H. and Whittaker, V.P. (1974) Effect of electrical stimulation on the yield and composition of synaptic vesicles from the cholinergic synapses of the electric organ of *Torpedo*: a combined biochemical, electrophysiological and morphological study. *J. Neurochem.*, 22, 435–450.

Zimmermann, H. and Whittaker, V.P. (1977) Morphological and biochemical heterogeneity of cholinergic synaptic vesicles. *Nature (Lond.)*, 267, 633–635.

Zimmermann, H., Dowdall, M.J. and Lane, D.A. (1979) Purine salvage at the cholinergic nerve endings of the *Torpedo* electric organ; the central role of adenosine. *Neuroscience*, 4, 979–993.

S.-M. Aquilonius and P.-G. Gillberg (Eds.)
Progress in Brain Research, Vol. 84
© 1990 Elsevier Science Publishers B.V. (Biomedical Division)

CHAPTER 45

Physiological cholinergic functions in the CNS

Alexander G. Karczmar

Department of Pharmacology, Loyola University Medical Center Maywood, IL 60153, and Research Services,
Edward J. Hines V.A. Hospital, Hines, IL, U.S.A.

Introduction and Antecedents

This is the seventh Meeting of the Informal International Cholinergic Club [IICC], its first Meeting having taken place almost 20 years ago, in 1970, in Skokloster.

In the course of these Meetings, we have considered the important aspects of the central cholinergic function; to list them is to emphasize the versatility and the richness of the field; this will be done, assigning the various subjects to the Meetings at which they were first approached.

Second, the highlights and the definitive accomplishments of these Meetings will be selected and stressed — there cannot be any doubt that these accomplishments are important and dramatic; however, the selection of the highlights is my own and it may differ from that which would be made by somebody else. These highlights will be related to some of the topics of this Meeting and to the conclusions reached by the presenters.

Third, these highlights will be commented upon, particularly by emphasizing the topics which were, perhaps, insufficiently stressed in the course of our Meetings and which should be stressed and brought to fruition at our future Meetings.

Before starting, let us state the obvious, and that is, that the central cholinergic system and its functions did not spring, suddenly, from our collective brow, like Athena from that of Zeus. Two examples of this truism must suffice, as it would

be impossible, at this time, to refer in any detail to the history of this field (see Karczmar, 1970, and Holmstedt and Liljestrand, 1963).

The first example illustrates the precocity of cholinergic studies as it shows that central cholinergic effects were known and studied long before there was any notion of acetylcholine (ACh) as a neurotransmitter — in fact, before the birth of the concept of chemical transmission — and of the cholinergic system, as defined by Dale (1938; see also McGeer et al., 1987). The illustration in question concerns central actions of physostigmine and atropine, and their antagonism; these actions have been known since the investigations of Kleinwachter, Bourneville, Fraser, Hudson and Bartholow in the sixties and seventies of the past century (cf. Karczmar, 1970, for references). The first — but not last in this field — controversy arose at that time, as Roberts Bartholow, a Cincinnati physician and Professor in the Cincinnati School of Medicine, claimed priority over the other workers, particularly Fraser, stating that in "1869, I distinctly announced the discovery of an antagonism between Atropia and Physostigma" (Bartholow, 1873; Fig. 1). In describing the actions of the two drugs in frogs and "warm-blooded animals" and their antagonism, Bartholow referred to a number of their central effects, including those on central reflexes and respiration.

The second illustration concerns what may be considered as the birth of the central cholinergic studies, defined as such, i.e., studies dealing with

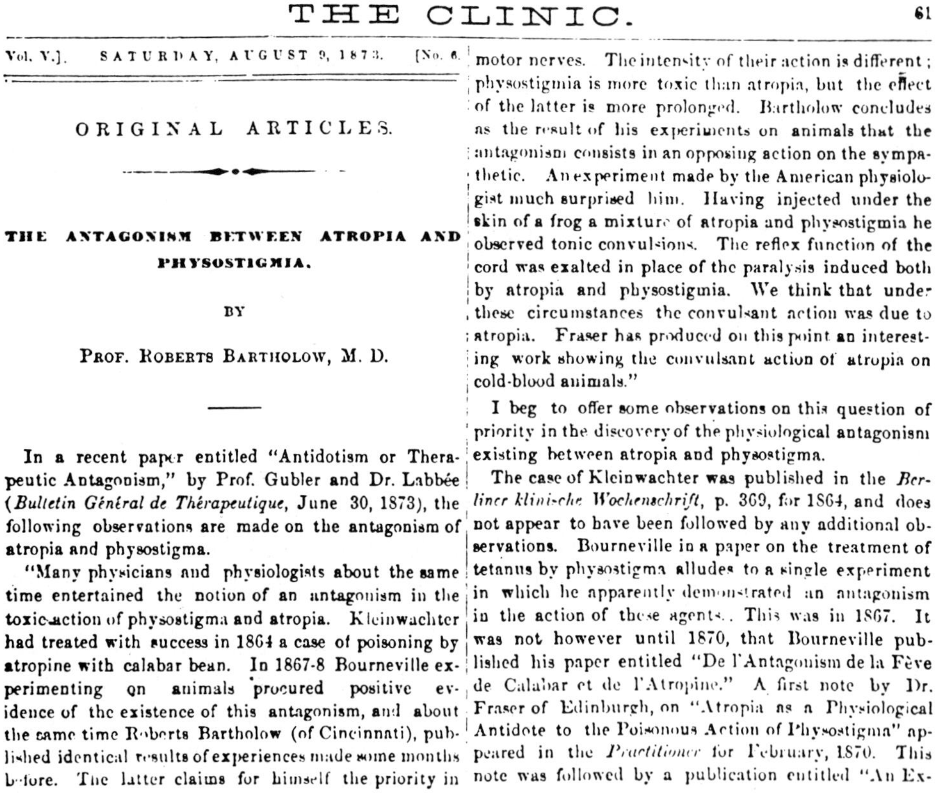

THE CLINIC. 61

Vol. V.]. SATURDAY, AUGUST 9, 1873. [No. 6.

ORIGINAL ARTICLES.

THE ANTAGONISM BETWEEN ATROPIA AND PHYSOSTIGMIA.

BY

PROF. ROBERTS BARTHOLOW, M. D.

In a recent paper entitled "Antidotism or Therapeutic Antagonism," by Prof. Gubler and Dr. Labbée (*Bulletin Général de Thérapeutique*, June 30, 1873), the following observations are made on the antagonism of atropia and physostigma.

"Many physicians and physiologists about the same time entertained the notion of an antagonism in the toxic-action of physostigma and atropia. Kleinwachter had treated with success in 1864 a case of poisoning by atropine with calabar bean. In 1867-8 Bourneville experimenting on animals procured positive evidence of the existence of this antagonism, and about the same time Roberts Bartholow (of Cincinnati), published identical results of experiences made some months before. The latter claims for himself the priority in motor nerves. The intensity of their action is different; physostigmia is more toxic than atropia, but the effect of the latter is more prolonged. Bartholow concludes as the result of his experiments on animals that the antagonism consists in an opposing action on the sympathetic. An experiment made by the American physiologist much surprised him. Having injected under the skin of a frog a mixture of atropia and physostigmia he observed tonic convulsions. The reflex function of the cord was exalted in place of the paralysis induced both by atropia and physostigmia. We think that under these circumstances the convulsant action was due to atropia. Fraser has produced on this point an interesting work showing the convulsant action of atropia on cold-blood animals."

I beg to offer some observations on this question of priority in the discovery of the physiological antagonism existing between atropia and physostigma.

The case of Kleinwachter was published in the *Berliner klinische Wochenschrift*, p. 369, for 1864, and does not appear to have been followed by any additional observations. Bourneville in a paper on the treatment of tetanus by physostigma alludes to a single experiment in which he apparently demonstrated an antagonism in the action of these agents. This was in 1867. It was not however until 1870, that Bourneville published his paper entitled "De l'Antagonism de la Fève de Calabar et de l'Atropine." A first note by Dr. Fraser of Edinburgh, on "Atropia as a Physiological Antidote to the Poisonous Action of Physostigma" appeared in the *Practitioner* for February, 1870. This note was followed by a publication entitled "An Ex-

Fig. 1. The photograph of the first page of the 1873 paper of Roberts Bartholow; also see text. Reprinted by permission from A.G. Karczmar (1970).

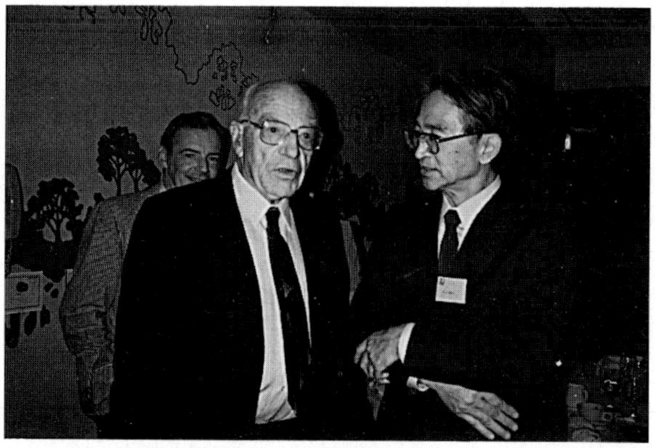

Fig. 2. J.C. Eccles (left) and K. Koketsu at a recent (1987) Meeting. Behind them, Robert L. Myers, an important investigator of the behavioral effects of drugs and transmitters, applied to and within, the animal brain.

central transmittive action of ACh. This beginning is due to the classical demonstration by Eccles, Fatt and Koketsu (Fig. 2) — none of whom, although still hale and alive, appeared as yet at our Meetings, not, I am sure, because of the lack of interest on the part of our organizers — of the cholinergicity of the synapse between the motoneurone collateral and the Renshaw cell. The earlier version of the studies in question appeared in an Australian journal (Eccles et al., 1953); as this paper is less well known than the subsequent paper published in London (Eccles et al., 1954), it may be of interest to show its frontispiece (Fig. 3; see also Eccles, 1987).

So, in our endeavors, we do not lack antecedents, and those described constitute but a frac-

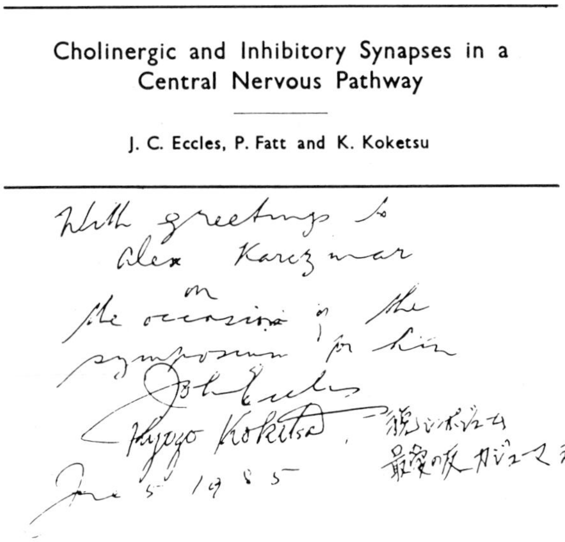
Cholinergic and Inhibitory Synapses in a Central Nervous Pathway

J. C. Eccles, P. Fatt and K. Koketsu

With greetings to Alex Karczmar on the occasion of the symposium for him
JC Eccles
Kyozo Koketsu
June 5 1985

Fig. 3. The frontispiece of a reprint of the 1953 paper by Eccles, Fatt and Koketsu; also see text. Reprinted by permission from A.G. Karczmar (1987).

TABLE I

Skokloster, 1970: Conference on the Effects of Drugs on Cholinergic Mechanisms in the CNS (E. Heilbronn and A. Winters)

Section A: Determination of acetylcholine and its precursors

Recent development in the determination of acetylcholine — D.J. Jenden

Environmental and technical preconditions influencing choline and acetylcholine in rat brain — I. Hanin, R. Mussarelli and E. Costa

Section B: Biosynthesis of acetylcholine II

On the turnover of acetylcholine in the brain — J. Schuberth, B. Sparf and A. Sundvall

The origin and turnover of choline in the brain — G.B. Ansell and S. Spanner

Choline acetyltransferase from mammalian brain — L.T. Potter and V.A.S. Glover

Subcellular localization of enzymes generating acetyl-CoA and their possible relation to the biosynthesis of acetylcholine — S. Tucek

tion of discoveries made before our first, 1970, Meeting with respect to the central cholinergic system by such luminaries as Henry Dale, David Nachmansohn, William Feldberg, Fred Schueller, Mikhail Michelson, Albert von Muralt, Martha Vogt, Henry McIntosh and many others; and, in fact, by some of those present here. This notwithstanding, the contributions made at these Meetings are many and outstanding, and this will be demonstrated and described presently.

Subjects of our seven Meetings

1. Skokloster Meeting. Our very first Meeting, the 1970 Meeting in Skokloster, illustrates the diversity of topics raised with regard to the central cholinergic system — and, in turn, the abundance of the field itself — and the importance of the concepts raised (Tables I–III).

A few of the topics and concepts should be commented upon. First, the Meeting addressed the methodology, developed actually by the presentors in question, concerning chemical determination of ACh and choline. This achievement, important as it was per se, became even more important by its consequences, as it made it possible to attack the important problems of the central turnover of ACh and of the central origin of ACh and of its precursor, choline. Indeed, the concept of the turnover of ACh as the significant marker of cholinergic function, initiated at that

TABLE II

Section C: Storage and release of acetylcholine

An analysis of the stimulatory action of atropine on release and synthesis of acetylcholine in cortical slices from rat brain — R.L. Polak

Investigations into the increase of acetylcholine output from the cerebral cortex — G.C. Pepeu, A. Bartolini and G. Deffenu

Effects of oxotremorine and atropine on choline acetylase activity — B. Holmstedt and C. Lundgren

Choline in the cerebrospinal fluid as a marker for the release of acetylcholine — S.-M. Aquilonius, J. Schuberth and A. Sundvall

Chemically induced changes in the acetylcholine uptake and storage capacity of brain tissue — E. Heilbronn and E. Cedergren

The compartmentalization of acetylcholine in cholinergic nerve terminals — L.A. Barker, M.J. Dowdall, W.B. Essman and V.P. Whittaker

The content of material with acetylcholine-like activity in the brain of animals following thiamine deprivation and treatment with pyrithiamine — P. Stern and R. Igic

440

TABLE III

Section D: Cholinergic receptors and active sites [a]

Improvement in the accuracy of histochemical localization of acetylcholinesterase. Facts and Artifacts — G.B. Koelle
The conformation of molecules affecting cholinergic nervous system — P. Pauling
Investigation of the chemical nature of acetylcholine receptor — A. Karlin
Proteolipid cholinergic receptors isolated from the central nervous system and electric tissue — E. DeRobertis, S. Fiszer de Plazas, J.L. La Torre and G.S. Lunt

Sections C and D: Behavioral and related phenomena

Acetylcholine and the morphine abstinence syndrome — J. Crossland
Effects of drugs which interact with central muscarinic receptors — R.W. Brimblecombe
Evidence of a central cholinergic mechanism functioning during induced excitation in avoidance behavior — M.H. Aprison and J.N. Hintgen

[a] Mixture of presentations on AChEs, behavior, receptors, tremorigenics and antiChEs.

Meeting, stayed with us for many years, till the complexity of its measurement and the arrival of the new methodologies concerning cholinergic receptors, choline acetyltransferase (ChAT) and ACh release seem to have diminished the interest in the measurement of ACh turnover.

The splendid contribution to this field, particularly to the story of metabolic generation of ACh, at the 1970 Meeting of our late friend, Brian Ansell (Table I; Ansell and Spanner, 1970; Ansell et al., 1987), must be emphasized, as should be the address of Stanislaus Tucek concerning the generation of acetylated co-enzyme A (Table I); furthermore, Paul Stern and R. Igic initiated at the Meeting in question the discussion of ACh precursors (Table II), a problem which is still with us.

Some of the participants initiated — and presented at the 1970 Meeting — another important subject, and that is, the matter of the dynamics of the ACh in the nerve terminal, and of the control of its central release (Table II). We will return many times in the course of this review to the question of the dynamics of the cholinergic vesicles and of vesicular and cytoplasmic ACh of the nerve terminals; similarly, the matter of the auto- and

hetero-control of the release of ACh — initiated by George Koelle in the late fifties (see Koelle, 1963, for "percussive" hypothesis of the release of ACh) continues to be the subject of interest and controversy.

Another important subject, initiated by some of the participants and presented for the first time at a major Meeting in Skokloster, was that of cholinergic receptors (Table III); the stereochemical structure and the possibility of the subdivision of the nicotinic and muscarinic receptors were discussed. The contribution to this area of the late Eduardo De Robertis (De Robertis et al., 1970), who introduced at that time the methodology still valid in the field of chemical isolation of the receptors, must be recognised.

The matter of behaviors dependent on central cholinergic transmission and of behavioral effects of cholinergic drugs was also addressed at the 1970 Meeting (Table III). This subject was not broached for the first time at Skokloster since, as already intimated in this paper, it indeed antedates the notion of cholinergic transmission; however, the theoretical basis of the cholinergic effects on conditioned learning (Table III; Aprison and Hintgen, 1970; see also Hintgen and Aprison, 1976), and the possibility of cholinergic correlates of addiction (Table III; Crossland, 1970) were first posited at that Meeting.

Finally, brief allusions were made at the Skokloster Meeting to the matter of cholinergic pathways — as explored in terms of the acetylcholinesterase stain (Table III; Koelle, 1970), effects of diet and dietary deprivation on ACh synthesis (Table III; Stern and Igic, 1970), etc.

2. Subsequent Meetings. At our subsequent Meetings, including the present, seventh Meeting, the topics addressed in Skokloster were expanded and emphasized, and several new topics were added (Tables IV–VIII).

The actions, pharmacological and toxic, of anticholinesterases were broached at the second, Boldern Meeting (Table IV). This subject was discussed at the subsequent Meetings, including the actions of anticholinesterases, particularly of

TABLE IV

CNS topics added or expanded upon at Meetings II–VII, 1974–1989: **Boldern, 1974 (P.G. Waser)**

AntiChE poisoning
Axonal transport
Cholinergic–dopaminergic interaction
Behavioral and related aspects of central cholinergic function
  REM sleep
  aggression
  memory and learning
  arousal and desynchronization
  appetitive and hypothalamic behaviors
Cholinergic receptors
Synthesis and turnover of ACh

TABLE V

CNS topics added or expanded upon at Meetings II–VII, 1974–1989: **LaJolla, 1977 (D.L. Jenden)**

Second messengers (cAMP and cGMP)
Central cholinergic pathways
Behavior
  nociception
  ACNMB
Treatment of mental disease
  cholinergic agonists
Mental disease and cholinergic system
Cholinergic–serotonergic interaction
Neurotoxins (peripherally acting)

the organophosphorus type, which do not depend on the inhibition of cholinesterases and accumulation of ACh; among these actions are the morphopathological effects, sometimes temporary, some-

TABLE VI

CNS topics added or expanded upon at Meetings II–VII, 1974–1989: **Florence, 1980 (G. Pepeu and H. Ladinsky)**

Cholinergic system of the eye
Cholinergic–peptidergic interactions
Trans-synaptic regulation
Trophic factors (gangliosides)
Modulation of transmission (peripheral)
Therapy of diseases with cholinergic implications
  treatment of mental disease – ACh precursors
  other clinical conditions
SDAT and aging, and cholinergic system
Cholinergic markers of disease
Neurotoxins (centrally acting)

TABLE VII

CNS topics added or expanded upon at Meetings II–VII, 1974–1989: **Oglebay Park, 1983 (I. Hanin)**

Central cholinergic system and cardiovascular function
Trophic factors (TFs acting on ChEs)
Second messengers (phosphotidylinositol turnover)
Scanning methods (PET)
Cholinergic–GABA interactions and modulation of transmission (central)

times of long duration, whether at the neuromyal junction or in the CNS (see also Karczmar, 1984).

The matter of the second messengers of the cyclic nucleotide and phosphatidyl inositol type was approached at our third and fifth Meetings, respectively (Tables V and VII). This subject was pursued at the subsequent Meetings, including the present one (see the presentations of Lambert and Nahorski, Joan Brown, and Michael Schimerlik) and further comments on this matter will be made subsequently.

Central neurotransmitter interactions and both pre- and post-synaptic modulations were first discussed at our second Meeting in Boldern, where the question of cholinergic-dopaminergic ineraction was broached (Table IV), and the interactions between the cholinergic system and other neurotransmitter systems including serotonergic, peptidergic and GABA-ergic systems, as well as mod-

TABLE VIII

CNS topics added or expanded upon at Meetings II–VII, 1974–1989

Buxton, 1986 (M.J. Dowdall and J.N. Hawthorne)
  Subclasses of nicotinic and muscarinic receptors and their molecular biology (see also Meetings I and II)
  Cholinergic system and development
  Trophic factors, including NGF
  Psychotropic drugs and the cholinergic system
  Cytoplasmic ACh and nerve terminal dynamics

Lidingo, 1989 (S.-M. Aquilonius)
  Spinal cholinergic mechanisms
  Cholinergic system and movement disorders
  Cholinergic system and anesthesia
  Cholinergic system and sleep
  Neurophysiology of hippocampal cholinergic system

ulation of cholinergic transmission were discussed at the subsequent Meetings (Tables V–VIII).

Trophic factors were first addressed at the Florence, 1980, Meeting, and this subject, particularly its central aspects, was rather sparingly addressed subsequently, as trophic factors affecting cholinesterases were described at the Oglebay Meeting of 1983, while studies of trans-synaptic regulations and of the trophic actions of gangliosides were presented at the Florence Meeting (Tables VI and VII). The effects of the NGF and the very important subject of the role of trophic factors in development and of the possibly trophic role of the cholinergic system in ontogenesis were, again, represented rather briefly (at the 1986 Buxton Meeting in 1986; Table VIII). A comment will be made on this matter subsequently.

Neurotoxins and their use in modelling diseases which present cholinergic implications, particularly SDAT, were referred to first at the La Jolla Meeting of 1977 and addressed again at the subsequent Meetings (Tables V and VI), including the present one. It is of interest in this context that the important subject of the clinical and therapeutic implications of the central cholinergic system was not referred to at our first, Skokloster Meeting; this subject was first attacked at our third, La Jolla Meeting (Table V) as well as at our subsequent, including the present, Meetings. Mental disease was particularly considered, but other diseased states were also addressed (Table VI), including, at the present Meeting, the movement disorders as well as the use of cholinergic agents in anesthesia (Table VIII). Don Jenden reviewed this matter most interestingly, particularly from the viewpoint of the development of pertinent drugs, at this Meeting.

Several topics, initiated at our first, Skokloster Meeting, were expanded and emphasized subsequently. Thus, the question of central cholinergic pathways was discussed at several Meetings, beginning with the La Jolla Meeting (Table V) and including this Meeting. The related subject of behaviors with cholinergic implications was discussed at several Meetings including the present one (Tables IV, V and VIII); yet certain important aspects of this matter remain to be discussed, and some comments will be made as to this problem subsequently. Similarly, the matter of central, particularly muscarinic receptors was pursued further, beginning with our second, Boldern Meeting (Table IV) and including our present Meeting. Also, the important matter of synthesis of ACh, the role of ACh precursors, and the relationship of this metabolism to that of phospholipids was discussed at several of our Meetings, including the Boldern Meeting (Table IV), and this subject was masterfully reviewed at the present Meeting by Stanislaus Tucek.

Finally, sporadic references were made at our Meetings to a number of matters, such as the axonal transport of ACh (Table IV), the role of the central cholinergic system in the regulation of the cardiovascular funtion (Table VII), synaptic mechanisms (Table VIII), etc.

Altogether, this listing of the topics broached at our seven Meetings constitutes the proof that, indeed, as stated earlier, an astounding versatility and richness of topics characterizes the central cholinergic system. Furthermore, several of these topics were pursued from one Meeting to another; thus, important conclusions can be reached as to several of the subjects in question, and this matter will be addressed in the next section of this review.

Highlights and gaps

The highlights of our seven Meetings are shown in Tables IX and X. Some of these highlights take the form of definitive statements, as certain problems referred to at our Meetings may be considered, perhaps optimistically, as essentially resolved; other highlights concern work which is still in progress. Finally, certain topics were broached to a limited extent at our Meetings and should be considered as representing gaps in the cholinergic lore; these are listed in Table XI, although this list should not be considered exhaustive.

Among the problems which may be considered as resolved — in terms of the work carried out by

TABLE IX

Highlights of CNS research generated at the seven meetings of IICC

Definition of central cholinergic pathways
their relation to REMS, Ag and memory
Dynamics of cholinergic vesicles and of ACh in the cholinergic terminals
Definition of subclasses of muscarinic and nicotinic receptors
molecular biology and cholinergic receptors
channel-receptor macromolecules
Elucidation of mechanisms of pre- and post-synaptic transmission
ionic mechanisms of synaptic potentials

the participants at these Meetings and in terms of research carried out elsewhere — is the problem of central cholinergic pathways. To a great measure, our knowledge of supraspinal central cholinergic pathways is well-nigh complete, and, at this Meeting, this state of the art was emphasized by Marsel Mesulam and Jose Palacios (Table IX). This accomplishment has a long history, as will be emphasized subsequently.

Several past contributors to our Meetings, particularly the McGeers (see McGeer et al., 1986, 1987), emphasized the role of such central cholinergic subsystems as the medial forebrain complex, parabrachial complex and the cholinergic reticular formation, while Mesulam described the central cholinergic system in terms of radiations originating from 7 cholinergic neuronal groupings; yet these groups of investigators are in good agreement with respect to the cholinergic innervation of the limbic system and the hippocampus via the septal and diagonal band radiation of the medial

TABLE X

Highlights of CNS research generated at the sevent Meetings of IICC

Identification of modulatory mechanisms at synapses and pathways
plurichemical modulation and transmission
Description of choline, ACh and phospholipid metabolism
what do ACh precursors accomplish?
Identifying animal models and therapy of cholinergic disease

forebrain system, of the thalamus and the sub-thalamus via the pediculopontine tegmental nucleus of the parabrachial system, and of the reticular formation via the giganto- and magno-cellular tegmental fields. Nor is there any controversy as to the interneuronal cholinergic fields or networks of the eye, the striatum, the vestibular system, etc.

This definition of the central supraspinal cholinergic pathways is fascinating per se, and also as it relates to specific behaviors, such as aggression, REM sleep (see Chapter 42 of this volume) and memory. The cholinergic implications of these and many other behaviors were discussed at several of our past Meetings (see Tables IV, V and VIII), and their cholinergic implications were clarified to a great extent; yet interesting aspects of this matter still remain to be explored, and this will be commented upon in the next section of this review.

At this Meeting, Per-Goran Gillberg addressed the matter of the spinal cholinergic system or systems; this subject is still incomplete, and this matter as well as certain special aspects of the supra-axial cholinergic system will be commented upon subsequently.

The condition of the subject of the cholinergic receptors (Table IX) may be considered as being half-way between the status of a definitive accomplishment and that of an unfinished task.

Indeed, this matter was discussed severally at our Meetings, beginning with the presentations of Peter Pauling and A. Karlin at our first, Skokloster Meeting (see Table III). At the subsequent Meetings both the pre- and post-synaptic receptors and the subtypes of the muscarinic and nicotinic receptors were defined and discussed, and the differences between the peripheral and the central nicotinic and muscarinic receptors were emphasized by several groups of investigators (see, for example, Nordstrom et al., 1986; Larsson and Nordberg, 1986; cf. also Karczmar, 1986); it is important, in this context, to refer to the demonstration at our 1986 Meeting of the presence of central nicotinic presynaptic receptors (Schwartz and Kellar, 1986), and to the molecular biology approach utilized by Eric Barnard with respect to chick brain receptors (Barnard et al., 1987) as presented by him at our Buxton Meeting.

This matter was expanded at the present Meeting, as Joan Brown and Michael Schimerlik associated the muscarinic receptors with the second messenger mechanisms, and as Schimerlik discussed the mapping of the receptor and of the receptor-G protein macromolecule. Furthermore, Herbert Ladinsky continued his discussion, presented at our earlier Meetings, of the heterogeneity of the muscarinic receptors (M_1–M_7) and of the pharmacological characteristics of the cloned receptors; the recent book which concerns particularly the pharmacology of the muscarinic receptors, edited by Joan Brown (Brown, 1989), should be mentioned in this context.

Altogether, the concept and the pharmacological — not necessarily structural and chemical — definition of the heterogeneity of both the nicotinic and muscarinic receptors are well established today, as is the concept of their pre- and post-synaptic location. Yet much work remains to be carried out; furthermore, certain advances made elsewhere were not sufficiently considered at our past and the present Meetings (see, however, the presentation by Barnard et al., 1987, at the Buxton Meeting). Thus, most of the studies presented at our Meetings concern the peripheral rather than the central, and the muscarinic rather than the nicotinic, receptors; yet some progress was made recently in several laboratories with respect to the central nicotinic receptors (see Schmidt, 1988). More importantly, the molecular biology of the receptors and their mapping which was and is being explored by several laboratories was insufficiently discussed at our Meetings; a comment will be made on this matter later.

Matters which are closely related to the definition of the cholinergic, post- and pre-synaptic receptors are those concerning the mechanisms underlying the pre- and post-synaptic function, their ionic fluxes, and the modulation of central cholinergic transmission (Tables IX and X). Again, these matters, while not completely resolved, par-

ticularly in the case of the CNS, were clarified to a large extent, and the current thinking on this problem was presented at this Meeting by James Halliwell and David Colquhoun. Both these investigators stressed the heterogeneity of particularly the muscarinic responses, the hippocampal muscarinic responses being quite similar in this respect to those described for the periphery by such workers as Paul Adams (cf. Adams et al., 1982), Nishi and the Kurume group (see Nishi, 1974), Libet (1970) and the Gallaghers (Schinnick-Gallagher et al., 1987); this heterogeneity is due mainly to the multiplicity of potassium currents, which include the so-called M-current, and to the involvement of calcium currents.

It must be stressed that these currents may have either a transmittive or a modulatory function (Koketsu, 1987), the other mechanisms which underlie modulatory processes being the interaction between various transmitters and, perhaps most importantly, the coexistence and co-release of two (or more!) neurotransmitters from the same neuron, as stressed at this Meeting by Bjorn Lindh and Tomas Hokfelt, one of the pioneers in the research concerning the multipresence of transmitters in the same neurons.

Still another area where much was accomplished and much was clarified since the early presentations on this matter in the course of our first, Skokloster Meeting (see above, and Table I) is that of ACh, choline and phospholipid metabolism, choline uptake and synthesis of ACh; in fact, much of this clarification is due to the research presented at out subsequent Meetings (Table IV), as reviewed at this Meeting by one of the pioneers of this research, Stanislaus Tucek. What is important in this area is the demonstration that brain phospholipids may generate choline, a notion which is a novel one, as before the research of Brian Ansell (Ansell and Spanner, 1970), Blusztajn and Wurtman (1983), Zeisel (1986) and Tucek (this Meeting, and Tucek, 1983) it was postulated that the brain is provided with choline via the blood, this choline being generated by the diet and peripheral metabolism. Furthermore, it was shown at our Meetings and elsewhere that there is a relationship between phospholipid metabolism and the choline generation via the phosphatidylcholine pathway on the one hand and the uptake and the metabolism of choline generated by its uptake on the other, and that there is considerable flexibility and feedback between the various compartments and pathways which are involved (see also Blusztajn and Wurtman, 1983; Blusztajn et al., 1986; Wecker, 1986; Zeisel, 1986). What needs further exploration and clarification is the capacity of exogenously applied precursors such as choline and phosphatidylcholine to generate ACh.

These Meetings, including the present one, shed much light on still another area, which is that of the biodynamics of the nerve terminal (Table IX). Much definitive knowledge was contributed to this subject at our Meetings, beginning with the presentation by Victor Whittaker, Michael Dowdall and their associates at our very first Meeting in Skokloster (Barker et al., 1970). At present, the efforts of that group as well as that of Maurice Israel (this Meeting; see also Israel, 1986) resolved much of the pertinent problems, and Victor Whittaker, in his elegant and thorough summary, described dynamics of vesicular ACh and its subtypes, the mechanisms of the nerve terminal choline uptake, the pathways of choline and the acetate, as well as the cycling of the vesicles to and from the nerve terminal membrane; this, and the contribution of Israel's group to the understanding of the dynamics of the cytoplasmic ACh gives us a well-nigh complete picture of the biodynamics of the nerve terminal. Of course, certain problems remain to be solved, such as the contribution to the pathways in question of choline uptake versus that of the metabolically derived choline, and, what is particularly pertinent for this review, the validity for the CNS of the model of the nerve terminal dynamics derived mostly from the studies of *Torpedo*.

Still another area of research may be also considered as being in a state of flux. Since our first consideration at these Meetings of neurotoxins (Tables V and VI) and their use as models for central disease with cholinergic implications much progress was made in this area, as exemplified by the presentations of Israel Hanin and Vahram Haroutunian at this Meeting with respect to useful models of SDAT. Progress was also made with the models of peripheral disease, such as myasthenia gravis, and Stanley Appel described at the present Meeting the development of a possible model of ALS (Lou Gehrig Disease). Yet the models available at this time for central diseases with cholinergic implications are not ideal. More importantly — and this was already emphasized above (see also the presentation of Don Jenden at this Meeting) much knowledge was gained but little clinical progress was made with respect to the therapy of central diseases with clear cholinergic implications such as SDAT, or of mental conditions which have less obvious cholinergic implications (see Karczmar, 1988).

Now, let us turn to the gaps in the progress of the central cholinergic research and/or lacunae in the coverage of certain subjects at our Meetings (see Table XI).

First, there is the question of the molecular biology of the constituents of the cholinergic system (Table XI). In this context, Stanislaus Tucek stressed in his review of the synthesis of ACh (see above) that an important advance in this area is constituted by the application of the methods of molecular biology to the mapping of ChAT and elucidation of the mechanisms underlying the action of ChAT. Yet in the course of our past Meetings the references to this important matter

TABLE XI

Gaps and topics insufficiently covered at the seven Meetings of IICC

Mechanisms of function and NGF and NFs
retro- and antero-trophins
Molecular biology of cholinergic constituents
Phosphatidyl inositol, nucleotides and neuronal phospho-proteins
their physiological role in signal mediation
their interactions

were very sparse, particularly with respect to the CNS. Only at this Meeting, Hermona Soreq presented data on the molecular biology of acetyl- and butyrylcholinesterase, and her presentation culminated her long and fruitful research along these lines; Michael Schimerlik described some aspects of the molecular biology of the muscarinic receptor; and Jaques Mallet and the Gif-sur-Yvette group spoke of the DNA encoding of ChAT. Nevertheless, this constitutes limited coverage of an area which is being intensely investigated, and this relative lack of molecular biology approaches in the case of the cholinergic receptors was already stressed (see above). This latter matter and its current status will be commented on subsequently.

Second, the question of neurotropic factors must be considered as a "gap" or, at least, a flux area; while some of the actions of gangliosides and certain other trophic factors were briefly considered at our fourth and fifth Meetings (see Tables VI and VII), and while the effects of these and additional trophic factors, particularly the NGF, were described at the sixth Meeting (see Table VIII; cf., particularly, Thoenen et al., 1987; Cuello et al., 1987; and Appel et al., 1987) as well at our present Meeting by Cuello and his associates, still the current activity in this area is intense, and further review of this subject is appropriate; a comment on this matter will be made subsequently.

Finally, there is the matter of the second messengers. Remarks as to the role in the central cholinergic function of cyclic nucleotides and phosphatidyl inositol were initiated at the third and fifth Meetings (see Tables V and VII), and brief references particularly to the phosphatidyl inositol cascade were made at our sixth, Buxton Meeting; however, the pertinent studies concerned mostly peripheral tissues (see, for example, Hawthorne et al., 1987; Loffelholz et al., 1987). As already alluded to, Stefan Nahorski and David Lambert, Joan Brown, and Michael Schimerlik also referred to the matter at this Meeting — Brown and Schimerlik were, again, concerned essentially with peripheral tissues, and only Lambert

and Nahorksi studied a tissue more pertinent to this review, a neuroblastoma. Obviously, much material, particularly the question of the physiological role of the second messenger systems and the problem of the interactions between these systems, was not covered at our present or past Meetings, and comments as to this important subject will be made in the next section of this review.

Comments on the highlights and gaps

CNS and spinal pathways

It was already pointed out that our present, quite complete understanding of the cholinergic pathways of the mammalian — including, to an extent, human — brain constitutes the culmination of many past efforts. Some of this long history is due to the investigations of the past presenters at these Meetings, particularly the McGeers (McGeer et al., 1986), Larry Butcher (Butcher and Woolf, 1986) and H.C. Fibiger (Fibiger and Lehman, 1981). Their work was — and is — based mainly on tracing the best marker for cholinergic neurons, ChAT, by means of the immunohistochemical and immunocytochemical methodology developed by Kimura, the McGeers, and their associates (Kimura et al., 1980).

Much earlier mapping of the central cholinergic system, dating in fact from the fifties and sixties, was accomplished by using AChE as the cholinergic marker and employing the histochemical stain for AChE developed by George Koelle; of course, because of certain peculiarities of its location described by Koelle at our first Meeting (cf. Koelle, 1963 and 1970, and Karczmar, 1969), AChE is not as reliable a marker of the cholinergic neurons as is ChAT; all the more remarkable is that the mapping provided by Koelle and Shute and Lewis (1967) is consistent with the definitive mapping based on the ChAT immunocytochemistry method, as exemplified by the painstaking identification by means of the AChE stain of presumably cholinergic central neurons by Koelle (Fig. 4; Koelle, 1963) and by the elegant and thorough description, based on the same method combined with an

Table 3. *Regions of the rat central nervous system exhibiting intense staining for AChE* (Neurons giving rise to peripheral motor and preganglionic autonomic fibers omitted; see text for method; from KOELLE 1954)

Region	Stained structures
Reticular formation (medulla)	Scattered neurons and fibers throughout
Nuc. of lateral funiculus (medulla)	Larger neurons most heavily stained
Nuc. of Roller	Scattered neurons and fibers
Ventral nuc. of reticular formation	Neurons and fibers show fairly consistent heavy staining
Nuc. of trapezoid body	Numerous scattered neurons and fibers
Dorsal and median nuc. of the raphe (midbrain)	Small clusters of heavily stained neurons and fibers
Dorsal, caudal ventral and rostral ventral nuc. of lateral lemniscus (midbrain)	Small, scattered, heavily stained neurons and fibers
Cerebellar cortex	Scattered cells in granular layer, mostly of large type; few stellate cells in molecular layer; numerous fibers of medulla
Pontine nuc.	Numerous scattered neurons and fibers very heavily stained
Nuc. interpeduncularis	Thickly clustered very heavily stained neurons and fibers of pars lateralis; occasional neurons of pars medialis
Superior colliculus	Densely-packed, moderately heavily stained neurons of stratum griseum; scattered fibers of non-optic layer of stratum opticum
Fasciculus retroflexus of Meynert	Most fibers heavily stained in cross section
Zona incerta	Few neurons and scattered fibers
Lateral habenular nuc.	Few small neurons and fibers; majority moderately stained
Anterior nuc. of thalamus	Few scattered neurons and numerous fibers of ventro-lateral portion
Lateral nuc. of thalamus	Heavily stained neurons and fibers interspersed with un-stained tracts
Caudate nuc.	Very heavily stained, closely-packed neurons and fibers; interspersed bundles of internal capsule largely unstained
Putamen	Densely packed, heavily stained neurons and fibers
Central nuc of amygdala	Scattered, very heavily stained fusiform neurons and fibers
Lateral nuc. of amygdala	Scattered, very heavily stained smaller globular neurons and fibers
Nuc. of lateral olfactory tract	Occasional neurons and fibers (majority unstained)
Tuberculum olfactorium	Densely packed small neurons and fibers
Diagonal band of Broca	Scattered neurons and fibers, many unstained
Nuc. accumbens septi	Numerous neurons and fibers

Fig. 4. Regions of the rat central nervous system exhibiting intense staining for AChE (neurons giving rise to peripheral motor and preganglionic autonomic fibers omitted). Reprinted by permission from Koelle (1963).

appropriate lesion technique, of the limbic and reticular cholinergic pathways by Shute and Lewis (Shute and Lewis, 1967; Lewis and Shute, 1967).

As certain as we are at this time of the essentials of the supraspinal cholinergic pathways, we are unclear as to the spinal cholinergic pathways, whether descending and ascending, or segmental; this is somewhat ironic as the first demonstration of a central cholinergic synapse concerned the spinal synapse at the Renshaw cell. Sten-Magnus Aquilonius and Per-Goran Gillberg demonstrated at this and at the previous Meeting (Aquilonius et al., 1987) the presence of the muscarinic receptors and ChAT-rich neurons in the spinal cord; indeed, their work as well as the earlier pharmacological evidence (Koketsu et al., 1969; Dun and Karczmar, unpublished data), strongly suggests that many cholinergic synapses are involved, including cholinergic neurons and interneurons, and that these synapses and pathways contribute to the well-known cholinergic pharmacological characteristics of the spinal DR-VR and DR-DR reflexes (Koketsu et al., 1969) — yet the knowledge of the organization of the pathways in question still eludes us: this is all the more regrettable in view of the potential importance of this knowledge with respect to the treatment of motoneuron disease (Aquilonius et al., 1987).

One additional comment is appropriate in this context; Gillberg, Askmark and Aquilonius presented, at this Meeting, indirect evidence indicating the presence in the posterior horn of muscarinic, presynaptic receptors in the spinal cord; the electrophysiological proof of the presence of such receptors in the ventral horn and the demonstration of their role in regulating the release of excitatory, non-ACh transmitter or transmitters was delivered recently by Jiang ad Dun (1986), and the pertinent data are shown in Fig. 5.

Cholinergic system and behavior: cholinergic implications of the organism–environment interaction

It has already been stressed that the presence of cholinergic radiations in the limbic, parabrachial and reticular systems underlies the multiplicity of behaviors with cholinergic implications; a number of such behaviors were discussed at our Meetings, including the present one (Tables III, IV and IX, and Chapter 42 of this volume).

Two points deserve emphasis in this context. First, there is no overt or covert (mental) behavior known to us which does not exhibit cholinergic implications, and it is of interest to list the behaviors and functions that were studied — and measured! — in animals and, in part at least, in man, categorizing them, somewhat arbitrarily, into organic and "mental" (Tables XII–XIV; cf. Karczmar, 1984). Among those, there are many which were studied extensively and presented at our Meetings, such as aggression, learning and hunger-seeking activities (see Table IV), and many which deserve further exploration, particularly with respect to their mechanisms, such as fear, brain excitability, and others (Tables XIII and XIV; Karczmar, 1979 and 1984).

Control

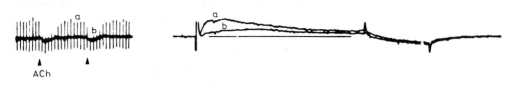

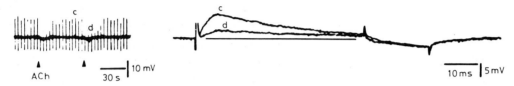

Fig. 5. Hyperpolarization of the postsynaptic membrane and suppression of evoked EPSPs by ACh in an unidentified ventral horn neuron. The recording was obtrained in a thin transverse neonatal rat spinal cord slice preparation. Intracellular recordings; ACh was applied by pressure ejection. Slow chart recordings are shown on the left of the figure. Upward deflections represent EPSPs evoked by stimulation of dorsal rootlets; downward deflections represent hyperpolarizing electrotonic potentials elicited by constant current pulses (not shown). Pressure ejection of ACh (arrowheads, 10 ms pulse duration, 40 psi) in this case produced a hyperpolarization and a marked decrease of EPSPs. Individual EPSPs and hyperpolarizing electrotonic potentials taken at the times marked by "a", "b", "c" and "d" on the left are shown on the right of the Figure. A 60% reduction was detected between recordings "a" and "b", whereas the electrotonic potentials remained unchanged. After superfusing the slice with strychnine (1 micro M) for 10 minutes, pressure ejections of ACh which now caused a much smaller hyperpolarization were ineffective in suppressing the EPSPs. Reprinted by permission from Jiang and Dun (1986).

Second, some of these behaviors may be linked together and described as a syndrome, and this concept has not been presented, so far, at our

TABLE XII

CNS (organic) effects of cholinergic drugs

  I. Motor behavior and related neurological syndromes
    A. Catalepsy
    B. Locomotor and related actions: gnawing, self biting, head motion, sniffing; compulsive circling; hypo-kinesia
    C. Tremor
    D. Convulsions

 II. Respiration

III. Appetitive behavior
    A. Hunger and feeding: effect dependent on brain site and species
    B. Thirst and drinking: effect dependent on brain site and species

IV. Thermocontrol
    A. Heat production
    B. Heat loss

For references to Tables XII–XIV, see Karczmar, 1978 and 1984. Table XII–XIV reprinted by permission from Karczmar, 1984.

Meetings. The behaviors and functions in question may be observed in awake, unanesthetized animals and they include cholinergic facilitation of learning, cholinergic EEG alerting and evocation of hippocampal theta activity, and cholinergic suppression or inhibition of motor activity, including the antagonism of motor effects of brain lesions or

TABLE XIII

CNS (organic) effects of cholinergic drugs

  V. EEG and brain excitability

 VI. Sleep
    A. REMS
    B. SWS

VII. Chronobiology
    A. Diurnal rhythms
    B. Hibernation, seasonal changes
    C. Aging

VIII. Sensorium
    A. Nociception
    B. Audition
    C. Vision

 IX. Sexual activity

TABLE XIV

Behavioral "psychological" and "mental" functions in animals with cholinergic connotations

---

I. Aggression
   A. Emotional (affective)
   B. Predatory
   C. Irritable

II. Learning and related phenomena
   A. Conditioning
   B. Memory (short and long term)
   C. Habituation
   D. Retrieval

III. Emotional behavior and fear

IV. Addiction, dependence, withdrawal syndrome
   A. Opiate addiction
   B. ETOH addiction

V. "Schizoid" behavior

VI. Organism–environment interaction (OEI)

---

amphetamine (Karczmar, 1979 and 1989). It should be added that, in anesthetized animal, cholinergic agonists produce REM sleep as demonstrated some 20 years ago (Karczmar et al., 1970; for further references, see Karczmar, 1979, Baghdoyan et al., 1988, and Chapter 42), and the cholinergic nature of the latter both in man and in animals was described at this Meeting by Chris Gillin (Ch. 42). Indeed, it was suggested in the past that the central cholinergic effects in the unanesthetized animal take the form of "awaken REM sleep" and include, indeed, mild muscle relaxation and a type of rapid eye movement (REM; Karczmar, 1970, 1979, 1989); the syndrome in question was termed Cholinergic Alert Non-Mobile Behavior (CANMB, Table XV; Karczmar, 1979; see also Vanderwolf, 1975).

TABLE XV

Cholinergic alert non-mobile behavior (CANMB)

Motor activity blockade muscle tonus diminution	Hippocampal theta rhythm (4–14 Hz)
	Cortical desynchronization
Behavioral alertness	Occasional eye movement
Learning facilitation	Analgesia

Another pertinent concept should be stressed: it may appear that learning and good perception of environment are linked, almost synonymous phenomena, yet this link may be quite spurious. Indeed, it was stressed (Karczmar, 1988, 1990) that the cholinergic facilitation of learning can be dissociated from behavioral counterparts of cholinergically evoked alerting, facilitation of goal-directed behavior, and improvement in the recognition of environmental changes such as novelty, this latter improvement resulting in cholinergic augmentation of habituation to trivial or no longer vital stimuli (see also Marczynski, 1978). Altogether, it was hypothesized that CANMB reflects cholinergic improvement in the Organism–Environment Interaction (OEI; see Table XIV and Karczmar, 1990); this concept should be pursued further at our future Meetings.

Trophic factors

While the trophic factors, particularly the NGF and the gangliosides, were discussed at our past meetings (see Thoenen et al., 1987; Cuello et al., 1987; Table VIII) and while Cuello and his associates discussed at this Meeting the central immunoreactive sites for NGF as well as the interaction between the ganglioside GM1 and NGF with respect to damage repair following appropriate central lesions, much additional work particularly with regard to other than NGF and ganglioside neurotrophic factors was and is being carried out.

It must be stressed that, of the many factors (Tables XVI–XX) which exhibit demonstrable trophic actions and which were identified chemically at least to some extent, only relatively few were shown to exert trophic actions on central cholinergic sites; these agents and their targets are listed in Table XVI. Two types of factor must be considered in this context, retrophins (Hendry and Iversen, 1973), i.e. trophic substances generated by the targets of various neurons and exerting their actions, retrograde fashion, on neurons in question, and antero-trophins which act in the opposite direction.

TABLE XVI

Retrophins and antero-trophins acting on cholinergic CNS

Substance	Target
Nerve growth factor (NGF)	Septo-hippocampal pathway, basal forebrain pathway
Neuroleukin (NLK; phospho-glucose isomerase)	MNs, septo-hippocampal pathway
Epidermal growth factor (EGF)	Basal forebrain pathway
Sialogangliosides (GM_1)	Basal forebrain and septo-hippocampal pathway
Fibroblast growth factor (FGF)	Septo-hippocampal pathway
Retina cognin	Amacrine cells

For references to Tables XVI–XX, see the text, and Gutmann, 1976; Guth, 1986; Gage and Bjorklund, 1987; Buznikov, 1984; Black et al., 1979; Dennis, 1981; Peng, 1987; Hendry, 1976; Harper and Thoenen, 1981; Salpeter, 1987; Meisami and Brazier, 1979; Riopelle and Riccardi, 1987; Stein et al., 1983; Porcellati et al., 1975; Walker et al., 1982; Walicke, 1989; Trisler, 1987; Greene and Shooter, 1980; Fox et al., 1982; Appel et al., 1987; Gospodarowicz, 1981.

TABLE XVII

Neurotropic factors with possible action on cholinergic ANS and CNS targets

Substance	Target
Cell adhesion (CAM), substrate adhesion, aggregation and clustering factors	Neural crest and ganglionic development, NMJ, spinal cord, DRG, olfactory tracts
Ciliary ganglion factor	Ciliary ganglia
ACh	NMJ, ganglia, CNS(?)
Trans-synaptic trophins	Ganglia, AdMe, CNS

TABLE XVIII

Neurotrophic factors with non-established action on cholinergic CNS target

Substance	Target
Calcitonin gene-related peptide (CGRP)	NMJ (muscle cholinergic receptor)
cAMP	NMJ
Neurogenic (MN) substance related NMJ-acting trophic substances	Muscle cholinergic receptors
Glycyl-L-glutamine or related TF	Ganglionic AChE
Glycoproteins (sciatin)	AChRs, AChE (NMJ)
Extracellular matrix components (ECMs)	ACh, AChE (NMJ)

TABLE XIX

Neurotrophic factors with non-established action on cholinergic CNS targets

Substance	Target
Brain derived neurotrophic factor (BDNF)	DRG
Purpurin	Retina (photoreceptors)
Apolipoprotein E and glial trophins	PC12, astrocytes, Schwann cells
Nexin	Neuroblastoma, sympathetic ganglion cells
S100b	Astrocytes, CNS neurons (?)
Nerve-dependent regeneration factor (mitotic factor)	Amphibian limb regeneration

Few other trophic factors may exhibit trophic actions on the cholinergic sites, but the definitive demonstration of such effects is still pending (Table XVII); there are many more trophic factors the actions of which on the central cholinergic sites were, essentially, not tested, and these are listed in Tables XVIII–XX.

Still one general comment should be made with respect to the substances in question. The discovery by Rita Levi-Montalcini (cf. Levi-Montalcini and Angeletti, 1968; see also Bueker, 1948) of the NGF concerned particularly its role in the mammalian development of the sympathetic ganglia; subsequently, its role in the development of the central cholinergic system was demonstrated by Hans Thoenen and his associates (Gnahn et al., 1983; Thoenen et al., 1987). There is ample evidence that the other trophic factors

TABLE XX

Neurotrophic factors with non-established action on cholinergic CNS targets

Substance	Target
Laminin–heparan sulfate proteoglycan (HSPG) complex	Retina (ganglion, cells) sciatic nerve, ciliary ganglion
Proteoglycans	Brain neurons?
Insulin and insulin-like growth factors (IGF-I and II)	Sympathetic, parasympathetic, cortical and cerebellar neurons
Oncogenes	PC12

also play a role in development, such as for instance the Neurogenic (MN) Substance, the Cell Adhesion Factor (CAM) and other trophic factors (Tables XVII and XVIII) which are needed for the ontogenesis and patterning of the cholinergic endplate receptors. On the other hand, it begins to be clear that NGF, gangliosides and other trophic or "neuronotrophic" (McGeer et al., 1987) factors are also effective when applied after damage or lesions to the peripheral and central nervous system. This is, of course, a new and most important concept, as until the sixties, "the mammalian brain has been regarded as a structure oriented to degeneration with a negligible capacity for regeneration" (McGeer et al., o.c.).

It appears that a number of factors exert proven trophic effects on the developing and adult central cholinergic structures, particularly the basal forebrain pathway (Table XVI), some factors being capable of exerting trophic actions on localized central cholinergic networks such as constituted by the amacrine cells of the retina (Table XVI); on the other hand, certain factors exert demonstrable effects on the peripheral cholinergic system, such as the ciliary ganglion factor and the CAM, already referred to, but their effects on the central cholinergic systems remain to be proven.

Other trophic substances warrant a comment. First, there are substances that may form a matrix needed for patterning and organization of cholinergic receptors, and, as such, related functionally to CAM; here can be included certain glycoproteins and Extracellular Matrix Components (ECMs; Table XVIII). All these factors may prove to be important in the developmental organization of the central cholinergic neurons and/or receptors. Then, there are factors important for the trans-synaptic trophic action and perhaps, for the activation of second messengers that may be involved in the trans-synaptic phenomena. These phenomena, described originally by Erminio Costa, Alessandro Guidotti and their coworkers and presented by them at one of our earlier Meetings (Costa et al., 1978), underlie the maturation of cholinergic postsynaptic structures and of the coupling between the latter and the appropriate transmitters in the ganglia and in the adrenal medulla; anologous processes may be discovered in the future with respect to the CNS.

Many of these and additional trophic factors were not studied thoroughly or not at all with respect to their possible effects on the central cholinergic sites (Tables XVIII–XX), and yet they may have such actions in view of their demonstrated effects on, for instance, cholinesterases, as in the case of proteoglycans and glycoproteins (Tables XVIII and XX). It is of interest that second messengers and ACh itself may be included here (Tables XVII and XVIII), and we should be reminded of the controversy, still alive, with respect to the role of ACh in muscle and neuromyal atrophy which follows skeletal muscle denervation (Albuquerque et al., 1972; Gutmann, 1976; Held et al., 1987). Finally, a factor of considerable interest to one of the present authors is the nerve-dependent regeneration factor (mitotic factor) which controls the regeneration of amputated urodele limbs (Table XIX); this factor seems to be generated by peripheral nerves irrespective of their anatomical and biochemical nature (Schotte and Karczmar, 1944; Karczmar, 1946); this chemically poorly identified factor was never tested with respect to nervous structures.

Cholinergic receptors and their molecular biology

It was pointed out above that the molecular biology of the constituents of the cholinergic system such as ChAT, AChE and cholinergic receptors, whether muscarinic or nicotinic and whether pre-or post-synaptic, and the related field of the mapping and structure of these constituents constitute areas of intense current research, and these areas seem to have been insufficiently addressed at our Meetings. Certain aspects of molecular biology and of the mapping of cholinergic receptors will be commented upon at this time.

1. *Structure of cholinergic receptors as it pertains to evolution.* As pointed out by Paul Salvaterra and his associates (Mori et al., 1987), "chemical neurotransmission requires gene products to act in

a coordinated manner during the synthesis, degradation and reception of a neurotransmitter". Thus, ontogenesis and genetics combine to provide the adult organism with effective and harmoniously acting, within themselves and also as they interact with each other, transmitter systems. What really constitutes the basis of this coordination is the structural homology and a lock-and-key fitness of the constituents of these systems.

Salvaterra and his associates (op. cit.; see also Salvaterra et al., 1987) considered this question with respect to ChAT of *Drosophila melanogaster*, the alpha subunit of the rat neuronal nicotinic receptor, and *Torpedo* AChE, and they came up with the concept of two lines of evolution concerning these three constituents of the cholinergic system (Fig. 6). First, they speculate that these cho-

linergic constituents evolved along the line of limited convergent (segmental) evolution presumably from several ancestral proteins; this line concerns sequential amino acid segments (Fig. 6) and may be valid particularly for the ChAT of *Drosophila* and the alpha subunit of the rat neurons.

Second, they note a global homology between major domains of *Drosophila* ChAT and *Torpedo* AChE (Fig. 6), and they also note the resemblance of the domains in question to those of the rat thyroglobulin; altogether, they suggest that the ChAT and AChE antedate thyroglobulin, as the common ancestral gene underlying the evolution of these two cholinergic constituents had "differentiated about 800 million years ago, when vertebrates and invertebrates were evolving separately" (Mori et al., 1987).

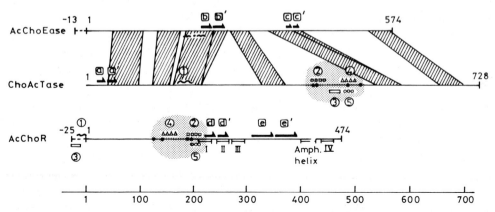

Fig. 6. Schematic representation of structural homologies within and among *Drosophila* ChAT (ChoAcTase), *Torpedo* AChE (AcChoEase), and rat neuronal nicotinic cholinergic receptor (AcCoR), alpha subunit. Each sequence is represented as a line, while a dashed line indicates the signal sequence or the sequence only included in precursors. The amino-terminal position of the *Drosophila* ChAT has not yet been identified; therefore, position 1 only indicates the furthest upstream residue so far sequenced (Itoh et al. (1986)). Homologous regions between ChAT and AChE are indicated by hatching between the two sequences (see also Fig. 1, Mori et al. (1987)). The active-site peptide for AChE is marked by a large asterisk between two thick wavy lines. The circled numbers denote the five homologous segments between ChAT and cholinergic receptor alpha subunit, distinguished by different symbols at approximate positions along each sequence (see also Fig. 2, Mori et al. (1987)). Thick arrows indicate internally duplicated sequences. The four extracellular cysteine residues characteristic of the nicotinic cholinergic receptor alpha subunit (Boulter et al. (1986)) are marked by closed (filled) circles. Also shown by closed (filled) circles are the four cysteine residues in ChAT. These residues are located in the vicinity of the homologous clustered segments 2–5 when comparing ChAT with the cholinergic receptor alpha subunit. The two regions enclosed by stippled ovals include all four cysteine residues and the homologous segments of ChAT and the cholinergic receptor alpha subunit. The transmembrane regions of acetylcholine receptor (I–IV) and the ampipathic helix (Finer-Moore and Stroud (1984); see also the Fig. 7 of this review) are indicated. Amino acid residues are numbered below the lines. With small modifications, this legend is that shown for their Fig. 3 in the Mori et al. (1987) paper. Reprinted by permission from Mori et al. (1987).

The speculative nature of these suggestions must be emphasized. Indeed, systemically and evolutionarily speaking, the forms selected by Salvaterra and his associates are very distant, there are many missing links, and much work with intermediate forms is needed before accepting the speculation in question; this does not subtract from its interest and from the heuristic nature of the molecular approach employed by these investigators.

2. *Structures and mapping of cholinergic receptors*. As already suggested, the subtypes of the nicotinic and muscarinic receptors discussed at our past Meetings as well as at our present Meeting concerned peripheral rather than central receptors. Furthermore, the molecular biology approaches to their mapping and sequencing (see, for example, Raftery et al., 1985) and the encoding of the segments of the receptor-channel macromolecule such as the channel itself (an approach embraced by the Jans (see, for example Timpe et al., 1988, and Schwarz et al., 1988), and additional methodology used to define their membrane spanning regions (cf., for example, Leonard et al., 1988) and their amphipathic, hydrophobic and hydrophilic domains were not presented in any detail at our Meetings.

The latter approach is, perhaps, the one that at this time provided the most definitive — albeit controversial as to its details — picture of the nicotinic receptor and its topography within the neuronal membrane. This picture is due to the researches of Michael Raftery (see Raftery et al., 1985), Changeux (1978; Popot and Changeux, 1984), Eric Barnard (as presented at our last Meeting; Barnard et al., 1987) and Jon Lindstrom and his associates (see Ratnam et al., 1986, and Kubalek et al., 1987). The model proposed by Lindstrom and his associates is presented (Fig. 7; see Ratnam et al., 1986), with the understanding that it may not be definitive. The model, proposed in this case for the alpha subunit of the nicotinic receptor of the *Torpedo*, accounts for the amphipathic, hydrophilic and hydrophobic domains, the polar groupings and the site of the channel, the ACh binding site and the NH$_2$ terminus and its

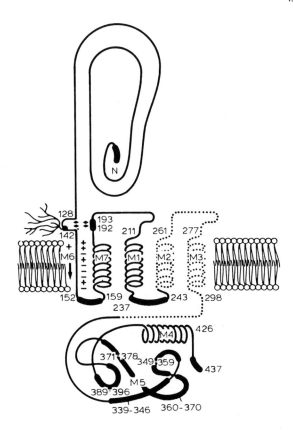

Fig. 7. Diagrammatic representation of a hypothetical model for the transmembrane structure of the alpha subunit of the nicotinic cholinergic receptor of the *Torpedo*. The line depicts the polypeptide backbone on which the positions of some residues is indicated by the appropriate numbers. Thick-line segments indicate sequences whose transmembrane orientation has been explicitly determined by a variety of methods (see Ratnam et al. (1986). Thin-line segments indicate sequences whose transmembrane orientation seems very likely due to constraints placed by the location of surrounding sequences. Dotted-line segments indicate sequences whose transmembrane orientation has yet to be demonstrated. Mi–M7: transmembrane domains. M1–M4 domains are proposed to be hydrophobic; M5 and M7 may be amphipathic alpha helix domains, M7 constituting possibly the lining of the cation channel, regulated by ACh binding at a site near the extracellular surface of this domain; M6 is presumably a hydrophilic domain. N-terminus is represented as extracellular, while C terminus is shown as cytoplasmic. This legend was reconstituted by the present author from the text of the paper of Ratnam et al. (1986) in which the figure originally appeared (see Fig. 9, Ratnam et al., 1986). As pointed out in the text of the paper in question, some of the suggestions described above are speculative and/or controversial. Reprinted by permission from Mori et al. (1986).

position with regard to the cytoplasmic and extracellular neuronal membranes. It must be emphasized in the present context that this model may not, at least in detail, be valid for the central nicotinic receptors, that the anologous studies of the muscarinic, particularly central, receptors are even further from being complete, and that generally much of the research referred to in this paragraph concerns non-mammalian species and other than central cholinergic receptors.

Second messengers, their role and interactions

1. *Second messengers and their function.* The beginning of the story of the two second messenger systems antedates these Meetings, as the pertinent work of the late Sutherland (cf. Sutherland et al., 1968) with cyclic nucleotides and of the Hokins (cf. Hokin and Hokin, 1960) with the phosphatidyl inositol cascade was initiated in the fifties and sixties. At our 1978 Meeting in La Jolla a session was devoted to the cyclic nucleotides as second messengers (see Table V), and their activation via nicotinic and muscarinic stimulation and the character of the "message" (Woody, 1978) were discussed; this subject and that of phosphatidyl inositol was referred to also, rather briefly, at the 1983 Meeting in Oglebay (see Table VII). Thus, the involvement of cAMP-dependent protein kinase in the phosphorylation of the *Torpedo* nicotinic receptor was discussed by Eriksson et al. (1983); Brown and Masters (1983) proposed that the activation in the chicken heart of a single subtype of muscarinic receptor leads, depending on the agonist, to the inhibition of cAMP and/or to the hydrolysis of the phosphatidyl inositol; while Hawthorne and Swilem (1983) pointed out that the phosphatidyl inositol system is exceptional in the case of the bovine adrenal medulla, as its activation in the latter does not mobilize Ca^{2+}, and may have a physiological role which is not yet clearly understood.

There was a hiatus in the discussion of the second messenger systems at the 1987 Buxton Meeting; but at the present Meeting three groups of investigators presented the results of their perti-

nent studies. Joan Brown pursued her studies, referred to above, of the physiological role in the parasympathetic, cardiac ganglia of the two pathways of phosphatidyl inositol hydrolysis, the diacylglycerol (diacyl glycol, DAG) and phosphatidyl inositol triphosphate (IP_3) pathway. The phospatidyl inositol cascade was also investigated by David Lambert and Stephan Nahorski as they dealt with human neuroblastoma cells, that is, a system more akin to the subject of this review; they concluded, similarly to Brown, that a single muscarinic receptor subtype, M_3, subserves the phosphatidyl inositol hydrolysis, its activation resulting in the release of Ca^{2+} and opening of the Ca^{2+} channel. Michael Schimerlik, studying a similar, peripheral muscarinic receptor, that of porcine atria, emphasized the mechanism of the muscarinic activation of a G protein coupler, G_i, as well as suggesting that muscarinic receptor subtypes may differentiate between responses activating cGMP and phosphatidyl inositol systems; it is noteworthy that Schimerlik referred to the interactions between the nucleotide and phospolipid systems.

Three comments should be made at the onset of further discussion of this important and exciting subject. First, besides the two second messenger systems referred to above, other second messenger systems, particularly that activated by Ca^{2+} and mediated by calmodulin and calmodulin-dependent protein kinases, may be distinguished today (see Greengard, 1987); these additional second messenger systems were barely referred to at our Meetings. Second, most of the studies presented so far at our Meetings, including those referred to above, concerned the peripheral rather than the central mechanisms which constitute the prime subject of this presentation; third, full knowledge of the physiological role of the two second messenger systems is still lacking.

Of course, we have a general understanding of that role, and it may be stated summarily that neurotransmitter actions and their modulations (Karczmar, 1987) are mediated by second messengers which initiate kinase-mediated phosphorylations, thus regulating receptor responses, ionic channel closings and openings, and ionic movements, particularly those of Ca^{2+} (cf. Greengard, 1978, 1987); at another level, second messengers seem to mediate trophic and developmental activities, as referred to at this Meeting by Brown (see also Changeux, 1983, and Laufer and Changeux, 1989; see also Table XVIII).

Two specific examples of the possible physiological role of the mechanisms dependent on second messengers and phosphorylations will be adduced, as they are specific, of considerable interest, possibly active centrally, and as the work of Maurice Israel, presented at this Meeting, has a bearing on one of these instances.

The first example concerns the role of a phosphoprotein, synapsin I (previously referred to as protein I), a major substrate for c-AMP-dependent protein kinase; Paul Greengard, a noted investigator for many years now in the area of nucleotide second messengers (Greengard, 1978) must be credited with elucidating its role as a regulator of release of transmitters, including ACh. In the present context, an interesting feature of this protein (see Table XXI) is that it is a major component of the synaptic fractions of the central and peripheral nervous system, concentrating particularly in the nerve terminals. Grengard proposes that the transmitter release is mediated by synapsin I via alteration of its phosphorylation state; this occurs at two regions of this protein and it depends, depending on the region, on calmodulin-Ca^{2+} and c-AMP-dependent kinases.

TABLE XXI

Synapsin I (Protein I) after Greengard (1987): Synapsin Ia; M_r 80,000: Synapsin Ib: M_r 86,000

Present only in central and peripheral neurons
Concentrated in NTs, including cholinergic
Associated with synpatic vesicles
Function: Bridge between cytoskeleton or plasma membrane
        and synaptic vesicles
   Phosphorylation opens up the bridge and/or Synapsin I
   binding to synaptic vesicles
   Consequence: transmitter release (Llinas et al., 1985)

In fact, these processes are initiated by presynaptic activation as well as the drugs which facilitate transmitter release, and Llinas and Greengard (Llinas et al., 1985) were able to demonstrate directly that, in the squid giant synapse at least, injection of synapsin I or of Ca^{2+}-calmodulin-dependent kinase facilitates neurotransmitter release.

As already stated, Greengard hypothesizes that synapsin I constitutes a general mechanism regulating the release of several transmitters. All the more interesting is the work of Maurice Israel (Israel et al., 1987), the latest results of this work being presented at this Meeting, as Israel demonstrates the presence in the nerve terminal membrane of the electric organ of the *Torpedo* as well as of the rat brain synaptosomes of a protein which he calls the mediatophore which is distinct from synapsin I and which is specifically involved in the regulation of the release of ACh — particularly in the nonquantal release.

The second example to be adduced concerns the role of second messenger systems in generating the synaptic processes of desensitization or inactivation of the nicotinic receptor. The phosphorylations of the nicotinic receptor are pertinent here; of course, these processes are immensely interesting on their own. As demonstrated by Raftery and his associates (Vandlen et al., 1979; Raftery et al., 1985), Karlin and his coworkers (Reynolds and Karlin, 1978; Karlin, 1980), Changeux (1981) and others, cholinergic receptor consists of four subunits, alpha, beta, delta, gamma, the alpha unit appearing twice (Fig. 8); the subunits are organized in a rosette, which is not shown in the figure. Subsequently, Huganir and Greengard (1983; for additional references see McGuinness and Greengard, 1987, and Greengard, 1987) demonstrated the presence of three kinases in the *Torpedo* postsynaptic membrane and, importantly, they were able to show that each of them is capable of catalysing one or more of the subunits of the nicotinic receptor of the *Torpedo*, as shown in Fig. 8. Furthermore, ACh does not induce the activation of the kinases

456

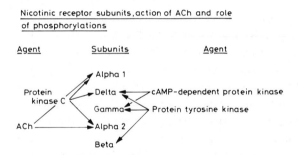

Nicotinic receptor subunits, action of ACh and role of phosphorylations

Fig. 8. Diagrammatic representation of specific phosphorylations evoked by the action of unidentified transmitter or transmitters on the nicotinic receptor of the Torpedo. The subunits of the receptor represented are actually arranged in a rosette to form the ionic channel (see text, and Greengard (1987), Huganir and Greengard (1983), and Ochoa et al. (1988)) — this is not represented in this diagram. Three specific kinases are shown as affecting the subunits in question. ACh is shown as acting on the two variants of the alpha subunit.

in question, and Greengard (1987) proposes that unidentified neurotransmitter or neurotransmitters is or are involved in the phosphorylations in question. It must be added that there is a bit of speculation in this proposal, and there is some controversy particularly with regard to the cAMP-dependent phosphorylation (see, for example, Smilowitz et al., 1981).

What would be the role of these phosphorylations if indeed they do not subserve the transmitter action of ACh? It appears that both in the case of the *Torpedo* receptor (Huganir et al., 1986) and in that of mammalian neuromyal junction (Albuquerque et al., 1986; for further references, see Ochoa et al., 1989, 1988) the phosphorylations underlie the process of desensitization, possibly via allosteric transitions of the receptor structure, particularly in the gamma and delta subunits (see Ochoa et al., 1989; and McNamee, personal communication). While Greengard hypothesized that non-ACh transmitters are involved in the phosphorylations in question (see above, Greengard, 1987; and Fig. 8), it must be noted that ACh itself is a powerful desensitizer (Kim and Karczmar, 1967), as are nicotinic agonists (see Perlman et al., 1987), and further exploration of ACh-mediated desensitization is needed.

Interestingly enough, the other messenger system, the phosphatidyl inositol cascade, may be also involved in desensitization, as the activation of phospholipase C, and the resulting phospholipid breakdown and the generation of the protein kinase activator, DAG, may contribute to desensitization; actually, so may also the generation of IP_3 and the resulting mobilization of Ca^{2+} (Ochoa et al., 1989; Jones et al., 1988). However, the contribution of this typically muscarinic phenomenon to nicotinic desensitization is speculative at this time.

A few additional words are needed with regard to desensitization. Some of us who are present at this Meeting are pioneers in this area, particularly Stephen Thesleff (see Thesleff, 1955; Katz and Thesleff, 1957). The phenomenon is of utmost importance, as it probably serves as a safety valve which protects transmission at the neuromyal junction and elsewhere (Karczmar et al., 1972). Hence, besides Thesleff and Katz, other outstanding investigators such as Magazanik, Vyskocil, Rang and Ritter, Changeux, Albuquerque, Nastuk and Parsons addressed this phenomenon and its mechanism (for references, see Ochoa et al., 1989; Barrett and Magleby, 1976; Karczmar et al., 1972; Karczmar, 1967).

What is significant in the context of this presentation is that desensitization, whether of the cholinergic receptor or of receptors activated by other transmitters, occurs both peripherally and centrally. Actually, Eccles introduced early on the concept of the central cholinergic desensitization as he proposed that the weak muscarinic response of the Renshaw cell (on the muscarinic response of the Renshaw cell, see the interesting paper of Ryall and Haas, which was presented at our 1975 Meeting) may be made apparent by desensitizing the primary response of the Renshaw cell, its nicotinic response (Fig. 9; Eccles, 1964, and personal communication). In fact, a useful maneuver for the identification of centrally acting transmitters consists of attempting to desensitize the site in question to presynaptic stimulation by applying by iontophoresis or pressure injection the

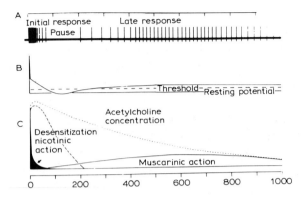

Fig. 9. Diagrammatic representation of the mechanism possibly underlying the overt appearance of the muscarinic response at the Renshaw cell. The initial, nicotinic rapid frequency response is illustrated under A; after a silent period, it is followed by a low-rate, muscarinic response. This triphasic response is related to changes in the response threshold and in the membrane potential (under B); it is also related (under C) to the desensitization that occurs with respect to the nicotinic response at the time of the presence at the membrane of high concentrations of ACh. As desensitization and ACh concentration diminish, the muscarinic response appears (C). From J.C. Eccles, personal communication, reprinted by permission.

suspected transmitter to that site (Dun and Karczmar, 1979).

One additional aspect of the matter at hand must be emphasized, and that is that there exists a reciprocal process, namely the process of sensitization, which was discovered during one of the early studies of the desensitization of the neuromyal junction (Karczmar, 1957, 1967). It subsequently became clear that this process exists with respect to the central cholinergic system as well (Koketsu, 1966; Koketsu and Karczmar, 1966). What is of interest is that, of the many substances studied, many are able to desensitize, including organophosphorus anticholinesterases (this effect of OP anticholinesterases is independent of the desensitizing action of these compounds due their capacity to accumulate ACh), while very few exert a sensitizing action, one of these agents being NaF (Karczmar et al., 1961, 1968; Karczmar and Ohta, 1981). It should be emphasized that NaF is active in the processes of transmethylation and the regulation of membrane fluidity, and in phospholipid metabolism (Hirata and Axelrod, 1978). An im-

portant action of NaF, its sensitizing effect at a central synapse, is illustrated in Fig. 10.

Of course, besides underlying such physiological processes as desensitization and trophic or developmental activities (vide supra), second messengers must fulfill additional physiological phenomena. Some of these, such as the processes of synaptic modulation, were discussed intensely elsewhere (see Karczmar, 1987; Costa et al., 1987), but were barely discussed at our Meetings. The second messengers must play additional, specific roles, and these, indubitably, will be considered at our future Meetings.

2. *Interaction between second messengers.* Are the various second messenger systems functioning independently of each other, or do they interact? If it existed, such interaction should be important as it could provide a point-to-point control of

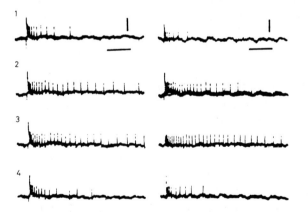

Fig. 10. Facilitation of the cat Renshaw cell discharge by NaF. Records with slower sweep speed are shown in the left hand column. The Renshaw cell discharges were evoked by antidromic stimulation of the ventral root. Tetraethyl pyrophosphate (TEPP), a potent organophosphorus anticholinesterase which penetrates readily into the CNS was given i. v. at a dose (0.05 mg/kg) which inhibits, completely and irreversibly, the central AChE. Records 1 and 2 were obtained before and 20 min after TEPP injection, respectively. NaF (20 mg/kg) was given i.v. immediately after record 2 was taken; records 3 and 4 were obtained 90 s and 3 min, respectively, after NaF administration. Note increase in the spike discharge frequency after TEPP (record 2) and further increase in frequency after NaF (record 3), which was followed by a marked decrease in discharge (record 4). Calibration: 1 mV (right- and left-hand columns); 20 (right hand column) and 40 (left-hand column) ms. Reprinted by permission from Koketsu (1966).

transmission that would include positive and negative feedback regulations. It should be pointed out that the neurotransmitters are involved in such interactions, as several types of the effects of transmitters — both pre- and post-synaptic — underlie the modulations of transmission (see above; Karczmar, 1987); presumably, second messenger systems are involved in these modulations.

Actually, that interactions between second messengers do exist was already intimated above, as such an interaction was described with respect to the phenomenon of desensitization; in this case, protein kinase C may be activatable not only by a specific non-ACh neurotransmitter as suggested by Greengard (see above; Greengard, 1987), but also by the breakdown of inositol phospholipids initiated by the activation of phospholipase C, and the resulting generation of DAG and IP_3 (Nishizuka, 1984 and 1986). Yet the important subject of interactions between second messengers was barely broached at our Meetings, although at this Meeting Schimerlik spoke of the relationship between the activation of the phosphatidyl inositol cascade and adenylate cyclase inhibition.

In fact, if one wishes to demonstrate the interaction between second messengers via showing that certain drugs and endogenous agents affect more than one second messenger system, and, more specifically, both the nucleotides and inositol phospholipids, a multitude of pertinent examples can be adduced, and just about any type of combined effect seems possible (Tables XXII and XXIII).

Actually, the phenomenon described at this Meeting by Schimerlik, i.e., the negative feedback exerted by the activation of the phosphatidyl inositol system on adenylate cyclase, was described by several investigators (Jakobs et al., 1979; Birdsall and Hulme, 1983; Horwitz, 1989; Horwitz and Perlman, 1987), although the mechanism of this negative feedback is uncertain (Horwitz, 1987).

As already stated, the relation between the effects of various compounds on the two systems may have just about any sign, depending on the site and compound; in the case of certain sites or

TABLE XXII

Interaction between cyclic nucleotides (cAMP and cGMP) and phosphatidyl inositol (PI) second messenger systems

---

I. Compounds activating both systems
  forskolin, isoproterenol, LH, TSH (chick myotubes, thyroid cells, cortex, endocrines)
  CGRP (chick myotubes)
  ACh (bronchiolar smooth muscle)

II. Compounds activating cAMP and/or cGMP systems which block PI turnover
  dibutyryl cAMP; theophylline; prostaglandins E_1, E_2; prostacyclin; alpha$_1$-adrenoceptors (rat, kidney, human platelets and neutrophils)

For references to Tables XXII and XXIII, see the text, and Laufer and Changeux, 1989; Nishizuka, 1984, 1986; Horwitz, 1989; Perlman et al., 1987; Hollingworth et al., 1985; Berridge, 1987; Neylon and Summers, 1988; Watson et al., 1984; Rhee et al., 1988; Labarca et al., 1984; Smith and Harden, 1985.

agents, the activation of inositol phospholipid metabolism may ultimately result, following early inhibition, in the activation of adenylate cyclase, or, indeed, lead to cyclic AMP accumulation not preceded by inhibition of adenylate cyclase (Table XXIII; cf., for example, Hollingworth et al., 1985; Laufer and Changeux, 1989). There may be also a separate group of compounds which seem to stimulate both systems simultaneously (Table XXII; cf. Berridge, 1987). Conversely, there are compounds such as theophylline and certain prostaglandins which activate the nucleotide systems

TABLE XXIII

Interaction between cyclic nucleotides (cAMP and cGMP) and phosphatidyl inositol (PI) second messenger systems

---

III. Compounds activating P.I. turnover
  (1) Inhibit and subsequently sensitize adenylcyclase
    ACh muscarinic agonists (pituitary tumor, heart)
  (2) Inhibit adenylcyclase and cAMP accumulation
    oxotremorine, muscarine (PC12)
  (3) Accumulate cAMP
    beta agonists, adenosine, VIP, 5-HT$_1$ and 5-HT$_2$ agonists (brain, pineal gland, RBCs);

    Positive feedback action on P.I. turnover
    VIP
  (4) Activate cGMP system via eicosanoid release
    leucotrienes, prostaglandins (platelets, erythrocytes)

---

while they block the phosphatidyl inositol turnover (Table XXII; for references, see Berridge, 1987, and Zigmond et al., 1989).

Can one make sense of these multiple interactions? At least, it seems possible to classify these events and suggest the primary events. Thus, the discoverer of the protein kinase C, Yasutomi Nishizuka (see Takai et al., 1977), stresses the role of this kinase and its activation of DAG as both a second messenger for growth and related processes, and an important link in the positive and negative feedback processes regulating the interaction between the two second messenger systems (Nishizuka, 1984, 1986). Nishizuka juxtaposes "bidirectional control systems", where cAMP-dependent protein kinase A and DAG-dependent protein kinase C exert a negative feedback on each other, and "monodirectional control systems", in which case the two kinases synergize with each other (Fig. 11). While the scheme proposed by Nishizuka is based particularly on the results obtained with platelets, lymphocytes and pituitary and developing cells (see Fig. 11), it may also hold for neurotransmitter action on the cardiac muscle as well as

the cortex and hippocampus, Na/K ATPase function, and channel processes (Berridge, 1987; Nishizuka, 1984, 1986).

However, the exact mechanisms underlying these interactions and regulations are unknown; several important areas may be cited in this context. First, the molecular mechanism underlying the activation of the G proteins — the first step in activating the two second messenger systems — is largely unknown. Second, precise knowledge of the pathways of the nucleotide and inositol phospholipid metabolism is still lacking. For example, DAG may be generated via the muscarinic activation of lipases other than phospholipase C, and be formed from other phospholipid sources than inositol diphosphate (IP2).

Finally, only speculations may be adduced with respect to the modes of the interaction between the second messenger systems. One such mode may concern the G proteins, as they exhibit common subunits, namely the subunits beta and gamma; the activation of one G protein may free these subunits, which can then bind to the alpha subunits of another G protein, thus affecting its

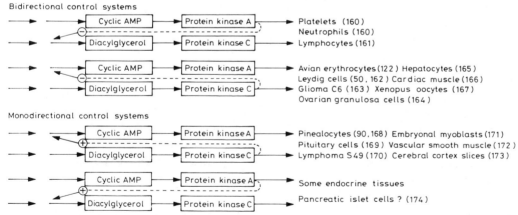

Fig. 11. Diagrammatic presentation of the modes of interaction of two major signal-transducing (second messenger) systems, phosphatidyl inositol–protein kinase C system and a cyclic nucleotide system, the cAMP-dependent protein kinase A system. Two types of interaction are indicated, interactions resulting in a negative feedback (bidirectional control systems), and interactions resulting in synergisms or potentiations (monodirectional control systems). Tissues exhibiting the effects in question are shown on the right; the effects concern mostly — but not always — trophic and related actions; see also Text. Numbers in parenthesis indicate references cited in the original paper (Nishizuka (1986)). The legend for the original figure (Fig. 3, Nishizuka, 1986) was slightly expanded. Reprinted by permission from Nishizuka (1986).

function (Perlman, personal communication). Also, phosphorylations mediated by one system may modulate the function of the other system, whether via phosphorylation of G protein, receptors or effector enzymes. In addition, Ca^{2+}-dependent processes and Ca^{2+} mobilization, generated by a second messenger system or a particular transmitter, may modulate the function of another second messenger system. Thus, the marked rise in intracellular calcium characteristically mediated by nicotinic stimulation may activate both the inositol phospholipid cascade and adenylate cyclase.

These important problems, largely untouched at our Meetings and, for that matter, unresolved elsewhere, should be emphasized at our next Meeting.

Envoi

As stressed in this review and as emphasized at this Meeting by Nordberg, Mesulam, Gottfries and Appel in their Session on the Future Prospects of Research on Central Cholinergic Mechanisms, the central cholinergic system has come a long way since the sixties of the last century and since our first Meeting in Skokloster, and it has a long way to go!

The "cholinergikers" are notoriously resourceful and creative; it is not easy to predict the areas which they will attack in the future and, by definition, it is impossible to foresee the discoveries which they will make. However, perhaps the areas which seem to offer most promise may be listed without too much risk.

First, much attention will indubitably be paid to molecular aspects of the central cholinergic system; the molecular investigations of the genetic and ontogenetic control of the synchronization of the appearance of the constituents of the central cholinergic system during development of transmission and function will gain additional impetus in the years to come, as will the investigations of the molecular and structural aspects of these constituents, including particularly the central nicotinic and muscarinic receptors.

Second, much remains to be done to identify *all* the trophic factors which may be involved in the development of the central cholinergic system as well as in the processes of regeneration and plasticity of that system — the concept of its plasticity being, indeed, new and revolutionary.

Third, there is the question of the interaction between cholinergic and non-cholinergic transmission. What must be further explored in this case is the morphology and the circuitry which underlie this interaction, as well as the transmittive and functional consequences of this interaction. Investigations of the related topic of the modulation of cholinergic transmission and function will be similarly expanded.

Fourth, much was done in the last thirty years in the area of second messengers, and much more must be still accomplished. The identification of *all* second messengers, the definiton of the metabolic pathways involved and the clarification of the phosphorylation sites and mechanisms are needed. Another related area is that of the physiological significance of the second messenger systems, with regard to both central transmission and other central processes, including sensitization, desensitization and modulation of transmission and function. What promises to be the exciting related area of research is the area of interactions between the second messenger systems, their mechanisms, and their relation to the interactions between central neurotransmitters.

Fifth, the formation of ACh and choline must be further explored, and, particularly, the role of the precursors of both ACh and choline in the synthesis of ACh in the CNS, and the relation between ACh and phospholipid metabolism must be better understood, as these matters are important both on the basic level and for the treatment of diseases related to central cholinergic deficit. In this context, the question of the treatment of Alzheimer dementia and other central diseases with cholinergic correlates is wide open, or more precisely, completely unresolved!

Sixth, there is a question of the development of cholinergic or anticholinergic drugs which may be useful centrally, and the review presented at this Meeting by Don Jenden constitutes a heuristic departure in this regard. Indeed, there is a paradox here: while cholinergic and anticholinergic drugs are widely used for the treatment of peripheral disease and in anesthesia, and while the central cholinergic system is important in an array of functions, behaviors and diseases — as emphasized in this review — yet cholinergic and anticholinergic drugs that may be useful for the pertinent therapy have not been developed so far.

Finally, much remains to be done for elucidating in terms of these various central mechanisms and processes the multiple phenomena of behavior. In this context, the sadly neglected area is that of the role of the cholinergic system in the OEI — a role important for both learning and perception — and, indeed, consciousness!

Altogether, it seems that we will have our hands full, prior to and at our next Meeting in Montreal, and in fact, for many Meetings to come.

Acknowledgements

Some of the research from this laboratory and Dr. N.J. Dun's laboratory referred to in this review was supported by NIH grants NS06455, NS15858, RR05368, NS16348 and GM77, VA Grant 4830, grants from Potts and M.E. Ballwebber Foundations, and Senior Fullbright (1987–1988) and Guggenheim (1969–1970) Fellowships.

Dr. R. L. Perlman of the U. of Chicago and Dr. J. Nawrocki of Hines VA Hospital discussed with this author certain portions of this review; their help is gratefully acknowledged, as is that of Ms. J. Mixter, Reference Librarian, Loyola U. Medical Center. Special thanks are due to Ms. Corrine Arthur for expert secretarial help.

References

Adams, P.R., Brown, D.A. and Constanti, A. (1982) M-currents and other potassium currents in bullfrog sympathetic neurones. *J. Physiol. (Lond.)*, 330: 537–572.

Albuquerque, E.X., Warwick, J.E., Tasse, J.R. and Samsone, F.M. (1972) Effects of vinblastine and colchicine on neural regulation of the fast and slow skeletal muscles of the rat. *Exp. Neurol., 38:* 607–634.

Albuquerque, E.X., Deshpande, S.S., Aracava, Y., Alkondon, M. and Daly, J.W. (1986) A possible involvement of cyclic AMP in the expression of desensitization of the nicotinic acetylcholine receptor. *FEBS Lett.,* 199: 113–120.

Ansell, G.B. and Spanner, S. (1970) The origin and turnover of choline in the brain. In E. Heilbronn and A. Winters (Eds.), *Drugs and Cholinergic Mechanisms in the CNS*, Forsvarets Forskningsanstalt, Stockholm, pp. 143–162.

Ansell, G.B., Soppitt, A.J. and Spanner, S. (1987) The effect of lithium and physostigmine on levels of glutamate, aspartate and gamma-aminobutyrate in rat brain. In M.J. Dowdall and J.N. Hawthorne, (Eds.), *Cellular and Molecular Basis of Cholinergic Function*, pp. 789–193, Ellis Horwood, Ltd., Chichester.

Appel, S.H., McManaman, J.K., Smith, R.G., Vaca, K.W. and Bostwick, J.R. (1987) Cholinergic trophic factors from skeletal muscle and hippocampus. In M.J. Dowdall and J.N. Hawthorne (Eds.), *Cellular and Molecular Basis of Cholinergic Function*, pp. 401–410, Ellis Horwood, Ltd., Chichester.

Aprison, M.H. and Hintgen, N.J. (1970) Evidence of a central cholinergic mechanism functioning during drug induced excitation in avoidance behavior. In E. Heilbronn and A. Winters, (Eds.), *Drugs and Cholinergic Mechanisms in the CNS*, pp. 543–562, Forsvarets Forskningsanstalt, Stockholm.

Aquilonius, S.-M., Askmark, H., Ebendal, T. and Gillberg, P.-G. (1987) Neuropharmacology of motor neuron disease. In M.J. Dowdall and J.N. Hawthorne (Eds.), *Cellular and Molecular Basis of Cholinergic Function*, pp. 729–735, Ellis Horwood, Ltd., Chichester.

Baghdoyan, H.A., Rodrigo-Angulo, M.L., McCarley, R.W. and Hobson, J.A. (1987) A neuroanatomical gradient in the pontine tegmentum for the cholinoceptive induction of desynchronized sleep signs. *Brain Res.,* 414: 245–264.

Barker, L.A., Dowdall, M.J., Essman, W.B. and Whittaker, V.P. (1970) The compartmentalization of acetylcholine in cholinergic nerve terminals In E. Heilbronn and A. Winter (Eds.), *Drugs and Cholinergic Mechanisms in the CNS*, pp. 193–224, Forsvarets Forskningsanstalt, Stockholm.

Barnard, E.A., Beeson, D.M.W., Cockroft, V.B. Darlison, M.G., Hicks, A.A., Lai, F.A., Moss, S.J. and Squire, M.D. (1987) Molecular biology of nicotinic acetylcholine receptors from chicken muscle and brain. In M.J. Dowdall and J.N.H. Hawthorne (Eds.), *Cellular and Molecular Basis of Cholinergic Function*, pp. 15–32, Ellis Horwood, Ltd., Chichester.

Barrett, E.F. and Magleby, K.L. (1976) Physiology of cholinergic transmission. In A.M. Goldberg and I. Hanin (Eds.), *Biology of Cholinergic Function*, pp. 29–100, Raven Press, N.Y..

Bartholow, R. (1973) The antagonism between atropia and physostigmia. *Clinic,* 5: 61–63.

Berridge, M.J. (1987) Inositol triphosphate and diacylglycerol: two interacting second messengers. *Annu. Rev. Biochem.,* 56: 159–193.

462

Birdsall, N.J.M. and Hulme, E.C. (1983) Muscarinic receptor subclasses. *Trends Pharmacol. Sci.,* 4: 459–463.

Black, I.B., Coughlin, M.D. and Cochard, P. (1979) Factors regulating neuronal differentiation. *Soc. Neurosci. Symp.,* 4: 184–207.

Blusztajn, J.K. and Wurtman, R.J. (1983) Choline and cholinergic neurons. *Science,* 221: 614–620.

Blusztajn, J.K., Licovitch, M., Richardson, U.I. and Wurtman, R.J. (1987) Phosphatidylcholine as a precursor of choline for acetylcholine synthesis. In M.J. Dowdall and J.N. Hawthorne (Eds.), *Cellular and Molecular Basis of Cholinergic Function,* pp. 341–346, Ellis Horwood, Ltd., Chichester.

Boulter, J., Evans, K., Goldman, D., Martin, G., Heinemann, S. and Patrick, J. (1986) *Nature,* 319: 368–374.

Brown, J.H., (Ed.) (1989) *The Muscarinic Receptors.* Humana Press, Clifton, N.J..

Brown, J.H. and Masters, S.B. (1983) Differential effects of carbachol and oxotremorine on muscarinic receptors, cyclic AMP formation, and phosphoinositide turnover in chick heart cells. In I. Hanin, (Ed.), *Dynamics of Cholinergic Function,* pp. 939–946, Plenum Press, New York.

Bueker, E.D. (1948) Implantation of tumors in the hind limb field of the embryonic chick and the developmental response of the lumbosacral nervous system. *Anat. Rec.,* 102: 369–389.

Butcher, J.L and Woolf, N.J. (1986) Cholinergic systems in the central nervous system: Retrospection, anatomic distribution, and functions. In I. Hanin (Ed.), *Dynamics of Cholinergic Function,* pp. 1–10, Plenum Press, New York.

Buznikov, G.A. (1984) The action of nuerotransmitters and related substances on early embryogenesis. *Pharmac. Ther.,* 25: 23–59.

Changeux, J.-P. (1981) The acetylcholine receptor. An allosteric membrane protein. *Harvey Lect.,* 75: 85–255.

Changeux, J.-P. (1983) Concluding remarks: on the "singularity" of nerve cells and their ontogenesis. *Progr. Brain Res.,* 58: 465–478.

Costa, E., Chuang, D.M., Guidotti, A. and Hollenbeck, R. (1978) Control of nuclear function in chromaffin cells by persistent activation of nicotinic receptors. In D.J. Jenden, (Ed.), *Cholinergic Mechanisms and Psychopharmacology,* pp. 267–283, Plenum Press, N.Y..

Costa, E., Hanbauer, I. and Guidotti, A. (1987) Receptor-receptor interactions in the modulation of nicotinic receptors in adrenal medulla. In N.J. Dun and R.L. Perlman, (Eds.), *Neurobiology of Acetylcholine, Symposium Held in Honor of Alexander G. Karczmar,* pp. 355–368, Plenum Press, N.Y..

Crossland, J. (1970) Acetylcholine and the morphine abstinence syndrome. In E. Heilbronn and A. Winters (Eds.), *Drugs and Cholinergic Mechanisms in the CNS,* pp. 355–359, Forsvarets Forskningsanstalt, Stockholm.

Cuello, A.C., Stephens, P.H., Garofalo, L., Maysinger, D. and Tagari, P.C. (1987) Cortical damage and the effects of sialoganglioside GM1 on forebrain cholinergic neurons. In M.J. Dowdall and J.N. Hawthorne (Eds.), *Cellular and Molecular Basis of Cholinergic Function,* pp. 389–394, Ellis Horwood, Ltd., Chichester.

Dale, H.H. (1938) Acetylcholine as a chemical transmitter substance of the effects of nerve impulses. The William Henry Welch Lectures, *J. Mt. Sinai Hosp.,* 4: 401–429.

De Robertis, E., Fiszer de Plazas, S., La Torre, J.L. and Lunt, G.S. (1970) Proteolytic cholinergic receptors isolated from the central nervous system and electric tissue. In E. Heilbronn and A. Winters (Eds.), *Drugs and Cholinergic Mechanisms in the CNS,* pp. 505–520, *Forsvarets Forskningsanstalt,* Stockholm.

Dennis, M.J. (1981) Development of the neuromuscular junction: inductive interactions between cells. *Annu. Rev. Neurosci.,* 4: 43–88.

Dun, N.J. and Karczmar, A.G. (1979) Action of substance P on symapathetic neurons. *Neuropharmacol.,* 18: 215–218.

Eccles, J.C. (1964) *The Physiology of Synapses.* Springer-Verlag, Heidelberg.

Eccles, J.C. (1987) The story of the Renshaw cell. In *Neurobiology of Acetylcholine, Symposium Held in Honor of A.G. Karczmar,* N.J. Dun and R.L. Perlman (Eds.), pp. 189–194, Plenum Press, New York.

Eccles, J.C., Fatt, P. and Koketsu, K. (1953) Cholinergic and inhibitory synapses in a central nervous pathway. *Australian J. Sci., 16:* 50–54.

Eccles, J.C., Fatt, P. and Koketsu, K. (1954) Cholinergic and inhibitory synapses in a pathway from motor-axon collaterals to motoneurons. *J. Physiol. (Lond.),* 126: 524–562.

Eriksson, H., Salmonsson, R. Liljeqvist, G. and Heilbronn, E. (1983) Studies on cAMP-dependent protein kinase obtained from nicotinic receptor-bearing microsacs. In I. Hanin (Ed.), *Dynamics of Cholinergic Function,* pp. 933–937, Plenum Press, N.Y..

Fibiger, H.C. and Lehmann, J. (1981) Anatomical organization of some cholinergic systems in the mammalian forebrain. In G. Pepeu and H. Ladinsky (Eds.), *Cholinergic Mechanisms,* pp. 663–672, Plenum Press, N.Y..

Finer-Moore, J. and Stroud, R.M. (1984) *Proc. Natl. Acad. Sci. USA,* 81: 155–159.

Fox, C.F., Linsley, P.S. and Wrann, M. (1982) Receptor remodeling and regulation in the action of epidermal growth factor. *Fed. Proc.,* 41: 2988–2995.

Gage, F.H. and Bjorklund, A. (1987) Trophic and growth regulating mechanisms in the central nervous system monitored by intracerebral neural transplants. *CIBA Found. Symp.,* 126: 143–159.

Gerebtzoff, M.A. (1959) *Cholinesterases.* Pergamon Press, London.

Gilman, A.G. (1984) G proteins and dual control of adenylate cyclase. *Cell, 36:* 577.

Gnahn, H., Hefti, F., Heumann, R., Schwab, M.E. and Thoenen, H. (1983) MGF-mediated increase of choline acetyltransferase (ChAT) in the neonatal rat brain: Evidence for a physiological role of NGF in the brain? *Dev. Brain Res.,* 9: 45–52.

Gospodarowicz, D. (1981) Epidermal and nerve growth factors in mammalian development. *Annu. Rev. Physiol.,* 43: 251–263.

Greene, L. A. and Shooter, E.M. (1980) The nerve growth

factor: Biochemistry, synthesis and mechanism of action. *Annu. Rev. Neurosci.,* 3: 353–402.

Greengard, P. (1978) *Cyclic Nucleotides, Phosphorylated Proteins and Neuronal Function.* Raven Press, New York.

Greengard, P. (1987) Neuronal phosphoproteins. *Mol. Neurobiol.,* 1: 81–119.

Guth, L. (1986) "Trophic" influences of nerve on muscle. *Physiol. Rev.,* 48: 645–687.

Gutmann, E. (1976) Neurotrophic relations. *Annu. Rev. Physiol.,* 38: 177–216.

Harper, G.P. and Thoenen, H. (1981) Target cells, biological effects, and mechanism of action of nerve growth factor and its antibodies. *Annu. Rev. Pharamcol.,* 21: 205–229.

Hawthorne, J.N. and Swilem, A-M. F. (1983) Polyphosphoinositide and phosphoprotein reponses to muscarinic receptor activation in bovine adrenal medulla. In I. Hanin (Ed.), *Dynamics of Cholinergic Function.* pp. 947–951, Plenum Press, New York.

Held, I.R., Syers, S.T., Yeoh, H.C. and McLane, J.A. (1987) Role of cholinergic neuromuscular transmission in the neuroregulation of the autophosphorylatable regulatory subunit of cyclic AMP-dependent protein kinase type II and the acetylcholine receptor content in skeletal muscle. *Brain Res.,* 407: 341–350.

Hendry, I.A. (1976) Control in the development of the vertebrate sympathetic nervous system. In S. Ehrenpreis and I.J. Kopin (Eds.), *Reviews of Neurosciences,* vol. 2, pp. 149–194, Raven Press, New York.

Hendry, I.A. and Iversen, L.L. (1973) Changes in tissue and plasma concentrations of nerve growth factor following removal of the submaxillary glands in adult mice and their effects on the sympathetic nervous system. *Nature,* 243: 500–504.

Hintgen, N.J. and Aprison, M.H. (1976) Behavioral and experimental aspects of the cholinergic system. In A.M. Goldberg and I. Hanin (Eds.), *Biology of Cholinergic Function,* pp. 515–566, Raven Press, New York.

Hirata, F. and Axelrod, J. (1978) Enzymatic synthesis and rapid translocation of phosphatidylcholine by two methyltransferases in erythrocyte membranes. *Proc. Natl. Acad. Sci. USA,* 75: 2348.

Hokin, M.R. and Hokin, L.E. (1960) The role of phosphatidic acid and phosphoinositide in transmembrane transport elicited by acetylcholine and other humoral agents. *Int. Rev. Neurobiol.,* 2: 99–136

Hollingsworth, E.B., Sears, E.B. and Daly, J.W. (1985) *FEBS Lett.,* 184: 339–342.

Holmstedt, B. and Liljestrand, G. (1963) *Readings in Pharmacology.* Pergamon Press, Oxford.

Horwitz, J. (1989) Muscarinic receptor stimulation increases inositol-phospholipid metabolism and inhibits cyclic AMP accumulation in PC12 cells. *J. Neurochem.,* (in press).

Horwitz, J. and Perlman, R.L. (1987) Measurement of inositol phospholipid metabolism in PC12 pheochromocytoma cells. *Methods Enzymol.,* 141: 169–175.

Huganir, R.L., Delcour, A.H., Greengard, P. and Hess, G.P. (1986) Phosphorylation of the nicotinic acetylcholine recep-

tor regulates its rate of desensitization. *Nature,* 321: 774–776.

Huganir, R.L. and Greengard, P. (1983) cAMP-dependent protein kinase phosphorylates the nicotinic acetylcholine receptor. *Proc. Natl. Acad. Sci. USA,* 80: 1130–1134.

Israel, M. (1987) The release of acetylcholine: An approach to its molecular mechanism. In M.J. Dowdall and J.N. Hawthorne (Eds.), *Cellular and Molecular Basis of Cholinergic Function,* pp. 232–244, Ellis Horwood, Ltd., Chichester.

Israel, M., Meunier, F.M., Morel, N. and Lesbats, B. (1987) *J. Neurochem.,* 49: 975–982.

Itoh, N., Slemmon, J.R., Crawford, G.D., Morita, E., Itakura, K., Hawke, D., Shively, J.E., Williamson, R. and Salvaterra, P.M. (1986) *Proc. Natl. Acad. Sci. USA,* 83: 4081–4085.

Jakobs, B.H., Aktories, K. and Schultz, G. (1979) GTP-dependent inhibition of cardiac adenylate cyclase by muscarinic cholinergic agonists. *Arch. Pharmacol.,* 310: 113–119.

Jiang, Z.G. and Dun, N.J. (1986) Presynaptic suppression of excitatory postsynaptic potentials in rat ventral horn neurons by muscarinic agonists. *Brain Res.,* 381: 182–186.

Jones, O.T., Eubanks, J.H., Earnest, J.P. and McNamee, M.G. (1988) A minimum number of lipids are required to support the functional properties of the nicotinic acetylcholine receptor. *Biochem.,* 27: 3733–3742

Karczmar, A.G. (1946) The role of amputation and nerve resection in the regressing limbs of urodele larvae. *J. Exp. Zool.,* 103: 401–427.

Karczmar, A.G. (1957) Antagonism between a bis-quaternary oxamide, WIN 8078, and depolarizing and competitive blocking agents. *J. Pharmacol. Exp. Therap.,* 119: 39–47.

Karczmar, A.G. (1967) Multiple mechanisms of action of drugs at the neuromyal junction as studied in the light of the phenomenon of "reversal". *Laval Medical,* 38: 465–480.

Karczmar, A.G. (1969) Is the central cholinergic nervous system overexploited? *Fed. Proc.,* 28: 147–157.

Karczmar, A.G. (Ed.) (1970) Introduction: History of research with anticholinesterase agents. In *Anticholinesterase Agents,* vol. 1, Section 13, Interntl. Encyclop. Pharmacol. Therap., pp. 1–44, Pergamon Press, Oxford.

Karczmar, A.G. (1978) Multitransmitter mechanism underlying selected function, particularly aggression, learning and sexual behavior. In P. Deniker, C. Radouco Thomas and A. Villeneuve (Eds.), *Neuropsychopharmacology, Proc. 10th Congress CINP,* vol. 1, pp. 581–608, Pergamon Press, Oxford.

Karczmar, A.G. (1979a) Brain acetylcholine and animal electrophysiology. In K.L. Davis and P.A. Berger (Eds.), *Brain Acetylcholine and Neuropsychiatric Disease,* pp. 265–310, Plenum Press, N.Y..

Karczmar, A.G. (1979b) Possible mechanism underlying the so-called "Divorce" phenomena of EEG desynchronizing actions of anticholinesterases. Regional Midwest EEG Meeting.

Karczmar, A.G. (1984) Acute and long lasting central actions of organophosphorus agents. *Fund. Appl. Toxicol.,* 2: S1–S17.

Karczmar, A.G. (1986) Conference on dynamics of cholinergic function: overview and comments. In I. Hanin (Ed.), *Dynamics of Cholinergic Function*, pp. 1215–1259, Plenum Press, New York.

Karczmar, A.G. (1987) Introduction to the session on modulators. *Neuropharmacology*, 26: 1019–1026.

Karczmar, A.G. (1988) Schizophrenia and cholinergic system. In A.G. Sen and T. Lee (Eds.), *Receptors and Ligands in Psychiatry*, pp. 29–63, Cambridge University Pree, Cambridge.

Karczmar, A.G. (1990) Central cholinergic system, memory and environment-organism interactions. In L. Ravizza (Ed.), *La Memoria e le Memorie*, Torino-St Vincent (in Press).

Karczmar, A.G. and Ohta, Y. (1981) Neuromyopharmacology as related to anticholinesterase action. *Fund. Appl. Toxicol.*, 1: S135–S142.

Karczmar, A.G., Kim, K.C. and Koketsu, K. (1961) Endplate effects and antagonism of d-tubocurarine and decamethonium by tetraethylammonium and methoxyambenonium. *J. Pharmacol. Exp. Therap.*, 134: 199–205.

Karczmar, A.G., Koketsu, K. and Soeda, S. (1968) Possible reactivating and sensitizing action of neuromyally acting agents. *Int. J. Neuropharmacol.*, 7: 241–252.

Karczmar, A.G., Nishi, S. and Blaber, L.C. (1972) Synaptic modulations. In A.G. Karczmar and J.C. Eccles (Eds.), *Brain and Human Behavior*, pp. 63–92, Springer-Verlag, Berlin.

Karlin, A. (1980) In C.W. Cotman, C.W., G. Poste and G.L. Nicolson (Eds.), *The Cell Structure and Function*, pp. 191–260, Elsevier/North Holland, Amsterdam.

Katz, B. and Thesleff, S. (1957) A study of the "desensitization" produced by acetylcholine at the motor end plate. *J. Physiol. (Lond.)*, 138: 63–80.

Kim, K.C. and Karczmar, A.G. (1967) Adaptation of the neuromuscular junction to constant concentration of acetylcholine. *Int. J. Neuropharmacol.*, 6: 51–61.

Kimura, H., McGeer, P.L., Peng, J.H. and McGeer, E.G. (1980) Choline acetyltransferase containing neurons in rodent brain by immunohistochemistry. *Science*, 208: 1057–1059.

Koelle, G.B. (Ed.) (1963) Cytological distributions and physiological functions of cholinesterases. In *Cholinesterases and Anticholinesterase Agents*, pp. 187–298, Handbch. d. exper. Pharmakol., vol. 15, Springer-Verlag, Berlin.

Koelle, G.B. (1970) Improvement in the accuracy of histochemical localization of acetylcholinesterase. In E. Heilbronn and A. Winters (Eds.), *Drugs and Cholinergic Mechanisms in the CNS*, pp. 431–440, Forsvarets Forskningsanstalt, Stockholm.

Koketsu, K. (1966) Restorative action of fluoride on synaptic transmission blocked by organophosphorus anticholinesterases. *Int. J. Neuropharmacol.*, 5: 257–254.

Koketsu, K. (1987) Modulation by neurotransmitters of the nicotinic transmission in the vertebrates. In *Neurobiology of Acetylcholine, Symposium Held in Honor of Alexander G. Karczmar*, pp. 225–238, Plenum Press, New York.

Koketsu, K. and Karczmar, A.G. (1966) Action of NaF at various cholinergic synapses. *Fed. Proc.*, 25: 627.

Koketsu, K., Karczmar, A.G. and Kitamura R. (1969) Acetylcholine depolarization of the dorsal root terminals in the amphibian spinal cord. *Int. J. Neuropharmacol.*, 8: 329–336.

Kubalek, E., Ralston, S., Lindstrom, J. and Unwin, N. (1987) Location of subunits within the acetylcholine receptor by electron image analysis of tubular crystals from *Torpedo marmorata*. *J. Cell Biol.*, 105: 9–18.

Labarca, R., Janowsky, A., Patel, J. and Paul, S.M. (1984) Phorbol esters inhibit agonist-induced [^{3}H]inositol-1-phosphate accumulation in rat hippocampual cells. *Biochem. Biophys. Res. Commun.*, 123: 703–709.

Larsson, C. and Nordberg, A. (1986) Characterization of [^{3}H]-nicotine binding in rodent brain and comparison with the binding of other labelled nicotinic ligands. In I. Hanin (Ed.), *Dynamics of Cholinergic Function*, pp. 429–437, Plenum Press, New York.

Laufer, R. and Changeux, J.-P. (1989) Calcitonin gene-related peptide and cyclic AMP stimulate phosphoinositide turnover in skeletal muscle cells. *J. Biol. Chem.*, 264: 2683–2689.

Leonard, R.J., Labarca, C.G., Charnet, P., Davidson, N. and Lester, H.A. (1988) Evidence that the M2 membrane-spanning region lines the ion channel, pore of the nicotinic receptor. *Science*, 242: 1578–1581.

Levi-Montalcini, R. and Angeletti, P.U. (1968) Nerve growth factor. *Physiol. Rev.*, 48: 534–569.

Lewis, P.R and Shute, C.C.D. (1967) The cholinergic limbic syetm: Projections to hippocampal formation, medial cortex, nuclei of ascending cholinergic reticular system, and the subfornical organ and supra-optic crest. *Brain*, 90: 521–540.

Libet, B. (1970) Generation of slow inhibitory and excitatory postsynaptic potentials. *Fed. Proc.*, 29: 1945–1956.

Llinas, R., McGuinness, T.L., Leonard, C.S., Sugimori, M. and Greengard, P. (1985) Intraterminal injection of Synapsin I or calcium/calmodulin-dependent protein kinase II alters neurotransmitter release at the squid giant synapse. *Proc. Natl. Acad. Sci. USA*, 82: 3035–3039.

Marczynski, T.J. (1978) Neurochemical mechanisms in the genesis of slow potentials: A review and some clinical implications. In D. Otto (Ed.), *Multidisciplinary Perspectives in Events Related to Brain Potential Research*, pp. 23–35, Environmental Protection Agency, Washington, D.C.

McGuinness, T.L. and Greengard, P. (1987) Protein phosphorylation and synaptic transmission. In L.C. Sellin, Libelius, R. and Thesleff, S. (Eds.), *Neuromuscular Junction*, pp. 111–124, Elsevier Science Publs., Amsterdam.

McGeer, P.L., McGeer, E.G., Kimura, H. and Peng, J.-F. (1986) Cholinergic neurons and cholinergic projections in the mammalian CNS. In I. Hanin (Ed.), *Dynamics of Cholinergic Function*, pp. 11–22, Plenum Press, New York.

McGeer, P.L., Eccles, J.C. and McGeer, E.G. (1987) *Molecular Biology of Mammalian Brain*. Plenum Press, New York, 2nd Edition.

Meisami, E. and Brazier, M.A.B. (Eds.) (1979) *Neural Growth and Differentiation*. Raven Press, New York.

Mori, N., Itoh, N. and Salvaterra, P.M. (1987) Evolutionary origin of cholinergic macromolecules and thyroglobulin. *Proc. Natl. Acad. Sci. USA*, 84: 2813–2817.

Neylon, C.B. and Summers, R.J. (1988) Inhibition by cAMP of the phosphoinositide response to alpha adrenoceptor stimulation in rat kidney. *Eur. J. Pharmacol.*, 148: 441–444.

Nishi, S. (1974) Ganglionic transmission. In J.I. Hubbard (Ed.), *The Peripheral Nervous System*, pp. 225–255, Plenum Pree, N.Y., 1974.

Nishizuka, Y. (1986) Studies and perspectives of protein kinase C. *Science, 233:* 305–311.

Nishizuka, Y. (1984) The role of protein kinase C in cell surface signal transduction and tumour promotion. *Nature*, 308: 693–697.

Nordstrom, O., Unden, A., Grimm, V., Frieder, B., Ladinsky, H. and Bartfai, T. (1986) In vivo and in vitro studies on a musscarinic presynaptic antagonist and postsynaptic agonist: BM-5. In I. Hanin (Ed.), *Dynamics of Cholinergic Function*, pp. 405–422, Plenum Press, New York.

Ochoa, E.L.M., Medrano, S., deCarlin, M.C. and Dilonardo, A.M. (1988) Arg-Lys-Asp-Val-Tyr (thymopeptin) accelerates the cholinergic-induced inactivation (desensitization) of reconstituted nicotinic receptor. *Cel. Mol. Neurobiol.*, 8: 325–331.

Ochoa, E.L.M., Chattopadhyay, A. and McNamee, M.G. (1989) Desensitization of the nicotinic acetylcholine receptor: molecular mechanisms and effect of modulators. *Cel. Mol. Neurobiol.*, 9: 141–178.

Peng, H.B. (1987) Development of acetylcholine receptors clusters induced by basic polypeptides in cultured muscle cells. In N.J. Dun and R.L. Perlman (Eds.), *Neurobiology of Acetylcholine, Symposium Held in Honor of Alexander G. Karczmar*, pp. 17–26, Plenum Press, New York.

Perlman, R.L., Cahill, A. and Horwitz, J. (1987) Protein phosphorylation and phospholipid metabolism in the superior cervical ganglion. In N.J. Dun and R.L. Perlman (Eds.), *Neurobiology of Acetylcholine, Symposium Held in Honor of Alexander G. Karczmar*, pp. 111–120, Plenum Press, New York.

Popot, J.-L. and Changeux, J.-P. (1984) Nicotinic receptor of acetylcholine: structure of an oligomeric membrane protein. *Physiol. Rev.*, 64: 1162–1239.

Porcellati, G., Ceccarelli, B. and Tettamanti, G. (Eds.) (1975) *Ganglioside Function: Biochemical and Pharmacological Implications*. Plenum Press, New York.

Raftery, M.A., Conti-Tronconi, B.M. and Dunn, S.M.J. (1985) Structural and functional aspects of the nicotinic receptor. *Fund. Appl. Toxicol., 5:* S39–S40.

Ratnam, M., Le Nguyen, D., Rivier, J., Sargent, P.B., and Lindstrom, J. (1986) Transmembrane topography of nicotinic acetylcholine receptor: Immunochemical tests contradict theoretical predictions based on hydrophobicity profiles. *Biochemistry*, 25: 2633–2643.

Reynolds, J. and Karlin, A. (1978) *Biochemistry*, 17: 2035–2038.

Rhee, S.G., Suh, P.-G., Ryu, S.-H. and Lee, S.Y. (1988) Studies of inositol phospholipid-specific phospholipase C. *Science.*, 244: 546–550.

Riopelle, R.J. and Riccardi, V.M. (1987) Neuronal growth factors form tumours of Van Recklinghausen neurofibromatosis. *Can. J. Neurol. Sci.*, 14: 141–144.

Ryall, R.W. and Haas, H.L. (1975) On the physiological significance of muscarinic receptors on Renshaw cells: A hypothesis. In P.G. Waser (Ed.), *Cholinergic Mechanisms*, pp. 335–342, Raven Press, New York.

Salpeter, M.M. (Ed.) (1987) *The Vertebrate Neuromuscular Junction*. Alan Liss, Inc., New York.

Salvaterra, P.M., Bournias-Vardiabasis, N., Nair, T., Hou, G. and Lieu, C. (1987) In vitro differentiation of *Drosophila* embryo cells. *J. Neurosci., 7:* 10–22.

Schmidt, J. (1988) Biochemistry of nicotinic acetylcholine receptors in the vertebrate brain. *Int. Rev. Neurobiol.*, 50: 1–38.

Schotte, O.E. and Karczmar, A.G. (1944) Limb parameters and regression rates in denervated amputated limbs of urodele larvae. *J. Exp. Zool.*, 97: 43–70.

Schwartz, R.D. and Kellar, E.J. (1986) Nicotinic cholinergic recpetors labeled with [3H]acetylcholine in the brain: characterization, localization and in vivo regulation. In I. Hanin (Ed.), *Dynamics of Cholinergic Function*, pp. 467–479, Plenum Press, New York.

Schwarz, T.L., Tempel, B.L., Papazian, D.M., Jan, Y.N. and Jan, L.Y. (1988) Multiple potassium-channel components are produced by alternative splicing at the Shaker locus in *Drosophilia. Nature*, 331: 137–142.

Shinnick-Gallagher, P., Hirai, K. and Gallagher, J.P. (1987) Muscarinic receptor activation underlying the slow inhibitory postsynaptic potential (S-I.P.S.P.) and the slow excitatory postsynaptic potential (S-E.P.S.P.). In N.J. Dun and R.L. Perlman (Eds.), *Neurobiology of Acetylcholine, Symposium Held in Honor of Alexander G. Karczmar*, pp. 245–254, Plenum Press, New York.

Shute, C.C.D. and Lewis, P.R. (1967) The ascending cholinergic reticular system: Neocortical, olfactory, and subcortical projections. *Brain*, 90: 497–520.

Smilowitz, H., Hadjian, R.A., Dwyer, J. and Feinstein, M.B. (1981) Regulation of acetylcholine receptor phosphorylation by calcium and calmodulin. *Proc. Natl. Acad. Sci. USA*, 78: 4708–4712.

Smith, McH. M. and Harden, T.K. (1985) Muscarinic cholinergic receptor-mediated attenuation of adenylate cyclase activity in rat heart membranes. *J. Cyclic Nucleot. Prot. Phosphoryl. Res.*, 9: 197–210.

Stein, D.G., Finger, S. and Hart, T. (1983) Brain damage and recovery: Problems and perspectives. *Behav. Neur. Biol.*, 37: 185–222.

Stern, P. and Igic, R. (1970) The content of material with acetylcholine-like activity in the brain of animals following thiamine deprivation and treatment with pyrithiamine. In E. Heilbronn and A. Winters (Eds.), *Drugs and Cholinergic Mechanisms in the CNS*, pp. 419–427, Forsvarets Forskningsanstalt, Stockholm.

Sutherland, E.W., Robinson, G.A. and Butcher, R.W. (1968) Some aspects of the biological role of adenosine 3′, 5′-monophosphate (cyclic AMP). *Circulation*, 37: 279–306.

Takai, Y., Kishimoto, A., Inoue, M. and Nishizuka, J. (1977) Studies on a cyclic nucleotide independent protein kinase and its proenzyme in mammalian tissues. I. Purification and characterization of an active enzyme from bovine cerebellum. *J. Biol. Chem.*, 252: 7603–7609.

Thesleff, S. (1955) The mode of neuromuscular block caused by acetylcholine, nicotine, decamethonium and succinylcholine. *Acta Physiol. Scand., 34:* 218–231.

Thoenen, H., Auburger, G., Hellweg, R., Heumann, R. and Korsching, S. (1987) Cholinergic innervation and levels of growth factor and its mRNA in the central nervous system. In M.J. Dowdall and J.N. Hawthorne (Eds.), *Cellular and Molecular Basis of Cholinergic Function*, pp. 379–388, Ellis Horwood, Ltd., Chichester.

Timpe, L.C., Schwarz, T.L., Tempel, B.L., Papazian, D.M., Jan, Y.N. and Jan, L.Y. (1988) Expression of functional potassium channels from Shaker cDNA in Xenopus oocytes. *Nature,* 331: 143–145.

Trisler, D. (1987) Synapse formation in retina is influenced by molecules that identify cell position. *Cur. Topics Develop. Biol.,* 21: 277–308.

Vanderwolf, G.H. (1975) Neocortical and hippocampal activation in relation to behavior: Effects of atropine, phenothiazines and amphetamine. *J. Comp. Physiol. Psychol.,* 88: 300.

Vandlen, R.L., Wu, W.C.-S., Eisenach, J.C. and Raftery, M.A. (1979) Studies of the composition of purified *Torpedo californica* acetylcholine receptor and of its subunits. *Biochem.,* 18: 1845–1854.

Walicke, P.A. (1989) Novel neurotrophic factors, receptors and oncogenes. *Annu. Rev. Neurosci.,* 13: 103–126.

Walker, P., Weichsel, M.E., Eveleth, D. and Fisher, D.A. (1982) Ontogenesis of nerve growth factor and epidermal growth factor in brains of immature male mice: correlation with ontogenesis of serum levels of thyroid hormones. *Pediat. Res.,* 16: 520–524.

Watson, S.P., McConnell, R.C. and Lapetina, E.G. (1984) The rapid formation of inositol phosphates in human platelets by thrombin is inhibited by prostacyclin. *J. Biol. Chem.,* 259: 13199–13203.

Wecker, L. (1986) The utilization of supplemental choline by brain. In I. Hanin (Ed.), *Dynamics of Cholinergic Function*, pp. 851–858, Plenum Press, New York.

Woody, C.D. (1978) If cyclic GMP is a neuronal second messenger, what is the message. In D.J. Jenden (Ed.), *Cholinergic Mechanisms and Psychopharmacology*, pp. 253–260, Plenum Press, New York.

Zeisel, S.H. (1986) Factors which influence the availability of choline to brain. In I. Hanin (Ed.), *Dynamics of Cholinergic Function*, pp. 837–850, Plenum Press, New York.

Zigmond, R.E., Schwarzschild, M.A. and Rittenhouse, A.R. (1989) Acute regulation of tyrosine hydroxylase by nerve activity and by neurotransmitters via phosphorylation. *Annu. Rev. Neurosci.,* 12: 415–461.

S.-M. Aquilonius and P.-G. Gillberg (Eds.)
Progress in Brain Research, Vol. 84
© 1990 Elsevier Science Publishers B.V. (Biomedical Division)

CHAPTER 46

The synthesis of acetylcholine: twenty years of progress

Stanislav Tuček

Institute of Physiology, Czechoslovak Academy of Sciences, 14220 Prague, Czechoslovakia

Introduction

The organization by Edith Heilbronn (Heilbronn and Winter, 1970) in February 1970 of the Cholinergic Symposium at Skokloster (which was to become the first in a series of highly stimulating and successful scientific sessions) was not incidental: It was a consequence of the surge of interest in the biochemistry of cholinergic neurons and synapses which occurred during the 1960s and which brought cholinergic research into the forefront of neuroscience. Recalling what happened in the research on the synthesis of ACh during the two decades following the Symposium at Skokloster, one realizes that this was a period of unremitting activity, which has borne fruit in terms of hundreds of findings of long-lasting significance. It would be difficult to review all of them, but it may be of interest to look backwards to retrace at least some of the most important approaches to the investigation of ACh synthesis, considering not only what has been achieved but also what has *not* been achieved and remains to be clarified in future decades. More systematic reviews of the research on choline acetyltransferase and on the synthesis of ACh may be found in other publications (Tuček 1978, 1983, 1984, 1985, 1988); studies on the turnover of ACh, performed in the early 1970s, have been reviewed by Hanin and Costa (1976).

The synthesis of ACh proceeds according to the equation

$$\text{Acetyl-CoA} + \text{Choline} \rightleftharpoons \text{CoA} + \text{Acetylcholine}$$

and is catalysed by the enzyme choline acetyltransferase (ChAT, EC 2.3.1.6). All the components of the reaction had been identified by the 1960s (Hebb 1963, 1972), but the sources of both substrates used for the synthesis of ACh, the chemical nature of ChAT, the mechanism of its action, its distribution in neurons and between neurons, the factors affecting its expression and the effects of diseases upon the synthesis of ACh and upon the cholinergic neurons are much better understood today than they were twenty years ago.

Choline acetyltransferase and the expression of cholinergic features in neurons

The main concern of neurochemists regarding ChAT in the 1970s was the purification of the enzyme, performed with two aims in mind: (1) to characterize the enzyme (to determine its primary structure), and (2) to use the purified enzyme as the antigen in order to obtain pure antibodies. Both aims have been achieved, but both of them in ways different from those anticipated twenty years ago: The primary structure was not revealed by the analysis of a purified enzyme (except for short sequences) but, rather, by the analysis of complementary DNAs; and the purest antibodies were obtained thanks to the introduction of techniques for the production of monoclonal antibodies (Levey et al., 1981). These qualifications notwithstanding, the purification was a necessary precondition for progress, and the effort spent on

TABLE I

Purification of choline acetyltransferase from mammalian tissues

Source	μmol ACh /min/ mg protein	Authors
Human placenta	2.4	Morris (1966)
Rat brain	1.9	Rossier et al. (1973)
Rat brain	4	Malthe-Sørenssen et al. (1973)
Rat brain	20	Rossier (1976)
Bovine caudate nucl.	28.5	Malthe-Sørenssen et al. (1978)
Human placenta	92.7	Hersh et al. (1978)
Bovine caudate nucl.	54	Ryan and Clure (1979)
Bovine caudate nucl.	120–160	Cozzari and Hartman (1980)
Pig brain	135	Eckenstein et al. (1981)
Bovine caudate nucl.	142	Cozzari and Hartman (1983)

its achievement was enormous. Many laboratories contributed to gradual improvements of the purification procedures; selected data in Table I make it clear how great an increase in purity was achieved within little more than 10 years.

As in so many areas of neurobiology, genetic and molecular genetic approaches have been applied to the study of ChAT in the 1980s. The gene for ChAT was identified as early as 1980 in polytene chromosomes of Drosophila by Greenspan (1980). Messenger RNAs from the brain or spinal cord have been shown to induce the synthesis of ChAT after injection into oocytes by Gundersen et al. (1985) and Berrard et al. (1986). Finally, complementary DNAs for ChAT have been cloned by Salvaterra's group (Itoh et al., 1986; Salvaterra, 1987) for the enzyme from Drosophila and by Mallet and colleagues (Berrard et al., 1987) for the enzyme from the pig. As a result, the primary structure of ChAT is now known for two species, and a comparison of the sequences in Drosophila and the pig indicates considerable stability of the enzyme during phylogenetical development (Berrard et al., 1989). The structure of the active centre still awaits clarification.

Contradictory interpretations of the kinetic mechanism of the catalytic action of ChAT were being offered over a long period of time. The controversy seems to have been resolved by the finding of Hersh (1982; Hersh and Peet, 1977), indicating that the reaction catalysed by ChAT follows a random Theorell-Chance mechanism in which a low but finite number of ternary complexes exists.

There is no doubt that ChAT produces ACh mainly in the close vicinity of sites from which ACh is being released, i.e. in the nerve terminals (Hebb and Whittaker, 1958; Whittaker et al., 1964; Tuček, 1967a), although, like all neuronal proteins, the enzyme itself is being synthesized in the nerve cell bodies. Axonal transport of ChAT was investigated in many laboratories in the 1970s (for references see Tuček, 1978, and Dahlström, 1983) and the most likely conclusion from these studies was that the transport is slow (2–17 mm/day in mammals) and unidirectional. The assumption of such slow rates of transport raises the question, however, of how ChAT survives the long period of time which is necessary for transport in long nerves; as much as 250 days would be needed for the transport at a rate of 4 mm/day (Tuček, 1975) along a nerve which is 1 m long. No mechanism is known which would protect the enzyme against inactivation.

For more than a decade, it appeared that an earlier serious controversy on the localization of ChAT within the nerve terminals had been resolved by the work of Fonnum (1968), showing that, in the presence of a physiological concentration of salt, most of the enzyme is soluble and is probably dissolved in the cytoplasm. In the mid-1980s, however, attention was drawn to the neglected part of the enzyme which remains associated with membranes during subcellular fractionation even in the presence of high concentrations of salt. Three lines of evidence now support the view that the presence of a membrane-bound pool of ChAT (existing in parallel with the larger cytoplasmic pool) is a regular feature of cholinergic nerve terminals:

(a) Data indicating the presence of a high-salt insoluble (detergent-soluble) pool of ChAT in membranes obtained after the disruption of synaptosomes (Benishin and Carroll, 1983; Eder-Colli and Amato, 1985; but see Bruce and Hersh, 1987).

(b) Data obtained with Triton X-114, a detergent apparently capable of separating hydrophobic from hydrophilic proteins (Eder-Colli et al., 1986; Docherty and Bradford, 1988).

(c) Data from Bradford's group, indicating that cholinergic nerve terminals are lysed in the presence of antibodies against ChAT and of the complement, which suggests that the antibodies against ChAT bind to an epitope on the outer surface of the synaptosomes (Docherty et al., 1982; Docherty and Bradford, 1988). Each of these three lines of evidence has its weak points; taken together, however, the available data make the assumption of a membrane-bound pool of ChAT quite likely. The way in which ChAT is attached to the membrane remains to be determined; some data suggest that the enzyme may change its position and become alternately cytoplasmic and membrane-bound. Although it is easy to speculate about the function of the membrane-bound enzyme, no reliable evidence has been presented that it plays any specific functional role, different from that of the cytoplasmic enzyme.

Considering the synthesis of ACh, one had to ask not only in which parts of the neurons is ACh synthesized, but also in which neurons it is produced. One of the largest achievements, if not the largest achievement of the investigations of cholinergic neurons in the last two decades has been the elucidation of the origin of ACh in the brain cortex, i.e. the clarification of the arrangement of ascending cholinergic pathways and of the special position of the basal forebrain cholinergic nuclei in the cholinergic system. Twenty years ago, there was little clear information as to the kind of neurons or nerve terminals which contain ACh and ChAT in brain cortex. It was already suspected, however, that ACh and ChAT are mainly contained in extrinsic cholinergic nerve fibres rather than in intrinsic cholinergic neurons. Among the reasons for such an assumption was the observation made by Hebb, Krnjević and Silver (1963) that undercutting of the cortex greatly diminished the activity of ChAT within it.

The discovery that the cortex is cholinergically innervated from the nuclei of the basal forebrain cannot be ascribed to one or two researchers. Many studies have contributed to the gradual elucidation of the ascending cholinergic pathways in the brain, among them those by Divac (1975), Mesulam and Van Hoesen (1976), Wenk et al. (1980), and Mesulam et al. (1983a). Four methods have mainly assisted the progress in the field: histochemistry of cholinesterases, particularly that performed at intervals after the administration of a strong cholinesterase inhibitor; retrograde tracing of markers like horse radish peroxidase, fluorescent dyes and lectins; immunohistochemical detection of ChAT; and biochemical measurements performed after specific lesions.

The basic picture of the arrangement of ascending cholinergic pathways was established in the early 1980s (reviews Cuello and Sofroniew, 1984; Kása, 1986; Mesulam, 1988), and Mesulam and colleagues (1983b; 1988) introduced a practical nomenclature for cholinergic nuclei, designating them with letters and numbers Ch1–Ch8. More recent work has provided clarification of important details. More information is still needed with regard to the specificity of the cholinergic innervation of the cortex by basal forebrain cholinergic neurons. In the rat, individual basal nucleus neurons innervate cortical areas of no more than 1–1.5 mm in diameter (Price and Stern, 1983; see also Eckenstein et al., 1988), but these areas are probably larger in human brain because the number of cholinergic neurons is too small compared to the area of the cortex. Among other unclarified features the puzzle persists of why one can discover intrinsic cholinergic neurons in the brain cortex of rats (Levey et al., 1984) but not in the cortex of other animal species.

Simultaneously with the discovery of the basal forebrain cholinergic system another important finding was achieved: the discovery that Alzheimer's disease is accompanied by a profound decrease in the activity of ChAT in brain cortex and in the ability of cortical tissue to synthesize ACh (Davies and Maloney, 1976; Perry et al., 1977; White et al., 1977). This finding was of enormous importance. Although it did not reveal the etiology of the disease, it did uncover a key pathogenetic factor in the development of dementia and served as a powerful stimulus for further investigations both of dementia and of the cholinergic system in the brain. It was soon followed by the discovery that the number of cholinergic neurons is diminished in the basal nucleus of Meynert in patients with Alzheimer's disease, indicating that the cholinergic neurons are dying (Whitehouse et al., 1982; Arendt et al., 1983; Tagliavini and Pilleri, 1983; Wilcock et al., 1983). The reason why the cholinergic neurons of the basal forebrain are preferentially affected in Alzheimer's disease awaits clarification (review Candy et al., 1986).

A new direction of cholinergic research was opened by the publication by Patterson and Chun (1974) of data bearing on the question of why certain neurons become cholinergic. Patterson and Chun reported that sympathetic neurons from new-born rats developed the expected adrenergic properties when they were grown in culture in the absence of other cells, but that they became cholinergic when they were grown together with certain non-neuronal cells. Soon afterwards, it was shown that the development of cholinergic properties in cultured sympathetic neurons could also be induced by culture media conditioned by certain non-neuronal cells (review Patterson, 1978). The effect of environmental factors on the development of the cholinergic phenotype in neurons was also revealed in experiments with heterotopic transplantations (review Le Douarin, 1980). These findings raised the hope that it might soon become possible to explain the molecular mechanism responsible for the expression of cholinergic properties in nerve cells, but the progress proved to be difficult. Although it has been possible to isolate factors from conditioned media or from cell ex-

TABLE II

Factors inducing the expression of choline acetyltransferase in sympathetic neurons in culture

Weber M.J. (1981)
  Not fully identified component of glioma and heart cell conditioned media. M_r 40–45 kDa.
Weber M.J., Raynaud B., Delteil C. (1985)
  Glycoprotein form skeletal muscle cell conditioned media. M_r 21 kDa.
Fukada K. (1985)
  Glycoprotein from heart cell conditioned media. M_r 45 kDa.
Kessler J.A., Conn G., Hatcher V.B. (1986)
  Soluble brain protein with high affinity for heparin. M_r 50 kDa.
Wong V., Kessler J.A. (1987)
  Protein ionically associated with spinal cord membranes. M_r 29 kDa.
Adler J.A., Schleifer L.S., Black I.B. (1989)
  Protein ionically associated with spinal cord membranes. M_r 27 kDa.

tracts which induce the production of ChAT and the expression of other cholinergic features in cultured sympathetic neurons (Table II), it has been left for future decades to find out whether and which of these factors affect the development of the nerve cells in vivo, by what cells they are produced in vivo, and what is their mechanism of action.

In addition to factors which *induce* the expression of cholinergic features, other factors have been found to *enhance* their expression. Nerve growth factor (NGF) was for a long time believed to affect only the development of peripheral sensory and adrenergic neurons, and it came as a surprise when it was discovered that NGF also stimulates the development of brain cholinergic neurons in culture (Honegger and Lenoir, 1982) and, under in vivo conditions, of cholinergic neurons in the basal forenrain and, to a lesser degree, in the striatum during their normal development (Gnahn et al., 1983; Mobley et al., 1986; review Thoenen et al., 1987). NGF supports both the survival and the differentiation of cholinergic neurons in the basal forebrain and has been found to exert dramatic protective effects upon these neurons after they have been damaged by axotomy; it is also capable of diminishing the old-age atrophy of central cholinergic neurons and of supporting memory in old rats (Fischer et al., 1987). Data on the presence of NGF receptors in central neurons have been reviewed by Johnson and Taniuchi (1987). Since the molecular mechanism of action of NGF on the nerve cells is unknown, its unravelling is likely to represent one of the exciting chapters of neurobiology in future decades.

In addition to NGF, many other substances have been found to increase the activity of ChAT in neurons, including insulin (Kyriakis et al., 1987), triiodothyronine (Hayashi and Patel, 1987), trophic polypeptide isolated from skeletal muscle (McManaman et al., 1988) and a number of less well defined trophic factors detected in tissue extracts and conditioned cell culture media. Positive effects of co-cultured cells on the activity of ChAT in neurons were noted as early as 1973 by Giller et al. The mechanism by which hormones and trophic factors affect the survival, growth and differentiation of neurons and the expression of their cholinergic features awaits clarification.

Choline

As early as 1959, observations concerning the synthesis and release of ACh in perfused sympathetic ganglia led F. C. MacIntosh (1959) to the remarkably farsighted prediction that "cholinergic transmitter systems must include a fourth specific component in addition to the three we have been discussing (i.e., ACh, ChAT and cholinesterases): a choline carrier located in some membrane at the synapse". Concentrative uptake of labelled choline by the nervous tissue was first described in the mid-1960s (Hodgkin and Martin, 1965; Schuberth et al., 1966; Quastel, 1966) and immediately started to be widely investigated. In the beginning of the 1970s, however, the time was ripe for the discovery of the specific component of the cholinergic transmitter system predicted by MacIntosh, namely of the high-affinity carriers of choline. Haga (1971) concluded from indirect observations

that the uptake of choline into cholinergic neurons is probably mediated by a specific carrier, and within two years several groups of workers (Yamamura and Synder, 1972, 1973; Whittaker et al., 1972; Haga and Noda, 1973; Kuhar et al., 1973; Dowdall and Simon, 1973) reported data which clearly indicated that, in addition to the ubiquitous low-affinity carriers, a specific sodium-dependent high-affinity carrier for choline is present in the surface membranes of the cholinergic nerve terminals. Within a short period of time, sufficient data had been accumulated to justify the conclusion that the synthesis of ACh in the nerve terminals mainly occurs from the choline which is supplied by the high-affinity carriers.

Subsequent development was less dramatic. The questions to be asked concerning the carriers were, of course, what they look like and how they work. It proved possible to investigate their function after incorporation into liposomes (King and Marchbanks, 1980; Meyer and Cooper, 1982; Vyas and O'Regan, 1985), but it was only recently that promising reports appeared on the possibility of their affinity labelling (Rylett, 1988) and immunoaffinity purification (Knipper et al., 1989).

With regard to the function of the carriers, several important aspects still await clarification. One of them concerns the nature of their dependence on Na^+ ions: although it is suspected that the carriers effect a co-transport of Na^+ ions and choline, the co-transport of Na^+ has not yet been demonstrated. Another debatable point concerns the effect of functional activity of the nerve terminals on the activity of the carriers. Most observations indicating that the high-affinity uptake of choline is increased by the flow of nerve impulses can be explained as a result of a decrease in the concentration of ACh in the nerve terminals and of subsequent disinhibition of the carriers (Jenden et al., 1976), and as a result of post-stimulation hyperpolarization of the terminals. The view that other mechanisms may be involved in the post-stimulation activation of high-affinity choline carriers has been expressed repeatedly (e.g., O'Regan and Collier, 1981), and Saltarelli et al. (1988)

presented data suggesting that the carriers are also controlled by phospholipase A_2 and by free arachidonic acid in the membrane.

Dross and Kewitz (1972) published a seminal paper in which they have shown, inter alia, that radioactive choline from the blood mixes rapidly with choline in the brain, but that the radioactivity of brain choline never reaches that in the blood, probably because unlabelled endogenous free choline is constantly produced in the brain. The production of free choline in the brain was confirmed by data in the same paper indicating that the concentration of choline is higher in the blood leaving the brain than in that entering the brain in rats: the same was discovered by Aquilonius et al. (1975) in men.

The source of the free choline which is continuously produced in the brain has been the subject of much interest but a full and quantitative understanding of the economy of choline and choline-containing compounds in the brain has not been reached. There is little doubt that much of the free choline which is added to the blood by the brain originates from brain phosphatidylcholine. It was believed for a long time that the brain is unable to produce the choline moiety of phosphatidylcholine by adding methyl groups to phosphatidylethanolamine, but in the late 1970s several groups (Skurdall and Cornatzer, 1975; Blusztajn et al., 1979; Mozzi and Porcellati, 1979) succeeded in proving that some production of phosphatidylcholine from phosphatidylethanolamine does occur in the brain; the rate is so slow, however, that the de novo production of the choline moiety of phosphatidylcholine in the brain cannot account for the whole production of free choline in the brain. It is necessary to assume that the brain is permanently supplied not only with free choline, but also with phosphatidylcholine from the blood, and this assumption is supported by much indirect and a little direct evidence (review Ansell and Spanner, 1982); not enough information is available on the quantity of phosphatidylcholine supplied to the brain and on the ways in which it is treated in the brain. Possibly, future thinking about

the homeostasis of choline in the brain will be strongly influenced by the recent finding (Löffelholz, 1989b) that the brain takes up choline from the blood when its plasma concentration is high and releases it into the blood when the plasma concentration drops to "normal" low level.

ACh itself has been found to serve as an important source of choline for the synthesis of new ACh. In experiments on sympathetic ganglia, more than 50% of choline from the released ACh (which had been hydrolysed by cholinesterases in the synaptic clefts) was re-utilized for the synthesis of new ACh (Collier and MacIntosh, 1969; Collier and Katz, 1974). Similar conditions probably exist in cholinergic synapses in other locations.

Data have been presented indicating that the supply of choline may be rate-limiting not only in experiments in vitro (e.g., in the presence of an inhibitor of the choline carriers or in the absence of Na^+ ions), but also in vivo (Wecker and Schmidt, 1980). When brain slices are stimulated in the absence of free choline, the hydrolysis of phosphatidylcholine is speeded up and the choline released from it is used for the synthesis of ACh (Ulus et al., 1989). The activation of muscarinic receptors has also been found to be accompanied by an increased release of free choline from phosphatidylcholine (Corradetti et al., 1983; Doležal and Tuček, 1984; review Löffelholz, 1989a; the released choline may be utilized for the synthesis of ACh.

Acetylcoenzyme A

In 1968, the first study was published by Browning and Schulman investigating the source of acetyl groups in ACh with the use of radiolabelled precursors, and it was soon followed by a number of investigations performed both in vitro (Itoh and Quastel, 1970; Nakamura et al., 1970; Cheng and Nakamura, 1970; Sollenberg and Sörbo, 1970; Lefresne et al., 1973) and in vivo (Tuček and Cheng, 1970, 1974). These studies have established that, in mammalian brain, the acetyl-CoA which is used for the synthesis of ACh originates mainly from glucose and pyruvate. On the other hand, acetate appears to serve as the main source of acetyl groups in the acetyl-CoA which is used for the synthesis of ACh in the electric organ of electric fish (Israel and Tuček, 1974).

Since the acetyl-CoA which is produced from pyruvate is intramitochondrial, the question has been frequently considered of how this acetyl-CoA or its acetyl groups are transported across the inner mitochondrial membrane, but a definitive solution has not so far been found. Sollenberg and Sörbo (1970) proposed that the intramitochondrial acetyl-CoA is first transformed to citrate and, under the influence of ATP citrate lyase, is transformed back to acetyl-CoA in the cytosol. ATP citrate lyase can be inhibited, however, by means of (-)hydroxycitrate, and yet the synthesis of ACh from glucose is only diminished by about 30% after complete inhibition of the enzyme (Sterling and O'Neill, 1978; Gibson and Shimada, 1980; Tuček et al., 1981). It appears, therefore, that the citrate pathways are responsible for the supply of no more than a third of the total number of acetyl groups needed for the synthesis of ACh in mammalian brain tissue.

Two other pathways have been proposed for the transfer of acetyl-CoA or its acetyl groups across the inner mitochondrial membrane in cholinergic nerve endings. In one pathway, acetylcarnitine serves as the carrier of acetyl groups (Doležal and Tuček, 1981; Sterri and Fonnum, 1980). In the other pathway, acetyl-CoA is believed to cross the inner mitochondrial membrane through presumptive hydrophilic channels which are formed in the membrane in the presence of Ca^{2+} ions (Tuček, 1967b; Polak et al., 1978; Benjamin and Quastel, 1981; Říčný and Tuček, 1983; Benjamin et al., 1983); a related phenomenon has been described for polar compounds other than acetyl-CoA (see Haworth and Hunter, 1980, for references). Both mechanisms suggested in this paragraph still await confirmation.

It has been shown that the supply of acetyl-CoA has a regulatory influence on the synthesis of ACh in experiments in vitro (Gibson et al., 1975) and

perhaps also in vivo (Doležal and Tuček, 1982). The effects of a reduction in the availability of acetyl-CoA on the synthesis of ACh were particularly marked in experiments in which brain slices had been incubated in the presence of low concentrations of glucose (Říčný and Tuček, 1980) and of metabolic inhibitors (Říčný and Tuček, 1981). While the control of the production of acetyl-CoA from pyruvate in the mitochondria has been much investigated (reviews Wieland, 1983, and Yeaman, 1989), very little is known about the means whereby the cells achieve and maintain the desirable ratio between the concentrations of acetyl-CoA inside and outside the mitochondria. These mechanisms are of obvious interest with regard to the control of ACh synthesis, in which the maintenance of a constant ratio between the concentrations of the substrates and products of the reaction catalysed by ChAT plays a fundamental role (review Tuček, 1984).

References

Adler, J.E., Schleifer, L.S. and Black, I.B. (1989) Partial purification and characterization of a membrane-derived factor regulating neurotransmitter phenotypic expression. *Proc. Natl. Acad. Sci. USA*, 86: 1080–1083.

Aquilonius, S.-M., Ceder, G., Lying-Tunell, U., Malmlund, H.O. and Schuberth, J. (1975) The arteriovenous difference of choline across the brain of man. *Brain Res.*, 99: 430–433.

Arendt, T., Bigl, V., Arendt, A. and Tennstedt, A. (1983) Loss of neurons in the nucleus basalis of Meynert in Alzheimer's disease. *Acta Neuropathol.*, 61: 101–108.

Benishin, C.G. and Carroll, P.T. (1983) Multiple forms of choline-O-acetyltransferase in mouse and rat brain: solubilization and characterization. *J. Neurochem.*, 41: 1030–1039.

Benjamin, A.M. and Quastel, J.H. (1981) Acetylcholine synthesis in synaptosomes: mode of transfer of mitochondrial acetyl coenzyme A. *Science*, 213: 1495–1496.

Benjamin, A.M., Murphy, C.R.K. and Quastel, J.H. (1983) Calcium-dependent release of acetyl-coenzyme A from liver mitochondria. *Can. J. Physiol. Pharmacol.*, 61: 154–158.

Berrard, S., Faucon-Biguet, N., Gregoire, D., Blanot, F., Smith, J. and Mallet, J. (1986) Synthesis of catalytically active choline acetyltransferase in Xenopus oocytes injected with messenger RNA from rat central nervous system. *Neurosci. Lett.*, 72: 93–98.

Berrard, S., Brice, A., Lottspeich, F., Braun, A., Barde, Y.-A. and Mallet, J. (1987) cDNA cloning and complete sequence of porcine choline acetyltransferase: In vitro translation of

474

the corresponding RNA yields an active protein. *Proc. Natl. Acad. Sci. USA,* 84: 9280–9284.

Berrard, S., Brice, A. and Mallet, J. (1989) Molecular genetic approach to the study of mammalian choline acetyltransferase. *Brain Res. Bull.,* 22: 147–153.

Blusztajn, J.K., Zeisel, S.H. and Wurtman, R.J. (1979) Synthesis of lecithin (phosphatidylcholine) from phosphatidylethanolamine in bovine brain. *Brain Res.,* 179: 319–327.

Browning, E.T. and Schulman, M.P. (1968) (^{14}C)Acetylcholine synthesis by cortex slices of rat brain. *J. Neurochem.,* 15: 1391–1405.

Bruce, G. and Hersh, L.B. (1987) Studies on detergent released choline acetyltransferase from membrane fractions of rat and human brain. *Neurochem. Res.,* 12: 1059–1066.

Candy, J.M., Perry, E.K., Perry, R.H., Court, J.A., Oakley, A.E. and Edwardson, J.A. (1986) The current status of the cortical cholinergic system in Alzheimer's disease and Parkinson's disease. *Progr. Brain Res.,* 70: 105–130.

Cheng, S.-C. and Nakamura, R. (1970) A study on the tricarboxylic acid cycle and the synthesis of acetylcholine in the lobster nerve. *Biochem. J.,* 118: 451–455.

Collier, B. and Katz, H.S. (1974) Acetylcholine synthesis from recaptured choline by a sympathetic ganglion. *J. Physiol. (Lond.),* 264: 489–509.

Collier, B. and MacIntosh, F.C. (1969) The source of choline for acetylcholine synthesis in a sympathetic ganglion. *Can. J. Physiol. Pharmacol.,* 47: 127–135.

Corradetti, R., Lindmar, R., Löffelholz, K. (1983) Mobilization of cellular choline by stimulation of muscarinic receptors in isolated chicken heart and rat cortex in vivo. *J. Pharmacol. Exp. Ther.,* 226: 826–832.

Cozzari, C. and Hartman, B.K. (1980) Preparation of antibodies specific to choline acetyltransferase from bovine caudate nucleus and immunohistochemical localization of the enzyme. *Proc. Natl. Acad. Sci. USA,* 77: 7453–7457.

Cozzari, C. and Hartman, B.K. (1983) Choline acetyltransferase. Purification procedure and factors affecting chromatographic properties and enzyme stability. *J. Biol. Chem.,* 258: 10010–10013.

Cuello, A.C. and Sofroniew, M.V. (1984) The anatomy of the CNS cholinergic neurons. *Trends Neurosci.,* 7: 74–78.

Dahlström, A. (1983) Presence, metabolism, and axonal transport of transmitters in peripheral mammalian axons, In A. Lajtha (Ed.), *Handbook of Neurochemistry,* Vol. 5, Plenum Press, New York, pp. 405–441.

Davies, P. and Maloney, A.J. (1976) Selective loss of cholinergic neurons in Alzheimer's disease. *Lancet,* 2: 1403.

Divac, I. (1975) Magnocellular nuclei of the basal forebrain project to neocortex, brain stem, and olfactory bulb. Review of some functional correlates. *Brain Res.,* 93: 385–398.

Docherty, M. and Bradford, H.F. (1988) Choline acetyltransferase in mammalian synaptosomes: evidence for an integral membrane-bound form. *Neurochem. Int.,* 13: 119–127.

Docherty, M., Bradford, H. and Anderton, B. (1982) Lysis of cholinergic synaptosomes by an antiserum to choline acetyltransferase. *FEBS Lett.,* 144: 47–50.

Doležal, V. and Tuček, S. (1981) Utilization of citrate, acetyl-carnitine, acetate, pyruvate and glucose for the synthesis of acetylcholine in rat brain slices. *J. Neurochem.,* 36: 1323–1330.

Doležal, V. and Tuček, S. (1982) Effects of choline and glucose on atropine-induced alterations of acetylcholine synthesis and content in the brain of rats. *Brain Res.,* 240: 285–293.

Doležal, V. and Tuček, S. (1984) Activation of muscarinic receptors stimulates the release of choline from brain slices. *Biochem. Biophys. Res. Commun.,* 120: 1002–1007.

Dowdall, M.J. and Simon, E.J. (1973) Comparative studies on synaptosomes: Uptake of (N-Me^{3}H) choline by synaptosomes from squid optic lobes. *J. Neurochem.,* 21: 969–982.

Dross, K. and Kewitz, H. (1972) Concentration and origin of choline in the rat brain. *Naunyn-Schmiedeberg's Arch. Pharmacol.,* 274: 91–106.

Eckenstein, F., Barde, Y.-A. and Thoenen, H. (1981) Production of specific antibodies to choline acetyltransferase purified from pig brain. *Neuroscience* 6: 993–1000.

Eckenstein, F.P., Baughman, R.W. and Quinn, J. (1988) An anatomical study of cholinergic innervation in rat cerebral cortex. *Neuroscience* 25: 457–474.

Eder-Colli, L. and Amato, S. (1985) Membrane-bound choline acetyltransferase in Torpedo electric organ: a marker for synaptosomal plasma membranes? *Neuroscience* 15: 577–589.

Eder-Colli, L., Amato, S. and Froment, Y. (1986) Amphiphilic and hydrophilic forms of choline-O-acetyltransferase in cholinergic nerve endings of the Torpedo. *Neuroscience* 19: 275–288.

Fischer, W., Wictorin, K., Björklund A., Williams, L.R., Varon, S. and Gage, F.H. (1987) Amelioration of cholinergic neuron atrophy and spatial memory impairment in aged rats by nerve growth factor. *Nature,* 329: 65–68.

Fonnum, F. (1968) Choline acetyltransferase binding to and release from membranes. *Biochem. J.,* 109: 389–398.

Fukada, K. (1985) Purificarion and partial characterization of a cholinergic neuronal differentiation factor. *Proc. Natl. Acad. Sci. USA,* 82: 8795–8799.

Gibson, G.E., and Shimada, M. (1980) Studies on the metabolic pathway of the acetyl group for acetylcholine synthesis. *Biochem. Pharmac.,* 29: 167–174.

Gibson, G.E., Jope, R. and Blass, J.P. (1975) Decreased synthesis of acetylcholine accompanying impaired oxidation of pyruvic acid in rat brain minces. *Biochem. J.,* 148: 17–23.

Giller, E.L., Schrier, B.K., Shainberg, A., Fisk, H.R. and Nelson, P.G. (1973) Choline acetyltransferase activity is increased in combined cultures of spinal cord and muscle cells from mice. *Science,* 182: 588–589.

Gnahn, H., Hefti, F., Heumann, R., Schwab, M.E. and Thoenen, H. (1983) NGF-mediated increase of choline acetyltransferase (ChAT) in the neonatal rat forebrain; evidence for a physiological role of NGF in the brain? *Dev. Brain Res.* 9: 45–52.

Greenspan, R.J. (1980) Mutations of choline acetyltransferase and associated neural defects in Drosophila melanogaster. *Comp. Physiol.,* 137: 83–92.

Gundersen, C.B., Jenden, D.J. and Miledi, R. (1985) Choline

acetyltransferase and acetylcholine in Xenopus oocytes injected with mRNA from the electric lobe of Torpedo. *Proc. Natl. Acad. Sci. USA,* 82: 608–611.

Haga, T. (1971) Synthesis and release of (^{14}C)acetylcholine in synaptosomes. *J. Neurochem.,* 18: 781–798.

Haga, T. and Noda, H. (1973) Choline uptake systems of rat brain synaptosomes. *Biochim. Biophys. Acta,* 291: 564–575.

Hanin, I. and Costa, E. (1976) Approaches used to estimate brain acetylcholine turnover rate in vivo; effects of drugs on brain acetylcholine turnover rate. In A.M. Goldberg and I. Hanin (Eds.), *Biology of Cholinergic Function, Raven Press, New York,* pp. 355–377.

Haworth, R.A. and Hunter, D.R. (1980) Allosteric inhibition of the Ca^{2+}-activated hydrophilic channel of the mitochondrial membrane by nucleotides. *J. Membrane Biol.* 54: 231–236.

Hayashi, M. and Patel, A.J. (1987) An interaction between thyroid hormone and nerve growth factor in the regulation of choline acetyltransferase activity in neuronal cultures, derived from the septal-diagonal band region of the embryonic rat brain. *Dev. Brain Res.* 36: 109–120.

Hebb, C. (1963) Formation, storage, and liberation of acetylcholine, In G.B. Koelle (Ed.), Cholinesterases and Anticholinesterase Agents, Handbuch d. exper. *Pharmakologie, Ergänzungswerk,* Vol. 15, Springer Verlag, Berlin, pp. 55–88.

Hebb, C. (1972) Biosynthesis of acetylcholine in nervous tissue. *Physiol. Rev.,* 52: 918–957.

Hebb, C.O. and Whittaker, V.P. (1958) Intracellular distributions of acetylcholine and choline acetylase. *J. Physiol.,* 142: 187–196.

Hebb, C.O., Krnjević, K. and Silver, A. (1963) Effect of undercutting on the acetylcholinesterase and choline acetyltransferase activity in the cat's cerebral cortex. *Nature,* 198: 692.

Heilbronn, E. and Winter, A. (Eds.) (1970) *Drugs and Cholinergic Mechanisms in the CNS,* Almquist and Wiksell, Stockholm.

Hersh, L.B. (1982) Kinetic studies of the choline acetyltransferase reaction using isotope exchange at equilibrium. *J. Biol. Chem.,* 257: 12820–12834.

Hersh, L.B. and Peet, M. (1977) Re-evaluation of the kinetic mechanism of the choline acetyltransferase reaction. *J. Biol. Chem.,* 252: 4796–4802.

Hersh, L.B., Coe, B. and Casey, L. (1978) A fluorimetric assay for choline acetyltransferase and its use in the purification of the enzyme from human placenta. *J. Neurochem.,* 30: 1077–1085.

Hodgkin, A.L. and Martin, K. (1965) Choline uptake by giant axons of Loligo. *J. Physiol. (Lond.),* 179: 26P–27P.

Honegger, P. and Lenoir, D. (1982) Nerve growth factor (NGF) stimulation of cholinergic telencephalic neurons in aggregating cell cultures. *Dev. Brain Res.,* 3: 229–238.

Israël, M. and Tuček, S. (1974) Utilization of acetate and pyruvate for the synthesis of "total", "bound" and "free" acetylcholine in the electric organ of Torpedo. *J. Neurochem.,* 22: 487–491.

Itoh, T. and Quastel, J.H. (1970) Acetoacetate metabolism in infant and adult rat brain in vitro. *Biochem. J.* 116: 641–655.

Itoh, N., Slemmon, J.R., Hawke, D.H., Williamson, R., Morita, E., Itakura, K., Roberts, E., Shively, J.E. and Crawford, G.D. (1986) Cloning of Drosophila choline acetyltransferase cDNA. *Proc. Natl. Acad. Sci. USA,* 83: 4081–4085.

Jenden, D.J., Jope, R.S. and Weiler, M.H. (1976) Regulation of acetylcholine synthesis: does cytoplasmic acetylcholine control high affinity choline uptake? *Science* 194: 635–637.

Johnson, E.M. and Taniuchi, M. (1987) Nerve growth factor (NGF) receptors in the central nervous system. *Biochem. Pharmac.* 36: 4189–4195.

Kása, P. (1986) The cholinergic systems in brain and spinal cord. *Progr. Neurobiol.,* 26: 211–272.

Kessler, J.A., Conn, G. and Hatcher, V.B. (1986) Isolated plasma membranes regulate neurotransmitter expression and facilitate effects of a soluble brain cholinergic factor. *Proc. Natl. Acad. Sci. USA,* 83: 3528–3532.

King, R.G. and Marchbanks, R.M. (1980) Solubilization of the choline transport system and re-incorporation into artificial membranes. *Nature,* 287: 64–65.

Knipper, M., Boekhoff, I. and Breer, H. (1989) Isolation and reconstitution of the high-affinity choline carrier. *FEBS Lett.,* 245: 235–237.

Kuhar, M.J., Sethy, V.H., Roth, R.H. and Aghajanian, G.K. (1973) Choline: selective accumulation by central cholinergic neurons. *J. Neurochem.,* 20: 581–593.

Kyriakis, J.M., Hausman, R.E. and Peterson, S.W. (1987) Insulin stimulates choline acetyltransferase activity in cultured embryonic chicken retina neurons. *Proc. Natl. Acad. Sci. USA,* 84: 7463–7467.

Le Douarin, N.M. (1980) The ontogeny of the neural crest in avian embryo chimaeras. *Nature,* 286: 663–669.

Lefresne, P., Guyenet, P. and Glowinski, J. (1973) Acetylcholine synthesis from (2-^{14}C)pyruvate in rat striatal slices. *J. Neurochem.,* 20: 1083–1097.

Levey, A.I., Aoki, M., Fitch, F.W. and Wainer, B.H. (1981) The production of monoclonal antibodies reactive with bovine choline acetyltransferase. *Brain Res.,* 218: 383–387.

Levey, A.I., Wainer, B.H., Rye, D.B., Mufson, E.J. and Mesulam, M.-M. (1984) Choline acetyltransferase-immunoreactive neurons intrinsic to rodent cortex and distinction from acetylcholinesterase-positive neurons. *Neuroscience,* 13: 341–355.

Löffelholz, K. (1989a) Receptor regulation of choline phospholipid hydrolysis. *Biochem. Pharmacol.,* 38: 1543–1549.

Löffelholz, K. (1989b) Communication on the Symposium *Pharmacological Interventions on Central Cholinergic Mechanisms in Senile Dementia (Alzheimer's Disease),* Berlin, July 28–30.

MacIntosh, F.C. (1959) Formation, storage, and release of acetylcholine at nerve endings. *Can. J. Biochem. Physiol.,* 37: 343–356.

Malthe-Sørenssen, D., Eskeland, T. and Fonnum, F. (1973) Purification of rat brain choline acetyltransferase; some immunochemical properties of a highly purified preparation. *Brain Res.,* 62: 517–522.

Malthe-Sørenssen, D., Lea, T., Fonnum, F. and Eskeland, T.

476

(1978) Molecular characterization of choline acetyltransferase from bovine brain caudate nucleus and some immunological properties of the highly purified enzyme. *J. Neurochem.*, 30: 35–46.

McManaman, J.L., Crawford, F.G., Steward, S.S. and Appel, S.H. (1988) Purification of a skeletal muscle polypeptide which stimulates choline acetyltransferase activity in cultured spinal cord neurons. *J. Biol. Chem.*, 263: 5890–5897.

Mesulam, M.-M. (1988) Central cholinergic pathways: Neuroanatomy and some behavioral implications. In M. Avoli, T.A. Reader, R.W. Dykes and P. Gloor (Eds.), *Neurotransmitters and Cortical Function,* Plenum Publishing Corporation, New York, pp. 237–260.

Mesulam, M.-M. and Van Hoesen, C.W. (1976) Acetylcholinesterase-rich projections from the basal forebrain of the rhesus monkey to neocortex. *Brain Res.*, 109: 152–157.

Mesulam, M.-M., Mufson, E.J., Levey, A.I. and Wainer, B.H. (1983a) Cholinergic innervation of cortex by the basal forebrain: cytochemistry and cortical connections of the septal area, diagonal band nuclei, nucleus basalis (substantia innominata) and hypothalamus in the rhesus monkey. *J. Comp. Neurol.* 214: 170–197.

Mesulam, M.-M., Mufson, E.J., Wainer, B.H. and Levey, A.I. (1983b) Central cholinergic pathways in the rat: An overview based on an alternative nomenclature (Ch1–Ch6). *Neuroscience,* 4: 1185–1201.

Meyer, E.M. and Cooper, J.R. (1982) High-affinity choline transport in proteoliposomes derived from rat cortical synaptosomes. *Science,* 217: 843–845.

Mobley, W.C., Rutkowski, J.L., Tennekoon, G.I., Gemski, J., Buchanan, K. and Johnston, M.V. (1986) Nerve growth factor increases choline acetyltransferase activity in developing basal forebrain neurons. *Mol. Brain Res.* 1: 53–62.

Morris, D. (1966) The choline acetyltransferase of human placenta. *Biochem. J.* 98: 754–762.

Mozzi, R. and Porcellati, G. (1979) Conversion of phosphatidylethanolamine to phosphatidylcholine in rat brain by the methylation pathway. *FEBS Lett,* 100: 363–366.

Nakamura, R., Cheng, S.-C. and Naruse, H. (1970) A study on the precursors of the acetyl moiety of acetylcholine in brain slices. *Biochem. J.,* 118: 443–450.

O'Regan, S. and Collier, B. (1981) Factors affecting choline transport in the isolated retina. *Brain Res.,* 93: 548–551.

Patterson, P.H. (1978) Environmental determination of autonomic neurotransmitter functions. *Ann. Rev. Neurosci.,* 1: 1–17.

Patterson, P.H. and Chun, L.L.Y. (1974) The influence of non-neuronal cells on catecholamine and acetylcholine synthesis and accumulation in cultures of dissociated sympathetic neurons. *Proc. Natl. Acad. Sci. USA,* 71: 3607–3610.

Perry, E.K., Perry, R.H., Blessed, G. and Tomlinson, B.E. (1977) Necropsy evidence of central cholinergic deficits in senile dementia. *Lancet,* 1: 189.

Polak, R.L., Molenaar, P.C. and Braggaar-Schaap, P. (1978) Regulation of acetylcholine synthesis in rat brain. In D.J. Jenden (Ed.), *Cholinergic Mechanisms and Psychopharmacology,* Plenum Press, New York, pp. 511–524.

Price, J.L. and Stern, R. (1983) Individual cells in the nucleus basalis-diagonal band complex have restricted axonal projections to the cerebral cortex of the rat. *Brain Res.,* 269: 352–356.

Quastel, J.H. (1966) Molecular transport at cell membranes. *Proc. R. Soc. B.,* 163: 169–196.

Říčný, J. and Tuček S. (1980) Relation between the content of acetylcoenzyme A and acetylcholine in brain slices. *Biochem. J.* 188: 683–688.

Říčný, J. and Tuček, S. (1981) Acetylcoenzyme A and acetylcholine in slices of rat caudate nuclei incubated in the presence of metabolic inhibitors. *J. Biol. Chem.,* 256: 4919–4923.

Říčný, J. and Tuček, S. (1983) Ca^{2+} ions and the output of acetylcoenzyme A from brain mitochondria. *Gen. Physiol. Biophys.,* 2: 27–37.

Rossier, J. (1976) Purification of rat brain choline acetyltransferase. *J. Neurochem.,* 26: 543–548.

Rossier, J., Baumann, A. and Benda, P. (1973) Improved purification of rat brain choline acetyltransferase by using an immunoabsorbent. *FEBS Lett.,* 32: 231–234.

Ryan, R. and McClure, W.O. (1979) Purification of choline acetyltransferase from rat and cow brain. *Biochemistry,* 18: 5357–5365.

Rylett, R.J. (1988) Affinity labelling and identification of the high-affinity choline carrier from synaptic membranes of Torpedo electromotor nerve terminals with (^{3}H)choline mustard. *J. Neurochem.,* 51: 1942–1945.

Saltarelli, M.D., Yamada, K., Coyle, J.T. (1988) Phospholipase A_2 and the regulation of high-affinity choline uptake in rat striatum: correlation between (^{3}H)arachidonate release and (^{3}H)hemicholinium-3 binding. *Neurochem. Int.* 13, suppl. 1, 167.

Salvaterra, P.M. (1987) Molecular biology and neurobiology of choline acetyltransferase. *Mol. Neurobiol.,* 1: 247–280.

Schuberth, J., Sundwall, A., Sörbo, B. and Lindell, J.-O. (1966) Uptake of choline by mouse brain slices. *J. Neurochem.,* 13: 347–352.

Skurdal, D.N. and Cornatzer, W.E. (1975) Choline phosphotransferase and phosphatidyl ethanolamine methyltransferase activities. *Int. J. Biochem.,* 13: 887–892.

Sollenberg, J. and Sörbo, B. (1970) On the origin of the acetyl moiety of acetylcholine in brain studied with a differential labelling technique using ^{3}H-^{14}C-mixed labelled glucose and acetate. *J. Neurochem.,* 17: 201–207.

Sterling, G.H. and O'Neill, J.J. (1978) Citrate as the precursor of the acetyl moiety of acetylcholine. *J. Neurochem.,* 31: 525–530.

Sterri, S.H. and Fonnum, F. (1980) Acetyl-CoA synthesizing enzymes in cholinergic nerve terminals. *J. Neurochem.,* 35: 249–254.

Tagliavini, F. and Pilleri, G. (1983) Neuronal counts in basal nucleus of Meynert in Alzheimer's disease in simple senile dementia. *Lancet,* 1: 469–670.

Thoenen, H., Bandtlow, C. and Heumann, R. (1987) The physiological function of nerve growth factor in the central nervous system: Comparison with the periphery. *Rev. Physiol. Biochem. Pharmacol.,* 109: 145–178.

Tuček S. (1967a) Observations on the subcellular distribution of choline acetyltransferase in the brain tissue of mammals and comparisons of acetylcholine synthesis from acetate and citrate in homogenates and nerve-endings fractions. *J. Neurochem.,* 14: 519–529.

Tuček, S. (1967b) The use of choline acetyltransferase for measuring the synthesis of acetylcoenzyme A and its release from brain mitochondria. *Biochem. J.,* 104: 749–756.

Tuček. S. (1975) Transport of choline acetyltransferase and acetylcholinesterase in the central stump and isolated segments of a peripheral nerve. *Brain Res.,* 86: 259–270.

Tuček, S. (1978) *Acetylcholine Synthesis in Neurons,* Chapman and Hall, London, 259 pp.

Tuček S. (1983) The synthesis of acetylcholine. In A. Lajtha (Ed.), *Handbook of Neurochemistry,* 2nd edn., Vol. 4, Plenum Press, New York, pp. 219–249.

Tuček S. (1984) Problems in the organization and control of acetylcholine synthesis in brain neurons. *Prog. Biophys. molec. Biol.,* 44: 1–46.

Tuček S. (1985) Regulation of acetylcholine synthesis in the brain. *J. Neurochem.,* 44: 10–24.

Tuček S. (1988) Choline acetyltransferase and the synthesis of acetylcholine. In V.P.Whittaker (Ed.), *The Cholinergic Synapse, Handbook of Experimental Pharmacology,* Vol. 86, Springer-Verlag, Berlin, Heidelberg, pp. 125–165.

Tuček, S. and Cheng, S.-C. (1970) Precursors of acetyl groups in acetylcholine in the brain in vivo. *Biochim. biophys. Acta,* 208: 538–540.

Tuček, S. and Cheng, S.-C. (1974) Provenance of the acetyl group of acetylcholine and compartmentation of acetyl-CoA and Krebs cycle intermediates in the brain in vivo. *J. Neurochem.,* 22: 893–914.

Tuček, S., Doležal, V. and Sullivan, A.C. (1981) Inhibition of the synthesis of acetylcholine in rat brain slices by (-)hydroxycitrate and citrate. *J. Neurochem.,* 36: 1331–1337.

Ulus, I.H., Wurtman, R.J., Mauron, C. and Krzysztof, J. (1989) Choline increases acetylcholine release and protects against the stimulation-induced decrease in phosphatide levels within membranes of rat corpus striatum. *Brain Res.,* 484: 217–227.

Vyas, S. and O'Regan, S. (1985) Reconstitution of carrier-mediated choline transport in proteoliposomes prepared from presynaptic membranes of Torpedo electric organ, and its internal and external ionic requirements. *J. Membr. Biol.,* 85: 111–119.

Weber, M.J. (1981) A diffusible factor responsible for the determination of cholinergic functions in cultured sympathetic neurons. *J. Biol. Chem.,* 7: 3447–3453.

Weber, M.J., Raynaud, B. and Delteil, C. (1985) Molecular properties of a cholinergic differentiation factor from muscle-conditioned medium. *J. Neurochem.,* 45: 1541–1547.

Wecker, L. and Schmidt, D.E. (1980) Neuropharmacological consequences of choline administration. *Brain Res.,* 184: 234–238.

Wenk, H., Bigl, V. and Meyer, U. (1980) Cholinergic projections from magnocellular nuclei of the basal forebrain to cortical areas in rats. *Brain Res. Rev.,* 2: 295–316.

White, P., Hiley, C.R., Goodhardt, M.J., Carrasco, L.H., Keet, J.P., Williams, I.E. and Bowen, D.M. (1977) Neocortical cholinergic neurons in elderly people. *Lancet,* 1: 668–670.

Whitehouse, P.J., Price, D.L., Struble, R.G., Clark, A.W., Coyle, J.T. and De Long, M.R. (1982) Alzheimer's disease and senile dementia; loss of neurons in the basal forebrain. *Science,* 215: 1237–1239.

Whittaker, V.P., Michaelson, I.A., Kirkland, R.J.A. (1964). The separation of synaptic vesicles from nerve-ending particles ('synaptosomes'). *Biochem. J.,* 90: 293–303.

Whittaker, V.P., Dowdall, M.J. and Boyne, A.F. (1972) The storage and release of acetylcholine by cholinergic nerve terminals: recent results with non-mammalian preparations. *Biochem. Soc. Symp.,* 36: 49–68.

Wieland, O.H. (1983) The mammalian pyruvate dehydrogenase complex: structure and regulation. *Rev. Physiol. Biochem. Pharmacol.,* 96: 123–170.

Wilcock, G.K., Esiri, M.M., Bowen, D.M. and Smith, C.C.T. (1983) The nucleus basalis in Alzheimer's disease: cell counts and cortical biochemistry. *Neuropathol. Appl. Neurobiol.,* 9: 175–179.

Wong, V. and Kessler, J.A. (1987) Solubilization of a membrane factor that stimulates levels of substance P and choline acetyltransferase in sympathetic neurons. *Proc. Natl. Acad. Sci. USA,* 84: 8726–8729.

Yamamura, H.J. and Snyder, S.H. (1972) Choline: high-affinity uptake by rat brain synaptosomes. *Science,* 178: 626–628.

Yamamura, H.I. and Snyder, S.H. (1973) High affinity transport of choline into synaptosomes of rat brain. *J. Neurochem.,* 21: 1355–1374.

Yeaman, S.J. (1989) The 2-oxo acid dehydrogenase complexes: recent advances. *Biochem. J.,* 257: 625–632.

S.-M. Aquilonius and P.-G. Gillberg (Eds.)
Progress in Brain Research, Vol. 84
© 1990 Elsevier Science Publishers B.V. (Biomedical Division)

CHAPTER 47

Achievements in cholinergic research, 1969–1989: drug development

Donald J. Jenden

Department of Pharmacology and Brain Research Institute, UCLA School of Medicine, Los Angeles, CA 90024-1735, U.S.A.

Introduction

During the last twenty years the emphasis in cholinergic drug development has shifted from anticholinergics to new strategies for the enhancement of cholinergic function. This shift has undoubtedly resulted from the recognition that the cognitive loss in Alzheimer's disease, one of the commonest causes of morbidity and mortality in older patients, is associated with and probably caused by a relatively specific loss of cholinergic projections from the basal forebrain to the neocortex and hippocampus (Whitehouse et al., 1982; Coyle et al., 1983). By analogy with the successful use of DOPA in Parkinson's disease, it seemed likely that cholinergic enhancement might be equally useful in Alzheimer's disease. This hope has not been borne out, although some marginal improvement has been demonstrated. However, it has led to a surge of interest in the promotion of cholinergic function, in the development of new ways of selectively interfering with cholinergic mechanisms to produce experimental models, and in the discovery of new chemical and instrumental probes which may be helpful in evaluating cholinergic function. The last two of these topics are dealt with elsewhere in this symposium; this brief review will focus on new ways of selectively enhancing cholinergic function.

Muscarinic receptor subtypes

The first indication that muscarinic receptors may be heterogeneous came from a report of a remarkable new compound with the code number McN-A-343 (Roszkowski, 1961). This compound is a potent ganglionic stimulant, causing among other effects a dramatic rise in blood pressure, but its actions are blocked by atropine and unaffected by nicotinic agents. It has little effect at conventional muscarinic sites such as gastrointestinal smooth muscle and peripheral blood vessels. These properties suggested that it activates a specific subset of muscarinic receptors which were subsequently referred to as M_1 (Goyal and Rattan, 1978), while those most sensitive to classical muscarinic agents were given the designation M_2. Another early indication of muscarinic receptor heterogeneity was the cardioselective antimuscarinic effect of gallamine (Riker and Wescoe, 1951; Clark and Mitchelson, 1976), a compound which in common with several other neuromuscular blocking agents is now generally believed to interact allosterically with the muscarinic receptor (Birdsall et al., 1981, 1984). It was not until 1980 that Hammer et al. (1980) described the relatively selective antagonistic actions of pirenzepine at M_1 sites. This distinction between M_1 and M_2 sites was subsequently confirmed by ligand binding studies (Hammer and Giachetti, 1982, 1984). However, it soon became apparent that neither M_1 nor M_2 receptors were homogeneous. M_1 receptors in sympathetic ganglia are more sensitive to blockade by hexahydrodiphenidol than are those in the hippocampus (Lambrecht et al., 1987), and probably represent a distinct subtype; similarly, M_2 receptors in the heart appear to be distinct from those in the ileum. Cardiac M_2 receptors are more sensitive than ileal receptors to AFDX-116 (Hammer et al., 1986; Giachetti et al., 1986; Micheletti et al., 1987) himbacine (Anwar-ul et al., 1986) and particularly methoctramine (Melchiorre et al., 1987, Melchiorre, 1988), while the reverse is true of 4-DAMP (Barlow et al., 1976) and hexahydrodiphenidol (Mutschler and Lambrecht, 1984).

The last decade has resulted in an avalanche of discovery on muscarinic receptor subtypes, which is exemplified by the proceedings of three international symposia on the subject (Hirschowitz et al., 1983; Levine et al., 1985, 1987). Five distinct muscarinic receptors have been cloned and sequenced (Kubo et al., 1986; Peralta et al., 1987a, 1987b; Bonner et al., 1987, 1988), their coupling mechanisms have been partially elucidated (for review see Nathanson, 1987), a number of relatively specific ligands have been described (for review see Mitchelson, 1988), and specific residues responsible for binding and coupling have been proposed (Hulme et al., 1987, Wheatley et al., 1988). For further information the reader is referred to several excellent reviews on the subject (Schimerlik, 1989; Ramachandran et al., 1989; Birdsall et al., 1988; Mitchelson, 1988; Goyal, 1988; Barnes et al., 1988; Melchiorre, 1988; Eglen and Whiting, 1986).

Muscarinic agonists

This has been an active field of investigation and has recently been reviewed (Ringdahl, in press). There has been particular interest in tertiary amines with potent muscarinic properties since these are likely to penetrate into the central nervous system and may therefore be of potential therapeutic value in Alzheimer's disease, but only partial success has been achieved in obtaining specificity for central sites as opposed to peripheral, for postsynaptic sites as opposed to presynaptic, and for cortical sites as opposed to those in other areas of the brain. New compounds representing progress toward these objectives include numerous analogues of oxotremorine (for review see Ringdahl and Jenden, 1983), arecoline (Mutschler and Hultzsch, 1973; Mutschler and Lambrecht, 1984), aceclidine (Fisher et al., 1987; Sanders et al., 1988) and pilocarpine. RS86 is an old compound which has been reevaluated in this new context (Palacios et al., 1986).

Receptor reserve as a factor in site specificity

Discrete receptor subtypes are not the only basis for specificity of agents acting on these receptors at different functional sites. It has long been recognized that distributional factors may play an important role, especially in determining relative potency in vivo in the central nervous system and in the periphery (Mayer et al., 1959; Brodie et al., 1960; Karlen and Jenden, 1970). In the case of partial agonists, an alternative mechanism for site specificity has more recently been pointed out (Kenakin, 1986). In studying a series of oxotremorine analogues on the isolated guinea pig ileum and guinea pig bladder, Ringdahl (1987a,b; Ringdahl and Markowicz, 1987) observed that the compounds fell into three groups: some were full agonists on both tissues; some were full agonists in the ileum but partial agonists in the bladder, while a third group were partial agonists in the ileum but behaved primarily as antagonists in the bladder. The ability to discriminate between the two tissues was clearly related to the intrinsic efficacy of the compound; agonists of low intrinsic efficacy stimulated responses in the ileum but blocked responses in the bladder. No corresponding differences were found between the dissociation constants or the relative efficacy in the two tissues. These partial agonists therefore displayed tissue selectivity without discriminating between tissue receptors.

Site specificity determined by intrinsic efficacy has also been demonstrated in vivo (Ringdahl et al., 1987; Ringdahl, 1988). Compounds with high intrinsic efficacy such as oxotremorine produced salivation, analgesia, hypothermia and tremor in mice. Agents with moderate intrinsic efficacy produced only the first two effects, and even antagonized the tremor produced by oxotremorine. BM 5, which has even lower intrinsic efficacy, was potent in producing analgesia, but was a partial agonist with respect to hypothermia and a potent antagonist of oxotremorine-induced tremor (Ringdahl et al., 1987; Ringdahl, 1988). BM 5 has also been reported to discriminate between presynaptic and postsynaptic muscarinic effects both in vitro (Nordstrom et al., 1983) and in vivo (Casamenti et al., 1986), presumably on the same basis.

Exploitation of site specificity on the basis of intrinsic efficacy is of course limited to agonists as opposed to antagonists; its practical value is also limited by the fact that relative agonist potency at different sites is determined by the receptor reserve at those sites, and cannot be manipulated at will pharmacologically.

Cholinesterase inhibitors

Inhibition of cholinesterase is one of the classic ways of enhancing cholinergic function, and it is not surprising that cholinesterase inhibitors have been extensively studied in dementia of the Alzheimer type (DAT), but this strategy is limited by several factors. There is strong evidence that cholinergic terminals in the cortex have undergone marked degeneration in DAT; for example there are marked reductions in both choline acetyltransferase (Rossor et al., 1984) and high-affinity choline transport (Rylett et al., 1983). A therapeutic response to cholinesterase inhibitors therefore depends upon the effective function of the surviving terminals. Unlike direct muscarinic agonists, which offer some hope of specificity be-

tween several functional sites, cholinesterase inhibitors are likely to have effects at all cholinergic synapses to which the drugs have access, and numerous side effects are to be expected such as disturbances of mood, posture, movement, sleep and neuroendocrine balance, in addition to effects mediated peripherally, although these can at least in principle be blocked by a peripherally acting anticholinergic agent such as N-methylatropine. Finally it is well established that there are autoreceptors on many cholinergic terminals which mediate an inhibition of acetylcholine release. Cholinesterase inhibitors can be expected to potentiate the effect of acetylcholine at these sites and therefore impede neuronal communication by inhibiting acetylcholine release. On the other hand, anticholinesterases can be expected to potentiate acetylcholine at nicotinic as well as muscarinic sites, which may be significant in the context of Alzheimer's disease (Whitehouse et al., 1986; Flynn and Mash, 1986; Perry et al., 1987).

Despite these limitations, physostigmine has received numerous trials in DAT, usually with some modest effect on memory. These have recently been reviewed (Becker and Giacobini, 1988). Physostigmine has a short half-life (about 30 min), and must therefore be administered in a sustained release formulation, by infusion or at short intervals. There has therefore been considerable interest in cholinesterase inhibitors with a longer duration of action. Some promising analogues of physostigmine (Brufani et al., 1986) and miotin (Enz et al., in press) have recently been described with this objective. Although measurement of erythrocyte cholinesterase levels is often advocated as a means of monitoring the clinical effect of physostigmine and other carbamate inhibitors, it should be noted that most conventional methods are likely to give spurious results because of the pseudo-irreversible inhibition of the enzyme that these inhibitors produce (Michalek and Stavinoha, 1978); moreover inhibition of the enzyme may outlast the presence of the intact drug, as in the case of organophosphates. Some older compounds with anticholinesterase properties have been reinvestigated in this new context. Galanthamine is a naturally occurring reversible inhibitor which is relatively specific for acetylcholinesterase (Thomsen et al., in press) and has a relatively long duration of action. Tacrine (1,2,3,4-(tetrahydro-9-aminoacridine)) has received a good deal of publicity as a result of a favorable report by Summers et al. (1986) and a laudatory editorial in the New England Journal of Medicine (Davis and Mohs, 1986). It is a centrally active, noncompetitive cholinesterase inhibitor (Heilbronn, 1961; Patocka et al., 1976) with a longer duration of action than physostigmine, but has several other actions in addition, including excitatory effects on hippocampal pyramidal neurones (Stevens and Cotman, 1987), inhibition of monoamine uptake (Drukarch et al., 1988), inhibition of high-affinity choline transport (Buyukuysal and Wurtman, 1989) and interaction with a PCP binding site (Albin et al., 1988). It is not clear to what extent these actions may contribute to the clinical effects. The validity of the study by Summers et al. (1986) has been questioned by a number of authors on methodological grounds (Pirozzolo et al., 1987; Tariot and Caine, 1987), and liver toxicity is a major problem, but tacrine is currently the subject of a large multicenter trial. HP029, the 1-hydroxy derivative of tacrin, has also received some attention (Puri et al., 1989).

There are, of course, innumerable cholinesterase inhibitors available with a much longer duration of action (Usdin, 1970). Most of these are lipophilic compounds that distribute rapidly in the body. Although a few have been applied therapeutically, most have been developed for toxicological purposes, and many produce a delayed neurotoxic effect (Cavanaugh, 1973; Johnson, 1975) which eliminates them from therapeutic consideration. Nor is it clear that such a prolonged effect is desirable, since it seems more likely to result in a self-defeating down-regulation (Ehlert et al., 1980) than a relatively short-acting drug which could be discontinued at night. Despite these problems, metrifonate has recently been proposed as a treatment for Alzheimer's disease (Becker and Giacobini, 1988). Metrifonate is an antihelminthic which undergoes spontaneous non-enzymatic conversion to dichlorvos (Nordgren et al., 1978), an irreversible organophosphate anticholinesterase used an insecticide. A delayed neurotoxic effect of dichlorvos is considered unlikely but not impossible (Johnson, 1981). In view of this hazard from long-term use, and the innumerable alternatives that exist, it is by no means clear that metrifonate is an optimal choice for long-acting cholinesterase inhibitor in Alzheimer's disease.

Acetylcholine release promoters

Enhancement of acetylcholine release is a logical alternative to the inhibition of cholinesterase. Ideally this could be accomplished at many sites by blocking muscarinic autoreceptors, but no agents are known that are sufficiently specific to be useful. However, there is a group of aminopyridines which enhance transmitter release by prolonging the depolarization associated with the action potential. This action is mediated by blockade of potassium channels and results in increased influx of Ca^{2+} (Bowman, 1982). These compounds have been shown to enhance performance experimentally in aging and in hypocholinergic states (Davis et al., 1983; Gibson and Petersen, 1983; Peterson and Gibson, 1983), but clinical results have not been consistent (Wesseling et al., 1984; Davidson et al., 1988). It is possible that this action contributes to the clinical effects of tacrin, since this drug has been reported to block potassium channels (Stevens and Cotman, 1987). Since Ca^{2+} influx may facilitate the synthesis of acetylcholine as well as its release (see Tucek, 1985), these release enhancers deserve further investigation. They should, however, be given with choline or lecithin to reduce the likelihood of inducing a functional choline deficiency.

Future prospects

The past two decades have seen a flood of new information on the components of cholinergic systems and the functional relationships between them. The techniques of molecular biology, ultrastructural morphology, radioligand binding and analytical chemistry have played major roles in these advances and in turn have depended on the availability of specific high-affinity or irreversible ligands, i.e. drugs. The emphasis on enhancement of cholinergic function which has characterized the past decade will at best yield drugs which are of temporary and symptomatic benefit; it seems likely that the years to come will provide a better understanding of the processes controlling development, differentiation, maintenance and repair of cholinergic (and other) neurones. This in turn will lead to a new generation of drugs which modulate these processes. The next 20 years may well see advances in neurochemistry and pharmacology which will allow presymptomatic diagnosis and even prophylaxis of the progressive degenerative diseases that threaten the present generation.

Acknowledgements

Work by the author reported in this chapter was supported by USPHS grant MH17691. The author is grateful to Holly Batal for excellent bibliographic and editorial assistance.

References

Albin, R.L., Young, A.B. and Penney, J.B. (1988) Tetrahydro-9-aminoacridine (THA) interacts with phencyclidine (PCP) receptor site. *Neurosci. Lett.*, 88: 303–307.

Anwar-ul, S., Gilani, H. and Cobbin, L.B. (1986) The cardioselectivity of himbacine: a muscarine receptor antagonist. *N-S Arch. Pharmacol.*, 332: 16–20.

Barlow, R.B., Berry, K.J., Glenton, P.A.M., Nikolaou, N.M. and Soh, K.S. (1976) A comparison of affinity constants for muscarine-sensitive acetylcholine receptors in guinea-pig atrial pacemaker cells at 29°C and in ileum at 29°C and 37°C. *Br. J. Pharmacol.*, 58: 613–620.

Barnes, P.J., Minette, P. and Maclagan, J. (1988) Muscarinic receptor subtypes in airways. *Trends Pharmacol. Sci.*, 9: 412–417.

Becker, R.E. and Giacobini, E. (1988) Mechanisms of cholinesterase inhibition in senile dementia of the Alzheimer type: clinical pharmacological and therapeutic aspects. *Drug Dev. Res.*, 12: 163–195.

Birdsall, N.J.M., Burgen, A.S.V., Hulme, E.C. and Stockton, J.M. (1981) Gallamine regulates muscarinic receptors in the heart and cerebral cortex. *Br. J. Pharmacol.*, 74: 798P.

Birdsall, N.J.M., Hulme, E.C., Stockton, J.M. and Wong, E.H.F. (1984) The occurrence of allosteric interaction between binding sites on muscarinic receptors. In C. Melchiorre and M. Gianella (Eds.), *Highlights in Receptor Chemistry*, Elsevier, Amsterdam, pp. 217–223.

Birdsall, N.J.M., Curtis, C.A.M., Eveleigh, P., Hulme, E.C., Pedder, E.K., Poyner, D. and Wheatley, M. (1988) Muscarinic Receptor Subtypes and the selectivity of agonists and antagonists. *Pharmacology*, 37 (suppl. 1): 22–31.

Bonner, T.I., Buckley, N.J., Young, A.C. and Brann, M.R. (1987) Identification of a family of muscarinic acetylcholine receptor genes. *Science*, 237: 527–532.

Bonner, T.I., Young, A.C., Bram, M.R. and Buckley, N.J. (1988) Cloning and expression of the human and rat M_5 muscarinic acetylcholine receptor genes. *Neuron*, 1: 403–410.

Bowman, W.C. (1982) Aminopyridines — their pharmacological actions and potential clinical uses. *Trends Pharmacol. Sci.*, 3: 183–185.

Brodie, B.B., Kurz, H. and Shanker, L.S. (1960) The importance of dissociation constant and lipid solubility in influencing the passage of drugs into the cerebrospinal fluid. *J. Pharmacol. Exp. Ther.*, 130: 20–25.

Brufani, M., Marta, M. and Pomponi, M. (1986) Anticholinesterase activity of a new carbamate, heptylphysostigmine, in view of its use in patients with Alzheimer's dementia. *Eur. J. Biochem.*, 157: 115–120.

Buyukuysal, R.L. and Wurtman, R.J. (1989) Tetrahydroaminoacridine but not 4-aminopyridine inhibits high-affinity choline uptake in striatal and hippocampal synaptosomes. *Brain. Res.*, 482: 371–375.

Casamenti, F., Cosi, C. and Pepeu, G. (1986) Effect of BM 5, a presynaptic antagonist-postsynaptic agonist, on cortical acetylcholine release. *Eur. J. Pharmacol.*, 122: 288–290.

Cavanagh, J.B. (1973) Peripheral neuropathy caused by toxic agents. *Crit. Rev. Toxicol.*, 2: 365–417.

Clark, A.L. and Mitchelson, F. (1976) The inhibitory effect of gallamine on muscarinic receptors. *Br. J. Pharmacol.*, 58: 323–331.

Coyle, J.T., Price, D.L. and DeLong, M.R. (1983) Alzheimer's disease: a disorder of cortical cholinergic function. *Science*, 219: 1184–1190.

Davidson, M., Zemischlany, Z., Mohs, R.C., Horvath, J.B., Powchik, P., Blass, J.P. and Davis, K.L. (1988) 4-aminopyridine in the treatment of Alzheimer's disease. *Biol. Psychiat.*, 23: 485–490.

Davis, H.P., Idowu, A. and Gibson, G.E. (1983) Improvement of 8-arm maze performance in aged Fischer 344 rats with 3,4-diaminopyridine. *Exp. Aging Res.*, 9: 211–214.

Davis, K.L. and Mohs, R.C. (1986) Cholinergic drugs in Alzheimer's disease. *N. Engl. J. Med.*, 315: 1286–1287.

484

Drukarch, B., Leysen, J.E. and Stoof, J.C. (1988) Further analysis of the neuropharmacological profile of 9-amino-1,2,3,4-tetrahydroacridine (THA), an alleged drug for the treatment of Alzheimer's disease. *Life Sci.,* 42: 1011–1017.

Eglen, R.M. and Whiting, R.L. (1986) Muscarinic receptor subtypes: a critique of the current classification and a proposal for a working nomenclature. *J. Auton. Pharmacol.,* 5: 323–346.

Ehlert, F.J., Kokka, N. and Fairhurst, A.S. (1980) Altered [^{3}H]-quinuclidinyl benzilate binding in the striatum of rats following chronic cholinesterase inhibition with diisopropylfluorophosphate. *Mol. Pharmacol.,* 17: 24–30.

Enz, A., Hofmann, A., Gmelin, G. and Kelly, P.H. (in press) Pharmacological properties of SDZ ENA713, a novel acetylcholinesterase inhibitor. *Proceedings of a Symposium on Pharmacological Interventions on Central Cholinergic Mechanisms in Senile Dementia,* Berlin, July 28–30, 1989.

Fisher, A., Heldman, E., Brandeis, R., Pittel, Z., Dachir, S., Levy, A. and Karton, I. (1987) Restoration of cognitive functions in an animal model of Alzheimer's disease. In M.J. Dowdall and J.N. Hawthorne (Eds.), *Cellular and Molecular Basis of Cholinergic Function,* Ellis Horwood, Chichester, pp. 913–927.

Flynn, D.D. and Mash, D.C. (1986) Characterization of 1-[^{3}H]-nicotine binding in cerebral cortex: comparison between Alzheimer's disease and the normal. *J. Neurochem.,* 47: 1948–1954.

Giachetti, A., Micheletti, R. and Montagna, E. (1986) Cardioselective profile of AF-DX 16, a muscarine M_2 receptor antagonist. *Life Sci.,* 38: 1663–1672.

Gibson, G.E. and Peterson, C. (1983) Pharmacologic models of age-related deficits. In T. Crook, S. Ferris and R. Bartus (Eds.), *Assessment in Geriatric Psychopharmacology,* Mark Powley Associates, Connecticut, pp. 323–343.

Goyal, R.K. (1988) Identification, localization and classification of muscarinic receptor subtypes in the gut. *Life Sci.,* 43: 2209–2220.

Goyal, R.K. and Rattan, S. (1978) Neurohumoral, hormonal, and drug receptors for the lower esophageal sphincter. *Gastroenterology,* 74: 598–619.

Hammer, R. and Giachetti, A. (1982) Muscarinic receptor sybtypes: M_1 and M_2 biochemical and functional characterization. *Life Sci.,* 31: 2991–2998.

Hammer, R. and Giachetti, A. (1984) Selective muscarinic receptor antagonists. *Trends Pharmacol Sci.,* 5: 18–20.

Hammer, R., Berrie, C.P., Birdsall, N.J.M., Burgen, A.S.V. and Hulme, E.C. (1980) Pirenzepine distinguishes between different subclasses of muscarinic receptors. *Nature,* 283: 90–92.

Hammer, R., Giraldo, E., Schiavi, G.B., Monferini, E. and Ladinsky, H. (1986) Binding profile of novel cardioselective muscarine receptor antagonist, AF-DX 116, to membranes of peripheral tissues and brain in the rat. *Life Sci.,* 38: 1653–1662.

Heilbronn, E. (1961) Inhibition of cholinesterases by tetrahydroaminacridine. *Acta Chem. Scand.,* 15: 1386–1390.

Hirschowitz, B.I., Hammer, R., Giachetti, A., Keirns, J.J. and

Levine, R.R. (1983) *Subtypes of Muscarinic Receptors,* Elsevier, Boston, 103 pp.

Hulme, E.C., Wheatley, M., Curtis, C. and Birdsall, N.J.M. (1987) The muscarinic acetylcholine receptors: structure, function and location of the ligand binding site. In S. Cohen and M. Sokolovsky (Eds.), *International Symposium on Muscarinic Cholinergic Mechanisms,* Freund Publishing House, Ltd., London, pp. 192–211.

Johnson, M.K. (1975) The delayed neuropathy caused by some organophosphorus esters: mechanism and challenge. *Crit. Rev. Toxicol.,* 3: 289–316.

Johnson, M.K. (1981) Delayed neurotoxicity — Do trichlorphen and or dichlorvos cause delayed neuropathy in man or in test animals? *Acta Pharmacol. Toxicol.,* 49 (Suppl. V): 87–98.

Karlen, B. and Jenden, D.J. (1970) The role of distribution as a determinant of central anticholinergic specificity in a series of oxotremorine analogs. *Res. Comm. Chem. Path. Pharmacol.,* 1: 471–478.

Kenakin, T.P. (1986) Tissue and receptor selectivity: similarities and differences. *Adv. Drug Res.,* 15: 71–109.

Kubo, T., Fukuda, K., Mikami, A., Maeda, A., Takahashi, H., Mishina, M., Haga, T., Haga, K., Ichiyama, A., Kangawa, K., Kojima, M., Matsuo, H., Hirose, T. and Numa, S. (1986) Cloning, sequencing and expression of complementary DNA encoding the muscarinic acetylcholine receptor. *Nature,* 323: 411–416.

Lambrecht, G., Moser, U., Riotte, J., Wagner, M., Wess, J., Gmelin, G., Tacke, R., Zilch, H. and Mutschler, E. (1987) Heterogeneity in muscarinic receptors: evidence from pharmacological and electrophysiological studies with selective antagonists. In S. Cohen and M. Sokolovsky (Eds.), *International Symposium on Muscarinic Cholinergic Mechanisms,* Freund Publishing House, Ltd., London, pp. 245–253.

Levine, R.R., Birdsall, N.J.M., Giachetti, A., Hammer, R., Iversen, L.L., Jenden, D.J. and North, R.A. (1985) *Subtypes of Muscarinic Receptors II,* Elsevier, Boston, 97 pp.

Levine, R.R., Birdsall, N.J.M., North, R.A., Holman, M., Watanabe, A. and Iversen, L.L. (1987) *Subtypes of Muscarinic Receptors III,* Elsevier, Boston, 93 pp.

Mayer, S., Maickel, R.P. and Brodie, B.B. (1959) Kinetics of penetration of drugs and other foreign compounds into cerebrospinal fluid and brain. *J. Pharmacol. Exp. Ther.,* 127: 205–211.

Melchiorre, C. (1988) Polymethylene tetramines: a new generation of selective muscarinic antagonists. *Trends Pharmacol Sci.,* 9: 216–220.

Melchiorre, C., Cassinelli, A. and Quaglia, W. (1987) Differential blockade of muscarinic receptor subtypes by polymethylene tetramines. Novel class of selective antagonists of cardiac M-2 muscarinic receptors. *J. Med. Chem.,* 30: 201–204.

Michalek, H. and Stavinoha, W.B. (1978) Effect of chlorpromazine pre-treatment on the inhibition of total cholinesterases and butyryl-cholinesterase in brain of rats poisoned by physostigmine or dichlorvos. *Toxicology,* 9: 205–218.

Micheletti, R., Montagna, E. and Giachetti, A. (1987) AF-DX 116, a cardioselective muscarinic antagonist. *J. Pharmacol. Exp. Ther.*, 241: 628–634.

Mitchelson, F. (1988) Muscarinic receptor differentiation. *Pharmacol. Ther.*, 37: 357–423.

Mutschler, E. and Hultzsch, K. (1973) Uber Struktur-Wirkungs-Beziehungen von ungesattigten Estern des Arecaidins und Dijydroarecaidins. *Arzneim. Forsch./Drug Res.*, 23: 732–737.

Mutschler, E. and Lambrecht, G. (1984) Selective muscarinic agonists and antagonists in functional tests. *Trends Pharmacol. Sci.*, (Suppl.) 5: 39–44.

Nathanson, N.M. (1987) Molecular properties of the muscarinic acetylcholine receptor. *Annu. Rev. Neurosci.*, 10: 195–236.

Nordgren, I., Bergstrom, M., Holmstedt, B. and Sandoz, M. (1978) Transformation and action of metrifonate. *Arch. Toxicol.*, 41: 31–41.

Nordstrom, O., Alberts, P., Westlind, A., Unden, A. and Bartfai, T. (1983) Presynaptic antagonist-postsynaptic agonist at muscarinic cholinergic synapses. N-methyl-N-(1-methyl-4-pyrrolidino-2-butynyl)acetamide. *Mol. Pharmacol.*, 24: 1–5.

Palacios, J.M., Bolliger, G., Closse, A., Enz, A., Gmelin, G. and Malanowski, J. (1986) The pharmacological assessment of RS86 (2-ethyl-8-methyl-2,8-diazaspiro-[4,5]-decan-1,3-dion hydrobromide). A potent, specific muscarinic acetylcholine receptor agonist. *Eur. J. Pharmacol.*, 125: 45–62.

Patocka, J., Bajgar, J., Bielavsky, J. and Fusek, J. (1976) Kinetics of inhibition of cholinesterases by 1,2,3,4-tetrahydro-9-aminoacridine *in vitro. Coll. Czech. Chem. Comm.*, 41: 816–824.

Peralta, E.G., Winslow, J.W., Peterson, G.L., Smith, D.H., Ashkenazi, A., Ramachandran, J., Schimerlik, M.I. and Capon, D.J. (1987a) Primary structure and biochemical properties of an M_2 muscarinic receptor. *Science,* 236: 600–605.

Peralta, E.G., Ashkenazi, A., Winslow, J.W., Smith, D.H., Ramachandran, J. and Capon, D.J. (1987b) Distinct primary structures, Ligand binding properties and tissue-specific expression of four human muscarinic acetylcholine receptors. *EMBO J.,* 6: 3923–3929.

Perry, E.K., Perry, R.H., Smith, C.J., Dick, D.J., Candy, J.M., Edwardson, J.A., Fairbairn, A. and Blessed, G. (1987) Nicotinic receptor abnormalities in Alzheimer's and Parkinson's diseases. *J. Neurol. Neurosurg. Psychiat.*, 50: 806–809.

Peterson, C. and Gibson, G.E. (1983) Amelioration of age-related neurochemical and behavioral deficits by 3,4-diaminopyridine. *Neurobiol. Aging*, 4: 25–30.

Pirozzolo, F.J., Baskin, D.S., Swihart, A.A. and Appel, S.H. (1987) Oral tetrahydroaminoacridine in the treatment of senile dementia, Alzheimer's type. *N. Engl. J. Med.*, 316: 1603.

Puri, S.K., Hsu, R.S., Ho, I. and Lassman, H.B. (1989) Single dose specificity, tolerance and pharmacokinetics of HP029 in healthy young men: A potential Alzheimer agent. *J. Clin. Pharmacol.*, 29: 278–284.

Ramachandran, J., Peralta, E.G., Ashkenazi, A., Winslow, J.W. and Capon, D.J. (1989) The structural and functional interrelationships of muscarinic acetylcholine receptor subtypes. *Bioessays,* 10: 54–57.

Riker, W.F., Jr. and Wescoe, W.C. (1951) The pharmacology of Flaxedil with observations on certain analogs. *Ann. N.Y. Acad. Sci.,* 54: 373–394.

Ringdahl, B. (1987a) Structural requirements for affinity and efficacy of N-(4-amino-2-butynyl) succinimides at muscarinic receptors in the guinea pig ileum and urinary bladder. *Eur. J. Pharmacol.*, 140: 13–23.

Ringdahl, B. (1987b) Selectivity of partial agonists related to oxotremorine based on differences in muscarinic receptor reserve between the guinea pig ileum and urinary bladder. *Mol. Pharmacol.*, 31: 351–356.

Ringdahl, B. (1988) 5-methyl-2-pyrrolidone analogues of oxotremorine as selective muscarinic agonists. *J. Med. Chem.*, 31: 683–688.

Ringdahl (in press) Structural determinants of muscarinic agonist activity. In J.H. Brown (Ed.), *The Muscarinic Receptors,* The Humana Press Inc., New Jersey.

Ringdahl, B. and Jenden, D.J. (1983) Minireview: Pharmacological properties of oxotremorine and its analogs. *Life Sci.,* 32: 2401–2413.

Ringdahl, B. and Markowicz, M.E. (1987) Muscarinic and antimuscarinic activity of acetamides related to oxotremorine in the guinea pig urinary bladder. *J. Pharmacol. Exp. Ther.,* 240: 789–794.

Ringdahl, B., Roch, M. and Jenden, D.J. (1987) Regional differences in receptor reserve for analogs of oxotremorine in vivo: implications for development of selective muscarinic agonists. *J. Pharmacol. Exp. Ther.,* 242: 464–471.

Rossor, M.N., Iversen, L.L., Reynolds, G.P., Mountjoy, C.Q. and Roth, M. (1984) Neurochemical characteristics of early and late onset types of Alzheimer's disease. *Br. Med. J.,* 288: 961–964.

Roszkowski, A.P. (1961) An unusual type of sympathetic ganglion stimulant. *J. Pharmacol. Exp. Ther.,* 132: 156–170.

Rylett, R.J., Ball, M.J. and Colhoun, E.H. (1983) Evidence for high affinity choline transport in synaptosomes prepared from hippocampus and neocortex of patients with Alzheimer's disease. *Brain Res.,* 289: 169–175.

Saunders, J., Showell, G.A., Snow, R.J., Baker, R., Freedman, S.B. (1988) 2-Methyl-1,3-dioxaazaspiro [4,5] decanes as novel muscarinic cholinergic agonists. *J. Med. Chem.,* 31: 486–491.

Schimerlik, M.I. (1989). Structure and regulation of muscarinic receptors. *Annu. Rev. Physiol.,* 51: 217–227.

Stevens, D.R. and Cotman, C.W. (1987) Excitatory actions of tetrahydro-9-aminoacridine (THA) on hippocampal neurons. *Neurosci. Lett.,* 79: 301–305.

Summers, W.K., Majovski, L.V., Marsh, G.M., Tachiki, K. and Kling, A. (1986) Oral tetrahydroaminoacridine in long-term treatment of senile dementia, Alzheimer type. *N. Engl. J. Med.,* 315: 1241–1245.

Tariot, P.N. and Caine, E.D. (1987) Oral tetrahydroaminoacridine in the treatment of senile dementia, Alzheimer's type. *N. Engl. J. Med.,* 316: 1605.

Thomsen, T., Fischer, J.P. and Kewitz, H. (in press) Inhibition of acetyl- and butyryl-cholinesterase by galanthamine; in vivo and in vitro investigations. *Proceedings of a Symposium on Pharmacological Interventions on Central Cholinergic Mechanisms in Senile Dementia,* Berlin, July 28–30, 1989.

Tucek, S. (1985) Regulation of acetylcholine synthesis in the brain. *J. Neurochem.,* 22: 11–24.

Usdin, E. (1970) Reactions of cholinesterases with substrates, inhibitors and reactivators. In A.G. Karczmar (Ed.), *International Encyclopedia of Pharmacology and Therapeutics, Vol. 1, Section 13: Anticholinesterase Agents,* Pergamon Press, Oxford, pp. 47–353.

Wesseling, H., Agoston, S., Van Dam, G.B.P., Pasma, J., de Witt, H.J. and Haringa, H. (1984) Effects of 4-amino-pyri-dine in elderly patients with Alzheimer's disease. *N. Engl. J. Med.,* 310: 988–989.

Wheatley, M., Hulme, E.C., Birdsall, N.J.M., Curtis, C.A.M., Eveleigh, P., Pedder, E.K. and Poyner, D. (1988) Peptide mapping studies on muscarinic receptors: receptor structure and the location of the ligand binding site. *Trends Pharmacol. Sci. Suppl.,* 9: 19–24.

Whitehouse, P.J., Price, D.L., Struble, R.G., Clark, A.W., Coyle, J.T. and DeLong, M.R. (1982) Alzheimer's disease and senile dementia: loss of neurons in the basal forebrain. *Science,* 215: 1237–1239.

Whitehouse, P.J., Martino, A.M., Antuono, P.G., Lowenstein, P.R., Coyle, J.T., Price, D.L. and Keller, K.J. (1986) Nicotinic acetylcholine binding sites in Alzheimer's disease. *Brain Res.,* 371: 146–151.

Subject Index